1998

REDESIGNING HEALTHCARE DELIVERY

REDESIGNING HEALTHCARE DELIVERY

A practical guide to reengineering, restructuring, and renewal

Peter Boland, Editor

BOLAND HEALTHCARE • BERKELEY

This handbook was a complex undertaking that benefited from the advice, criticism, and encouragement of content experts throughout the country. In addition, a number of internal staff and editorial team members were instrumental in guiding and shaping this publication: Laurie Mayhew, lead copy editor and production supervisor; Aileen Kantor, initial-stage copy editor; Candace Coar and Patty Hammond, proofreaders; Carl Wikander, indexer; Claire Linden, manuscript and production coordinator; and Ann Anton, administrative coordinator. Seventeenth Street Studios provided design and composition.

This publication is designed to provide accurate and authoritative information in regard to the subject matter covered. It is sold with the understanding that neither the authors nor the publisher is engaged in rendering legal, accounting, or other professional service. If legal advice or other expert assistance is required, the services of a competent professional person should be sought. (From a *Declaration of Principles* jointly adopted by a Committee of the American Bar Association and a Committee of Publishers and Associations.)

The Capitation Sourcebook: a practical guide to managing at-risk arrangements
edited by Peter Boland
Library of Congress Catalog Card Number: 96-85377
ISBN: 0-9652717-1-4

To Sierra

Contents

■ Part IV
MANAGEMENT TOOLS

Preface

REDESIGNING HEALTHCARE DELIVERY is intended to meet the strategic and day-to-day needs of varied practitioners, operational managers, and healthcare executives for improving care delivery. Successful reengineering methodologies are presented as examples of what healthcare organizations are doing to dramatically enhance performance and document value. The book provides step-by-step methodologies for redesigning inpatient, outpatient, and ambulatory care. The authors propose a fundamental rethinking of how care is organized and provided based on the premise that many notions about management reengineering and operational restructuring may be too limited to sufficiently increase competitiveness and produce substantial improvements in healthcare delivery.

In order to reduce costs significantly without undermining quality, providers and payers must develop new approaches to care delivery that are based on customer needs, anticipated market conditions, and collaborative redesign principles. The analytical methods and management techniques in this volume reflect practical considerations and operational benchmarks, such as cost reduction targets, clinical quality criteria, and customer service objectives.

Documenting cost, quality, and service performance is the key to accountability and is becoming the standard for judging health plans and medical care. This message is a wake-up call for the entire healthcare industry. What healthcare purchasers have made clear is the need to significantly cut the cost of providing medical care so that health plan premiums are more affordable. In short, employers and payers want the healthcare industry to operate within specific price parameters. Therefore, customer loyalty will require price-competitive services.

The healthcare industry's greatest challenge is to meet market-based demands for better care at lower cost. To accomplish this objective, providers and payers must redesign delivery systems and clinical treatment to better meet the needs of patients, employers, and local communities. This will require a large allocation of capital to retool current operations, a serious commitment to rethink care delivery, and the political will to embrace fundamental change. How this change is designed and led is the key to success.

This book is written for practitioners by practitioners as a guide to restructuring and refocusing care while revitalizing healthcare organizations. Each chapter addresses difficult problems and offers detailed solutions that can be used by hospitals, medical groups, and managed care organizations. By taking a "best practices" approach, the book demonstrates how others have been able to

- Prepare organizations for change and then lead and manage it

- Develop growth strategies to generate new revenue and opportunity

- Involve stakeholders in planning and implementation methodologies

- Align vision, strategies, and resources to achieve performance targets

- Customize reengineering approaches for internal and external customers

- Manage the human aspects of change during redesign and reengineering activities

- Design workforce reduction as a positive step in redefining employees' new roles and expectations

- Refocus services around customer requirements rather than organizational priorities

- Create "virtual" organizations in addition to vertically integrated delivery systems

- Rethink fundamental assumptions about core business strategies, functions, and services

- Align management functions and responsibilities with core activities

- Restructure operations to improve efficiency and clinical quality

- Apply best practices for clinical reengineering

- Develop clinical care maps to guide care and reshape organizational culture

- Improve employee productivity through cross training

- Use information technology to restructure work and redesign operations

Redesigning Healthcare Delivery is organized into four sections, each of which builds a knowledge base for reengineering healthcare delivery. Section one discusses the market forces propelling systemwide transformation, the need for repositioning medical care, and the necessary emphasis on outpatient rather than inpatient services in light of changing utilization patterns.

Section two presents a number of change management principles and techniques, such as how to lead organizational change; identify business priorities before reengineering; link reengineering to revitalizing an organization; align business purpose and operations; relate strategy to tactics; and balance market, cost, and quality issues. Additional material on systemwide transformation focuses on new core competencies, performance reengineering methodologies, work redesign activities, and different implementation approaches.

Section three develops a number of case studies on business process redesign techniques including operations improvement, resource management, cost recovery, service mix, information systems support, organizational culture, quality management, patient flow, continuous quality improvement, treatment protocols, and clinical care paths. Three case studies on patient-focused care detail how hospitals can streamline management, restructure patient care sites, and use collaborative design principles. Three additional health plan examples explain how to increase customer satisfaction, reframe member services, and integrate financing and delivery components.

Section four highlights management tools such as communication to engage employees and gain physician support; teamwork and training programs to improve productivity; and information systems and technology innovation to restructure work, organizations, and services.

The goal of this publication is to stimulate critical thinking and initiate a dialogue among industry stakeholders about how to lead and manage fundamental change, promote revitalization and renewal of healthcare organizations, and increase the value of care to patients and customers. Reader feedback is an essential ingredient in this process and is highly valued by Boland Healthcare. Readers should point out what further learning material would enhance their knowledge base, job skills, and career development and are encouraged to send their suggestions to:

Peter Boland, PhD
President and Publisher
BOLAND HEALTHCARE, INC.
1551 Solano Avenue, 2nd Floor
Berkeley, California 94707
Telephone: 510-524-4521
Fax: 510-524-4607
E-mail: bolandinfo@aol.com

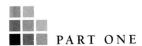

PART ONE

INTRODUCTION

1

The role of reengineering
in healthcare delivery

Peter Boland, PhD
President
Boland Healthcare, Inc.
Berkeley, California

THERE IS A FINANCIAL CRISIS facing the healthcare industry. It is not simply a problem of cost containment or operational streamlining. This is far deeper and demands a keen understanding of what is at stake and the types of values that can encourage or inhibit profound change throughout the healthcare community.

The healthcare industry is at a watershed moment. It can either embrace fundamental change and rethink the meaning of health on an individual and systemwide basis, or it can simply continue on its present course. Today, the conventional wisdom represents a continuing investment of healthcare capital, staff, and philosophy in an approach to care that does not markedly improve community health status, which is the ultimate indicator of health system effectiveness. The current approach also represents an outdated professional culture ill suited to cope with the massive impact of societal forces, such as economic restructuring, technological innovation, aging, and consumerism.

In order to measurably increase health status, quality, or cost effectiveness, there must be a serious national dialogue among stakeholders about the goals and limits of healthcare delivery in this country. Society's expectations about what the health system should do and for whom must be clearly defined in terms of priorities and accountabilities, because limited funding compels choices among competing services, approaches, and ideologies.

It is time for the healthcare industry and the public to grapple together with conflicting values about the appropriate role of government, individual and group responsibility, and the capacity of institutions to assure better healthcare in the future. This calls for an explicit public-private dialogue and a commitment to develop a new social contract for healthcare. It must delineate what government should and should not do and how to structure accountability between public agencies and private healthcare plans in order to improve the health status of local communities. It is in everyone's interest to establish meaningful parameters for accountability.

To this end, healthcare organizations must initiate a profound transformation to meet the needs of patients, employers, insurers, and the government. Healthcare organizations will increasingly be held accountable by purchasers and payers for improving the health status and functioning of individuals and groups, decreasing overall healthcare spending, and improving customer service to their health plan members. Reengineering is an essential methodology for meeting these needs. It is also a powerful mechanism for improving organizational performance and building better relationships among key stakeholders. Successful reengineering boils down to a few key ingredients: simplifying and redesigning how people work, improving their job skills, motivating them to perform better, and providing the necessary equipment, technology, and facility support.

There are at least eight related factors that help explain the magnitude of change taking place in the industry. These include: market forces, structural redesign and reengineering phases, organizational culture, customer focus, population-based risk management, systemwide reengineering, health status factors, and chronic care management. Each of these elements is described in this chapter. When taken together, they suggest a fundamental shift in the future direction of healthcare delivery.

Market forces

Reengineering represents a methodology for thinking about work, organizational purpose, and performance. It is not an answer or an end in itself but a means to an end. Its success depends on an organization's commitment and ability to manage fundamental change. The need for reengineering and the parameters for how much and how fast organizations must change is determined by local markets.

As market forces define stringent cost and performance targets for healthcare organizations, reengineering methodologies become essential survival tools to manage change and improve service. Cost reduction demands by purchasers and payers have been driving down provider reimbursement rates each year, but this is not a viable long-term strategy. Rates can only be ratcheted down so far before payment no longer covers real costs and provider resentment negatively affects the physician-patient relationship. At that point, quality is jeopardized. Fundamental delivery system redesign is therefore necessary, because healthcare organizations cannot sufficiently reduce their ongoing operating costs without sustained effort.

The market's need for substantially lower healthcare premiums compels providers—including hospitals, physicians, and other practitioners—to face the stark reality that industrywide consolidation will result in few clear winners and many losers. At a minimum, there will be much more service integration between health plan administration and patient care delivery functions, among facilities and practitioners, and within institutions through comprehensive case management and individualized care protocols. Widespread merger and acquisition activity will leave few organizations untouched and will provide further rationale to integrate fragmented services and operations using reengineering tools and to change management techniques. Therefore, just sustaining current practices will not meet customer demands for significant cost reduction and improved service quality, which means doing more for less.

Reengineering healthcare delivery is not limited to institutional pro-viders and organizations. Using a systems approach to reduce costs, improve quality, and increase customer satisfaction, employers and employees must be involved in redesigning care delivery. Health plans must encourage and enable customers to assume more responsibility as partners to reduce the need for costly care and improve medical outcomes. This responsibility applies to benefits design, worksite safety, and injury prevention and can be extended to include lifestyle risk management programs, employee incentives, and early screening and referral mechanisms such as employee assistance programs.

Market forces and industry dynamics are generating an unprecedented level of change, resulting in reduced need for acute care facilities, providers, and healthcare vendors. Managed care has cut the utilization rate for inpatient services to such an extent that most markets now have a significant excess of hospital beds and physician specialists. Thus, both successful and challenged organizations are being forced to reassess their future in light of decreasing revenue, increasing competition, and the demand for more accountability and documented results. These factors make fundamental change a requirement for survival; incremental change on a piecemeal basis will not enable healthcare organizations to succeed. Much more serious intervention is required. Organizations must rapidly rethink what they do and how they do it to remain competitive.

One of the most important factors is how technology is used to improve the quality of care and overall system performance. Advances in technology, particularly management information systems, provide people and organizations with new and better ways to communicate, analyze data, structure organizations, and reduce the cost of doing business. Although technology helps drive change and is a prerequisite for successful reengineering, reengineering is primarily about people. Managing the human side of organizational change is now the biggest challenge facing the healthcare industry. Technology is a necessary but insufficient tool for redesigning how people and organizations work. Staff skills, knowledge, and work roles must be expanded and integrated to meet customer needs.

Managed care is the most powerful force responsible for reshaping healthcare today. Reengineering initiatives and change strategies do not exist in a vacuum; they must be approached with the knowledge of where the industry is moving and how managed care is evolving. Its stages of development vary across different markets, and the type and pace of change is defined locally. As shown in Table 1, cost control, network management, accountability, and customer focus are potent forces that drive change depending on the stage of the particular market.

DEVELOPMENT STAGES

During the past two decades, there has been a concerted effort by health plans to decrease costs by using techniques such as preauthorization, case management, and negotiated discounts from fee schedules. These techniques were followed by the development of primary care provider networks and exertion of more systematic cost and quality controls on them and on physician specialists, hospitals, allied health professionals, and ancillary services vendors. Payers have placed increasing financial risk on individual providers by implementing capitated or budget-based reimbursement.[1]

TABLE 1
Managed care industry development cycle

Driving forces	Stage one	Stage two	Stage three
Cost control	Contain specific costs case by case	Consolidate vendors and distribution channels:	Manage at-risk groups
	Achieve economies of scale:	■ hospitals	Integrate patient care delivery and health plan administration functions
	■ membership	■ medical groups	
	■ geographic concentration	■ ancillary services	
	■ service volume	■ health plans	
	Transition fee-for-service to budget-based reimburesment	Contain continuum of cost throughout care delivery	
Network management	Build primary care networks	Integrate continuum of services and providers through multidisciplinary care teams:	Establish interdependent alliances across and within industry sectors
		■ primary care	
		■ specialty care	
		■ behavioral healthcare	
		■ allied healthcare	
Accountability	Develop aggregate cost reports	Document service and clinical quality	Consolidate information services and reporting functions:
			■ administrative
			■ clinical
			■ financial
Customer focus	Offer comprehensive employee benefits packages and covered services	Increase customer value:	Document treatment outcomes
		■ medical management	Improve health status:
		■ treatment outcomes	■ members
		■ member focus	■ population groups
			■ community

As cost pressure intensified and reimbursement levels decreased, providers and health plans began to consolidate for economic survival. Hospitals and health plans increasingly purchased physician practices. Many hospitals merged or were purchased by larger hospital management companies that, in turn, pressured suppliers for lower prices as a trade-off for greater volume. This activity led to increasingly streamlined distribution channels. Another benefit of this consolidation was the opportunity to use multidisciplinary patient care teams to integrate a continuum of services across providers and, thereby, improve quality and cost control. But again, this progression did not occur in lockstep fashion in every locale, and some markets have not yet experienced all of these developments.

Today, purchasers are increasingly demanding more value from their providers, and this has elevated quality to a high priority. Purchasers and large employers have demanded it, and clinicians have embraced continuous quality improvement methodologies to improve and document care provided. Clinical and service quality are now the objects of data collection and reporting efforts for providers and health plans in addition to cost profiles. Perceived value, not just cost control, has become an important criterion for judging health plan adequacy. Value means effective medical management, better treatment outcomes, and improved customer satisfaction—all of which must be documented as a justification for purchasers' premiums and ongoing business trust.

A growing emphasis on accountability dictates that delivery systems consolidate most of their data repositories, information services, and reporting functions. This consolidation will enable them to better integrate administrative, clinical, and financial data into easy-to-understand yet comprehensive reports. Still, employers need more "actionable data" to make better decisions about designing employee benefits. What health plans need are more flexible and focused information systems to manage provider networks and document the effect of services on the health of enrollees.

Structural redesign

Reengineering is a developmental and evolutionary process. It follows a logical sequence of events, but organizations do not simply go through it in a linear manner. The process generally creates a particular momentum and direction, depending on how aggressively senior management pushes reengineering and on the extent of change an organization can withstand and manage. Once reengineered activities are implemented, the organization adapts and the project then enters a new phase of refinement. Additional core business functions are often targeted for redesign, thus further expanding the circle of reengineering projects.

Each layer of management may need to be restructured again at different points in the process.

Typically, organizations experience a series of lesser changes before they recognize that fundamental change, more radical than incremental, is necessary. An organization may start by analyzing how business is conducted and identifying problems and potential solutions and then reworking a particular function, product line, or organizational component. The analysis and redesign activity often results in changing work roles to lower costs and improve productivity. This activity is referred to as rightsizing or downsizing an organization because it generally involves laying off or reassigning staff. Downsizing is not a long-term strategy, however. It does not increase revenue or create new products and opportunities for growth.

Often, senior management must lead reengineering efforts by example and restructure itself before clinical reengineering; otherwise, management will not have the credibility or demonstrated expertise to tackle clinical redesign. Clinical process reengineering is one type of reengineering that emphasizes the development of standardized treatment protocols for specific types of patients. In time, this can lead to the realization that standardized protocols, where appropriate, should be developed for whole groups of patients. This approach will enable delivery systems to focus on disease management approaches for groups of patients, not just individual episodes of illness.

Redesign efforts that target clinical services sometimes begin with a continuous quality improvement program and standardized patient care protocols. Although this approach may improve the clinical quality of care, it does not dramatically increase savings or service quality. Substantial cost savings and breakthroughs in member satisfaction require rethinking the full continuum of care and individual services. The goal of reducing costs inevitably leads to aligning the economic incentives of providers with those of the health plan. Unless these reimbursement incentives are similar and encourage cost-effective behavior by providers, the health plan will not succeed in the long run.

Management restructuring, in contrast, tries to reduce the number of layers between top management, practitioners, and patients, thus giving more responsibility and authority to individuals who have direct contact with patients and plan members. This approach leads to greater accountability, reduced cost, better service quality, and increased patient satisfaction. Likewise, it is important to automate as many administrative functions as possible in order to increase efficiency and customer service. Cost reduction efforts usually lead to management restructuring and clinical service redesign, as shown in Table 2. Without the major components of a delivery system or health plan acting in concert, significant cost savings will not be realized.

Among the biggest challenges of reengineering is developing a strong member focus for all organizational activities. If the overall goal is to better serve health plan members and patients, then an organization must redesign its administrative and caregiving services around its members' health needs and cultural sensitivities. Part of developing a member focus and redesigning clinical care is creating personal care plans for all enrollees and their dependents. Personal care plans should address members' current and expected healthcare needs based on demographic characteristics and identifiable risk factors, including family history.

Another reengineering goal is to increase customer satisfaction through seamless delivery of care among different services and vendors. Making patient care and members' services truly seamless requires rethinking and redesigning the individual components of the current delivery system. Purchasers and plan members want fully integrated services across the continuum of care to be user-friendly and transparent in

TABLE 2
Healthcare reeengineering phases

Phase one	Phase two	Phase three	Phase four
Analyse business: ■ problems ■ opportunities Redesign work roles Reduce costs	Restructure management Automate functions Redesign clinical services and standardize treatment protocols Align provider financial incentives: ■ physicians ■ other practitioners ■ hospitals ■ ancillary services	Develop a member focus Create personal care plans Integrate information components: ■ administrative ■ clinical ■ financial ■ member ■ demographic Standardize care for patient groups	Integrate clinical disciplines and functional departments Integrate core functions: ■ patient care delivery ■ health plan administration ■ community-based services

terms of coordination. This challenge means integrating each clinical discipline with each functional department, thereby replacing a traditional departmental approach with an interdisciplinary cross-departmental approach to patient care. Likewise, it means integrating health plan administration and patient care functions with community-based services. Community-based services must be included because they help reduce the incidence and prevalence of disease, illness, and injuries. Early intervention by schools, social service agencies, and self-help organizations educates plan members and the community about preventing many accidents and injuries and some illnesses.

In order to reduce costs and create seamless delivery from a member's perspective, providers and health plans need to redefine service priorities and decide which duplicate services and functions to eliminate. For example, utilization management responsibilities and activities are often administered separately—and redundantly—by health plans, hospitals, medical groups, allied health practitioners, and numerous third-party vendors. Each overlapping activity must be critically evaluated to determine whether it should be provided at all—and if so, by whom and where.

At present, there is not enough emphasis on integrating and consolidating providers' and health plans' roles to reduce operating costs and improve service quality. Redundancy is a critical shortcoming of many delivery systems and, if corrected, could generate dramatic systemwide savings. However, this requires partnering organizations to relinquish certain administrative functions—even those that generate revenue. This challenge is very difficult, but there is little alternative if healthcare delivery systems are committed to substantially increasing value.

Purchasers and payers want a significant level of cost taken out of healthcare delivery and will choose vendors that can do this. It is unclear whether most health plans or hospital systems have the organizational resources in terms of capital, information technology, and management depth—in addition to the political will—to streamline and coordinate potentially overlapping functions. Thus, there is an emerging need for "system integrators" to play this role in each market. The most likely candidates may be technology companies, advanced provider organizations and delivery systems with substantial capital access, or joint venture arrangements created among these stakeholders.

The first generation of system integrators, largely technology companies, are developing flexible information platforms that will enable different stakeholders to redefine and restructure their service functions as shown conceptually in Figure 1. This new management tool will help delivery systems and practitioners coordinate administrative and clinical activities in a way that greatly enhances member service and patient care. Administrative transactions that may improve include such diverse functions as eligibility verification, referral authorization, utilization review, admissions and discharges, and claims processing. Improved clinical activities will include managing and coordinating patient care among different types of practitioners and facilities, collecting and analyzing diagnostic data, assisting patients and families with rehabilitation and recovery, and managing the full range of ambulatory care services for patients. As a result of consolidating and streamlining operations through this use of information technology, system integrators can

FIGURE 1
Overlapping service functions

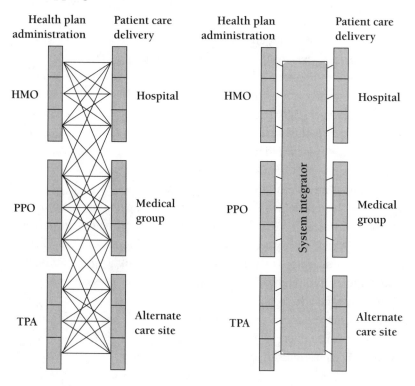

remove significant costs from the entire caregiving process. This is a fundamental corporate strategy that goes far beyond ad hoc staff reductions and operational efficiency projects. It also necessarily entails considerable disruption and subsequent realignment within an organization, all of which may create additional short-term expense and anxiety.

Organizational culture

Successful reengineering involves transforming an organization's culture —its guiding principles, values, and behavior patterns. Organizational culture largely determines how and even whether an organization redesigns and integrates decision making with operational requirements. Reengineering fundamentally changes an organization because it addresses basic questions about values, vision, mission, and work in relation to the customer. Since reengineering entails fundamental changes, the values embodied in an organization and by its leaders determine the type and extent of change undertaken. Reengineering requires stakeholders to rethink their roles and responsibilities. It also requires a tangible change in individual behavior (e.g., team-oriented collaboration), group performance (e.g., shared decision making), and organizational culture (e.g., customer focus). As a result, the corporate culture of an organization, as well as the subculture of its divisions and departments, must be examined for potential obstacles to reengineering activities. Moreover, such changes should be presented to people as a restatement and expression of the organization's culture.

For example, measuring improvement in member health status as an indicator of performance suggests large-scale organizational change but not a change in values. A change of this magnitude, however, does require a fully developed cultural strategy to implement a new way of doing business. A cultural strategy centers on changing how people think and act and overcoming their resistance to change in order to better meet customer needs. This is particularly true of the physician component in healthcare. Physicians are often the most challenging group to involve in reengineering efforts; but once motivated to participate, they make a significant contribution to improving clinical efficiency, quality, and patient satisfaction.

Organizational change is often impeded by cultural factors that are less tangible than technical ones and far more difficult to successfully manage. Changing the structure of an organization will have limited effect unless it is predicated on restating and adapting the traditional beliefs of those in the organization while changing their longstanding behaviors. Thus, a cultural change strategy is needed that embraces and reinforces the organization's and department's values as well as its business strategy (i.e, where it is going as an organization), operational strategy (i.e., how the organization is going to accomplish its goals and objectives), and payment strategy (i.e, types of payer contracts and reimbursement mechanisms) while trying new methods to meet the continuing mission.

In any healthcare organization, there are often numerous voices for change but little agreement on the specifics or pace. Moreover, administrators, technical staff, physicians, and customers all have different perspectives on how an organization should change. These views may reflect an organization's, department's, or individual's beliefs—particularly if the organization has not explicitly reinforced its own values in writing and in action. Even when values are reinforced, there is little initial constituency for radical change in most organizations despite the fact that it is required to survive. However, there is almost always overwhelming support for maintaining the status quo because organizational change is disruptive and often personally threatening to staff.

Healthcare leaders must develop a unified, compelling vision and rationale for change—whether incremental or radical—that links market demands for lower costs and better service to two critical categories of factors: the organization's cultural values and mission and a road map on how to get there. Change initiatives are more likely to succeed if a practical blueprint is agreed upon by senior management regarding what needs to be accomplished, how to do it, and the expected benefits for the organization and its customers. This calls for sponsoring as well as actively leading change. Leading change requires top management to collaborate with middle management and technical support staff at every step in the redesign initiative. Individuals are most likely to support what they help create, and this becomes a prerequisite for effective implementation.

Shared values and trust are the most important resources an organization has to draw upon in repositioning itself through reengineering. They are the basis for collaborative decision making across all organizational levels and professional disciplines and are a prerequisite for changing an organization's corporate culture. The organizational and personal turbulence often caused by this transition must be acknowledged and factored into redesign strategies. Moreover, it must be orchestrated and managed in such a way as to reflect and maintain both shared values and trust. However, this process calls for new leadership and change management skills not commonly found in organizations patterned on a command-and-control management style, which is typical of healthcare institutions.

When healthcare organizations are restructured based on reengineering principles—such as work redesign, customer focus, service integration, management restructuring, and cross training—their form and function change accordingly. Thus, traditional organizational charts with lines and boxes are modified and complemented by role relationships that explain how individuals and business units must support each other in meeting customer service goals and financial targets. These new interrelationships stress partnership, accountability, and an explicit customer service orientation. Senior management must support frontline staff who have the most contact with customers, including physicians, and remove bureaucratic obstacles for them to better serve patients and members.

Customer focus

Streamlining operations, increasing departmental efficiency, and cost-cutting techniques alone are not powerful enough to produce more than 15 to 20 percent of the cost reductions that payers want. The balance of these savings requires a new awareness of customer needs and priorities.

The focus of attention among healthcare organizations is gradually shifting from the provider to the purchaser and end user—the patient. This reflects the fact that customers now largely set the agenda for change in terms of funding and reimbursement parameters, meaning how much will be spent on healthcare in the future and where. A new set of customer expectations is created when the patient becomes the real focus of the delivery system. Payers and patients alike want to feel that their unique needs are uppermost in providers' minds. This frame of reference requires across-the-board reinterpretation of organizational purpose as well as changes in attitudes, behavior, and services. This is part of what population-based care means. Practitioners' roles and responsibilities and health plans' accountability to members are being redefined in response to this dynamic.

Health plans and providers must reconfigure service delivery to provide a full continuum of care for members. For many, this means putting together a virtually integrated company rather than a vertically or horizontally integrated one. That does not necessarily mean merging the assets of the participants but instead managing their service components through contractual relationships. The virtual approach suggests a different organizational structure and management orientation to care delivery. Regardless of the approach, however, the newly created continuum of care must have as its purpose the improvement of members' health status.

Healthcare reengineering should be driven by what the customer wants and what the market needs. As a result, customers' issues and concerns are gaining prominence and even preeminence in day-to-day operations of delivery systems. Healthcare organizations of all types are struggling to resolve six fundamental business issues that will determine their success or marketplace failure. They are trying to

1. Determine what services should be performed by the organization or in conjunction with others through virtual relationships or subcontracts

2. Identify when services should be performed according to a personal care plan for each member, one that projects healthcare needs throughout a member's life and serves as a frame of reference for episodic care as well

3. Analyze services that should be performed in order to reduce cost and improve quality—both clinical and service dimensions—through restructured relationships within and among delivery systems, hospitals, subacute facilities, medical groups, and allied health professionals

4. Determine who should perform the service, based on redesigned patient care teams—multidisciplinary, primary care-based—and self-care management guidelines and instructions, in conjunction with patient care team coordinators

5. Decide where the service should be performed based on patient convenience, treatment efficacy, and availability of subacute services and settings

6. Develop a compensation structure for providers to increase motivation and reward performance for meeting patient needs, customer expectations, and organizational goals

This programmatic reorientation from a provider-based to a customer-driven philosophy represents a fundamental shift in ideology, institutional priorities, and direction for the healthcare industry. It embodies a change in values that affects everyone's daily roles and responsibilities. This questioning is especially threatening because it forces hospitals and physicians to reevaluate their services from a patient's point of view. Likewise, this process forces managed care organizations to judge their services from a member and employer perspective. Each role change represents a break from the past and business as usual.

Reengineering is based on the premise that delivery systems and affiliated vendors will embrace radical change to better meet customer needs. It assumes that many healthcare organizations will adapt and change in order to survive and gain market share, regardless of how wrenching change is for them. If this assumption is not correct, then the most likely alternative is to lose business, fall behind in terms of product innovation, and be forced to merge with a stronger partner on the latter's terms.

Population-based risk management

Managed care organizations evolve and change in response to underlying market trends, financial constraints, and innovative ways to treat patients. Payers are forcing providers to more aggressively manage risk as a means of rendering better care. Some delivery systems are also shifting from a focus on individual episodes of acute care to include broader population-based attempts to improve the health status of enrolled groups. This is an important step because payers and patients are best served when their delivery systems adopt a systematic approach to manage overall health risk for a defined population.

Managing populations requires a broader perspective than caring for individuals. It means changing the emphasis from being event driven to risk driven—reducing the likelihood of illness with preventive services or intervening sooner in the illness cycle through early detection and screening services. It also requires matching specific medical and social services to specific target groups. The objective is to better manage the health risk of target groups, which is a strategy that extends well beyond acute care patients and chronically ill members. To identify and manage population-based risk, new information systems, tracking mechanisms, and medical management procedures must be developed and established. At the same time, to better manage aggregate costs as well as unit costs, multidisciplinary care teams must focus on the drivers of acute care episodes—the underlying psychological, economic, and sociological factors that affect the incidence and prevalence of disease and injuries. Care teams can then use treatment protocols that identify the least costly and most clinically appropriate settings to direct patient care.

This shift in treatment strategy calls for delivery systems to take more responsibility for providing care in three ways: providing care that best fits the medical, social, and cultural profile of the enrolled population; maintaining and improving the health status of at-risk groups; and lowering the cost of care for individuals and the community, as shown in Figure 2.

As more risk continues to be transferred from public payers and employers to health plans and providers, plans and providers will be called upon to manage the care of high-risk, high-cost groups such as the frail elderly, AIDS patients, and chronically ill children on a capitated basis. Here, an emphasis on risk management encourages delivery systems to concentrate on containing and monitoring the impact of care, which includes measuring plan members' health status and patient functioning.

The role of delivery systems and partnering organizations, such as

FIGURE 2
Community-focused care model

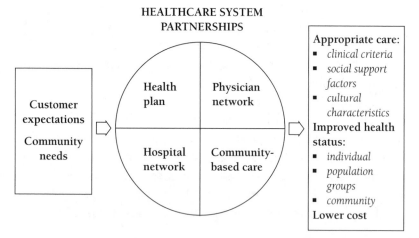

medical groups, hospitals, ancillary services vendors, and other providers, must change in order to intervene in illness sooner and more effectively. It is too costly for customers and health plans, particularly capitated arrangements, to wait until a member is acutely ill or in need of chronic care services. At the same time, it is not known how long it takes for most illness prevention services to pay off in terms of reduced need for acute care services. Prompt preventive care makes sense to patients because it is perceived as enhancing their quality of life, which is a further rationale for health plans to invest in it.

Risk management also calls for increased care coordination among provider organizations and delivery systems—seamless patient care along a service continuum—to reduce overlapping functions and duplicated services. This requires increased functional integration and tighter working relationships among employers, insurers, delivery systems, and providers. These interdependencies are created among stakeholders for a reason: such seamless care is more cost effective and increases the value to customers.

Systemwide reengineering

Because hospitals and most physicians only treat patients once they are sick, practitioners have little occasion to influence the course of events that lead up to the episode of care itself. Therefore, an effective reengineering objective is to avoid the need for high-cost medical services such as hospital admissions. By influencing the underlying causes of acute care episodes that can be controlled, such as preventable accidents and injuries and behaviorally linked illnesses, health plans can realize financial savings and members maintain better quality of life. This requires intervening early on a systemwide basis before acute or chronic care management is necessary, as shown in Figure 3.

The progression from "healthy" to "chronic" is partly a function of controllable factors and factors beyond an individual's direct control. However, with appropriate and early intervention, an individual's health status can be influenced toward the healthy end of the continuum even if his or her current status is at-risk or acute. As the current demographic bulge passes from middle age into the 65-plus age group, delivery systems will be overwhelmed by the prevalence of chronic illness and the accompanying cost burden. Reengineering the current approach to care now is an economic necessity for healthcare delivery systems and society.

FIGURE 3
Life cycle stages and health status factors[2]

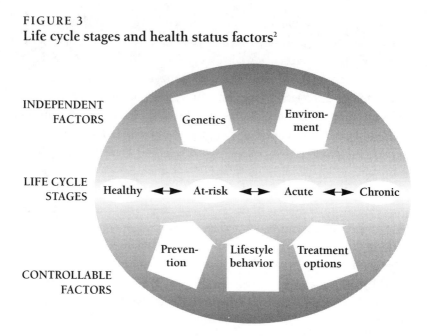

Chronic care management

Managed care delivery systems are deeply rooted in the acute care model of medicine. This model is not geared to an aging population whose chronic illnesses cannot be cured and who need relief of symptoms and prevention of further dysfunction. It calls for a biopsychosocial model (i.e., medical, social, and community orientation) that encompasses far more than physiological factors commonly associated with acute care treatment. The goal of chronic care management is not curative; the emphasis is on quality of life and level of function. A multidisciplinary team is required to integrate primary and specialty care with home-based and community-based services. Both patient and family perspectives must be integrated into the care process for treatment to be effective and valued. This approach means reengineering and reorienting current medical management practices that are often based more on the needs of healthcare organizations and providers than on patients or health plan members.

At the same time, organizations must have sufficient management depth, skills, and knowledge to be successful as market demands evolve.

Challenging institutional beliefs and assumptions is not enough; organizations need to know how to accomplish new tasks and redesign existing programs. If organizations lack basic core competencies like change management, project management, and customer management, for example, they will need to develop such skills.

One of the most important competencies an organization must demonstrate is helping its employees master new technical and process skills. This forces many healthcare organizations to realize the critical and unavoidable role of continuing education for employees. Acquiring such skill calls for a human resources strategy well integrated with the organization's strategic goals and operational objectives. An effective human resources strategy includes ongoing training for employees who want to acquire appropriate skills to fit new work responsibilities that occur as a result of redesign and reengineering efforts. Both the employee and the employer must be clear on what their mutual responsibilities are during each phase of reengineering and as a result of organizational restructuring. Without resolving this issue, organizations will undercut a key potential of reengineering: learning faster than the competition. Healthcare organizations must demonstrate the critical linkage between human resources, organizational learning, and overall business strategy to be successful and profitable.

Conclusion

The healthcare industry is going through a dramatic redesign process. Price competition, capacity consolidation, and capitated risk arrangements are powerful market forces responsible for restructuring the healthcare industry from top to bottom.

The most pressing agenda for healthcare delivery systems is meeting customer needs, improving health status, and lowering costs. Reengineering is a powerful methodology that helps healthcare organizations reorder institutional priorities, provide more cost-effective care, and increase value to customers. Reengineering is not a panacea; it is a critical core competency and requisite skill for healthcare organizations if they are to succeed under managed care in the future.

To be successful, reengineering initiatives must be propelled by an accurate reading of healthcare industry trends and dynamics as well as by an organization's unique vision of its ongoing role and mission. Furthermore, the initiative must be supported by a senior management team willing to embark on a course of action that will significantly affect how management and staff work and what they do as healthcare professionals.

Systemwide reengineering encompasses a broad view of healthcare integration that includes three levels of activity: managing community and health plan partnerships; consolidating overlapping delivery system functions among participating providers and vendors; and redesigning administrative functions, clinical services, and caregiving programs to improve health status. The current approach to reengineering is limited, for the most part, to gaining operational efficiencies (i.e., part of the third level of activity). Winning healthcare delivery systems in the future will embrace all three levels of change in order to maximize improvements in health status, organizational performance, and customer service.

The scope and pace of this change is profound. It affects all aspects of healthcare delivery and is forcing stakeholders to realize and accept the need for continuous change and adaptation. That is the essence of successful reengineering; it is an ongoing process that never ends.

NOTES

1. P. Boland, "The Power and Potential of Capitation," in *The Capitation Sourcebook* (Berkeley: Boland Healthcare, 1996).
2. This model is adapted from New Century Healthcare Institute, San Francisco, California.

2

Repositioning medical services for managed care

Cheryl Robbins
Partner
Deloitte & Touche Consulting Group
Los Angeles, California

Hospitals in the united states have traditionally operated with a reliable, uncapped source of revenue. Indemnity insurance companies paid the hospital bill for insured Americans, covering the high costs of state-of-the-art hospital care. Indemnity insurance allowed both patient and physician to take advantage of the latest in diagnostic testing, treatment, and facilities.

In 1965, the government developed Medicare and Medicaid programs to finance healthcare for the nation's elderly and medically indigent. These financing mechanisms increased funding and utilization for most hospitals; new hospital facilities opened and others expanded, sparing no cost in the process.

The introduction of prospective payment provided hospitals with their first major limitations on Medicare funding. Now, with the emergence of managed care, hospitals see inpatient utilization diminish as the percentage of capitated revenues grow. Many Medicaid programs now follow the managed care industry's lead, creating initiatives to move Medicaid recipients into managed care plans. Empty beds and facilities are forcing hospitals to consolidate or close. Others remain open but with downsized services and staff.

In response, innovative hospitals have introduced ambulatory care services as a low-cost alternative to traditional hospital care. Mainstream hospitals are matching this innovation in ambulatory care in an attempt to offset falling demand for inpatient care.

The medical industry itself continues to produce technological innovations that will have major impact on healthcare. In the not-too-distant future, genetic testing, performed any time during a person's life or even before birth, will predict important lifelong requirements for medical care. The test will be easy, inexpensive, and fast, and it may revolutionize the way diagnostic work is done by both physicians and hospitals.

The result? Hospital teams, formed in times of expansion and affluence, must now compete for shrinking healthcare dollars. At the same time, medical innovations are diminishing the need for facility-based services that have defined American hospitals for centuries. This dynamic environment has left hospital management teams with two questions: How to compete today? How to confront a future of unpredictable, escalating change?

New physician role

In markets with high managed care penetration, financial incentives create demand for lower-cost medical care, forcing physicians and hospitals to rethink fundamental strategies for healthcare delivery.

Today, managed care insurers pay primary care physicians (PCPs) a predetermined amount per month for each member served in the managed care network. In these cases, physicians are forced to reduce the cost of primary care to less than the per member per month (PMPM) amount. If this is achieved, the physician's personal income is sustained. If patients become sick or are chronically ill, requiring more care, the physician loses personal income. PCPs cannot sufficiently lower costs by improving physician office activities or by changing the form of treatment. A new primary care operating model is required.

To reduce the cost of primary care, some physicians are developing practice models that redistribute work normally done by the PCP. For example, some private physicians and physician groups have chartered nurses to call chronically ill patients on a daily or weekly basis. Caregivers check to see that medications are taken, exercises are done, and medical diets adhered to. They answer patient questions and provide moral support. With patients actively managed, the PCP sees fewer patients each day but spends more time planning each patient's care.

With this model, cost per patient is lowered in two ways. Nursing calls are less expensive than calls made by physicians. In addition, by reducing the need for acute care visits, physicians see patients less often, and the physicians' costs are further reduced. Because fewer acute care visits are required, physicians may also expand the size of their practice to serve more patients. Each new patient brings additional monthly capitated revenues.

At the same time, costs are reduced by dealing with lifestyle issues that block patients' progress or by preventing acute illness episodes in chronically ill patients. For example, if an emphysema patient smokes, the patient will require a higher rate of ongoing care. By pointing the patient to groups that can help break the smoking habit, a persistent barrier to health improvement is removed and the requirement for care reduced. In another example, diabetic patients, prone to complications such as circulation problems, can be scheduled for more frequent checkbacks. By spotting warning signs early, the potential for medical complications—and the requirement for care—is reduced.

What is the result? PCPs, once dedicated to treatments and compensated for seeing as many patients as possible in a given day, now focus on health maintenance and reducing the need for acute care physician visits. In addition to lowering their own costs, PCPs are beginning to help patients reduce their total cost of healthcare. When patients require hospitalization, PCPs and their staffs will increasingly serve as the patient's care manager, counseling the patient on low-cost alternatives to traditional hospital care. In this way, PCPs will drive further demand for lower-cost ambulatory services and hospital care. In a few states, regulators have allowed PCPs to accept full capitation for medical care spending. In these states, PCPs make final decisions on hospital selection and spending. Other states are expected to follow.

To survive financially, physicians are looking beyond their current models of delivering healthcare to find lower-cost delivery methods. The physician's new mission? First, create and maintain healthier patients. Second, keep patients out of expensive delivery units.

New hospital role

How does this shift in medical priority—from treatment to health maintenance—affect traditional hospital care? In the near term, hospitals must cope with fixed cost and excess capacities, which are difficult to change. Hospitals have already reduced variable costs—for personnel, supplies, and services—by squeezing departmental budgets. To reduce costs further, some hospitals have downsized by consolidating treatment facilities and reducing administrative costs. Others have implemented "patient-focused care." In this approach, nurses, ancillary staff, and support staff are trained in multiple skill sets to eliminate duplicate tasks performed by specialized staff. For example, a nurse may periodically check a hospital patient's blood pressure. A respiratory therapist may again take the patient's blood pressure along with other monitoring tests already performed by the nurse. In patient-focused care, these tasks are performed by one caregiver with a broadened skill set.

Unfortunately, these efforts are not enough. In markets with high managed care penetration, price competition demands further reduction in acute care costs. As capitated physicians find new ways to reduce hospital days per 1,000, inpatient days will continue to fall at an alarming rate. At the beginning of the decade, the hospital industry maintained four hospital beds for every 1,000 Americans. Analysts forecast that in the future, hospitals will maintain one hospital bed for every 1,000 Americans.

At the same time, medical advances are changing fundamental approaches to healthcare. Surgeons are adopting techniques that can be performed on an outpatient basis. Disease specialists are experimenting with treatments that can be extended to and completed in the patient's home. Home products allow patients to monitor blood pressure, glucose levels, and other conditions, reducing medical costs and increasing patient convenience.

What used to require hospitalization now requires a physician visit. What used to require a physician visit now requires a self-administered home test. To participate in these healthcare advances, hospital teams must think differently about hospital facilities, technology, and home services as vehicles for delivering medical care.

To compete for referrals, hospitals must support surgeons and specialists in providing these new low-cost services. With new equipment, such as laser technology, surgery becomes less invasive, allowing hospitals and specialists to shorten patient stays and perform surgeries as ambulatory services. As hospitals compete for referrals with low-cost alternatives to traditional hospital care, they will themselves reduce the need for traditional facilities-based medicine.

With these trends on the horizon, hospital staffs must leave behind the idea that their business is hospitals. Instead, management, clinical professionals, and supporting staff must recognize their core competency is providing a specific portfolio of healthcare services to a set of managers of patient populations.

This core competency requires management processes and information systems that

- Identify target populations (e.g., hypertensive patients) that can be served profitably by the hospital. These target populations are secured by establishing mutually beneficial relationships with PCPs who manage the target population's overall health. Hospital services are delivered by establishing relationships with specialists who specialize in treatments these populations require

- Monitor the health trends of the populations managed by each PCP to identify how quickly medical advances must be put into place. For example, if a physician group has a large number of hypertensive patients, there may be an opportunity for the hospital to help with a disease management program

- Monitor and integrate medical advances into traditional facilities-based hospital services as needed to meet the demands of target populations. For example, the hospital may develop an information-sharing program between the hospital pharmacy and the PCP to monitor results of the new disease management program

- Replace facilities-based services with new forms of medical care. For example, the hospital may offer a new home-monitoring program to assist in the disease management effort

This is not a one-time change in cost structure or care delivery process. It is a fundamental repositioning of hospitals to a new kind of healthcare enterprise that can evolve its services as medical technologies evolve and population needs change. This repositioning gives hospitals competitive strength, whether operating on their own or within an integrated delivery system.

A hospital team can begin the transformation by

- Clearly defining its target customers and understanding requirements from each customer's point of view

- Expanding market strategies and programs to meet target customers' needs

- Reengineering to take full advantage of streamlined processes and medical and technological advances that reduce the need for facility-based medical care

- Becoming competent at reporting outcomes to prove the organization's value to its customers

Customer redefined

In indemnity insurance markets, hospitals design and scale services to meet the needs of local communities. A local community comprises people who live within a defined radius of the hospital facility. The hospital's relationship with its community is the focus of hospital management and clinical staff.

In managed care, the hospital's customers must include the PCP. Patients are referred to a specialist and hospital by PCPs working inside or outside the traditional service area. For example, physicians in a managed care network may refer all cancer patients to a regional specialist and hospital known for its cost-effective cancer treatment expertise. Or local physicians may refer expectant parents to a local birthing center instead of the local hospital for new baby delivery.

Geographic presence no longer serves as the automatic selection criteria for hospitals and their specialists. From the patient's perspective, nonemergency managed care is obtained from the best physicians and facilities within a managed care network. In managed care, to attract as well as retain a desirable customer base, hospitals must provide proven, cost-effective services. To do so, the hospital must know what the network requires.

Population-based management is the study and treatment of patient populations managed by PCPs. In these studies, hospitals analyze the needs of these patient populations to establish the most cost-effective medical management possible. For example, if a group of physicians practices in an area with a young population and a hospital is targeting these physicians, then effective low-cost maternity services, pediatrics, and drug abuse prevention may be important. If a physician group manages patients with chronic respiratory illness and a hospital is targeting these physicians, then specialized monitoring and prevention programs may be important.

What is the managed care hospital's number one priority? Shifting its focus toward PCPs as key customers. This shift is handled by adjusting the hospital's culture to recognize both the new role of PCPs in determining the hospital's financial success and the new role of specialists as "partners" of PCPs. By shifting focus toward PCPs as key customers, new partnership models emerge. For example, PCPs have found that sending nurse practitioners to a chronically ill patient's home to assess lifestyle risks and to establish active monitoring can prevent trips to the specialist. When patients are hospitalized, the primary care team works inside the hospital to speed recovery and transition the patient back to home care. Hospitals and specialists provide service to the primary care provider by helping to design the risk assessment and care plan.

In managed care, hospitals must partner with PCPs to plan new services and to forecast demand. The hospital's potential patient base can no longer be measured by the number of people living in the local community. Instead, it is measured by adding up the patient populations of each PCP with whom the hospital has or is targeting a relationship and estimating its share of these populations. After primary care relationships are established, the patient populations' needs are assessed. Armed with this information, hospitals can design services, attract specialists, and scale capacity to meet the needs of PCPs and their patients. This population-based management approach replaces traditional hospital forecasting and planning methods.

To implement population-based management, some hospitals are envisioning information systems that will report to each PCP the real-time status of patients throughout their hospital stay. A PCP, in turn, will enter into the information system comments or recommendations based on long-term experience with the patient's care. In this way, the hospital, physician, and specialists work as a team to monitor and plan each patient's care. At the same time, the hospital earns favor with its most important customer—the PCP—with services tailored to the needs of the physician's patients.

A hospital using population-based management techniques can work with physicians to integrate medical innovations and migrate traditional services to new forms of healthcare, at a rate appropriate to the physicians' needs. For example, laser surgery quickly and dramatically reduced inpatient procedures, forcing hospitals to react quickly by expanding outpatient surgical services. If patient populations of PCPs were thoroughly understood, the impact of laser surgery could have been predicted and planned for in advance, giving the hospital a "first mover" advantage.

Because medical innovation and patient populations change dramatically over shorter and shorter periods of time, population-based management must be the hospital's new core competency in the twenty-first century. How can hospitals develop this new competency? A hospital reengineering project can be used to put the required operational foundation into place.

Operations strategies for managed care

Hospitals are questioning if reengineering will provide the answers needed to survive in dynamic times. They have struggled to realize the promise of dramatic change, without much success to date.

Why is dramatic change so elusive? Primarily because reengineering is confused with cost cutting. Transformation opportunities emerging from strategic forces introduced by managed care, medical advances, and information technology are overlooked or ignored. For example, a hospital targeted maternity services for a 30 percent reduction in cost. Focus was on variable cost such as skill mix and productivity. A 20 percent cost reduction was achieved. After the project was complete, the hospital suddenly found that neither 20 nor 30 percent reductions were enough. Competitors were gaining market share with 12-hour birthing centers, midwives, and home nursing services. Cost cutting targeted an existing healthcare service, eliminated cost, and assumed the basic operating model stayed in place. While this may have produced results, the effort did not tap into the strategic opportunities offered by reengineering.

Delivery system reengineering looks at customers' needs, now and in the future, and identifies ways in which work can be done to create a stronger position in the managed care market. Cost structures are radically altered by asking hospital teams to rethink their fundamental approach to medical care.

What is the result? The reengineering process challenges everything about today's medical care. It migrates hospitals from inpatient services to other types of medical care where opportunities exist. It identifies other uses—such as hospice and rehabilitation services—for empty hospital facilities. And it helps management make tough decisions to shed services that require more fixed cost than service revenues warrant.

How will a hospital know if it is time to reengineer for managed care? It is time to reengineer if a hospital team can answer these seven questions positively:

- "Has the time come when we must compete, or prepare to compete, on cost in the managed care marketplace?"

- "Do we understand how the PCP's shift in priority—from treatment to health maintenance—affects referrals for our services?"

- "Do we understand the populations we will serve as a result of these referrals, the medical needs of these populations, and population and medical trends over the next 5 to 10 years?"

- "Do we require dramatic change if we are to compete effectively in this changing market?" (Dramatic change is a 30 percent or more improvement in financial strength, market share, or customer service.)

- "Are market pressures severe enough that the board, management, clinicians, and medical community recognize and agree that we must change?"

- "Are incentives in place to support nurses and physicians in creating new approaches to medical care?"

- "Do we have a strong leader capable and willing to lead the enterprise through dramatic change?"

Reengineering phases

Reengineering a hospital for managed care starts with a four-phase project. If done correctly, these four phases help hospital teams answer two critical concerns; how to compete in a low-cost managed care market and how to confront a future of unpredictable escalating change.

The following reviews each phase, highlighting the special challenges associated with reengineering hospitals for managed care.

PHASE ONE: ESTABLISH THE CHANGE IMPERATIVE

In phase one, the hospital team pinpoints specific needs for change and supports the analysis with qualitative information and statistical data. Hospital teams quickly recognize that the future market can support only one half of current hospital beds. They realize that winners must offer the best quality for the lowest cost and that only the sickest patients will require hospital care. In many cases, hospital professionals, for the first time, look at hospital services from this strategic market perspective. Often, leadership engages reengineering experts to develop a fact base with which to define the change imperative, to help conduct benchmarking, and to define and select the processes to reengineer.

Key steps are to

- Define the impact of managed care penetration on the hospital

  Identify how many hospital patients and potential patients belong to capitated health plans

  Estimate the penetration of managed care patients over the next three to five years

  Estimate the impact of managed care revenue on the hospital's total revenue stream over the next three to five years

  Identify the cost structure required to cover operating costs and achieve targeted margins

  Compare the required cost structure to the hospital's current cost structure to show the need for dramatic change

- Identify core processes and competencies that are critical to competing in the managed care market and to operating under new cost structures. Core processes might include

  Information sharing with PCPs

  Population-based management

New forms of low-cost medical care such as dramatic shifts to home care

- Profile the customer base and critical target customers, including PCPs and specialists

- Analyze healthcare needs of patient populations and population growth trends over the next 5 to 10 years

- Identify how much of competing hospital business is capitated and review the transformations hospitals are making in response

- Identify best practices in related industries

- Forecast probable market scenarios and the hospital's future if it does not reengineer. Scenarios might include

An experienced managed care provider buys a hospital competitor

One HMO locks the hospital out

Five or six HMOs consolidate into two or three and sign exclusive hospital arrangements

In many organizations, this is the first time a team of managers and staff work together to gain a broader market perspective. By clarifying the impact of medical advances and managed care, reengineering teams pave the way to up-front executive commitment and down-the-road staff support.

What is the top hospital reengineering risk? Eliminating this phase and starting with the simple objective of lowering cost. For example, a community hospital looked at next year's operating budget and decided it needed a 10 percent reduction in cost and reengineering to improve business processes. When the reengineering team examined managed care trends, it realized the hospital would require a 30 to 60 percent cost reduction within five years to compete. The team also realized these numbers could be achieved only by replacing traditional inpatient services with new forms of medical care. After the change imperative phase, the reengineering team reset its requirements for change.

What are the top reengineering challenges? Keeping leadership drive and commitment and developing strong change management capabilities. When dramatic change is required, both the medical decision-making model and the care delivery model must be challenged and placed in the context of the total care delivery continuum. Primary care gatekeeper physicians face dramatic changes in their medical decision-making model as HMOs obtain better outcomes information. Already, HMO panels question the medical necessity of decisions that fall outside of preset parameters. As the need for cost reduction increases, HMOs will search for better practices to further challenge the decision model. The hospital equivalent of this has been utilization management.

Hospitals have begun challenging the care delivery model with the institution of clinical pathways. Caregivers develop care delivery plans around the existing medical decision-making model. They fail to challenge the medical decision-making model itself.

The true power of reengineering hospital service is in the integrated reengineering of both the medical decision-making model and the care delivery model. Positive results are being achieved by bringing physicians and caregivers together to challenge assumptions about hospitalization. For example, bone marrow transplants that used to require weeks of hospitalization are being followed on an outpatient and home care basis because physicians, nurses, and ancillary clinicians are together rethinking how care can be delivered.

If physicians and nurses are brought in early to identify and understand the need for change, their talent can be applied to create innovative approaches to medical care. In turn, these innovations can radically lower cost, while maintaining the physician's control over the total continuum of the patient's care.

Hospitals face several other unique challenges when reengineering. If nursing, clinical, and clerical staff are represented by unions, the unions must be enfranchised early. By including union leaders in the change imperative phase, leaders can be made aware of economic pressures behind managed care and the consequences of not embracing radical future change.

At the end of the change imperative phase, the following are defined and documented:

- Why change is needed

- How much change is needed

- The hospital's managed care strategy

- Customer profiles

- The impact of the hospital's managed care strategy on physicians, nurses, and clinical and support staff, and how change will be shaped to benefit each

- A process model of the enterprise

- Core clinical and management processes targeted for change

- Benchmarking results

PHASE TWO: CREATE VISION AND TARGETS

In phase two, reengineering leaders work to envision new approaches to medical care that can position the hospital for long-term success in a managed care market.

This phase brings management, administrative staff, nurses, physicians, and other clinical leaders together to envision approaches to deliver high-quality, low-cost medical care. For example, to support and strategically position specialists, hospitals may decide to provide new medical technology, lower-cost structures with fast process cycle times, and accurate customized information about treatment. The reengineering experts often conduct team building in this phase. They challenge organizational tendencies to be timid and incremental in visions and targets. The team shifts its focus away from this year's reality to the challenges they will face in a three- to five-year time frame. They establish new, aggressive performance targets that help specify their new processes and programs.

Key steps are to

- Define service and performance targets from each customer's perspective. Targets might include the following:

    PCPs—easy access to patient information throughout the hospital stay and participation with the hospital team in patient planning and monitoring

    Specialists—instant response when requesting patient tests

    Patients—comfort and a feeling of personal care

    Health plans—low cost and good reputation

- Identify how current operations are viewed from each customer's perspective. Hospitals may find the following

    PCPs—patients drop into a "black hole" when they visit the hospital. The episode of care is taken over by the specialist and hospital

    Specialists—tests are often late or missing

    Patients—often feeling isolated and afraid, patients must interact, on average, with more than 150 hospital staff in a typical stay.

    Health plans—rising costs and no information about quality

- Identify the gap between customer performance targets and customer perceptions

- Define and prioritize what is to be done to close the gap

- Create a vision for how to do the work

    Brainstorming is encouraged. Feasibility and evaluation discouraged

    Ask, "if we had a new business and could start from scratch, what would we design?"

- Identify potential enablers of change: streamlined service, medical advances, new types of facilities, information technology, new medical expertise, and new approaches to administrative tasks

- Adjust the change management plan to account for changes resulting from new visions

When reengineering a hospital for managed care, the team imagines new services, redefines existing ones, and makes use of facilities in new ways. Visioning may include delivering care using new methods and medical technology to shorten hospital stays. It may include developing new ambulatory and home health services. Additionally, it may include launching new hospice or rehabilitation services to make use of empty hospital facilities. It may include involving families as caregivers. It may include new relationships and medical care processes involving PCPs and their clinical staff.

For example, in response to intense economic and competitive pressures, both low-cost and high-end providers have already implemented radical new approaches to medical care. Organizations serving the poor found facility-based services costly and inadequate. They now provide services to special community populations using mobile pediatric units, mobile dental units, and mobile mammogram units. Dermatologists specializing in hair transplants are replacing methods that required one physician and numerous visits with a transplant process that uses teams of physicians and one patient visit.

What is the top visioning risk? Too often, hospital reengineering teams view physicians as adversaries rather than partners in creating new visions for medical care. As a result, project teams create visions for the care delivery model only. They consolidate treatment facilities, reduce administrative costs and streamline nursing tasks. With this focus, they fail to redesign the delivery of care and the medical decision-making model that is the major driver of delivery. By including physicians and investigating the medical decision-making model early in the visioning phase, hospital visions can encompass dramatic change in medical care.

A formal business case is developed to compare the degree of change required (from the change imperative) with the projected results of the reengineering effort. This will help validate the commitment of focus and resources to the effort. It will also help determine if the vision is too timid or not specific enough.

At the end of the vision phase, the following are defined and documented:

- "As is" baseline information

- New visions for clinical and management processes

- New performance targets

- Formal business case

PHASE THREE: REDESIGN, BUILD, AND IMPLEMENT

Phase three is the heart of the hospital reengineering process. In this phase, administrative staff, clinical staff, and outside experts come together to redesign, build, and implement the way administrative work is done and the way medical care is delivered. New medical technologies are acquired, information systems are created or purchased, medical expertise is updated, and medical facilities replanned.

Design teams consist of the visioning team, plus managers and frontline staff. Individuals respected for their frontline expertise, those admired by colleagues, those who understand the way work is currently done, and those who bring outside experiences are critical to the redesign effort. Reengineering experts typically provide the specific methods and tools for designing, building, and implementing new processes.

Key steps are to

- Acquire new medical technology and methods expertise

- Design, develop, and implement information systems

- Plan and implement medical facility changes

- Design, develop, and pilot new clinical and management processes

- Design and launch education and training programs

- Transition hospital management, clinical staff, and administrative staff

- Launch reengineered services

What is the top design and implementation risk? Underestimating the impact of change on the people who comprise the hospital's expertise. When the impact is underestimated, the potential resistance to change is underestimated. The change management challenge is to strike the critical balance between the urgency of the need and the time and training needs of the people most affected by reengineering. A significant amount of change involves tasks performed by physicians and nurses. Hospital teams must understand and work with medical professionals to align the timing of administrative change with the time needed for medical practice changes to occur. More importantly, hospital teams must understand that change will be the rule in the future. Learning to change quickly will be an important organization competency in order to thrive in managed care.

At the end of the redesign, build, and implement phase, the following are complete:

- New medical technology

- Purchased or constructed information systems

- Refurbished (or divested) medical facilities

- New performance measures

- Trained personnel

- New managed care services

- Performance at or above target levels

PHASE FOUR: MONITOR AND RESPOND

In phase four, the hospital team formalizes lessons learned to help the team plan for future changes in the managed care market.

These steps include

- Document and communicate lessons learned in the reengineering process

- Monitor hospital performance, comparing results to visions and goals

- Implement an ongoing process to monitor the needs of patient populations managed by PCPs

- Implement ongoing processes to monitor emerging regulations, advances in medicine, and new market trends

- Implement a process to update the hospital's managed care strategy every 12 months

What is the top risk? Viewing the hospital reengineering process as one-time change. When reengineering is viewed as one-time change, hospitals may experience initial success, but quickly fall behind managed care competitors. Hospital reengineering is a strategic repositioning of the traditional hospital to a new kind of healthcare enterprise that can evolve its services as medical technologies evolve and population needs change. This requires culture and management processes that monitor the market and support ongoing change. In this phase, these management processes are put into place and the management team begins to operate with a new future perspective.

For example, regulation plays a critical role in the managed care market. Scope of practice regulation is particularly important. Nurse practitioner coalitions are lobbying for the right to prescribe some medications, allowing them to perform work that is now reserved for physicians. By monitoring regulatory trends, hospitals can envision new opportunities for future reengineering designs and new processes.

At the end of the monitor-and-respond phase, the following processes are firmly in place:

- Reengineering results monitoring

- Medical innovations and competitive benchmark monitoring

- Regulation monitoring

- Population-based management

Future of healthcare

In the twenty-first century, virtual hospitals will consist of physical facilities, ambulatory services, and home-based hospital beds monitored by nursing control centers and attended to by home visiting nurses. As these trends emerge, winning hospitals will embrace these changes profitably and with successful medical outcomes.

To get started, hospitals must tackle short-term financial problems associated with facility costs and excess capacity. This may require closing or finding new uses for traditional facilities. At the same time, the cost of inpatient services must be lowered to maintain a competitive position in today's healthcare marketplace.

Once financially strong, hospitals can invest the time and resources required to reposition for managed care. This transformation's timing will be determined by managed care market penetration, regulation, and a hospital's readiness for change.

By starting now, hospitals can make today's services more competitive, while developing new skills and insights to guide their continuing transformation.

3

Becoming a market-focused healthcare organization

Kathryn Payne
Independent Consultant
Houston, Texas

Gennaro J. Vasile, PhD
Vice President
Gemini Consulting
Morristown, New Jersey

"BUILD IT AND THEY WILL COME—that is the way we used to think about growing our business," laments the president of a large healthcare organization, recalling the outdated approach of building hospitals as if they alone were the magnet for new patients and increased revenue. Hospital administrators now recognize that this era has ended. Institutions that once flourished now struggle to survive in their newly competitive industry. New and mounting pressures come from all sides: spiraling costs, managed care, demands for deep discounts from HMOs, price caps from third-party payers, changes in medical practice, requirements of participating in hospital networks, and even the desire of patients to take charge of their own health. Fees are being forced down, hospital stays are growing shorter, admissions and revenues are dropping. In short, the industry is undergoing a rapid and fundamental realignment that challenges the competitive ingenuity of even the best-managed hospitals.

Surviving or flourishing in the midst of such challenges will require an entirely new mind-set. Incremental change alone will not yield competitive advantage when competitors are equally pressured by market shifts and customer demands. Future leaders will develop a childlike sensitivity to the marketplace, observing through fresh eyes and addressing with naive energy the opportunities that are hidden in destabilized healthcare structures.

Organizations suddenly swept up in industrywide turmoil, however, have little time to deliberate over strategy. They must respond—and quickly—to the pressing demands of customers and competition. The themes and questions weighing heavily on the minds of leaders are

- *Impetus for change.* How do leaders ensure that their employees recognize market shifts that will force the organization to change?

- *Journey of change.* How might organizational change be broken into manageable stages while moving fast enough to keep up with (or outpace) competition? Are there traps along the way?

- *Others' experiences.* What can be learned from other firms that have traveled such a path?

- *Market targets.* What is the ultimate goal? Which market targets would provide the largest positive impact on the organization and its customers?

The future will be shaped by leaders who dare to challenge the status quo, chart a path for organizational change, and redefine healthcare services within the context of changing customer demands.

Impetus for change

Too often people are prisoners of their own knowledge. Understanding industry trends is necessary; however, ideas that jolt an organization out of its status quo often spring from less obvious trends. In fact, assumed knowledge can result in an arrogance that becomes the chief obstacle to creativity, binding organizations to traditional strategies in nontraditional times.

Consider, for a moment, a narrow, industry-based view of healthcare trends. Beginning in the 1970s and accelerating in the 1980s, several shifts destabilized healthcare structures. First, the traditional boundaries of the delivery system began to blur. Insurers integrated with providers, providers mimicked insurers, commercial insurers plunged into managed care, and providers linked with providers to establish powerful networks. Kaiser Permanente, once practically alone in the untapped field of managed care, became a household name in areas outside of its historical network; Sutter Health emerged in California; Allina appeared in Minnesota. Not-for-profit hospitals began to form partnerships with profit systems like Columbia/HCA Healthcare Corporation, seeking the advantage of deep corporate pockets. Mayo Clinic and other group practices expanded, acquiring physician groups and hospitals. Through a series of mergers, Harvard Community Health Plan expanded geographically from its exclusive Boston base to Rhode Island and New Hampshire.

Second, healthcare reform accelerated the reconfiguration of the customer base. Suddenly, large segments of the population—approaching 40 to 50 percent in some states—belonged to HMOs. In more than 20 states, Medicaid became managed care friendly, while integrated systems were practically forced on providers in Washington and Minnesota.

Industry leaders have begun deliberating over a system in which everyone shares the same revenue stream—the prepaid, capitated dollar. In such a system, the emphasis focuses on reducing the cost per covered life. The struggle shifts to who controls the capitated dollar and who bears what risk. Even in Boston, where hospital charges had been tethered to state regulations, providers have found that they are affected by employer demands and competition among HMOs and indemnity insurers.

Spurred on by media attention and President Clinton's agenda for health reform, the public grew increasingly hostile about soaring healthcare costs. Even philanthropic hospital campaigns to raise capital for new buildings and equipment met stiff resistance. The message was clear: focus on results, not buildings. Hospitals began to wrestle with increasingly familiar issues. The growth of contractual arrangements was forcing a fresh look at marketing approaches and customer needs. Reduced revenues and declining utilization were requiring new sources of growth. Financial risk from capitated contracts was demanding skills in cost control and risk management. Loss of medical staff and changing referral patterns were beckoning a new kind of management.

From an industry perspective, several competitive responses emerged:

- Integration and consolidation

- Cost reduction and price competition

- Redefinition of value and customer satisfaction

Not surprisingly, healthcare providers began to travel down similar paths.

INTEGRATION AND CONSOLIDATION

Mergers, acquisitions, and strategic alliances have proliferated throughout the industry. Experts estimate that the next five years will bring a 40 percent reduction in hospital days, one of the many indicators that most hospitals will be compelled to find partners for growth and economies of scale or to downsize and refocus.

COST REDUCTION AND PRICE COMPETITION

What hospital has not launched cost reduction initiatives? Within the last four years, cost pressures on indivdual hospitals have led to 30 to 40 percent staff reductions. Reflecting both a reduced tendency to hospitalize people and shorter stays, the number of acute care beds occupied each day has dropped by 25 to 30 percent in the most competitive managed care markets. (At roughly $1,000 per day for an acute care bed, this represents significant savings.) Economic pressures have taken their toll on specialist incomes as well, driving reductions of up to 40 percent. Specialty care units have been closed, laboratory work has been reduced, compensation systems have been restructured, and physician-to-nurse ratios have been driven down. No-holds-barred medical practices have been forced to become stringently controlled business enterprises.

REDEFINITION OF VALUE AND CUSTOMER SATISFACTION

With capitation looming, hospitals face a challenge that is more daunting than cost control: growth. The former paths to growth and solvency—building hospitals, securing licensed beds, keeping beds filled, and attracting more patients needing high-priced surgeries—amount to financial suicide in managed care. Instead hospitals must redirect their goals to keep people healthy and, in doing so, find new paths for growth. The pricing pressure that has already overtaken markets like southern California will continue to narrow pricing differentials, eventually leading to true competition based on value—only this time value will be defined by patients and buyer groups more than the medical community.

Forced to match the pace of competitors, many firms have adopted competitive responses: integration and consolidation and cost reduction and price competition. Fewer firms have endeavored to redefine value from the eyes of changing customer groups. Instead, organizations tend to get trapped in a death spiral: reducing cost, selling harder, measuring customer satisfaction, and circling back to cost reduction—all without changing the product.

As healthcare leaders come to grips with the changes spurred by market reform, they are looking for lessons in the journeys of other firms. Although there is no correct or incorrect order for the stages of change, experience across volatile industries teaches that competitive responses take an increasingly familiar route.

Journey of change

STAGE ONE: LOWER PRICES AND LOWER COSTS

Usually, the first change that organizations face squarely is cost control. The symptoms of trouble often follow times of unprecedented growth and profitability. After several cycles of unquestioned price increases, the organization notices that meeting customers' pricing expectations and service demands is more difficult. Competition is rampant and products and services begin to look the same. The most frequent response is to discount products and services. Lower prices inevitably require lower costs, forcing the organization to cut fat.

In stage one of the journey toward change, the emphasis falls on cutting costs, reengineering processes, and leveraging existing technology more efficiently. Cost cutting and internally driven reengineering work for a while, providing temporary relief, but only to the extent that competitors stand still. Stage one is useful; it is even mandatory because the competitors will certainly not stand still. However, this regimen inevitably reaches the point of diminishing returns. If an organization is unable to tune its product and service offering to the changing needs of the market, it inevitably enters the downward spiral of commoditization—discounting deeper and deeper with nowhere to turn for growth.

The trend seems to fit healthcare today: health benefit costs have dropped below inflation for the first time in two decades. HMOs are accepting contracts from leading insurers and employers for flat monthly fees that are 45 percent lower per person than they were a year or two ago. With the revenue stream per patient defined, healthcare leaders have to figure out how to more efficiently deliver care, run a hospital, and ensure quality outcomes with the same level of diligence and creativity that man-ufacturers of industrial commodities have been forced to apply for decades. In this competitive environment, reengineering—once a cost-reducing differentiator—will become a qualifier.

Eventually, successful organizations look outward, wondering how they can improve positioning in the marketplace and enter stage two of the journey—the turn toward sales and marketing.

STAGE TWO: ACKNOWLEDGING THE MARKET

The organization in stage two acknowledges that traditional channels for attracting customers do not work as well as they used to. The buying power or influence has shifted; the customer has become elusive. This feeling is pervasive in healthcare today as physicians and administrators battle over who customer are: patients? employers? employees and their families? health plan members? insurers? Some will even argue that the physicians are the end-users.

Reaching beyond organization walls, perhaps truly acknowledging the market for the first time, executives launch market studies, design promotional campaigns, and expand sales and marketing activities. Although organizations may boast of market focus, the emphasis in stage two often remains primarily internal in nature. Market studies are based on competitive benchmarking, comparing existing products and services to existing competitive options. Product features and prices are compared, but the products remain the same. Community demo-graphics may be researched, but the definition of "community" is rarely questioned.

For example, when Miami Baptist noticed a growing percentage of patients traveling from the Caribbean, its leaders saw an opportunity: What if they were more aggressive about courting those prospective cus-tomers? What barriers would they have to remove to make Miami Baptist an irresistible attraction for an international community? The solution was to create an international services center. By offering a long-distance appointment system, arranging travel and lodging for family members, and providing translation services, Miami Baptist enriched its service offering. It is a far cry from traditional healthcare services, yet a low-cost enhancement that secured new sources of healthcare revenue. Such bold strokes required more creativity than community demographics or benchmarking might have indicated.

Too often, firms in stage two miss the best opportunities. The sales and marketing activities and departments may be a bit more effective or efficient, but the customer response remains the same. Limited success soon brings on stage three: the drive for customer satisfaction.

STAGE THREE: DRIVING FOR CUSTOMER SATISFACTION

Seeking to recapture growth and price stability, organizations will look for ways to address a deeper customer need than cost. Initiatives will be launched to measure customer satisfaction with existing products and services: Is the physician acceptable? Is the price right? Was the waiting time okay? The aim in stage three is to let customer suggestions drive the organization. Unfortunately, few satisfaction surveys challenge the customers' real values and, therefore, allow little room for creative response. What if a large customer segment—wanting to take more personal responsibility for health maintenance—was seeking nutritional, fitness, and holistic healthcare coaches outside of the hospital system? Would a question like "Is the price right?" uncover the opportunity?

For example, Blue Cross-Blue Shield of Washington and Alaska's idea to pilot test an alternative care product was driven more by the unsolved demands of an emerging market segment than by satisfaction or dissatisfaction with current products. The new offering, which sold out within months of introduction, required open minds about the boundaries of traditional healthcare products and customer satisfaction.

Customer surveys that question satisfaction with existing service options leave the customer no recourse except to ask for more of the same for less. When this ultimately proves to be an impractical solution to the overall business problem, many organizations are driven back to the cost-cutting initiatives of stage one, disillusioned and discouraged to find that the path is circular.

STAGE FOUR: REGAINING SHARE WITH MARKET FOCUS

Ask most healthcare professionals and they will tell you that their goal is to be the low-cost, high-quality provider. Although customer satisfaction and quality leaders can capture market share and even profit margin, the competitive edge exists only until competitors duplicate the performance. Again, few competitors will stand still. Continuously "raising the bar" in this way provides new challenges: discovering emerging customer expectations; developing new solutions; and redefining products, services, and internal business practices to meet the new challenges. Such creative approaches to revitalizing the business can actually change the dynamics of an entire industry.

For example, recognizing that diagnostic guidelines would squeeze hospital reimbursements and force down hospital supply prices, Baxter reframed its hospital supply business (and raised the competitive challenge) by introducing supply management services. The move essentially allowed hospitals to outsource an administrative burden—a privilege for which they paid a premium—and Baxter to build a new source of revenue and profit.

Pharmacy Benefits Management (PBM) firms reframed the pricing, distribution, selection, and development of pharmaceuticals. Furthermore, they captured the underserved buyer-influencer group of employers by offering an expert service to reduce employees' pharmaceutical costs. In both of these examples, the product was broadened beyond the initial businesses of hospital supplies or pharmaceuticals and redefined to add more value to the buyer's business.

Successful journeys of change

At some time, all organizations travel through one or more of the stages of change: reduce cost, improve marketing and sales, boost customer satisfaction, or regain share with market-focused products and services. Regardless of the starting point, the primary challenge is to recognize the root cause of the problem, not just the symptoms. Maintaining the long-term health of an organization is no less complex than ensuring human health. Just as great physicians balance the needs of a patient's body, mind, and spirit, so too must the executive guide the organization. At play constantly are the organization's body (i.e., people, structure, infrastructure, and business practices), its mind (i.e., experience base, skills, beliefs, and know-how), and its spirit (i.e., willingness to change, energy, and attitude). Thus, the most successful journeys of organizational change are guided by a balanced set of rules:

- *Remember who makes change happen.* Mobilize and involve people

- *Establish priorities.* Balance needs for cost containment, competitive differentiation, and customer service

- *Expect and measure results.* Set targets, develop measurement systems, and insist on results

- *Follow a path lighted by the market.* Restructure business practices to deliver new value to the marketplace

None of these rules suffice alone. A strategy based on conventional conceptions of the customer will yield disappointing results in a market that changes almost daily. A business process (e.g., admissions, emergency care, procurement, materials management, innovation, care teams, or compensation and rewards) that has been reengineered to cut costs from an internal perspective is an empty victory if it provides no differentiating value in the emerging market. It is pointless to mobilize around a faulty strategy. Conversely, the best strategy and most enlightened business plans go unrealized if the organization cannot be mobilized to pursue them.

The following pages track a small community hospital through stages of change, focusing on how the four guiding rules shaped its approach. This fictitious hospital, Madison General, represents a composite drawing of solutions implemented across several hospitals facing similar challenges. Woven together, the experiences paint a picture of a holistic change program—linking market-focused strategies, operations improvements, information technologies, and human resources. It is the power of integration that executives across multiple industries have found to provide the soundest platforms for lasting organizational change. The purpose of the composite drawing is to enable healthcare professionals to imagine a more complete and inspiring journey of change and to design a path for integrating cost reduction, marketing and sales, customer satisfaction, and market focus.

CASE STUDY

With 900 employees and 225 beds, this East Coast, not-for-profit hospital traveled the entire path of competitive response, from stage one through stage four, over a period of years. Reaching for more than simple cost reduction, the CEO boldly sought to transform the hospital into a market-focused organization.

Madison General faced a predicament that is becoming increasingly familiar. Admissions were declining. Under pressure from third-party payers, the average length of stay per patient was also being driven down.

The state agencies responsible for administering Medicaid and Medicare were determining how many days of hospitalization they would pay for, regardless of the actual length of the stay, and forcing the extra cost back to the hospital. Allowing for differences by medical service, the average stay at Madison had previously hovered between six and seven days. Soon, that figure dropped to just five days. In obstetrics, for example, the normal delivery of a baby had required a three-day stay. In 1993, that had dropped to two days. In 1994, it would drop to one day and, in 1995, to eight hours. The combination of falling admissions and shorter stays meant a decline in revenue from 1992 to 1994 of 18 percent.

The drop in admissions also reflected a shift in influence from the patient to the payer. Formerly, the patient had some latitude in deciding where to give birth, have surgery, or undergo testing. Managed care changed all that. Such decisions were being driven by the payer with whom the physician was aligned. By insisting that the physician use the lower-cost hospital or by paying a set fee for a procedure regardless of what the hospital charged, payers were driving physicians to the lowest cost hospitals. The pressure was especially intense for Madison. Located in the seventh fastest growing area for managed care in the nation, Madison was competing not only for patients but also for physicians. Hospitals in the area were being urged by payers to end duplication of services. Furthermore, payers were influencing which services at which hospitals would survive. Madison definitely had an impetus to change.

Remember who makes change happen

Realizing the extent of change required to survive, the CEO involved employees in an effort to strengthen the hospital competitively. Focusing on the market forces, both threatening and promising, the CEO launched what was to become a two- to three-year change program. How Madison did it provides a vivid example of effectively mobilizing people to change.

Going far beyond incremental process improvements, the CEO challenged people to think, behave, and act differently to achieve entirely new ways of working. To do so, he had to mobilize 900 employees. In practice, Madison focused on the two top-down components of leadership development and large-scale mobilization and the two bottom-up components of work teams and the encouragement of individual change. In the absence of top-down leadership, Madison had seen that the organization would bristle with bottom-up initiatives but stay rooted in place. Without a bottom-up component, top-down directives would trickle down and trickle out.

Leadership development begins when the CEO first considers making large-scale changes to meet new competitive demands. The job of CEO is a lonely one, and often at this stage the top leader turns to someone outside the organization for a frank discussion of problems and options. In Madison's case, the CEO turned to a consulting firm. He first brought together consultants and top management to design a six-week effort to identify key priorities, quantify financial targets, and mobilize a somewhat sleepy workforce.

To ensure communication and involvement, a full-time joint team of Madison employees and consultants was formed. The team's makeup in itself communicated a powerful message. Three of the hospital's most respected and able people—the controller, the emergency room manager, and the radiology manager—were asked to lead the effort.

Over the ensuing six weeks, work teams from all levels analyzed how the hospital operated in the present; they also designed what it would be in the future. Cost containment certainly figured prominently in the analysis, but emerging market needs were equally important. The joint team designed a 10-month phase-one change program for reshaping the hospital in line with emerging market needs. It was an ambitious program, designed to move on many fronts at once and to deliver results quickly.

To inspire participation, the joint team launched new communication vehicles: town meetings (large meetings involving all levels of hospital employees), employee interviews, brown paper fairs (informal events to solicit input about the current and future states of Madison's business), a weekly newsletter, and an open-door policy.

Forty managers were convened to announce the change program in Madison's first town meeting. Questions, open discussion, and debate were encouraged. Commitment for the effort was spotty at first. Top management was clearly enthusiastic; however, middle managers remained leery, remembering previous experience with short-lived initiatives. Employees on the ground floor participated most energetically and contributed extensively. Enthusiasm bubbled up from the bottom, cascaded down from the top, and eventually engulfed the middle. This confirmed the necessity of mobilizing from the top down and the bottom up at the same time. Continuing their theme of open communication, team members attended departmental staff meetings to get the word out. Managers were also tasked with cascading word of the program to all of the hospital's 900 employees.

Interviews of 120 employees from all functions and levels—nurses, admissions clerks, physicians, administrators, community leaders, and patients—provided an early foundation for priority setting. Many of the priorities identified by employees were pushed to the next stage of analysis: "brown papers."

On long stretches of ordinary brown butcher paper, teams drew diagrams of the work steps involved in critical hospital procedures. Included were admissions, operating room scheduling, radiology and laboratory scheduling, medical records management, inpatient and outpatient care, emergency room management and patient flow, medical unit configuration, supplies procurement, inventory management, and pharmacy management. All of the people involved in the day-to-day work steps of each business practice were involved in building the brown papers. For example, admissions clerks, nurses, physicians, radiologists, laboratory technicians, records managers, administrators, and home health workers documented the inpatient and outpatient processes. Using markers, stickies, and colored pencils, employees threw themselves into representing the entire process, from admitting to seeing the doctor to leaving the hospital. People could come by at their convenience and make their contribution and come back again when inspiration struck. At night, when skeleton crews had to stay close to their posts, the brown paper was taken to each department so that all shifts could participate in the "as-is" analysis of the inpatient process.

The six-week mobilization culminated with a display of all the brown papers, graphs, charts, and studies that the work teams had produced. The documents highlighted the number of work steps, people, and departments involved, areas of duplication or delay, and cost of labor and materials. All employees were invited to add their comments and observations to the papers, hanging along an entire wall of a third-floor unit. The response was overwhelming. Hundreds of people turned out—everyone from the president to the physicians to hospital volunteers. The brown paper fair produced a real atmosphere of teamwork, communication, and trust. No one hesitated to offer comments and suggestions. By the end of the day, hospital personnel had identified more than 500 opportunities for improvement. Such results created an implicit and powerful argument for change, an argument that hospital employees had produced themselves.

Mobilization continued with a series of town meetings regarding implementation. The meetings (one of which was conducted in Spanish) drew 300 employees—twice the number that had attended in the past. Employees from all levels enthusiastically appeared in a video explaining why they thought Madison needed to change and establishing the timetable for achieving it. Such participation was a far cry from the days of executive fiat and was duly noted by the employees.

By engaging the emotions, the intellect, and the professionalism of each individual, Madison General had laid the groundwork for a more fundamental shift: people were beginning to transform. In a work session one day, the CEO, bewildered by the information confronting him, paused and made a frank admission: "I can't see it," he said. "It is just not clear to me what the future of this hospital is going to look like." "Well, it's clear to me," said an emergency room employee in a firm voice. All eyes in the room turned toward her. "I can see it perfectly clearly," she said. The president looked at her in astonishment and then laughed. "You better stay near me then," he said, "because I have to explain all this to the board of directors." It was a small but revealing moment. In the emerging atmosphere of trust, open communication, and learning, this employee had come to see the bigger picture and was perfectly comfortable adding her voice to the proceedings. The open exchanges, on the part of both the nurse and the CEO, signaled the beginning of a culture change that was to characterize the remainder of the change journey at Madison General.

Such active involvement of employees at all levels had an unexpected benefit: Madison employees began to build a competency for managing change. They designed the new business practices and procedures themselves, rather than having them dictated from on high or having them imposed mechanically from outside according to the latest management formula. They worked with a larger network of people, drawing on an extended pool of talent and ideas. Employees broadened their perspective to take in not only the hospital but the market as a whole. Most importantly, they learned how to transform the organization themselves, a new skill that will prepare them for the day when competitive conditions change again, as they inevitably will.

Establish priorities

Realizing that the hospital had to focus its limited resources on the critical few initiatives, the joint team used the brown paper results to help winnow down the priorities. The business practices that work teams subsequently reengineered would be those that provided the best opportunities for cost containment, competitive differentiation, or customer service advantage. Work teams would be launched to address each priority and to ensure that results would be achieved from the bottom up.

Later, Madison would be forced to deal with the tougher, more fundamental question of how to serve new customer segments, but, for now, driving down costs was key. Thus, the hospital started with stage one of their change program: cost containment. They moved swiftly. A layer of management was eliminated. The costs associated with various procedures and units were compared. Physicians incurring unusually high laboratory costs were asked to reconsider their lab practices.

Quality programs were designed to improve procedures and services while lowering costs. After finding that many of the duplications and delays occurred as patients flowed between departments and phases of care, the inpatient services team implemented a new database designed to follow the treatment and care of patients through the healthcare continuum: preadmission activities, admission (including financial screening), diagnostics (including radiology and laboratory), therapy (including inpatient and outpatient services and procedures), recovery, discharge, and follow-up. Previously, departments used disjointed and even incompatible systems, creating an independent patient record with each medical transaction. With information from the healthcare continuum database, the hospital eventually grouped patients by care needs, organized around cases instead of medical units, and reconfigured its services to match patient flow. The effort improved customer satisfaction while reducing time and duplication of effort. As a result the work team achieved two primary measurable targets: patient satisfaction increased (in some cases by as much as 10 percent) and average laboratory turnaround times (one of the primary reasons for delays in the beginning) decreased by 30 minutes.

In another quality initiative, monitoring medical imaging revealed that four out of five patients suffered severe headaches and nausea following myelograms at the hospital. Madison halted further myelograms until a new vendor could be found and new protocols established. Within one month the hospital reduced the rate of post-myelogram complications to zero. The quality program also discovered that blisters from the tape used in major orthopedic cases in the operating room were leading to infection. Substituting a special wrap around patients' dressings soon solved the problem. Similar improvements in quality and cost control were achieved throughout the hospital.

Expect and measure results

To maintain the pace and direction, each work team set an aggressive series of targets including financial results, achievement milestones, and customer satisfaction quotients unique to the process at hand. The financial benefits of overhauling the purchasing process, for example, were shaped when the work team persuaded key players to agree to a savings target. Initial calculations were worked up in cooperation with the controller and the purchasing manager. Then other relevant groups, including suppliers, physicians, managers, and support groups, were consulted until everyone agreed on a final range of possible savings. That final number carried great credibility: it had not been produced by the consultants, and all of the key people at every level believed it to be achievable. The agreed-upon range of savings was $1 to $3 million, the high end of which far exceeded the hospital's entire surplus of $2 million.

How could such a target be achieved? The initial analysis showed that Madison was building unnecessary inventory and losing virtually all of their negotiating leverage with suppliers by carrying inventory suited to the individual tastes and whims of every physician. The team could find few medical, business, or customer satisfaction justifications for carrying 16 different kinds of sutures or 18 different brands of plastic gloves. Early interviews with suppliers even indicated that some suppliers would consider working more closely with Madison, offering inventory management, on-line order entry, and even laboratory support. With nurses spending as much as 30 percent of their time on materials management, Madison stood to gain a lot from working with suppliers.

Another work team developed a tool for determining income generated by each medical service. It was the first time that Madison had viewed its medical units as a portfolio of products and services. Never before had they endeavored to decompose the revenue, contribution, and cost components of their products and services. The work teams began to understand the drivers of cost by looking at labor, materials, and turnaround time across the entire continuum of healthcare. These numbers, prosaic as they might seem, nevertheless generated great excitement. It was a new way of looking at things and it showed the staff the power they had in their hands to find the tools to transform the hospital.

These internally focused efforts did yield savings. But Madison could see that capitation would continue to produce ever-thinner margins. Getting the house in order was only a partial response to the new realities of managed care. Like most healthcare providers, Madison aspired to be the low-cost, high-quality provider. Thus, its initial internally generated efforts had focused on high-quality and, for a time at least, lower-cost healthcare. If the average stay was growing shorter, then it made sense to compensate by trying to increase the number of admissions.

In the second stage of competitive response, Madison emphasized market research, redoubled sales and marketing efforts, and nurtured physician channels in order to increase volume. Higher volume would compensate at least in part for plummeting price and overcapacity. The key was to reach out to the market.

In a radical departure from the traditional practices of the medical community, the hospital began to advertise in area newspapers in hopes of attracting more physicians and patients. The message was simple: discover Madison General. Seeking to educate the public about the great value in cost and quality that lay right on its doorstep, Madison was trying to differentiate itself from the seven other hospitals in the area. Attempting to attract more patients through the physicians as distribution channels, Madison even encouraged one physician to host a radio show regarding healthcare for ethnic groups in the community. Although a few new customers wandered through the door, Madison executives questioned whether marketing was a long-term answer to the powerful forces sweeping through healthcare.

Equally aggressive competitors were implementing similar varieties of reengineering, streamlining business procedures in order to save money, and competing with ever-declining prices. Further price wars would inevitably ensue, followed by more cost cutting, and so on in a vicious circle. The leaders at Madison knew that they had to avoid this trap.

Eager to go beyond the marketing stage, the hospital's leaders turned to the issue of customer satisfaction. Madison launched a work team to focus on customer needs. The watchwords of customer satisfaction were "listen," "be close," and "exceed expectations." Customer surveys, suggestion boxes, interviews, and other feedback loops were established to find out what customers wanted. The aim was to do anything, within reasonable budgetary constraints, that the customer suggested. Madison eliminated delays in admitting, cut down on paperwork, explained medical procedures clearly, processed insurance forms more efficiently, and trained medical staff to be more courteous. The approach began to orient people at all levels to customer satisfaction and simultaneously created excitement and energy.

Fourteen volunteers, drawn from many departments, went into the surrounding community and interviewed people at random about their use of healthcare facilities. Recent patients were surveyed by telephone. The survey turned up some interesting results. The overall conclusion was that patients were highly satisfied with Madison General. In fact, the hospital had long enjoyed a sterling reputation among people who had been patients there. Clearly, customer satisfaction, which the hospital had already achieved, was not going to reverse the decline in admissions. The findings did not really provide the impetus for change that the work team and executive steering committee expected.

Why not? Madison reviewed the types of questions posed. They asked patients for their impressions of Madison and its physicians. The survey listed Madison's services and asked which ones the respondent would recommend. For marketing purposes, it asked patients how they chose hospitals for specific services such as obstetrics, where they got their information about hospitals, and what kinds of physicians were needed in their communities. Questions included traditional probes about customer service and quality: How would you rank the quality of services at Madison General? How long did you have to wait to see your physician? Was the staff courteous and helpful? The results showed a customer satisfaction increase of about 10 percent over prior years.

Madison leaders still were not satisfied. The underlying theme was based on evaluating existing products and services, giving the customer and marketing department little creative license. Even the question asking about the kinds of physicians needed allowed the respondent to choose only from a traditional list of services the hospital already offered. Instead of focusing on emerging customer needs (which the current service offering may or may not have addressed) and then shaping the organization's products and services accordingly, Madison—like many institutions in stage three—was desperately trying to validate and widen the market for existing products and services.

As Madison proceeded down the path of customer satisfaction, it learned that

- Customers, unsure about medical and hospital practices, usually ask for more of what they are already receiving but at a lower price

- The hospital continues to concentrate its resources on current offerings, whether or not they are really appropriate for the emerging market

- What customers want is not necessarily driven by questions of hospital practice, but by quality of life issues (e.g., convenience, travel schedules) and intensely personal choices (e.g., stress management such as meditation, psychotherapy, Tai Chi, health spa retreats, and stress management courses; and alternative therapies such as massage, acupuncture, chiropractic, and naturopathy). The solutions are not always intuitively obvious, even to the customer

- Always acceding to customers' wishes deprives the hospital of the ability to make necessary trade-offs between cost and benefits, or ends and means

- In spite of programs of continuous improvement, competitors can achieve comparable levels of customer satisfaction, leading once again to a strategy of nondifferentiation

Madison General, finding that it already performed above the expectations of customers, would soon move on to a strategy that not only inspired enthusiasm at all levels but was a more compelling vision to mobilize around: building a market-focused organization.

Market-focused action

Madison's journey through stages one, two, and three embodied the "inside-out thinking" typical of the early responses of organizations that suddenly find themselves in the midst of intense competition: continue to make the product, figure out how to improve it incrementally, then figure out how to make people want it.

The president and management team knew that, unless they could find new opportunities for growth, the lower-price, lower-cost commodity spiral would lead to ever-declining revenues. Resisting their fear that a major misstep could hasten the very decline they were so eager to avoid, the team decided that it preferred the risk of revitalizing the institution to the safety of managing its slow decline.

First, the president added an outsider to the team, a proven manager with a reputation for innovation and risk taking. Next, the joint team decided to take a hard look at the market, regardless of Madison's current fit with it. The plan was to identify Madison's options and explore ways to integrate the hospital's activities around the most promising ones. Customer satisfaction had the advantage of great appeal to customers and employees, but as an overall strategy it prevented the organization from delving deeper into the more fundamental market shifts. Madison needed something more challenging to shake up the status quo.

The team recognized that caring for the medically indigent would continue to be an ethical obligation for the hospital but worried that capitated contracts limited their ability to shift costs. Looking for ways to support the indigent and to fund research, the team began to focus on building new sources of revenue. "How can we build revenue sources that are not necessarily attached to capitated contracts?" questioned one of the joint team members. "Or, at minimum, how can we enhance our services to secure better contracts from large buyer groups?" Appropriately challenged, the team went to work. They organized focus groups to question the end results sought by the customer. Some sessions were designed to explore large buyer-group needs. Others focused on individuals and families. The Madison team asked what customers valued most and what day-to-day issues were shaping their decisions. Did they value convenience, personal responsibility, time, cost containment, long-term relationships, or information? Did they travel a lot, suffer from stress, have trouble balancing family and career needs, invest in alternative or holistic healthcare products or services, work out of their homes, exercise, live in dual-income families, or struggle with single parenthood? What exactly did "healthcare" mean to them? If customers could have anything (and Madison could supply anything), would they want wellness programs, health information, personal health records, fitness centers, administrative support, a personal health or fitness consultant, stress reduction classes, acupuncture, homeopathic treatments, massage, or house calls? How much money did they spend per year, out of their own pocket, on managing their health?

The results began to reframe Madison's challenge. One large employer was suffering from a high incidence of injuries in one of its plants. Downtime and worker's compensation cases were increasing precisely as they were trying to drive excess cost out of the system. That particular customer wanted the convenience of (and was willing to pay for) a clinic on-site at the company's plant. Furthermore, they wondered if Madison's physicians might be willing to participate in a safety survey of the plant for health hazards.

A clear segment of individuals interested in alternative and preventive care also began to emerge. Many of these customers, Madison found, were spending up to $1,000 per year (of their own money, without reimbursement) on massage, acupuncture, relaxation courses, and homeopathic treatments.

Instead of trying to satisfy every whim of the customer, market-focused workshops began to hone in on product and service ideas: alternative care, health and safety on-site clinics, safety education, personal health and fitness consulting, expanded geographic coverage, and corporate house calls. Madison's next step would be to decide which strategic investments to make—capital investment, human resource development, alliance partners, recruiting, advertising, or facilities. Madison began developing a business case to explore the options.

To support their business plan and to test their new ideas, Madison extended the market-focused initiatives to include analysis of targeted geographic areas, competitors, and community needs. They surveyed payers on trends in reimbursement, regulation, reform, and capitation and constructed detailed payer profiles. This market research, together with the detailed as-is analysis done during mobilization, helped Madison redefine product and service offerings. The research confirmed a trend toward community care, which portended further decline in the number of inpatient admissions. But it also suggested opportunities such as wellness programs to bring the "well to the hospital" and outpatient care that "brings the hospital to the sick."

In addition to focusing on end-users, Madison began to think about their workforce as a market. Consequently, some of the hospital's future market focus will be built around physicians. Madison work teams are interviewing physicians and their office managers in order to understand the physicians' markets and their patients and to develop models of affiliation with the hospital. They will also be exploring ways to market their affiliated doctors rather than the hospital's name. And they will look for ways to improve their relationships with physicians by offering employee services that set Madison apart from other hospitals.

Madison's plan to differentiate itself for physicians provides a striking example of the difference between mobilizing for market focus and merely reengineering for cost savings. During the initial analysis, a Madison work team examined the operating room function. Among other things, a benchmarking study revealed that comparable hospitals nearby employed only two physician assistants in their high-volume operating room, while Madison employed seven with only half the volume. These highly paid professionals act as copilots in surgery, overseeing all of the operating room functions for the physician. Other hospitals in the area are phasing out this position. A simple, low-cost strategy would dictate that Madison follow suit, thus creating the kind of competitive parity. But Madison has decided not to view them as a potential source of savings, at least until the hospital's market-focus work can determine whether the service might be a significant strength in their relationships with physicians and patients. In short, Madison General's goal is to grow and thrive not merely survive.

Although Madison has not completed its journey of change, the early indicators of success are clear:

- Employees are more creative and open-minded about the possibilities for serving the community and gaining market share

- People are more adept at teamwork and reach out to those around them who offer new and unique perspectives

- New products and services are considered every day. Conversations are more likely to focus on market share, broadened customer needs, and revenue generation than on cost reduction and downsizing

- Customers are more interested in healthcare than they used to be. Some have even volunteered to help Madison launch new services

- Madison is seeking growth opportunities from nontraditional sources

In moving from worrying about the future to seizing it for themselves, Madison's people offer a useful lesson about the pattern of responses to new competitive conditions. Initially, unsettling changes inspire fear and drive the organization to look inward for ways to streamline, improve, and cut costs. The inadequacy of such an approach naturally produces the next stage—reaching out through marketing and sales. In almost cyclical fashion, the focus turns back inward through the lens of customer satisfaction with existing products and services. In many ways, all of these reactions are natural, each providing a zone of comfort, at least temporarily, for the organization. But none of them mobilizes the full potential of the organization as fully as market focus.

Madison General moved through the cycles quickly and ultimately chose to focus, without bias, on the market, consolidating the advantages of the earlier stages in a single, holistic transformation. As changes in healthcare continue to accelerate, other institutions will have to move along the path even faster, mobilizing their employees for market-focused action.

4

Rethinking outpatient strategies

William J. Leander, MBA
Cofounder and Director
PFCA
Atlanta, Georgia

THE FUTURE OF HEALTHCARE is in outpatient services.
This rising demand for outpatient care is fueled by technological advances and the shortening of inpatient hospital stays. Outpatient demand is also growing more complex as a broader range of interventions and diagnostics are performed on a come-and-go basis. In addition, the move toward more community-based preventive care further heightens the pivotal role of outpatient services. This increased demand puts outpatient services near the top of healthcare providers' lists of strategic imperatives for future success.

Mounting cost and service pressures will pose new challenges in meeting this demand. The introduction of a Medicare prospective payment system (PPS) for outpatient care will bring the same revenue contraction and cost reduction pressures that accompanied the introduction of the PPS for Medicare inpatients. Managed care organizations will award contracts based upon value—defined as Value = (Quality + Service) – Cost. For example, performance measures, such as average patient waiting time, will emerge as inputs into contractual decisions. In this environment, providers cannot sacrifice customer service (e.g., allowing wait times to increase) to reduce costs. Customers will demand both low cost and high service levels.

Most healthcare providers are poorly positioned to meet these future challenges. Their existing approach to providing outpatient services is still rooted in an inpatient model created for come-and-stay inpatients. This strategy dictates that each type of inpatient receives care from only one predetermined nursing unit. For example, heart patients go to the cardiac unit and pneumonia patients go to the general medical unit. Problems arise when all of the beds on a nursing unit are occupied and the heart patient is admitted to the general medical unit or the pneumonia patient to the cardiac unit. Neither unit is set up to properly care for other types of patients. There is no flexibility in terms of where inpatients are handled. However, this operating strategy does work well for inpatients coming to the hospital for a stay of several days.

Using this same strategy for outpatients means that only one area or department is set up to serve each type of arriving outpatient's total care needs. For example, outpatients requiring a routine chest x-ray, a few basic lab tests, and an EKG may have to travel to two or three different departments for these services. All patients requiring minor walk-in treatment only receive that care in the "fast-track" area of the emergency department. When the area or department needed by the outpatient is busy, there is only one choice available to the patient and to the provider: the customer waits.

This traditional operating strategy, created for inpatients but still used to serve outpatients, is "fixed" in that there is a rigid, predetermined relationship between the customer and where that customer receives care. This relationship holds firm during busy as well as slow weekdays and weekends. The various departments serving outpatients act as independent islands—like distinct circles with no overlap. Consequently, it offers no ability to adapt to fluctuations in demand. When a department or area is busy, its customers simply have to wait. The irony is that one department may be busy while another right down the hall is slow. As such, using an inpatient operating strategy to handle outpatients erodes the customer service levels that fuel patient and staff dissatisfaction.

This type of fixed strategy inflates costs as well. Each independent department staffs to peak demand in order to reduce customer waiting as much as possible during busy periods. However, it takes more than a 10 percent increase in staffing to keep service levels constant in the face of a 10 percent increase in outpatient demand. Thus, total operating costs rise faster than demand when independent departments staff to peak. This fact haunts providers facing predictions of escalating outpatient demand.

Serving outpatients under an inpatient strategy creates a severe performance dilemma. Service levels can be improved (e.g., less waiting) but only through an increase in costs and capacity (i.e., more staff, rooms, and equipment). Conversely, costs can be improved but only through a decrease in service levels such as more waiting. Under a traditional fixed strategy, providers can only offer high service levels or low costs, but not both.

In the future, not offering both high service levels and low costs will be fatal for providers. Thus, a fundamental rethinking of the strategy for providing outpatient services is required. This rethinking must be tailored to the unique nature and needs of outpatients or else the performance dilemma will be perpetuated. In general, rethinking outpatient services must introduce greater structural flexibility into the delivery system to meet the dynamic come-and-go challenges of outpatient services.

A more fluid strategy, allowing each type of outpatient to be served in more than one area or department, is required. When one department or area is busy, patients can immediately receive their care in another without having to wait.

This new strategy encompasses two initiatives. First, many outpatient departments are redesigned to meet a broader set of the patient's total care needs. For example, an outpatient needing an EKG, chest x-ray, and lab test would receive all of this care in a single area by a multidisciplinary team. Such redesign cuts down on patients traveling between different departments and eliminates costly red tape (e.g., coordination and redundant documentation) between these departments.

Second, this redesign calls for some shared responsibilities across departments (i.e., overlap among the circles). When demand backs up at a department, patients can be readily handled within another department (specifically designated as a secondary backup for that service). For instance, patients can receive a chest x-ray in the emergency department when the waiting time within the radiology department is too long and vice versa. This selective overlap controls patient waiting times by taking advantage of available resources outside of the department designated as the outpatient's primary service area. As such, it improves service levels without incurring additional costs. In fact, the fluid strategy can reduce costs by tempering the need for each department to always staff to peak.

The key to a successful fluid strategy is its design. The redesign must be highly selective, based upon detailed analyses of demand. It has to offer the right set of services within each department while establishing the right overlaps between departments. Too many services, the wrong ones, or too many overlaps build complexity and erode the value of the strategy. Properly designed, a more fluid strategy promises better service plus lower costs.

This chapter explores the fluid strategy for providing outpatient services in more detail. Through a case study, it contrasts the fixed and fluid strategies and describes the fluid approach's performance improvements, which include significant reductions in patient waiting and costs.

Strategic imperatives

In 1993, a 200-bed multispecialty provider in Wisconsin began to strategically rethink outpatient services. Its outpatient business was growing and profitable, and a new, street-level diagnostic clinic to serve both inpatients and outpatients was scheduled to open in 1994. Yet the hospital's leaders were troubled. Customers were increasingly dissatisfied with lengthy waiting times and disjointed service. Operating costs for outpatient services were already higher than anticipated and steadily rising. Freestanding clinics around the community were posing an increased competitive threat, and managed care was entering a previously insulated region.

The leaders knew that the new diagnostic clinic would help to improve customer entry and exit, yet they were still concerned. There was no reason to believe that customer waiting times would decrease significantly because of the new facility. They also realized the clinic would have many of its own administrative and support areas that might increase (or at best hold constant) the total cost of providing outpatient services. Thus, the new diagnostic clinic was not likely to offer the hospital an economic advantage in the marketplace.

Facing these mounting pressures, hospital leaders were convinced that the current strategy and operating structures would not work. They needed to rethink the strategy for outpatient services. To guide this rethinking, three strategic imperatives were established:

1. Provide exceptional service with no waiting and one-stop-shopping. Outpatients must receive everything they need in one place. They

must not travel to several different areas or departments. Customer waiting times will be continually monitored

2. Strive to enhance continuity across the continuum of care. Outpatients must receive care from the fewest number of caregivers possible. In the future, professionals delivering diagnostic and treatment care may also provide much of the preventive care (e.g., periodic testing, assessment, and education) for their outpatient customers

3. Reduce operating costs by maximizing flexibility of resources. The number of staff dedicated to outpatient services must be rigorously controlled. Staffing increases must be much less than the underlying increases in demand. At the same time, the new design must absorb unexpected fluctuations in demand in a real-time manner. Peak periods must be accommodated without eroding service levels (e.g., making customers wait longer)

Strategic mismatch

Achieving these strategic imperatives—better service and enhanced continuity at lower cost—may initially seem like an impossible goal. Adhering to an inpatient strategy to provide outpatient services kept the hospital (like other healthcare providers) from achieving this winning combination.

This mismatch between outpatient customers and an inpatient strategy can seriously hamper providers from rendering truly exceptional outpatient services; what works for patients admitted for four days does not work for those spending only four hours. The creation of stand-alone outpatient clinics, ambulatory surgery centers, and medical malls is an improvement. However, the mismatch remains. A new strategy and operating structure tailored to outpatient services is essential to future success.

Any fundamental rethinking of traditional approaches and beliefs is difficult because it entails both cultural and operational challenges. There is often more energy expended on why it will not work than on how it could work. Still, the Wisconsin hospital grappled with how to change because the alternative, clinging to a strategic mismatch, was a far more foreboding threat.

Fixed dilemma

The best way to describe the traditional inpatient strategy used to serve outpatient customers is fixed. Here, outpatient services are provided through a collection of independent and self-contained departments, each handling a very specific type of patient. These departments are islands of service separated by hallways, elevators, telephones, and computers.

Consider three typical outpatient locations within an acute care hospital: an outpatient nursing unit for postsurgical or postinterventional customers, a minor care area within the emergency department, and a diagnostic procedure and testing area within the outpatient admissions department. Each of these locations is an island. There is no sharing of resources, personnel, or capital. Each location is dedicated to a particular type of outpatient customer. They are managed separately and no one is aware of the demand or service level at each location.

At any time, the minor care area within the emergency department can be overflowing with waiting customers while the outpatient nursing unit is slow. The wait for x-rays could be an hour long within the outpatient admissions area while the satellite imaging area within the emergency department could be idle. Extend this illustration across many other outpatient locations—testing areas within ancillary departments, an ambulatory surgery department, a rehabilitation department—and the traditional fixed strategy results in a disjointed approach to outpatient care. Outpatient services, provided through a fixed strategy, is a cohesive product line in theory only.

Under a fixed strategy, the performance dilemma is that service levels and operating costs are always at odds. In each department, better service levels can be achieved only through higher costs once processes and procedures have been fine-tuned to maximize throughput. Conversely, significantly lower costs can be achieved only through reducing service levels. This win-lose penalty results from each outpatient service being its own island. Furthermore, continuity of care suffers. For example, many outpatients coming to a provider for routine diagnostic procedures and tests have to follow facility maps or colored tiles on the floor to guide them to and from various locations throughout the facility.

One of the greatest challenges facing outpatient service managers is to minimize such performance penalties. To do so, they have introduced complex staff scheduling systems, involving many shift options, and employed part-time personnel to match resources more closely with expected demand. They have used total quality management concepts and "systems thinking" to streamline activities and alleviate customer bottlenecks. Still, the fixed dilemma continues. These managers ultimately have to decide how much customer service they can afford to provide.

The Wisconsin hospital's leaders came face to face with this fixed dilemma in designing its new diagnostic clinic. Groups of staff and managers conducted extensive analyses to design the clinic in a restructured, patient-focused mode. It was designed to accommodate the range of needs of routine diagnostic outpatients to receive basic x-ray, mammography, ultrasound, and EKG services in the new facility. Phlebotomy would also be performed. For most of these outpatients, everything they needed would reside within the walls of the new clinic.

One hundred outpatients would visit the clinic each day. Several service areas were established on the floor plan. Each of these multifunctional areas could meet the entire set of needs of a routine diagnostic outpatient. The care of each arriving patient would be entirely provided in one of these areas. This design cut down on patient travel and inconvenience because patients no longer had to bounce between different departments.

Furthermore, a three-member team was designed to serve the patient from start to finish. At least one team member could perform all services, eliminating any reliance on outside staff. For example, one member of each team would be a radiological technologist (RT) cross-trained to perform phlebotomy and EKGs. This care team was largely self-sufficient despite the fact that Wisconsin law prohibits anyone other than an RT from performing x-rays. These same teams would also perform some of the administrative activities associated with the outpatient's visit. By providing the full range of services without external reliance, these teams reduce patient waiting and cut the costs associated with coordinating with other departments.

Through this initial design, the first two strategic imperatives for rethinking outpatient services—better service and enhanced continuity—were achieved. The hospital could now offer exceptional service, and most of the routine diagnostic outpatients received all of their care from one care team in one area.

The third strategic imperative of reduced operating costs posed a lingering challenge. The hospital wanted to virtually eliminate patient waiting. To provide this level of service to the clinic's outpatients, three care teams, representing nine staff members, were required. This staffing represented an annual wage-and-benefits expense of almost $450,000.

Unfortunately, this expense exceeded the aggressive target needed to make the clinic economically competitive. Even a restructured, patient-focused design fell victim to the fixed dilemma because of its self-contained approach. Service levels and operating costs were still at odds. Under this strategy, the only choice would be to consider sacrificing service levels in order to cut costs.

Fluid alternatives

The fixed dilemma arises from the rigidity of its underlying strategy—distinct circles with no overlap. This rigidity imposes the performance penalties that preclude healthcare providers from achieving their strategic imperatives to provide successful outpatient services in the future. More specifically, the fixed strategy forces providers to trade off service for cost; both cannot be achieved at the same time.

To eliminate these performance penalties, the traditional fixed strategy must be replaced with a more fluid one, tailored to outpatient services. A fluid strategy establishes some overlap of service between departments. This overlap allows resources within more than one area or department to handle each type of arriving outpatient. As such, there is a good alternative when demand backs up and waiting is a problem. This approach enables a department to relieve pressure in peak periods before service begins to crumble.

Under a fluid strategy, outpatient services as a cohesive product line become a network of interdependent resources rather than disjointed locations—circles with some overlap. The fluidity is essential given the nature of outpatient demand, especially the fluctuations in hourly and daily demand (which can never be totally predicted) and the need to provide more preventive care. The nature of outpatient demands calls for the flexibility of a fluid strategy, not the rigidity of a fixed one.

For example, the x-ray service within both the outpatient admitting and emergency departments could perform basic x-rays for either type of customer under a fluid strategy. When the outpatients in admitting back up, a few patients could be handled within the emergency departments. The odds that both departments are backed up at the same time are much less than one or the other being backed up.

The general rule of thumb under a fluid strategy is to draw upon resources from a secondary department if the alternative is to make the patient wait within the primary service. For example, a customer walking into the emergency department (primary service) in need of an x-ray would be served right then and there if the wait time is minimal. If there is a substantial wait due to lack of a qualified professional, a RT from admitting could come to the emergency area to perform the outpatient's x-ray. If the wait is caused by the lack of available equipment, the outpatient could go to the admitting area. As long as the travel time is less than the expected wait time, the patient is better off. High service levels are maintained without adding staff and cost to either department. Under a traditional fixed strategy, these departments have no overlap, which forces patients to wait unnecessarily.

Under a fluid strategy, this same patient arriving in an emergency department in need of treatment for a sprained ankle could be served by resources within the physical therapy department or the orthopedic nursing unit if waiting time in the emergency department is unacceptable. In the same way, a child coming into the emergency department for minor care could be served by resources from the pediatric nursing unit.

This same fluid strategy is leading some healthcare providers to consider an overlap in services between major care emergency departments and intensive care nursing units. In some cases, these two are being integrated into a single pool of resources, if not a single area.

A fluid strategy, which on the surface may seem like chaos, relies on highly selective design for control and long-term success. This design must be created using facts of detailed demand patterns, total care needs, competency requirements, capital costs, and license constraints. The outcome must not be a delivery system in which every type of outpatient is handled everywhere. This would almost certainly backfire, eroding quality and probably inflating costs through overcomplexity of coordination.

A fluid strategy provides selective overlap to maintain service levels even in peak periods. The patient or staff flow between departments must trickle, not flood, and it should be the exception, not the rule. Even a trickle between departments makes a very significant difference. The strategy calls for overlap, not total redundancy of services where every department can handle any type of outpatient. Typically, there are only one or two alternatives for serving any type of outpatient, not a dozen. The first choice is always to serve the customer right then and there within the primary service department.

The Wisconsin hospital turned to a fluid strategy to improve the cost effectiveness of the design of its new diagnostic clinic. The hospital leaders' goal was to decrease operating costs without cutting service levels. A design team scrutinized demand data and concluded that an entire three-member team could be eliminated if, on average, one in five arriving outpatients received their care outside of the clinic's outpatient service. This alternative reduced annual wage and benefit expenses by a third, for a $150,000 reduction.

Of course, most routine diagnostic outpatients received their care within the clinic, the primary choice. However, the occasional patients who would otherwise wait could receive their care either within the inpatient side of the clinic, the secondary choice, or the main radiology department of the hospital—the last resort. The x-ray capabilities were already in place in all three areas. Cross-training to perform EKGs and phlebotomy was needed as well as a communications system between the three areas. To minimize patient inconvenience, scheduled visits would be most frequently handled within the inpatient side of the clinic and the radiology department. Contacting these patients at home or work prior to their arrival would help them go directly to the right location. A call-in system could eventually be established where patients called in before leaving for the hospital.

Through a fluid strategy, the third imperative of minimizing costs through flexible resources now could be achieved. The outpatient design was flexible and could absorb fluctuations in demand in a real-time manner by accessing alternative resources (i.e., the second and third choices). This approach kept customer service consistently high, even during peak periods. Furthermore, the fluid strategy helped use resources better across the involved departments. In fact, the outpatient side of the clinic occasionally handled inpatients needing routine x-rays, too. The overlap works both ways.

Even on this small scale—the initial redesign involved only the routine diagnostic type of outpatient—rethinking outpatient services enabled the hospital to achieve its strategic imperatives. Patients receive no-wait, one-stop-shopping service. Continuity of care is enhanced, and costs were reduced by making resources more flexible. The performance dilemma of a fixed strategy was broken.

As expected, there were several implementation hurdles at the Wisconsin hospital. It took time to overcome concerns that the selective overlap of services—a challenge to both traditional practices as well as paradigms—could hurt quality or lead to patients and staff running all over the place.

Perhaps the greatest implementation hurdle at the Wisconsin hospital was an initial misconception by the second- and third-choice departments that a fluid design implied that they generally had too much time on their hands. This hurdle was overcome by explaining that the design was possible because of the combination of similar capabilities and off-setting patient arrival patterns. All three areas had similar capabilities in terms of x-rays, EKGs, and phlebotomy. However, inpatient demand for those services was concentrated in the early morning and early after-noon. Outpatient arrivals were less concentrated but exhibited almost the opposite pattern, peak periods in the late morning and late after-noon. Taken together, the two demand patterns smoothed into a more steady stream. The key to the fluid design was two demand patterns that fit together nicely and not the excess time of the staff.

Integration benefits

A fluid outpatient strategy establishes a network of interdependent and overlapping services within an institution. It can also extend across the various institutions of a healthcare system (e.g., HMOs, multihospital organizations, and affiliated clinic settings). In fact, the opportunities are even greater from a network of overlapping outpatient services among different institutions. The benefits grow as the number and diversity of outpatients and the number of potentially available services grow. This bodes well given the steady increase in outpatient demand and the importance of finding efficiencies through healthcare integration.

Pursuing a fluid strategy across a healthcare system entails two tiers of overlap in services. The first tier is across institutions, where the overlap of select services enhances performance at the system level. The design of this tier starts with decisions about which services will be performed at each institution. It concludes with the second tier, a determination of the overlap within each institution.

In the fluid strategy, overlapping services allow slow periods in one department to help offset busier periods in another. This flexibility helps maintain consistently high service levels despite fluctuations in demand. In the Wisconsin hospital case study, the focus is on treatment and interventional care (e.g., diagnostic testing). However, this same fluid strategy can also be used to provide preventive and wellness care also. Slow periods in providing treatment-oriented care can be used to deliver preventive care. This approach reduces the incremental costs of providing preventive care. For healthcare systems, a fluid strategy can lead to a more cost-effective way to manage a true continuum of care for all patients. The last thing a healthcare system should do is set up a preventive care division with dedicated, fixed resources, such as personnel.

Design methodology

The external and internal forces of each healthcare provider are unique. Therefore, no two fluid strategies and designs are exactly alike. However, the design and structure is typically founded on a set of eight major steps. The strategic visions and design process may be similar, but the resulting strategy and structure will be customized for each healthcare provider and system.

STEP ONE: DEFINE OUTPATIENT TYPES

The first major step in the design methodology is to define the various types of outpatients. Since these types will be the basis for determining how services will be provided under a fluid strategy, their definitions should center on the total care needs (i.e., interventional, treatment, diagnostic, preventive, and wellness) of those customers. This step can be difficult since many institutions place all outpatients into only one or two general groups. However, a focus on differences in needs can shed light on this initial step in the design process. For example, the Wisconsin hospital's outpatient population included eight distinct types, including the routine diagnostic population served in the new clinic. Other types included complex diagnostic, minor ambulatory surgery, and minor care walk-in.

STEP TWO: QUANTIFY DEMAND PATTERNS

The second step is to quantify the demand patterns of each patient type. These patterns reflect the characteristics of patient access to the health-care system or institution, including the schedulability of arrivals, arrivals by time of day and day of week, the total bundle of care needed during each arrival, and any interrelationships between arrivals. In quantifying these demand patterns, attention should be placed on what the patient's demand should or could be, not on what it is. This attention helps to avoid incorporating existing problems and biases into the future design.

STEP THREE: IDENTIFY CUSTOMER CONSTRAINTS

The third step in designing a tailored fluid strategy is to identify key customer-imposed constraints associated with each outpatient service. These constraints generally fall into two categories. The first category is buying constraints. For example, customers may buy or access some services based on proximity and convenience while technological sophistication may be more important for other services. Buying constraints have a strong marketing and patient focus.

The second category is care constraints. For example, the condition of some patient types, such as trauma patients, may be so unstable, urgent, or complex that this type of patient is not a good candidate for any degree of a fluid approach.

STEP FOUR: IDENTIFY SERVICE CONSTRAINTS

Step four identifies key service constraints in flexibility of delivery or performance. Services that are the best candidates for overlap can be readily replicated without incurring extensive capital expense or running into competency barriers. Therefore, each service is differentiated according to its capital intensity, license requirements, initial competency hurdles, and ongoing competency requirements.

These initial four steps provide most of the information needed to sketch out the fluid strategy and structure. In general, outpatient types and services facing few insurmountable constraints (e.g., routine diagnostic and minor treatment) are candidates for overlap. These services usually represent only 20 percent of all available outpatient services but 80 percent of demand volume. They are also the most unpredictable and routine. As such, designing these services under a fluid strategy gives a tremendous advantage in performance improvement.

STEP FIVE: DESIGN FIRST-CHOICE SERVICES

Once the strategy is sketched out, the subsequent step is to design the various first-choice services—the primary area for a particular type of outpatient. For example, the emergency department is the most likely first choice for serving minor walk-in patients. The Wisconsin hospital's new clinic was the first-choice service for its routine diagnostic outpatients. To better serve patients, these designs bring together services and skills traditionally found in separate departments. These designs include the floor plan, capital plan, role creation (e.g., multiskilled teams), and initial daily policies and procedures. They are detailed and complete so that a clear picture of each primary service emerges.

STEP SIX: DESIGN ALTERNATIVE SERVICES

Next, a plan for the second- and possibly third-choice service is put in place. The inpatient side of the Wisconsin hospital's clinic and its main radiology department are the second- and third-choice services, respectively, for the routine diagnostic outpatients. Resources from these services are called upon when the first choice is backed up. Alternative services are selected based upon how similar their existing capital and competencies are to the first-choice service. In other words, alternative services should be able to meet the majority of the patient's needs with their existing resources. The redesign of each alternative service, therefore, typically entails only minor augmentation. Demand patterns are also a pivotal consideration. The Wisconsin hospital's main radiology department only needed to augment its existing services with the ability to perform EKGs and phlebotomy. However, not all first-choice services need or should have second or third choices because creating overlap would be infeasible or undesirable.

STEP SEVEN: ESTABLISH DECISION-MAKING CRITERIA

The decision-making criteria for accessing these second- and third-choice services should then be clearly articulated and well documented. These criteria should include the priorities across alternative services. When the outpatient clinic (first choice) backed up at the Wisconsin hospital, the secondary choice was to serve the patient in the inpatient side of that same clinic. Customers were sent to the main radiology department only when this second choice was also unavailable. This priority minimized travel and inconvenience to the patient. Staff working in overlapping services must be clear about these priorities so that decisions are simple and well understood. Furthermore, they should know when to access an alternative service. For example, staff in the Wisconsin hospital's outpatient clinic used alternative services when the waiting time within the primary service reached 15 minutes.

Three factors keep any fluid strategy simple: clear decision-making criteria, creating only selective overlap in services across departments, and limiting the number of alternative services to only a second or third choice. A simple fluid design will yield significant and sustainable results. An overly complex one will fail.

STEP EIGHT: CREATE ENABLING SYSTEMS

The final step in the design methodology is to create enabling systems. First-choice departments must be able to schedule patients into second- and third-choice departments as needed. Direct, point-to-point communications between first-, second-, or third-choice departments is essential to determine the immediate availability within alternative services. Quality improvement mechanisms must extend to all services where the customers receive their care. In fact, an institution- or systemwide governance structure for outpatient services is needed to ensure consistency of practices and performance. These enabling systems help maximize the benefits of a fluid strategy.

Summary and recommendation

Healthcare providers must recognize and move away from the strategic mismatch between the traditional fixed, inpatient strategy, and the needs of its outpatients. This mismatch perpetuates the performance dilemma where service levels and operating costs are always at odds.

Successful providers of outpatient services will inevitably shift toward a more fluid strategy tailored to outpatient services. Structural flexibility is needed to provide high service levels and better continuity of care while minimizing costs.

There are cultural challenges in helping people shift from thinking of outpatient services as independent locations (i.e., islands) rather than a network of services (i.e., overlap). There are operational hurdles in planning, design, and the creation of enabling systems. Solving all challenges at once may be too much for some organizations. A prudent start is to select a single service and outpatient type—perhaps one in need of immediate improvement—in order to demonstrate the strategy and its benefits. This start builds the support and momentum needed to expand the fluid approach to the rest of the outpatient business.

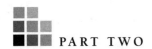
PART TWO

REDESIGN STRATEGIES AND METHODS

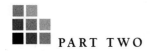PART TWO

Management principles

5

Principles for managing successful change

William Reeves
Partner, Managed Healthcare Consulting Practice
Price Waterhouse
St. Louis, Missouri

No one disputes that the American healthcare system is in the throes of massive change. Indeed, some assert that the system is being reformed privately from the bottom up by the actions of thousands of providers, payers, suppliers, and customers. There have been enormous bursts of both creativity and destruction as old realities have dissolved, replaced by startling new challenges. The royalty of healthcare, the teaching institutions with their myriad specialists, have seen their status and wealth erode while the humble family practitioner has risen in esteem and reward. Insurers have risen from mere bookkeepers to become the 900-pound gorillas of the system. Whole new businesses have been conjured into being: PBMs (pharmacy benefit managers), independent network managers, and disease managers. Fortune 500 executives have been forced to focus as much attention on their healthcare plans as on new product plans. The overall effect has been that healthcare—a historically localized, fragmented, some would even say a cottage industry—is going through its own industrial revolution, with standardization, integration, and automation being the favored instruments of change.

That unprecedented, systemwide levels of change will continue to occur is not in doubt. What is in doubt is exactly what healthcare managers should do about it. Specifically, every healthcare senior manager is asking two questions: In what direction should my organization change to be positioned for success? and How do I get there—how do I successfully guide my organization in making the change needed?

Each organization's situation—its markets, customers, competitors, capabilities, regulations—is unique and will require a rigorous, fact-based approach to set its direction in the marketplace. The real problem is that in the healthcare market, what to do is a moving target: what is appropriate for today is unlikely to hold true for tomorrow or the next day. This is why answering the second question (how to change?) is so important. Given that no strategy or capability is going to remain viable for very long, developing the capability to adapt to constantly changing circumstances is among the most important skills an organization and its managers can have. The research project that this chapter is based on is charged with outlining and understanding how organizations behave under the stress of change and how managers can improve the ability of their organizations to adapt and change when required. This research has led to certain conclusions or best practices regarding the nature of achieving organizational change.

Principles for change

The first conclusion is that there is not one answer: the circumstances surrounding individual change efforts are situation specific, and what must be done to transform an organization cannot be prescribed in advance. This is one of the key challenges of change: there is no explicit calculus, no prescriptive outline of the steps needed to drive change in an organization.

However, experience drawn from healthcare and other business sectors points out a finite set of principles that are key to achieving change. While no change effort has successfully applied all of these principles at the same time, by working toward them managers have substantially enhanced their ability to successfully implement change.

CONFRONT REALITY

Leaders and managers of successful organizations need to face a harsh reality: These structures—the products and services they offer, and the processes and technologies that support them—are not reality by tomorrow's standards. Leaders tend to be committed to the quaint notion that what they have built will continue to flourish indefinitely. However, the new reality sinks in as governments, competitors, and customers continue the process of "creative destruction" that has gone on throughout history.

FOCUS ON STRATEGIC CONTEXTS

The healthcare industry is experiencing explosive change. Driven by increasing intolerance of medical inflation and an increased willingness of governments and employers to innovate, this trend can only accelerate, and opportunities to profit (or fail) from the change will be endless. However, capital and energy are not. Knowing where to invest in change and where to seek improved performance will separate the victors from the vanquished. Most importantly, managers must look outside their own boundaries, seeking out opportunities for change beyond the traditional scope of their organizations. Efforts should be focused where the payback will be greatest.

SUMMON A STRONG MANDATE

Change must be supported by a strong mandate. This mandate is generally provided by top management, but it should be amplified by the voice of the customer. Without a mandate that is both strong and consistent, the level of resistance to change will soar, lessening its impact.

SET SCOPE INTELLIGENTLY

Setting an appropriate scope for a change effort is critically important. The focus should be on measurably improving performance in areas most important to the organization and its key stakeholders (i.e., owners, customers, and employees). The most important change in healthcare often must occur between organizations. However, overreaching the change sponsor's broadest possible sphere of influence can produce failure. If the definition of the scope is too limited, success may not matter.

BUILD A POWERFUL CASE FOR CHANGE

It cannot be assumed that others are prepared for change. It is seldom so, therefore a powerful case for change will need to be developed. The next step is to work relentlessly to generate consensus, beginning with executive management and radiating down and across the entire organization.

A case in point is a large Midwestern hospital that recently agreed to merge to improve its leverage and cost position. Unfortunately, the

hospital failed to build a compelling case for why the merger was necessary before it began. The result was enormous turmoil as the boards,
unions, physician-hospital organizations, and managements fought over
every conceivable issue. They had not been convinced of the necessity of
change.

LET THE CUSTOMER DRIVE CHANGE

The customer is an ally in building the case for change, both the paying
customer and the patient. Serving customers is a powerful common
denominator within organizations; customers are the raison d' être of the
organization. Their needs, rigorously examined, should dictate change.

Last year Alliance Blue Cross Blue Shield of Missouri (ABCBS) had a
difficult problem; competitors had introduced a new product into the
market. To respond in kind would require major organizational change.
Before they blindly imitated the competition, ABCBS carefully analyzed
the competitor's offering and asked customers and members to describe
what their needs were. Out of this came insights that allowed the company to develop a better targeted product, with less effort, more internal
buy-in and ultimately greater market success.

KNOW YOUR STAKEHOLDERS

Powerful individuals and groups have stakes in the contemplated
changes. This will create the need to segment, understand, and prioritize
the needs and motives of these stakeholders both within the organization and among key external groups.

One West Coast health plan learned the hard way about how stakeholders who have not bought in to the vision can thwart the best laid
plans. These plans had cultivated an image of being hard-nosed negotia-
tors, cutting very thin provider contracts. Some physicians became so
angry at the company's aggressiveness that they refused to contract with
the plan. There is speculation that this inability to develop a good working relationship with its physician stakeholders led to the plan's being
put up for sale.

COMMUNICATE CONTINUOUSLY

Communication with the stakeholder must actively continue as changes
are envisioned and implemented. The case for change and style of communication must resonate with them and convince them to act anew.

Clear, succinct messages will be understood. Honest messages will be believed.

RESHAPE MEASURES

In order to drive change and cause people to act anew, organizations must carefully examine their performance measures. First, an organization must build the vision, then design new measures consistent with its strategies and goals. It is importanat to take the time to reevaluate and, if necessary, dismantle old measures.

USE ALL OF THE LEVERS OF CHANGE

There are key points of application that repay all efforts—the levers of change. All of them should be used: target markets and customers, product and service offerings, the organizational structure, human resource systems (including reward programs, business processes, and supporting technologies). Large-scale change can be achieved only when all of these levers are brought to bear in a coordinated manner.

THINK BIG

The change leader must work tirelessly to persuade the change leadership team to think big and to draw positive innovations from people throughout the organization. Small thinking dominates many projects, with predictable results. People need to feel free to take the lid off, to think beyond traditional and accepted boundaries, and to surface dozens of ideas that may not work in order to come up with a few that are genuinely powerful.

As an example, a major managed care company's HMO was broken. The plan was losing money and had enormous operational, contractual, and customer problems. Instead of trying to reengineer their way out of a hopeless situation, the company decided to take a radical approach. They shut the plan down and outsourced a new HMO's operations to a proven regional HMO with a track record of success. The result of this high-risk strategy was the replacement of a liability with an asset that continues to be the centerpiece of the managed care organization's strategy.

LEVERAGE DIVERSITY

It is difficult to think beyond accepted boundaries, in part because these boundaries have become the accepted norm. An unparalleled opportunity for innovative thinking now awaits as increasing numbers of women, minorities, and foreign nationals enter healthcare organizations. Their experience can help managed care companies generate creative new solutions to meet the needs of diverse customers. These minds and perspectives will help shake the old paradigms and, where necessary, replace them.

BUILD SKILLS

No organization can overinvest in human capital. Build skills within all of the organization's levels. Skill building is a key performance measure for all employees. It means broadening the technical, problem-solving, decision-making, and leadership skills of those in the trenches. For managers, it means strengthening their own facilitation, delegation, listening, communication, and diversity skills.

PLAN

To drive change a documented and detailed action plan must be developed for change. It must cover all major actions required, including changes in processes, systems, people, organizational culture, the physical plant, the organizational structure, and training needs.

INTEGRATE THE INITIATIVES

Change programs bubble up continuously in high-performance organizations. Savvy executives strive to balance the entrepreneurship of high-initiative managers with the need to adhere to a focused strategy. As change programs emerge, define their objectives, and consume resources, it is critical to maintain a consistent, integrated rationale for the whole pattern of change. An unplanned patchwork of change initiatives will promote bitter competition for resources, confuse employees, and reduce the positive impact of any one initiative.

Change what?

Executives must consider how the organization currently operates and envision what it might be, could be, if all hopes are fulfilled. How might it operate far more successfully in the future? There is almost certainly a gap between the present and the future along a number of important dimensions. It is useful to formalize these dimensions through six "levers of change."

Markets and customers. The vision of present and future may include differences in the way an organization will or should view and segment its markets and customer base

Products and services. The refined market focus that is envisioned may be accompanied by changes in the scope and variety of products and services an organization seeks to bring to market. Perhaps a sense that there is a need to establish strategic alliances and partnerships with key customers and suppliers

Business processes. There will probably be a gap in the way an organization's business processes operate now and the way they will need to operate in the future to improve healthcare delivery. This change can be driven by introducing a new set of pointedly relevant performance measures at the corporate and business unit levels

People and reward systems. The vision may include differences in the kinds of people that will be needed, systems and measures for rewarding them, and the culture that sends them daily signals concerning "how we do business" and "what we are all about" as an organization

Structure and facilities. There is probably a gap between the organization's current structure and its best future configuration. New facilities may also show up in the vision of the kind of future worth having

Technologies. The vision may reveal a gap between the information-based technologies in place today and those needed to remain competitive in the future

The changes necessary to move the organization toward a vision of its strongest future are likely to involve change in all the above areas. This is so for the healthiest of organizations; the need to change is not necessarily a sign of poor corporate health. Stasis, on the other hand, is invariably a bad sign.

High-impact solutions

There is often an observed discrepancy between the results expected of specially appointed change project teams and the authority and freedom of action conferred on the teams by senior managements. Senior executives typically want and work hard to promote big results. But they will get only what they make possible. Hence, there are two important questions that change teams and senior executive sponsors need to clarify early: What is the scope of the project? and How many levers of change may the team actually access and alter?

For example, can the change team recommend and secure approval for significant changes in the organizational structure or is that option off limits? Can the team make substantial changes in the degree to which frontline employees are empowered or do union and human resource policy factors put this option out of bounds? Can the team suggest segmenting and serving customers in a brand-new construct? Can it consider discontinuing less attractive or conflicting product lines? Is it free to consider new performance measures and reward systems?

The answers to these questions, each of which tests the limit in relation to the six levers of change, will generate a realistic sense of the agreed scope of a change effort. This in turn will either enable or constrain the impact that can be expected.

The top executives of a major HMO recently attended a sophisticated seminar on business reengineering. All of them left the meeting excited about the breakthroughs possible through reengineering. To translate their excitement into action, they commissioned a team to lead a reengineering project with the objective of major performance improvement. However, the team was told, "Hands off organizational and incentive compensation issues." Performance measures were also just about off limits. By the time the ground rules were laid, the team was authorized to reengineer in only two of the six real levers of change.

The project was only a modest success. The team finished its work with the certainty that much more could have been achieved.

To achieve the best results from the change effort, it must have the right scope. However, setting scope and securing freedom of action appropriate to that scope are not simple matters. Is it a process, a department, or the whole organization that needs to be retooled? If a process, has it been examined well enough to be understood? What boundaries does the process cross? Who are the major stakeholders? Is the team genuinely empowered to think big and to lay hands on all the levers of change?

One-dimensional change typically generates either modest improvement in the bottom line or outright failure. Better change is always multidimensional. If people are expected to perform at higher levels, their work processes must be improved. They must have access to the right information and tools, have the authority to make decisions, be measured in new ways, and be rewarded for their better performance.

If organization structure is changed, then all the supporting activities and the line of command must be redesigned to give it the foundation necessary to succeed. This invariably requires a change in systems and technology infrastructure and performance evaluation and compensation systems.

If success requires redesigned processes, then job descriptions and training programs should be redesigned to reflect the new work requirements. Because if information technology investments are key, the people who will use the new technologies must be adequately trained and prepared.

High-performance organizations address change in all its dimensions. They involve people throughout the organization and beyond its boundaries. This multidimensional, comprehensive approach offers the potential for dramatic performance improvement in healthcare through solutions integrated across the healthcare delivery system.

The more successful healthcare systems are working with their hospitals, payers, and physicians to reengineer the multiple chains of activity. Forward-looking management teams recognize that the key to their success lies both within the company and outside in transforming relationships with key stakeholders. They know that an integrated solution will lower costs across the entire spectrum of healthcare delivery.

WHEN BAD THINGS HAPPEN TO GOOD PROJECTS

Broad-based change projects are complex, therefore much can go wrong, and some things will go wrong if only due to Murphy's Law. There are many solutions for overcoming the barriers to change. There will be setbacks, but the first thing that must be done is to understand them. The following is a list of the bad things that can happen to good projects.

Failure to deliver early, tangible results

Some would say the half-life of a change project is six months; that is, if there are no measurable results in six months, expect the support to halve and the barriers to double. While six months is not the half-life of an ambitious project, it may be the half-life of the support that is initially received. The worst thing that can be done is to design changes that require a huge investment and a long delivery time but offer no evidence of improved performance until a "big bang" implementation. Would such an effort be seriously supported? Would the effort be funded? The team should be pressured to come up with a generous handful of near-term wins. Those wins should be publicized upon arrival to build momentum and support. A few quick, adequately dramatic wins will also reassure the effort's sponsors.

The need for quick results is real if for no other reason than to keep hope alive. The discomfort of change eventually touches all involved and, as it does, change initiatives are likely to encounter resistance. When the discomfort reaches a stakeholder group, hope can be replaced with skepticism or agreement with cynicism as to whether the changes can or even should be achieved.

Drowning in details

While people often get excited about breakthrough possibilities at conferences, converting this excitement into sustained action back at the office on Monday morning is difficult. Even when breakthroughs are achieved on the conceptual level, implementation can be daunting. Yet breakthroughs are needed.

Breakthroughs are achieved by simplifying rather than complicating the way an organization operates. A simpler understanding of a problem and its solution, coupled with a sense of urgency to institute the simpler way quickly, can provide the breakthroughs of which so many companies are in need. Detailed analysis and justification are probably necessary but meticulous documentation, complete with overheads, must not be permitted to obscure or derail what is probably a step toward simplicity and an authentic breakthrough.

A large multihospital chain pursuing a project to uncover and cure problems in its patient accounting systems ultimately had to admit that the project had delivered little benefit. In the words of one executive, "The project team generated 180 feet of brown paper and not much else." Symptomatic of overemphasis on process mapping (and underemphasis on practical, results-oriented change), the team had mapped business processes until it and its organizational sponsors were exhausted. The process review had yielded no real change or performance improvement. The team decided to stow most of its brown paper and start over, this time focusing on the highest-priority problems. And it is meeting with success in a project now guided by a considered look at a very powerful lever of change—the system's performance measures.

Everything is high priority

Everything cannot be equally important; life is full of choices. Change teams must set a broad scope and work for a while at that gauge, then narrow in on choices that yield the most gain. While Pareto's Principle (the 80 to 20 percent rule) is generally true, administrative efficiency (which is the 20 percent) should not be focused on at the expense of developing the information and capabilities to improve care delivery (which is the 80 percent). Projects fail when priorities are not established early and refined throughout the effort.

Older performance measures block change

Fancy words cannot improve on the well-known assertion that what gets measured, gets done. All large-scale change efforts demand a reshaping of the performance measures that guide manager and employee actions. If the long-established measures are not disassembled, they will continue to drive behavior and block the changes that are intended. Attention should be focused on measures that truly drive the actions and affect the attitudes of employees. Most measures warp and distort behavior. Are these behaviors likely to change if they are not reshaped? Few policies are more effective in focusing employees' energies and attention than a properly designed performance management system. When measures are aligned with organizational strategies and goals, then the ability to drive change is greatly enhanced.

Failing to connect the dots

Ideas compete in business. Professional journals are rich in competing management techniques to improve business performance. While there are no pat solutions, many techniques (e.g., reengineering and total quality management) are legitimate; they should be tuned to specific organizational needs and put to work. However, failure to reconcile and integrate competing projects shaped by these methodologies can waste millions of dollars and exhaust the organization. The energy and loyalty of good people pitted against one another in efforts to protect turf or programs is largely wasted, and the disruption from strenuous battles of this kind can be so thoroughgoing that no single project delivers on its promise.

The voice of the customer is absent

What influence has the customer on the change process? The customer is typically a consistent voice and votes for what is valued when services are bought. While not institutionalized in healthcare, the concept of systematically listening to the customer (both payer and patient) is fundamental in qualifying for the Baldrige Award in the United States and in qualifying to be examined for certification under ISO 9000 (the global quality standard). But long before the advents of total quality management, reengineering, and the Baldrige Award, an organization's skill in listening to the customer and translating customer needs into action went a long way toward explaining why businesses succeeded or failed. Witness the emergence of the point-of-service concept. Not long ago large employers were trying desperately to move their membership into managed care. CIGNA listened to the customers' needs and built a product that worked and that no one else offered, thus accelerating the shift to HMOs in many markets. While this is a fundamental concept, few organizations systematically assess what the customer really wants. The voice of the customer is loud and clear in virtually every successful change effort. It is recommended that key customers and suppliers be invited to serve as liaisons on the change project team.

The voice of the employee is not heard

Winning in sports takes belief in the team's ability to execute and excel. During the course of a major sporting event, a single play or at-bat can change the entire momentum of competition. Change is a competition between the need for change and the barriers that resist it. Winning in a change project requires belief that barriers can be overcome and that the end result will be worth the price, and this belief must be widespread. If the manager in the dugout or pacing the sidelines in a headset believes but half the players have lost hope, the outcome is predictable. To achieve important, enduring, positive change, employee involvement is essential. Involving employees is messy. It is easier to form a small team, figure out the answers, and tell everybody else. But involvement builds commitment and significantly increases the likelihood of a successful transformation.

This has particular resonance in most healthcare reengineering. The leaders from the local physician and nursing groups should be invited to participate on the team. These leaders represent one of the largest constituencies in the delivery system. Their contributions and buy-in will work wonders toward translating plans into frontline results. Even if a physician presence is not feasible, it is essential that the leaders of departments who are involved and working with them be identified and act as their proxies.

Senior management wants to help, but doesn't know how

Every text and speech on change describes top management commitment as essential. Many bankrupt attempts at change result from failed efforts to maintain a visible level of support from the top. Top management typically means well but sometimes sends the wrong signals— often in the context of empowering employees. A new environment of empowerment is envisioned, but many executives cannot seem to let go. They destroy momentum by confusing the message about change. Their heads tell them, "share authority and we'll all win," but their emotions tell them, "share authority and I'll lose."

"What's in it for me" is unclear

People change when the case for change becomes a personal matter. Too many change programs are naively based on the premise that changes in employee or physician behaviors will occur "for the good of healthcare" or "for the benefit of future generations of patients." This is unlikely. Employees or physicians will change their behavior when management honestly promises to make things better and communicates persuasively that the coming change project is part of the solution for those individuals. The values in play are financial rewards, self-esteem, recognition, job satisfaction, career growth, and pride, as well as numerous other personal tangibles and intangibles.

Too much conventional wisdom

Successful change programs require a solid foundation in fact, and one company's facts will be quite different from another's. This means that exemplary solutions, even if they are reported in the most trusted business reviews, may not work for all. Facts may be different; conventional wisdom can kill.

Same old horses, same old glue

Failure to form a talented, diverse team representing all stakeholders is a cause of failure that often shows up too late to fix. Change means abandoning the current way of thinking. Teams that effectively drive change need to be populated with known innovators, not with status quo types. In other words, what it needs is new blood, without naiveté; diverse styles and backgrounds, but cooperative attitudes; and personalities that are brash, but not rash. Where conventional wisdom says, "it cannot be done here," real change teams will come up with breakthroughs.

Conclusion

The reality facing today's healthcare managers is stark. They cannot stop the merry-go-round and they cannot get off. All managers can do is predict, adapt, and take advantage of the very instability that gives them such discomfort. Those that cultivate this ability for better change will thrive, those that fail to adapt will die. This chapter has outlined the key common elements found by research to be present in successful change efforts and absent in failures. In addition, it has outlined the major pitfalls that commonly afflict large-scale organizational change. However, one inescapable fact bears repeating: there is no calculus, no single model for success, no one path to better change. It will take all the wit and wisdom that managers have to ride out this healthcare storm. Leaders must be as prepared as possible for better change.

NOTES

1. This chapter has been adapted from *Better Change: Best Practices for Transforming Your Organization*, (St. Louis: Burr Ridge, Irwin Professional Publishing, 1995). © Price Waterhouse LLP 1955, used with permission of the publisher.

6

Leading and transforming organizations

Mary Gelinas, EdD
Managing Director

Roger G. James, EdD
Managing Director
Gelinas James Akiyoshi
Oakland, California

A NUMBER OF ELEMENTS HELP transform an organization—a clear vision, motivated employees, attention to its customer focus, and an effective change process. One element, however, is of critical importance—the organization's leadership. Leaders are the critical players in transforming an organization. They are the linchpins of change.

Nowhere is leadership more critical than in healthcare organizations. Pressures to cut costs and maintain quality and the dual and frequently competing roles of physicians and administrators make decision making highly complicated.

Change always involves a substantial investment of time and resources. Leaders need to devote 20 to 50 percent of their time, or 8 to 20 hours per week, to a change effort if it is to be successful.[1] This chapter details what leaders need to do, say, and think to lead an effective change process, highlighting the basic phases of successful change efforts and the primary leadership tasks. Eliminating or poorly handling any of these tasks can undermine or negate the effort.

Phases of change

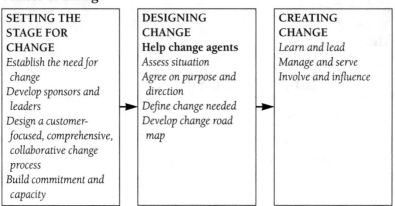

Phases of change

There are three phases of change: setting the stage for change, designing change, and creating change.

PHASE ONE: SETTING THE STAGE FOR CHANGE

In this first phase, leaders create the foundational cornerstones for change, which include

- Establishing the need for change

- Developing sponsors and leaders to lead the change process

- Designing a customer-focused, comprehensive, collaborative change process

- Building the organization's commitment and capacity to change

In this phase, leaders gather in a series of meetings to review relevant data from customers, competitors, and the marketplace. They then develop the case for change with other leaders and members, gathering information from key customers and major suppliers as they proceed. In addition to developing the case for change, leaders forge agreements with one another about the process they will use to change the organization and build their own and others' commitment to this process. As they do this, a collaborative relationship forms—a prerequisite to effectively leading change efforts.

First cornerstone: Make the case for change

The "case for change" includes five important elements: current and anticipated customer needs, market challenges and opportunities, the core purpose of the organization, the future direction of the organization, and the specific outcomes of the change initiative.

An organization performs through a series of explicit and implicit agreements among leaders and members. The most foundational of these agreements are those regarding the organization's purpose and direction (mission and vision). The mission describes why the organization exists, what unique products or services it provides to whom, and what unique value the organization adds to society. Its vision statement describes the desired future state of the organization. Such agreements should only be developed after an analysis of the organization's present and anticipated external environment and its internal strengths and weaknesses is conducted. The major challenges and opportunities in the environment and the organization's purpose and direction provide a common target for efforts to improve the organization.

Without a clearly articulated mission and vision for the organization, initiatives easily disintegrate into a series of competing and confusing projects that are not meaningfully connected and that divert time, resources, and attention from the critical job of improving the organization's performance and preparing it for new opportunities.

To effectively focus change, the vision statement should include the organization's primary goals, its strategy to achieve those goals, its values, its desired characteristics (i.e., business processes, structure, and systems), the desired characteristics of its members and leaders, and its ultimate culture.

Leaders must have a strong relationship or connection to the vision, and it should be manifested in their language, decisions, and actions. Leaders must also share their vision with all key stakeholders and incorporate the various stakeholders' views into the vision.

The desired outcomes for the change initiative are most effective when it is clear how the initiative will

- Support the mission's achievement and organization's vision

- Help the organization meet customers' needs

- Enable the organization to respond to current and anticipated demands of the marketplace

The desired outcomes are most effective when they are results oriented and inspiring to those who are expected to change. Concrete outcomes focus the initiative. For example, four of the desired outcomes from a recent organization redesign effort in a medical center of a health maintenance organization are

- Deliver healthcare services in a manner so overwhelmingly convenient that competitors will be eclipsed

- Increase the satisfaction and sense of self-worth of the providers and support staff

- Significantly increase member satisfaction; members (of the health maintenance organization) and staff remain with and feel pride in the program

- Become the "benchmark" for other medical centers in the HMO

Defining the mission, vision, and the specific desired outcomes of change initiatives in healthcare organizations can be challenging because the marketplace forces the organization to cut costs dramatically while maintaining and improving quality, customer service, and value. Often pressure to cut costs can be so intense it can overshadow other concerns. Change initiatives that focus primarily on cost cutting can achieve greater profits in the short run. However, organizations that take a longer-range view and focus on growth as well as efficiencies achieve higher revenue growth and market value.[2]

Thus, leaders must make agreements about the following:

- Major challenges and opportunities in the current and anticipated business environment

- Major strengths (including core competencies) and weakness of the organization

- Core purpose and organizational direction

- Important gaps between where the organization is and where it wants to be

- Purpose and outcomes of a change initiative

For example, managed care brought extraordinary challenges to one academic medical center with 700 beds and 450,000 annual ambulatory visits that primarily focused on fee-for-service and tertiary care. This organization's leadership team conducted a preliminary analysis of the current and future trends in healthcare, demographics, and financing in the region for which they provided tertiary care. Their higher-cost structure, required to maintain teaching programs, put pressure on them to reduce costs significantly as more managed care companies emerged and the pressure to use primary care physicians to maintain and limit access to more costly specialists increased. Fee for service was a thing of the past and managed care companies were contracting with them for discounted, predetermined, or capitated rates. It was a new world. The feedback from patients, families, and referring primary care physicians also alerted them to problems with customer service. The leaders concluded that profound change would be required in all aspects of the organization. The leaders needed to rethink the organization's current mission and outline the desired direction and future of the organization. The gaps between the organization's current state and its five-year vision created a compelling case for transforming the organization.

Second cornerstone: Develop sponsors and leaders

Sponsoring and leading change are two very different, yet important roles. Sponsors are the visionaries. They carry the big picture and pay the bills. They provide support and protection when the initiative treads into politically sensitive areas. The more senior the sponsors, the better the chances for success.

Leading change means daily leadership, including convening meetings, participating at key decision-making points (e.g., establishing the project budget and selecting consultants), and either acting as, or working closely with, a change agent. The chances for success also increase when the initiative is headed by the leaders of the organization and their direct reports. Although some leaders play both of these roles, in larger organizations these responsibilities are divided among two or more players.

For example, in the change effort at an academic medical center, the vice chancellor of the university and the CEO of the hospital and clinic sponsored the initiative. The CEO and his direct reports led the initiative, participated at key decision-making points, and championed the effort. A 10-person design team of physicians, senior nursing staff, and administrative leaders analyzed (along with hundreds of other stakeholders) the current organization and developed recommendations for organizational change. A physician, who was the head of a major department in the hospital and in the school of medicine, led the team.

As many senior executives know, the management layer just below them usually must be convinced that change is necessary and that working together more effectively is a critical aspect to create that change. Frequently accountable only for their individual function or department, these managers often find it challenging to take responsibility for leading an organizationwide initiative collectively. How they go about building the aforementioned agreements and put these cornerstones in place is important practice in collaboratively leading change.

Thus leaders must

- Agree on what they need to do to lead the change process

- Provide resources (e.g., budget, staff support, time)

- Develop their ability and that of other leaders to change and to lead change

- Put all the cornerstones into place

- Build understanding and support for the initiative among leaders at all levels

For example, in one change initiative in a primary care center that is part of a much larger HMO, the leaders negotiated support for the initiative with the key regional manager. The commitment to support the local initiative with money, staff, and verbal encouragement were critical to this initiative's success.

Third cornerstone: Design customer-focused, comprehensive, and collaborative change process

Although internal or external consultants can provide organizational change models, leaders must design change processes to work for their organization. If leaders do not understand or agree on the process, consultants or staff members can lead the initiative. This, however, may result in disaster. Consultants and staff lack a vested interest in seeing the organization succeed and change ceases to be a priority.

Agreeing on a change process includes making decisions about the depth and breadth of the initiative, the desired degree of participation by key stakeholders in the process, the process itself, and who will have primary responsibility for assessing the situation, developing recommendations for organizational change, and implementing those changes.

Change initiatives must focus on the customer and the business environment. "The more everyone in the company is imbued with knowledge of customers, the more likely that the organization can agree to change to serve them better."[3] Being customer-focused means understanding the needs and requirements of customers and the issues and challenges that face them. It also involves examining both the current and anticipated environment within which the organization and its customers are operating. This includes changes in technology, demographics, regulations, and market trends.

Change processes are also more effective when they are comprehensive. A comprehensive approach includes analyzing the breadth and depth of an organization to determine what is affecting the organization's performance. Breadth includes the following elements of organization. Figure 2 illustrates the interdependence of these elements and the importance of their alignment.

FIGURE 2
Elements of organization

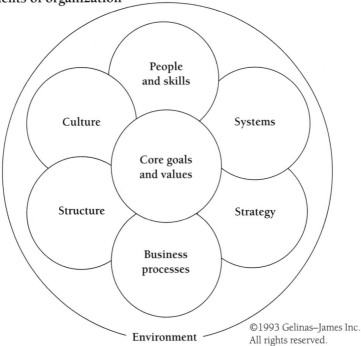

People and skills

Culture

Systems

Core goals and values

Structure

Strategy

Business processes

Environment

- Core goals and values—what the organization stands for and wants to achieve

- Strategy or basic approach to achieving its mission or purpose

- Business processes and relationships with customers and suppliers

- Structure—how people are organized in relation to one another (e.g., the definition of departments, units, and levels of supervision), as well as the physical layout

- Systems or the procedures that make the organization run, including information, planning, human resources, communication, evaluation, and renewal

- People and skills—the types of professions, knowledge, and skills

- Culture—the collective pattern of behaviors, values, and unwritten rules developed over time in an organization

- Environment—the customers, including their needs and requirements, as well as market trends, technological advances, regulations, and demographic shifts

Depth includes the organization's various components and levels.

Change processes are most effective when they are collaborative—they involve those who will be most affected by the change. The greater the degree of involvement in the first two phases of change, the less "selling" time needed prior to implementation. The proverbial wall that an organization can hit at the start of implementation becomes a smaller hurdle.

In addition to determining the appropriate depth and breadth of the initiative, leaders must define the extent and level of involvement of key stakeholders in the process. This involves leaders balancing a number of variables including time, potential impact, and the level of buy-in needed. Figure 4 can help leaders make conscious, informed choices about whom to involve and to what degree. Defining which decisions are open for participation is critical. Leaders do not want to involve others in a decision-making process if the decisions are already made.

Involving others in the process may include use of a variety of strategies, such as paper or electronic vehicles (e.g., memos, reports, posters, surveys, bulletin boards, e-mail, computer polling, newsletters, and videos); videotape presentations; teleconferencing via video or tele-

FIGURE 3
Components and levels of organizations—depth

1. Organization	Can be one organization; an umbrella organization (a holding company for a number of organizations), or a major unit of an umbrella organization (i.e., a subsidiary, an operating company, a group, a division).
2. Interdepartmental or cross-functional	The interface between two or more departments or units.
3. Departmental	A portion or subset of a major unit (e.g., a department).
4. Unit	A subset of a department (e.g., a unit or team).
5. Between units or teams	The interface between two or more units or teams.
6. Individual contributors	A manager of a unit or team.

Depth can also be interorganizational; the interface between two or more organizations, as in network organizations.

phone; one-on-one, small group (maximum of 15 participants), or large group meetings (15 to 100-plus participants).

For example, one medical center had attempted to improve quality and cut costs in various areas of the organization. It had, however, never taken a look at the entire organization—all elements, components, and levels. The leaders agreed that the changes in the business environment required a complete and comprehensive organizational change effort. Based on their experiences in implementing incremental changes, they also agreed the process needed to be collaborative and involve as many stakeholders (e.g., employees, physicians, insurers, and patients) in the

FIGURE 4
Desired degree of participation and level of involvement

Percentage of the organization (or customers-suppliers) you want to

Be kept informed	Provide feedback	Provide input	Participate in developing recommen-dations	Participate in decision making
_____ percent	_____ percent	_____ percent	_____ percent	_____ percent
_____ number	_____ number	_____ number	_____ number	_____ number

TIME AVAILABLE

< Little   Sufficient/expandable >

POTENTIAL IMPACT OF DECISION

< Low   Moderate   Great >

BUY-IN NEEDED

< Little   Moderate   A lot >

INFORMATION AND EXPERTISE OF STAKEHOLDERS

< Little   Sufficient   A lot >

DEVELOPMENTAL OPPORTUNITY

< Minimal   High   Maximum >

LEADER FLEXIBILITY

< Non-negotiable   Negotiable   Very flexible >

process as possible. By involving stakeholders in the process early, they hoped to minimize the strenuous and time-consuming task of selling changes needed prior to implementation. Their first step in collaboration was to solicit nominees from the top 40 managers in the organization for the team of change agents who would take the lead in determining what changes would be needed.

To execute this phase leaders must

- Agree on a change process to help the organization move from the current state to the desired future state

- Make sure that the process is focused on customers, is comprehensive enough to bring about the level of change needed, and includes appropriate involvement of all major stakeholders

- Agree on values and principles to guide the change process

- Identify change agents

- Agree on their role in the process

At the academic medical center noted earlier, the purview of the design team included the entire hospital and clinic. The team considered all elements (breadth), all components, and all levels (depth) of the organization. Although the hospital and clinic had implemented previous change initiatives, their approach had been piecemeal. The result was a level of transformation that was below what was needed for the organization to prosper.

In the medical center of the HMO noted earlier, the leaders agreed that a critical guiding principle was that the change process had to mirror the type of organization they wanted to create. They believed the future organization would need to provide a greater and more seamless continuum of services to patients and families using cross-functional teams to work collaboratively. Thus, this change initiative was led by a series of cross-functional teams representing medicine, nursing, diagnostics, and therapeutics. It examined the core processes of the healthcare system—from prevention through long-term care—and worked across the teams to develop organizational change recommendations.

Fourth cornerstone: Build commitment and capacity

Developing support throughout an organization is critical to the success of any change effort; without support from an organization's most influential leaders, a change initiative will fail. Although many transformation efforts start with only a handful of supporters, in the most successful ones the coalition of leaders supporting the initiative expands over time.[4]

The case for change, including the desired organization direction, is the instrumental component to create this commitment. The leaders of an organization must see themselves as the leaders of change, not as its victims. By taking this role, they are increasing the likelihood that the initiative will succeed. Equally important, they are preparing themselves for the roles they must continue to play in the future—anticipators, creators, and leaders of change.

Leading single- or multiple-change initiatives can present major challenges for teams at the top of organizations. If they have not seen themselves or functioned as an interdependent group with joint accountability for the organization's success, then they may have difficulties with these new responsibilities. They may not know how to manage current operations cooperatively while helping the organization transform itself. They will need to develop this know-how.

This is especially true in healthcare. Most administrators have managed change, but it rarely has been in partnership with physicians. Physicians, on the other hand, usually have little or no experience in leading organizational change or solving operational issues collaboratively. In recent years, physicians have seen themselves as the victims of change. Thus, administrators and physicians must take time to learn how to work together to lead change initiatives. The process through which physicians and administrators set the stage for change can serve as a laboratory in which to improve working relationships.

Physicians often face additional problems when leading change initiatives. Often for the first time, they must consider the effectiveness and future of the entire institution, not just the success of one practice or specialty area. Thinking in such balanced terms may be challenging for physicians who have traditionally practiced in environments where their priorities have been exclusively focused on the needs of their patients and their practice.

Thus, leaders must

- Build understanding and support within the organization about what the leaders believe is needed, why, how they plan to get there, and everyone's role in the process

- Build their and others' capacity to create change

At the academic medical center noted earlier, the CEO, his direct reports, and the design team held interactive sessions with midlevel managers, clinical chiefs, other physician-governing bodies, and several hundred employees. In these sessions, the leaders and change agents focused on building understanding and agreement on the case for change and the approach to change and on soliciting the hopes, concerns, and advice of all participants. Such meetings thereafter continued on a regular basis. Managers held themselves accountable for leading the change effort from inception through implementation.

PHASE TWO: DESIGNING CHANGE

In phase two, leaders and members of an organization determine how the organization needs to be transformed. Leaders have in place a team or teams of change agents (identified in phase one) who, with the guidance and active participation of the leaders, perform the following activities:

- Create a more in-depth understanding of the existing situation, including the strengths and weakness of the organization; opportunities and challenges (present and anticipated) in the environment; and customers' current, anticipated, and future needs. (This phase builds on and expands the preliminary assessment done by the leaders to define the purpose, desired outcomes, depth, breadth, and approach to a change initiative.)

- Refine or redefine the purpose, strategy, and direction of the organization

- Define and forge agreements on major changes the organization needs to make. Depending on the scope of the initiative, this could include business processes (including relationships with customers and suppliers), structure, systems, people and skills, and culture

- Develop a plan to implement the desired changes

During this phase, leaders have three primary responsibilities: communicating with key customers and stakeholders (e.g., major clients, key board members, and community leaders); participating at crucial decision-making points in the change process (e.g., agreeing on the critical strengths and weaknesses of the organization); and building understanding and agreement throughout the organization on the current situation, the desired direction, and the changes needed.

For example, at an academic medical center, the design team worked with the CEO and his top team to define and analyze the organization's core business processes and to conduct an in-depth assessment of customer needs and requirements. This top team helped conduct interviews with major employers, insurance companies, physician groups, and university leaders. The top team worked with the design team to redefine the organization's mission and vision in light of all the analytical findings. They participated with the design team in three major conferences where nearly 100 representatives of all key stakeholder groups participated. The purpose of these conferences was to build understanding and agreement on the findings, mission, and vision and redesign recommendations. These conferences provided invaluable feedback to the design and leadership teams and visibly demonstrated the commitment of these leaders to change.

Specifically, to design change leaders must see that understanding and agreements are built on the following:

- Current and anticipated situation—opportunities and challenges in the existing and projected environment, current and anticipated needs of customers, and strengths and weaknesses of the organization

- Purpose and direction—the mission and vision; vision includes core goals and values, strategy, and desired characteristics of business processes, structure, systems, people and skills, and culture

- What change is needed—changes needed in the business processes, structure, systems, people and skills, and culture

- Change road map—an implementation plan that describes who is responsible to do what when to implement the desired changes

Once these agreements are made, leaders play a critical role in building understanding and support for these agreements throughout the organization. Ideally, these agreements link directly to the case for change developed and communicated in phase one. If the agreements were originally built through highly participatory processes, this role will be less critical and time-consuming.

For example, in a comprehensive change process in a rural medical center, the leaders and members of the design team spent several months reviewing their findings, revising their mission and vision, and developing recommendations with hundreds of people in the organization. After a series of participatory meetings, they asked for volunteers to help develop implementation plans and serve on implementation teams. Several hundred people volunteered.

PHASE THREE: CREATING CHANGE

The purpose of this phase is to plan and implement the major organizational changes identified in phase two. This is the most challenging and fragile time in change initiatives. It is during this phase that initiatives get derailed, postponed, stalled, or eliminated for a new trend (e.g., "management by best seller"). Also, during this phase many people are uncomfortable and frightened. They may have to cope with a sense of loss as they let go of old work habits and roles and take on new responsibilities and challenges.

In this phase, leadership is most critical. In many cases, the leaders and their roles will have changed. During this phase leaders must continue to learn and lead, manage and serve, and influence and involve.

Learn and lead

Learning occurs by looking outside and inside the organization and listening to customers, studying competitors, and observing the patterns of the marketplace. This learning is pivotal to the effectiveness of each of the phases. By continuing to pay attention to the external environment during implementation, leaders ensure that changes being implemented will meet the ever-changing needs of customers and enable the organization to respond to marketplace challenges.

Leaders learn by listening to the observations, aspirations, and ideas of all in the organization and by listening to their own inner guidance and aspirations. A leader's commitment, values, and core purpose are an important part of the mix to successfully create change.

Leading implementation entails several tasks, including communicating, planning, tracking and evaluating, and championing.

Communicating is being willing to advocate the case for change over and over again with various constituencies; taking every available opportunity to talk about the organization's vision, including the change initiative in conversations and meeting agendas; and keeping the organization abreast of the changes as they occur and the impact of those changes. It also means rewarding people in the organization who are making significant improvements and treating with fairness those who are being negatively affected.

Planning necessitates developing a road map to guide the organization from its current state to its new one. This road map includes what needs to be done to implement the changes determined in phase two. It also describes processes through which critical stakeholders are involved in implementation.

For leaders, tracking and evaluating involves monitoring the progress and assessing the impact of the change initiative. Leaders must ensure that the original purpose and desired outcomes of the initiative are translated into more specific measures of success. Such an evaluation system should, as much as possible, use information-gathering systems already in place. Leaders must also pay as much attention to learning as they do to making progress and attaining success. What is learned along the way is at least as valuable as what is accomplished.

A leader's commitment gets fundamentally tested in this phase. Leading is being clear on what the leader stands for and making sure that his or her behavior and words are consistent.

In the tertiary care medical center, as the organization began to implement a series of major recommendations, it also began to explore a partnership with a primary care institution. This potential alliance seemed to make sense, but it diverted attention from the immediate changes needed. The CEO communicated in as many ways as he could the importance of pursuing both efforts. He described the implementation of the redesign recommendations as instrumental in the development of an effective partnership with the other organization.

Manage and serve

Managing requires keeping the organization functioning effectively as it reinvents itself. Many organizations call this "keeping the lights on while redesigning the organization." In redesign efforts of several power plants, this expression took on new meaning. The company literally had to keep the lights on for millions of customers while they transformed their plants.

Keeping the organization functioning while changing it remains an extremely challenging task in healthcare. Patients' need for care cannot stop while healthcare providers and administrators reinvent their institutions.

The primary challenge in organization improvement efforts is to ensure that everyone carries out their daily jobs effectively while preparing for new ways of work. However, if organizations only focus on day-to-day operations, they may be heading toward danger. Leaders must help the organization balance its focus between operating the day-to-day business and changing the organization. In one initiative, the COO had to clearly delineate to many department heads that they were required to sustain their current work as the organization changed.

Serving an organization and a change effort means removing obstacles, allowing people to create, and providing resources, time, and support for those who are transforming the organization. In healthcare this usually means freeing up providers for large blocks of time and providing backup to the physicians, nurses, clinical staff, and administrators so they can participate in improving the organization. Although this is expensive and challenging, it must be done. For example, in one hospital change initiative, administration provided backup services to replace those assigned full time for one year to the design team.

Influence and involve

Influencing is using both personal and positional power to get everyone in the organization to work toward common goals, be willing to take a stand in favor of a vision, and be willing to let it go as others build on it and make it theirs.

Leaders exert significant influence in an organization simply by focusing their attention on a given goal, area, or project. They influence the organization by what they say, what questions they ask, what items are on their meeting agendas, and where they spend their time. Each act is a message to the organization about what is important. Other leaders and members gauge the significance of a change initiative based on how much attention the leaders pay it.

People are committed to and support what they have participated in creating. To build support for change, leaders need to involve as many members of the organization as possible in the process of creating that change. Leaders have to make conscious choices about the degree of participation and level of involvement desired during implementation. The greater the possible impact and the higher the level of support needed for implementation, the more the process needs to engage the key players.

Participatory processes test leaders' beliefs and assumptions about people and what is possible. When leaders create processes through which they and the organization's members become navigators of their own future, organizational performance exceeds what leaders or members can create individually.

Leaders in healthcare have the challenge of engaging physicians in creating change. Since the role of physicians is unique—they are simultaneously customers and providers—their commitment is key to the success of any initiative. For example, at one academic medical center, all implementation teams are led by a physician and an administrator. Physicians make up one-third of the membership on all the teams. And, in a change initiative in an HMO, the steering committee is co-led by a physician and each of the four design teams (who are also responsible for implementation) is led by a physician.

Many of the physicians in the HMO were accustomed to a major share of the capitated market. For years, they had provided high-quality care for the lowest prices in their areas. Many of the physicians continued to ignore the flight of their members to the newly created HMO providing equal or better service for less. This lack of interest in the change initiative continued until the physician leader of the steering committee had a series of meetings with a number of influential practice leaders.

To create change leaders must

- See that a realistic and effective implementation plan is developed

- Define specifically how they will measure the success of the initiative

- Identify change agents who will have primary responsibility for implementing change

- Continue to educate organization members about why the organization needs to change

- Role model the new expectations regarding behaviors, attitudes, and values

- Describe personal challenges in the transition

- Absorb risks that accompany innovation and improvement

- Provide resources (i.e., time, staff, and budget) to those responsible for implementing change

- Lead and encourage

Summary

Leaders are the critical players in transforming organizations. Successfully balancing their attention between managing daily operations and leading a change initiative is no small feat. This task can be more complicated in healthcare because of the dual and sometimes competing roles of physicians and administrators. Leaders have roles in all three phases of a change initiative.

Table 1 summarizes the specific tasks for leaders in each phase of change in relation to the other critical players.

TABLE 1

Leading performance improvement initiatives

Players	Phases		
	Set the stage for change	*Design change*	*Create change*
With self (Leader)	Clarify personal hopes and dreams	Remember your intention and what you anticipated it would take	Focus attention and action on making it happen
	Assess what it will take personally and professionally to create dreams	Get support from family, friends, colleagues, consultants	Remember your intention and what you anticipated it would take
	Clarify intention	Remember that the difficult news is only part of the picture	Allocate resources to keep the organization going while transitioning into the new one
	Develop plan to build understanding and commitment of other leaders and key stakeholders	Anticipate what resources will be needed for implementation	
	Clarify decision-making process	Identify what changes you will need to make in your skills and behavior	
With top team	Conduct preliminary situation assessment	Keep team's attention focused on change initiative	Strategize how to manage current operations while leading organization transformation
	Define mission and "sketch" vision	Build agreement on team's role in change	Identify changes they need to make individually and collectively; personally and professionally
	Build capacity of leaders to lead change individually and collectively	Continue to develop top team's ability to lead change individually and collectively	
	Build agreements regarding purpose, scope, and process of change initiative(s)	Agree on performance measures	

TABLE 1 (CONTINUED)
Leading performance improvement initiatives

Players	Phases		
	Set the stage for change	Design change	Create change
With change agents	Identify team of change agents to play primary role in initiative Build understanding of and agreement on their charter	Provide resources, protection Cheerlead and encourage Participate at key decision-making points	Identify team(s) of implementors Build understanding of and agreement on their charter
With customers and other leaders	Enlist support and participation of leaders "above," "below," and "next door" Inform customers and major suppliers of pending initiative(s) and what support will be needed	Stay in close contact with customers and key leaders Clarify customer needs Clarify whether new markets, products, market penetration, or diversification is desired Check with them at key decision-making points	Stay in close contact with customers and key leaders Track impact of organization changes on customers and other relevant organizations
With the organization and key stakeholders	Communicate the "case for change" Communicate purpose, scope, and approach to change Define how "stake holders" will be involved	Lead process to build agreement on organization mission and vision Educate organization about business context (customer needs and requirements; shifts in market, technology, regulation, and demographics)	Communicate "case for change" Champion the changes Communicate new expectations to leaders and employees Educate organization about the current and anticipated business context

NOTES

1. G. Hall, J. Rosenthal, and J. Wade, "How to Make Reengeneering Really Work," *Harvard Business Review* 71, no. 6 (1993): 119.

2. M. Magnet, "Let's Go for Growth," *Fortune* (March 7, 1994): 60.

3. T. A. Stewart, "Rate Your Readiness to Change," *Fortune* (February 7, 1994): 109.

4. J. P. Kotter, "Leading Change: Why Transformation Efforts Fail," *Harvard Business Review* 73, no. 2 (1995): 62.

7

Reengineering to revitalize

Milan Moravec
President
Moravec and Associates
Walnut Creek, California

A NY HEALTHCARE ORGANIZATION—hospital, pharmaceutical company, or HMO—that is ready to embrace change in the way work is organized and how it gets done should place the following motto above the portals of its administration office: "Reengineer in haste, repent at leisure." Rushing into reengineering without a plan for revitalization sets an organization up for unintended and undesired results. Without a clear idea of what revitalization will entail, making necessary transitions can become extremely difficult.

What reengineering implies

It is important to clarify what reengineering really means. Many reengineering efforts fail to improve organizational performance because they are just glorified cost reduction programs, not new strategies for the future. Despite the popularity of the term, few leaders and managers are entirely clear on the differences between reeingineering, restructuring, and downsizing. These differences can be summed up briefly: *Downsizing,* the most popular form of organizational change during the early 1990s, refers to contraction—for example, divestments, closures, product or service curtailment, or personnel reduction. Organizations downsized because it was quicker and easier to make cuts than to ask (and answer) hard questions such as, "Do we need to transform the way we do business, and if so, what direction should we take?"

Since costs often were reduced, at least in the short term, these organizations were encouraged to downsize again. Some were overzealous, making further cuts even after profitability swung upward—and despite the fact that many downsized organizations were displeased with the overall results. Downsizing attempts to correct past mistakes rather than create future markets.

Restructuring, which often follows downsizing, can mean both expansion and contraction at the same time, and for that reason it is sometimes known as "rightsizing." It involves realigning the structure, adjusting the staffing mix, and focusing on areas of future growth. Thus, it requires considerable forethought and strategic planning. Still, it has more to do with catching up than moving forward.

Reengineering is a more fundamental, far-reaching, and future-oriented process than either downsizing or restructuring. It is not, as many believe, simply the elimination of certain types of work to gain efficiency. It involves redesigning the entire business system in order to gain competitive advantage in a particular industry.

Following is a brief summary of key steps in most reengineering efforts:

1. Position for change. Decide why the organization must change and envision what it should become. Develop focus and mobilize resources for implementation

2. Diagnose the way customers and patients are treated now, and how unstated rules and assumptions affect quality and cost. View the total process as a customer would

3. Redesign the organization and performance of work. Solicit input from stakeholders. Do not fix a part of the patient care process that management believes will not survive

4. Make the transition. Develop a transition strategy and identify phases, teams, responsibilities, and priorities. Manage resistance to change. Test new processes in limited areas. Evaluate for steady improvement

Reengineering begins with such questions as, "How do we want healthcare to look five years from now, and beyond?" "What must we do to ensure that our industry evolves in ways that are advantageous to our stakeholders—clients, employees, investors, suppliers, and neighbors?"

Reengineering an organization means revising assumptions about what it takes to be successful and competitive. This requires taking a whole-systems approach: looking at the interrelationships between business strategy, structure, technologies, culture, core processes, and mix of competencies needed to deliver more value to customers. Focusing on such imperatives for the future encourages innovation—an essential element in reengineering. Failure to promote innovation results in incremental change only, or "paddling faster" as one manager put it.

No matter which option the organization chooses—downsizing, restructuring, reengineering—its members and leaders will need to think about revitalization first and incorporate this concept into every step. Otherwise they will end up weaker than before. Sustainable vitality calls for new strategies, behaviors, and procedures to reinforce carefully crafted goals.

It is impossible to restructure or reengineer without breaking old patterns, and this is unsettling to everyone involved. To regain equilibrium and momentum, management and staff need a compelling vision and means of achieving that vision.

Organization readiness to change

Change, especially when it involves loss or transformation of jobs, brings people's fears to the surface. Distress signals include illness, lack of follow-through, burnout, slips in performance, and complaints from customers. Employees and professionals may focus on protecting themselves rather than on producing results; although they feel busier than ever, productivity sags.

A national study conducted by Symmetrix (a consulting firm) of 531 restructured companies concluded that there were two key barriers to change and revitalization: employee resistance and dysfunctional culture.[1] The term *culture* means "the way things are done around here." For example, physicians may stake out spheres of authority and control that persist while others are promoting the benefits of team care or regional collaboration. Even when people do not particularly like the way things are done, they may be resistant to striking out into the unknown, especially if they feel their jobs are at stake. Resistance to the change resulting from reengineering is likely to be widespread and even intense. One way some organizations have sensitized people to the need for change, and helped them clarify their respective roles in reshaping the culture, is by involving them in gauging the organization's readiness to change.

This exercise, which involves top management and representatives from other parts of the organization, focuses everyone on what needs to be done to make the revitalization successful. Before restructuring or reengineering, it is important that management and staff agree on "how we're doing" and "why we need to change." That baseline is a prerequisite for knowing how to proceed. The following is an excerpt from a diagnostic questionnaire that can be used as a blueprint to begin revitalization. Healthcare organizations can tailor it to their own specific situations and needs.

Organization readiness to change

With input from other stakeholders, assess the organization on the following elements of change readiness. For each item, use a scale of one point (low) to three points (high).

Sponsorship. Change will be easier if its sponsor and leader is a senior administrator (allow three points) or head of a unit (two points) rather than a staff member (one point).

Leadership. Successful change is more likely if leaders at all levels have direct responsibility for what is to be changed and have clear business results in mind. Score three points if administrators and unit heads lead change and communicate the reasons, two or one if they take (or are given) less responsibility.

Flexibility. Positive indicators include team decision making and plenty of upward and sideways communication. Negative indicators include a rigid structure, narrowly defined career paths, necessity of "going through channels," and a culture that discourages risk taking. Allow one to three points along this continuum.

Direction. Senior management should be committed to a future that looks different from the present. Score three points if the new vision, values, and mission are reflected in the words and actions of managers and professionals, one if they are not, two if they are sometimes.

Measurements. Score two points if the organization uses performance measures such as cost effectiveness of service and contract management, one point if not. Allow three points if performance and reward systems reinforce these measures.

Organization context. Allow three points if the proposed change supports strategic activities such as acquisitions or new services. Trouble may lie ahead if a change effort is isolated or if multiple change efforts are not aligned; allow one or two points.

Benchmarking. Allow two points if there is a continuing program that objectively compares the organization's performance to that of its competitors and systematically examines changes in the industry. Score three points if this benchmarking is used to challenge institutional assumptions and biases.

Processes and functions. Restructuring and reengineering will likely require redesigning business activities to cut across functions such as marketing and patient intake. If managers or physicians are rigidly turf conscious, change will be difficult. Allow more points if they are willing to change key procedures and sacrifice individual power for the good of the whole.

Learning mind-set. The key to revitalization is giving up the notion of total agreement on every aspect of change. Allow more points if the culture promotes constructive contention rather than denying conflicts and opposing points of view, and if the organization can modify its behavior quickly to reflect new knowledge and insights.

Experience with transformation. Allow three points if the organization has successfully implemented major changes in the last three years, fewer points if the changes were less significant, did not take hold, or did not occur.

The higher an organization's score, the more likely that change will succeed. If the score is, say, 24 to 30, signs are positive. To accelerate the process, focus resources on lagging factors (ones and twos). If the score is in the middle range change is possible but may be difficult. Bring ones and twos up to speed before attempting to implement large-scale change. If the score is below 15, change—until forced by catastrophe—will be extremely difficult. Focus first on building readiness and setting the stage for revitalization.

The rest of this chapter suggests ways to make these changes and improve organization performance.

Avoiding common pitfalls

The healthcare industry is vulnerable to the same kinds of restructuring, downsizing, and reengineering mistakes other organizations most frequently make. These fall into the following categories.

FAILURE TO ESTABLISH AND FOLLOW A CLEAR VISION

Too many organizations rush into restructuring or reengineering without a clear idea of where they need to go, and thus they base their decisions on past assumptions that may be counterproductive in the future. For example, such assumptions may ignore the increasing competitiveness of the healthcare environment. The organization's ability to access capital in the future and to price services to meet anticipated market demands for significantly lower rates should be central to the vision.

Leaders and managers may want to avoid the work it takes to establish a vision. The process is full of frustration, surprises, and unexpected delays. But until an organizational vision is established, leaders will be unable to inspire commitment or align strategies.

Before any kind of restructuring or reengineering begins, healthcare organizations need to answer the following questions:

Which customers will we serve in the future, and through what channels can we reach them?

What is required to meet the needs of those who use our services?"

Who will our competitors be in the future?

What will be the basis for our competitive advantage? What skills or capabilities will make us unique?

Where is the industry going, and what is our organization's role in this scenario?

What new technologies play a part in this trend? For example, which needs are served by formal mainframe data systems and which by distributed networks using personal computers?

What characterizes the best performers in our and other industries? Which practices can we adopt to set the standard in our industry rather than follow it?

How will downsizing, restructuring, or reengineering affect our ability to provide high-quality, accessible, and affordable healthcare?

What skills and competencies are going to be needed to compete in the future?

How will the organization obtain the performance needed from all employees?

Such questions illustrate the "what" of vision creation. But the "how" is just as important. While transformation cannot happen without the strong commitment of management, building commitment throughout the organization requires that management not dictate its vision, but allow the staff to take part in designing it. There is a great difference between, "Here's where we're going and why" and, "Let's create the future we individually and collectively want."

As people begin to work for what they want to build, rather than to please their boss, creativity and productivity will soar. One way to stimulate visionary thinking and build commitment is to convene a representative group of managers and nonmanagers and ask such questions as, "What would your ideal hospital look like?" or, "If you were starting a healthcare personnel system from scratch, how would you run it?" Individual visions can then be combined into a group vision. When people fulfill their internal needs, they become better able to evolve and change along with the organization.

It is important to consider which aspects of the business need incremental change and which need fundamental redesign. The latter require new assumptions, values, and perspectives. Many healthcare systems and hospitals have operated according to the "success begets success" theory, only to discover that success often begets failure. Continuing to do what made a business successful in the past can ruin it for the future, since industry parameters, from management of care to competition for patients and markets, are changing dramatically.

If the vision is sufficiently simple and compelling, all employees will be able to explain in their own words why the organization needs to change and in what direction. The vision will provide the necessary "pull" toward effective change. Of course, it is not enough just to have a vision sitting on the shelf. Management must become "vision apostles" and work teams must become "vision champions."

TAKING A PIECEMEAL APPROACH

Reengineering demands systems thinking, as does large-scale restructuring. Any change in one component—such as technology, learning processes, patient care procedures, or business strategies—will affect all the others, and planning must take such potential effects into account. Organizational culture and shared values translate into a set of common, expected behaviors. For example, people may feel subtle pressure to work at an unrelenting pace and be strongly oriented toward action rather than reflection, because that is the way certain key managers behave. Any major change effort that ignores this set of spoken or unspoken values will not take hold.

FAILURE TO CONSIDER ALL THE OPTIONS

This means not only choosing among downsizing, restructuring, and reengineering, but also asking such questions as "What are other, less dramatic ways to reduce costs or improve the skill mix?" The former might include hiring freezes, changes in benefits, voluntary separation and leaves without pay, and phased retirement. Improving skills could include expansion of volunteer programs and partnerships with community organizations. Specific cost figures are necessary to evaluate such options.

MANAGING THE TRANSITION POORLY

Like any other transition, downsizing, restructuring, or reengineering must be managed with great skill. Transition plans should prioritize all necessary business, personnel, and organization changes, how they will occur, who will be involved, and who will be responsible for results. Some business firms have smoothed the transition by establishing transition teams comprising representatives from many different functions—not just human resources, but also operations, legal, public relations, and marketing.

The emotional turbulence generated by downsizing, restructuring, and reengineering must be recognized and managed. Terminated workers, as well as remaining workers whose jobs have changed or expanded, need opportunities to vent their feelings without negative repercussions. Supervisors who will have to serve as the messengers need guidance, written materials, and role-playing practice as well as compassion. Their adeptness and sensitivity will have a profound effect on productivity, resilience, and the image of the organization.

INADEQUATE COMMUNICATION

Downsizing, restructuring, and reengineering demand constant, sharply focused communication from management, designed to

Develop a shared understanding of the situation that face the organization and the actions that are required to keep the business alive and competitive

Enlist the active involvement of the entire staff in the effort to plan these actions

Short-circuit rumors and unfounded concerns before they damage the commitment of the workforce

Communication needs to flow quickly upward (and sideways) as well. Different perspectives need to be aired. Individuals and teams will commit to changes more readily if they are allowed to challenge others' assumptions, even those of physicians and senior management. Without active dialogue, the changes will not be internalized or adopted.

IGNORING EFFECTS OF RESTRUCTURING OR REENGINEERING ON OTHER STAKEHOLDERS

Any healthcare business is a living system, continually affecting and being affected by other systems and subsystems, including clients, investors, vendors, and the community. Decisions on when and how to restructure and reengineer, as well as all public relations and external communication activities, need to take this fact into account. Thus, if hospital management decides to restructure and downsize, it needs to consider such questions as

What can we do to preserve our reputation for high-quality care and our position as a mainstay of the community?

Who needs to be informed of the restructuring plans, and when?

How will the transition affect each patient category, as well as patients' relatives?

What about relationships with suppliers?

The organization's board of directors should be involved in this part of the transition planning. A member of the board could join the transition team.

FAILURE TO MOBILIZE THE STRATEGIC WORKFORCE

After reengineering, particularly one involving significant downsizing, morale suffers and people are eager for something to look forward to. The new workforce, which includes not only members of the old organization but also new hires and part-time or contract workers, needs to be involved in restructuring the work. Their suggestions should be actively solicited, for they are the ones who will be responsible for the success of the newly structured enterprise.

NOT EVALUATING THE RESULTS

Reengineering is not a once-in-a-lifetime event. Since the healthcare industry is now characterized by constant, turbulent, and rapid change, structural and process reconfigurations will become an unavoidable part of working life. An organization that can learn to move past self-defined barriers to achievements it has not previously imagined will progress through continuing cycles of growth and transition (see Figure 1).

The selection of measures, quantifiable indicators related to goals, is essential to revitalization. The way the transition has been handled as well as the financial outcomes should be assessed: What specific aspects

FIGURE 1
Revitalization roller coaster

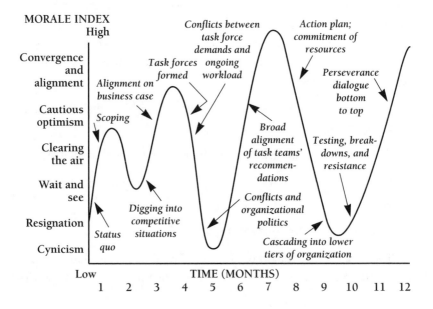

of the restructuring or reengineering produced value, as viewed by important stakeholders, including employees and clients? If certain goals were not met, why not? Answers to these questions set the stage for post-transition activities and prepare the organization for smoother transitions in the future.

Tools for the new enterprise

A reengineered organization is a new organization, requiring a shift in power. Especially if the organization is leaner, every member of its workforce must be mobilized to improve performance in relation to cost, quality, and customer satisfaction.

By now, many in the business world have come to acknowledge that the era of corporate paternalism is over. Since not even the most successful organization can honestly promise lifetime employment any longer, employees must take responsibility for their own careers. This means that the old concept of "loyalty" is dead, with neither the employer nor the employee having a long-term obligation to the other.

What, then, can ensure the commitment of employees, especially after reorganization and downsizing have left them fearful and confused? How can a workplace, especially one that has grown up under the assumption of paternalism and loyalty, shift the power dynamic and transform itself into an enterprise with revitalized communications, mutual trust and confidence, and initiative? Some organizations have adopted practices designed to dismantle rigid, hierarchical structures and to support individual responsibility and commitment. These innovations, described below, include dual career paths, culture change mechanisms, upward feedback, performance enhancement systems, and development of competencies.

DUAL CAREER PATHS

A typical career path is designed to reward only those employees who want to manage others. When a talented technical expert or professional, such as a nurse or scientist, reaches the top of the advancement ladder, management is the only place left to go. If the person does not want to be a manager or is not suited to be one, only three choices remain: stagnate in place, reluctantly move into a management position, or look for a better position in another organization or the consulting field.

Whatever choice the individual makes, the organization loses the contribution of a skilled professional. Also, by pushing so many people into management, the institution can end up with too many managers and too few people who are doing what they do best—just the opposite of what restructuring intends to do. A growing number of businesses have found a way out of this trap, and healthcare organizations should emulate their approach. To support the healthcare mission, especially when attempting to do more with fewer resources, it is essential to recognize the significance of nonmanagerial nurses and technical staff and allow them opportunities to grow professionally while rewarding them for their contributions.

One solution is to offer dual career paths: one track for would-be managers or administrators and another for individual contributors—people who want to enhance and apply their technical skills without supervising more and more layers in the hierarchy. The paths stay parallel, in terms of responsibility, influence, and compensation, all the way to the top of the organization.

In a healthcare institution, employees can grow through teaching and evaluating others, serving on recommendation committees, or leading advanced clinical teams while monitoring new team members. Dual career paths work best when they are flexible. For example, a research scientist who chooses the individual contributor track should be able to switch to the management track and back again as qualifications, patient care requirements, and career desires progress.

The parallel-path system can create a favorable climate for professional development and self-management while improving patient outcomes and broadening professional expertise in patient care activities and technologies. When employees' talents are used to best advantage, the organization gains greater productivity with a smaller and more committed staff, and more resources can be channeled into patient care services. Companies that have adopted the parallel-path system have also found it to be a valuable tool for recruiting, motivating, and retaining outstanding performers.

CULTURE CHANGE

Reengineering and revitalization inevitably require a change in an organization's culture. Some firms are addressing this issue directly by conducting workshops on culture change and how it relates to performance.

In such forums, participants determine what their current organizational culture is, how adaptive it is, and how it affects economic performance. They then identify, from their own experiences, the kinds of actions that have helped create culture change, as well as the obstacles to such efforts. They prioritize culture issues in the organization and specify steps they can take to create a healthier climate for success.

UPWARD FEEDBACK

This increasingly popular technique, which changes the way managers and staff members relate to each other, combines the advantages of effective communication, individual responsibility, and professional development. Essentially, upward feedback is a system by which staff members assess their supervisors on the way these supervisors manage people.

Understandably, the prospect of being evaluated by subordinates makes some managers nervous at first. But when everyone feels the need to improve communication and build trust, there is little resistance to upward feedback. Surveys of managers and staff, before the process is initiated, often reveal that both groups look forward to upward feedback as a much-needed opportunity for constructive communication and change.

Discomfort can be minimized without compromising candor if the process meets two criteria: (1) those who participate feel minimum pain and optimum gain, and (2) new awareness is translated into specific changes in behavior. When these two things happen, all members of the organization work more effectively in teams, and the workplace becomes both more efficient and pleasant.

PERFORMANCE ENHANCEMENT

Managers and staff of a manufacturing firm in the Northeast involved in restructuring decided to overhaul their performance management system in a way that would support the company's new goal of individual responsibility and initiative. A multilevel volunteer task force threw out the old performance appraisal system and replaced it with a process in which, among other things, employees can suggest who should assess their performance.

In this process, performance discussions are not used to control or reprimand but to promote a partnership between employee and supervisor. Together, the two define objectives, specify what each person needs to do, and review priorities periodically. Both receive training in communication and in seeking feedback.

This company's approach is just one way in which organizations are boosting performance and initiative at the same time. In a nonpaternalistic, loyalty-free business climate, employers can provide tools to help employees assume control of their own careers. For example, British Petroleum offers a voluntary do-it-yourself career and life development program that people use to improve their performance and satisfaction. A handbook tailored specifically to the organization takes them through self-assessment (e.g., skills, interests, values), goal setting, career planning, personal and professional development planning, and implementation. They are encouraged to conduct periodic career-focused discussions with their supervisors.

DEVELOPING COMPETENCIES

Traditional academic aptitude and knowledge tests do not necessarily predict job performance. Companies are confirming that certain competencies (i.e., general characteristics and capabilities such as relationship building, coaching, customer-service orientation, and flexibility) are better indicators of success. Many companies are beginning to identify the core competencies that contribute most to achieving their organization's goals and then to select and train employees for those competencies.

Competency assessment examines the people who perform well and defines the work in terms of the traits and behaviors of these people, rather than in terms of job descriptions. According to a study reported in the *Journal of Applied Psychology,* organizations that have focused on assessing and developing competencies have seen productivity increase by as much as 19 percent in low-complexity jobs and 48 percent in high-complexity jobs.[2]

The new leadership

Revitalization may call for reengineering management and leadership as well as the organization itself. Significant change means letting go of something, and in the case of reengineering, it means letting go of old "command and control" leadership practices. After a restructuring, which usually results in fewer managers, additional staff members need to develop and use leadership skills.

Although managers and leaders used to be essentially the same, the two roles have gradually diverged. The differences can be summed up as follows:

Managers initiate, administer, and maintain; leaders originate, innovate, and take risks

The good manager watches the bottom line and knows the cost of everything; the good leader focuses on the vision and knows the value of everything

The manager improves the efficiency of the status quo, asking how and when; the leader challenges the status quo, asking why

In innovative business organizations, leadership is cultivated among people at all levels. For example, Herman Miller, a furniture company, promotes "roving leadership," in which people step forward and take charge, on an as-needed basis, in their areas of competence, regardless of their place in the organization chart. Other companies have organization charts that look like floating, intersecting bubbles, continually being reconfigured to suit current needs.

Encouraging leadership through power sharing requires more than delegation. It means giving up power to someone else; for example, pushing decision authority down to the lowest possible level. Soliciting ideas is not enough. Those who come up with the innovations should be encouraged to act on them and thereby develop leadership competence.

In a revitalized healthcare organization, reengineered to provide the greatest possible opportunity and flexibility, even physicians and chief administrators need to give up certain decision-making powers; otherwise they become obstacles to revitalization. One key indicator of leadership is the ability to guide, listen, distill, champion, and inspire rather than dictate.

Hospital managers and physicians, traditional competitors for power and control, now need to engage one another as business partners and fellow team members. Mutual trust, not power over others, is the key ingredient in a revitalized organization. Authority should no longer be vested in a box on the organization chart, but in the ability to do a better job for a client, patient, or partner.

Karolinska Hospital in Stockholm took a risk when it created an administrative position for nurses called "nurse coordinator." This person's responsibilities include minimizing the number of visits patients must make—for example, by having them see a surgeon and an internist together. In such situations, nurses have authority over physicians. Although this has made some physicians uneasy, they realize that freedom from scheduling details enables them to concentrate on clinical work. The main advantage is better service to customers.

Getting started

How can a healthcare leader begin leading reengineering toward revitalization? Here are some recommendations derived from successful reengineering efforts in other industries:

1. Work on yourself first. Figure out how you are contributing to the status quo and then make visible changes. Be sure you are totally committed to the work ahead

2. Make sure the entire staff understands the current steps involved in managing patient care, and why things are currently done this way. This understanding provides the foundation for rethinking the total healthcare process in terms of what customers, rather than internal departments, need

3. Galvanize the commitment of others by encouraging active, intense dialogue, even argument. Every employee needs to walk an individual path to internalize and bond with the changes. Management cannot force reengineering

4. Align the changes to core business activities and results. Peripheral programs run by a staff unit will not accomplish much

5. Unify words and deeds. Unless decisions are viewed as consistent with the messages of change, cynicism will undermine the effort

6. Recognize role models. Promote and reward people who exemplify change

7. Do not transform everything immediately unless the organization is in dire condition. Some continuity with the past can be useful. For example, change can involve a return to essential values that will be important to future success

8. Never let up. Given all the resistance and difficulty of change, it is tempting to declare victory too early and stop or slow down. It is important to press ahead. Integrating changes takes time and many actions, and it is all too easy to return to the familiar when a barrier arises

9. Move as quickly as possible. Do not get stuck in analysis. Make up your mind and provide direction so you do not miss the window of opportunity. If movement is slow, resistance will build

10. If certain individuals are unable or unwilling to lead or participate actively in the change, allow them to leave. No one can be forced to be part of the process. Each employee will need to make a choice

Positive side of chaos

Change should begin before a crisis hits, such as a competitive or financial setback that may require severe downsizing. On the other hand, it is important to recognize that leaders can spearhead positive change even in the midst of chaos. A northern California utility, Pacific Gas & Electric, realized this when it suddenly had to deal with a new competitive environment. In the middle of reengineering its employee placement system, which was out of sync with its new vision and cost targets, a companywide reorganization threw everything, from budget-making authority to reporting structures, into uncertainty.

The employee placement reengineering team, however, forged ahead, making corrections along the way as needed. It discovered that disequilibrium actually accelerated the transformation. Time-wasting rules were suspended, turf wars were abandoned, and radical new ideas were generated and implemented in record time—because they had to be. Inaction was not an option and fast learning was essential.

Although chaos is certainly an uncomfortable state, it is a necessary stage in revitalization. With skillful leadership it becomes a crucible for innovation. Discomfort, high motivation, and a sense of urgency can be harnessed to generate solutions that were not evident before.

While downsizing, reengineering, and restructuring inevitably produce chaos, this can be constructive if the organization plans—from the beginning—with revitalization in mind. There is no point in radical change if revitalization does not follow. But it will not automatically follow without careful attention to the vision, competencies, processes, business strategy and culture, and continuous communication among stakeholders.

Reengineering involves changing the way people think about, organize, inspire, deploy, enable, measure, and reward work that adds value to clients. Work, managers, and employees all have to change if reengineering is to fulfill its promises.

A reengineering leadership team, like an aircraft pilot, should never consider taking off or landing without careful review of a checklist to ensure that all details are covered and aligned. Otherwise, the team will be attempting to touch down with the landing gear still up. It will be a very rough landing.

NOTES

1. Symmetrix, internal publication (Symmetrix, Boston, 1994, photocopied).
2. J. E. Hunter, F. L. Schmidt, and M. K. Judiesch, "Individual Differences in Output Variability as a Function of Job Complexity," *Journal of Applied Psychology* 75 (1990): 28–42.

8

Differentiating reengineering and continuous improvement

Tami Hechtel
Director, Organizational Development
The Bradford Group
Niles, Illinois

THE HEALTHCARE INDUSTRY has acknowledged that massive changes are imminent. The current debate centers around what those changes should be as well as how to accomplish them, not whether the changes are needed. Even though healthcare professionals may agree that large-scale change is needed, the methodologies are not quite as clear. Continuous quality improvement, patient care redesign, self-directed work teams—all are tools the healthcare industry has used to implement change.

Reengineering is the latest tool to be added to the list. However, identifying the need to reengineer is dramatically different from knowing how to actually do it. Organizations must invest a considerable amount of time and energy into understanding the use and limitations of reengineering as well as how it differs from other tools. In this chapter, 3 possible approaches to reengineering, streamlining, integrating, and transforming will be defined and examined along with 10 key issues that should be explored prior to reengineering including starting point, participation, customers' needs, type of change, frequency of change, typical scope, risk of failure, key enablers, organizational structure, and marketplace implementation.

A large number of healthcare organizations are still confused about the differences between reengineering and other performance improvement methodologies such as work redesign, total quality management

(TQM), and continuous quality improvement (CQI). The confusion exists, in part, because the interrelationships and mutual benefits of different improvement methodologies are not always well understood by the people attempting to implement them. It has also been difficult to quantify successful reengineering as the majority of examples are typically presented by consultants who are vested in success. "Reengineering" and words such as "reorganization," "redesign," and "restructuring" are consistently used interchangeably even though they have significantly different meanings and applications. In addition, with a reported 50 to 70 percent of reengineering initiatives failing, it becomes critical that healthcare organizations considering reengineering develop a working knowledge of the concept before implementing their reengineering efforts.[1] Many organizations ignore this basic advice and invest a minimal amount of time learning how to put a reengineering program into practice before jumping right in.

Although reengineering, redesigning, and quality initiatives typically have similar desired outcomes—productivity gains, increased marketplace competitiveness, cycle-time reductions, increased quality, and customer satisfaction—there are some significant differences. When comparing TQM/CQI with redesign, the differences really become those of degree rather than of methodology. Quality initiatives typically change approximately 10 to 20 percent of the work flow of a process, whereas redesign efforts change between 20 to 70 percent.[2] Quality initiatives use ongoing, incremental changes to impact process performance, whereas a redesign effort is more likely to be a one-time attempt for change of a more dramatic nature. Both methodologies, however, simplify and streamline the process based on its existing form.

Reengineering, on the other hand, requires organizations to create new procedures, using innovative and radical changes to the way work is performed to achieve dramatic improvements. In reengineering, typically 70 to 100 percent of a given process is altered. To be successful, a reengineering effort must first define the process to be reengineered in terms of cost or customer value. Secondly, the reengineered effort must penetrate to the company's core by challenging basic assumptions that affect issues such as roles and responsibilities, measurements and incentives, organizational structure, information technology, shared values, and skills.

Rethinking basic assumptions, whether implicit or explicit, about the best way to do work is at the heart of reengineering. It helps healthcare providers decide if they are doing the right things, not just doing things right by asking, "If we could recreate healthcare today, what would it look like?" Most organizations are driven by underlying, often unspoken assumptions. For example, the healthcare provider is the owner of the medical record, healthcare systems make the most money when people are the sickest, and specialists are required to do a majority of the services provided to the patient. These assumptions make up the very foundation upon which the current healthcare system is based. Of the three methodologies—reengineering, redesigning, or quality improvement—only reengineering requires healthcare to challenge basic assumptions.

Although challenging basic assumptions and starting over is a risky proposition because of the amount and impact of change required, many healthcare organizations have little choice. What were once common components of a traditional healthcare system—large numbers of inpatient beds, conservative management, stand-alone hospitals—are now obstacles to delivering healthcare with a more community-focused approach. Even though healthcare organizations may not have a choice about the need to change, they do have a choice about the tools and techniques they will use to implement it.

The healthcare system that can effectively challenge and respond to the industry's basic assumptions will, at least temporarily, gain a competitive advantage. Reengineering a minor process or a single activity can have a 1 percent impact on an organization's bottom line. However, reengineering a core process or business system in which basic assumptions are challenged can yield payoffs of 3 to 5 percent. Systematically reengineering all the core processes of an organization can yield returns as high as 30 percent.[3]

To understand the impact of reengineering, consider the following examples:

- After years of continually trying to improve their repair, billing, and marketing departments, GTE was determined to challenge the basic assumption that departments should act as separate functions. Instead of trying to improve them individually, GTE decided to reinvent its entire customer service process. GTE customers, it turned out, wanted one phone number to call, any time of the day, to request a repair, question a bill, sign up for a new service, or all three at once. By breaking down walls, retraining specialists to generalists, and using information technology, GTE is experiencing productivity gains as high as 30 percent.[4]

- In 1992, when Lotus Development Corporation surveyed its employees and learned that the human resource (HR) function was not seen favorably, they were not surprised. With over 6,000 worldwide employees initiating over 20,000 queries a year, it was not hard to see how the HR function had become buried in paperwork. The HR department at Lotus has changed dramatically since then. Instead of using reengineering to move its HR specialists to generalists, Lotus decided to take a different approach. There are no HR generalists. There is, however, a sophisticated phone service center that uses state-of-the-art technology to answer employee questions. The phone system combined with a group-ware product allows data sharing between different divisions worldwide. It has cut down dramatically on the number of calls that need to be handled by the HR staff. Using their personal computers (PCs), managers can look up organizational policies and procedures, read performance management guidelines, and learn more about their benefits packages. PCs are also strategically placed throughout the organization, in break rooms and cafeterias, so that any employee can initiate address changes, enroll in benefits, and get needed forms via the computer. With fewer calls and a more thoroughly educated customer, the HR staff was reduced from 56 employees to 42.[5]

While there is recognition of the need for a dramatic improvement in performance, too many healthcare organizations are making massive efforts to improve current systems and processes that will never have the capacity to meet their customers' future needs. A number of healthcare organizations mistakenly believe that by repackaging a portion of their quality or patient care redesign programs under the heading of reengineering, large-scale improvements will ensue. Al-though these organizations may see improvement in their current systems, it is highly unlikely that this approach to reengineering will give them a competitive advantage in a marketplace dominated by capitation and managed care. These efforts will more likely divert scarce resources away from the type of innovation that is critical. Even worse, such efforts could perpetuate the status quo, making it harder for organizations to implement meaningful change in the future.

Reengineering options

What approach should healthcare organizations use to challenge their basic assumptions and make the monumental leaps that could potentially ensue? Three possible approaches to reengineering include streamlining, integrating, and transforming.[6]

STREAMLINING

Streamlining offers a basic, segmented approach to reengineering that does not necessarily transform a process but rather cleans it up. For example, a critical care unit may reduce the length of stay for its coronary artery bypass patients from 10 to 5 days by establishing critical pathways and eliminating duplicate and nonvalue-added work.

Reengineering purists criticize this particular approach as nothing more than a repackaging of past methodologies devoid of challenging an organization's basic assumptions about how work is organized. This activity might eliminate several unnecessary jobs, improve customer satisfaction, and dramatically reduce length of stay, but it is not reengineering. Although this approach may make some healthcare organizations feel they are effectively managing change, the likelihood that this approach alone will allow an organization to be more competitive is unlikely. Unfortunately, this approach is being chosen by many healthcare systems unwilling to adequately prepare for the future.

INTEGRATING

The approach of replacing isolated, redundant, and inefficient tasks and procedures with a unified process has proven to be successful. A variety of industries and organizations such as the Ford Corporation and IBM Credit Corporation have reengineered inefficient procedures to effectively cut across functions and departments.[7]

As an industry, healthcare has tried to respond to the shift from inpatient to ambulatory care in a similar manner. Although many hospitals have been effectively moving the appropriate patients and procedures from inpatient beds into an outpatient system, ambulatory services still function in an environment where most assumptions, work processes, jobs, organizational structures, physical environment, and management practices support the inpatient side. The reality for most healthcare systems is that they must balance the implementation of reengineered activities within an environment currently not structured to support it.

TRANSFORMING

Transformational reengineering is about reexamining an organization's purpose. In essence, organizations are willing to gamble on a complete enterprise transformation in a relatively short amount of time. Typically, this approach is most often implemented by organizations that have very little to lose.

So what is wrong with this clean-sheet approach to transforming an organization? This idea may appeal to healthcare organizations that have become tired of dealing with cumbersome existing practices. Although, ideally, an organization might want to start from scratch, this approach ignores both its surrounding context and the purpose of a majority of reengineering projects—to gain dramatic leaps in improvement within an existing system. After reengineering, the position or role of the process in the company may have changed, but the rest of the company remains unchanged. Unless an organization has the resources and ability to rebuild all of its systems in a relatively short amount of time, the possibility of starting with a blank sheet is untenable. Although the most successful individual healthcare systems are likely to be the ones implementing radical change, the change within the healthcare industry as a whole is more likely to resemble an evolution rather than a revolution.

Another mistake of supporters of transformational reengineering involves the belief that the current process has little or no value in developing a successful reengineering initiative. The presumption that there is no value in using the way work is currently performed as input for reengineering is wrong. The process to be reengineered can show what adds value and what does not. Looking through the eyes of the customer and identifying what is valuable is one of the cornerstones upon which reengineering is based. The existing process serves as a source of knowledge about an organization's current customers. Combining this awareness of how customers' needs are currently met with large-scale innovation decreases the risk associated with scrapping an entire system and starting over.

While the approaches of streamlining, integrating, and transforming—are all possible, integrated reengineering is most likely to be successful in assisting the majority of healthcare organizations in adapting to the new marketplace. Streamlining is ineffective in challenging basic assumptions and meeting the needs of the new marketplace while transformational reengineering forces organizations to mobilize a massive amount of resources in a relatively short amount of time using a high-risk methodology.

There are numerous differences and similarities between reengineering and continuous improvement. The terms "process innovation" and "process improvement" are used to distinguish between "reengineering" and "quality improvement." Reengineering requires organizations and industries to challenge the assumptions upon which their business is based, using innovation and technology to build the ideal way in which business should be conducted. Reengineering is focused on large-scale innovation, and although innovation is most definitely a part of CQI efforts, it is traditionally on a smaller scale.[8]

Starting point

Reengineering initiatives start with a relatively clean slate, rather than from an existing process. The fundamental business objectives for the process may have been determined, but the means for accomplishing them has not. Designers of the process need to ask themselves, Regardless of how we have accomplished this objective in the past, what is the best possible way to do it now?

The starting point for healthcare is particularly challenging because assumptions must be examined on two levels—the way in which work gets done, and a reexamination of traditional healthcare services. Together these issues require fundamental rethinking of exactly what business a healthcare organization is in (i.e., is it a disease care system or a healthcare system?) and how to best service its customers.

Participation

Reengineering is typically implemented with a much greater top-down emphasis than the traditional bottom-up approach of past quality initiatives. The use of reengineering to simplify processes and reduce work that is not valuable from a customer's perspective can result in a more immediate and dramatic workforce reduction than with TQM or CQI. Any organization that expects its employees to support a process that could potentially eliminate their own jobs is being extremely naive. The impact of reengineering on issues such as employee morale, cross-training, and organizational loyalty can be overwhelming. However, by identifying and strategically planning for areas of potential growth prior to reengineering, healthcare organizations can reduce but not totally eliminate the impact of reengineering on their workforces.

Although reengineering is not the same as downsizing or restructuring, depending on the amount of nonvalue-added work that is eliminated, reengineering can result in a need to retrain employees and eliminate positions. A variety of organizations have found it helpful to offer other jobs within the organization to displaced workers or to cross-train their specialists into generalists who gain more control and influence over the reengineered process. Without proper planning, however, not all organizations may be able to be this generous. Not surprisingly, process owners may not work to eliminate their own jobs unless they have a reason to buy in to the reengineering effort. This makes the support and vision of the organization's leaders (along with the voice of the customer) critically important to reengineering success.

One of the most common errors made in reengineering is to use the process owners as the primary innovators in the reengineering effort. Interestingly, process owners typically are extremely uncomfortable with the idea of reengineering a process that directly impacts them. When 172 mid- and upper-level healthcare management professionals attending the 1994 International Quality and Productivity Center's national conference on reengineering in healthcare were asked to identify whether the processes they owned needed to be reengineered, continuously improved, or eliminated, the group had an interesting response. The entire group (the process owners) claimed their processes only needed to be continuously improved. When those same professionals were asked to respond to that question for the processes of which they were the customers, 56 percent said the process in question needed to be reengineered, 32 percent said the process needed to be continuously improved, and 12 percent said the process should be eliminated. In addition, the structures of most organizations do not reflect the cross-functional nature of the healthcare business. Most management professionals are in positions that require them to be responsible for either a small portion of a large process or a highly specialized process, making it difficult for them to identify opportunities for large-scale improvements. Only those in positions overlooking multiple functions (if such positions exist within a particular organization) may be able to see opportunities for large-scale innovation.

Thus, the lesson learned is not that process owners should not be included in the reengineering process but rather that external customers should have a stronger voice in reengineering if large-scale innovation is the expectation. One midwestern healthcare system addressed this issue by paying external customers to be active members on their reengineering teams. Having the voice of the customer in every meeting helped the internal reengineering team members challenge long-held beliefs about what customers want and how business should be conducted.

Customers' needs

Past quality initiatives have focused primarily on following customer needs based on feedback that organizations receive about their current processes, services, or products. Reengineering requires an organization to anticipate and predict customer needs in a more global context—many of which may be outside of the system's current limitations. Healthcare organizations have been particularly perplexed by the magnitude of involving the voices of the large number of customers, employees, physicians, and vendors they serve in a change initiative as complex as moving from a disease care to a healthcare system. A growing number of healthcare organizations are using "critical mass events" to implement large system change.

Critical mass events are large group meetings designed to bring a whole systems view of the organization into the room. Also known as future-search conferences, large-scale interactive processes, and open-space meetings, critical mass events ultimately assist organizations in compressing the amount of time needed to implement large system change. Typically participants number between 50 and 150, but groups as large as 5,000 have been successfully implemented.

Critical mass events are not about small-scale change but rather are used to analyze the organization on at least three different levels. Typically, external forces including the community, marketplace performance, competition, customers, and change are examined, followed by an observation of an organization's technical systems and processes and an analysis of the human side of the business—evaluation and rewards systems, training programs, motivation, and relationships. It is not the information that is being examined that makes these events so unusual, but rather who is involved and how the change is accomplished.

Companies like Ford, Levis Strauss, and Boeing along with healthcare organizations like the Sisters of Mercy Health System, St. Louis, and the Community Medical Center and Ocean County Health Department, New Jersey, have used critical mass events to attack a variety of system issues. In the case of Ford, the company needed to open a new plant quickly. Boeing's new airliner, the 777, is a result of a critical mass approach.[9] The Sisters of Mercy used a critical mass approach to plan for a multimillion-dollar reduction in operating expenses, at the same time renewing their eight-state, 15-institution system. The Sisters of Mercy brought together not only their system executives, employees, and customers but physicians, board members, government leaders, and heads of educational institutions as well. The Ocean County Health Department, Community Medical Center, and three other hospitals involved 150 people in changing the health status of their community.[10]

Critical mass events not only support but cultivate the innovation and creativity necessary to successfully reengineer. By bringing large, diverse groups together, healthcare organizations can decrease time and complexity of communicating large system changes. The use of critical mass events in a reengineering context is one option for healthcare organizations determined to anticipate the future, not only for themselves, but for their customers as well.

Type of change

True reengineering is about radical change. Many organizations find reengineering initiatives difficult to implement because of the potentially dramatic impact on other activities directly and indirectly connected with the reengineered process. The organizations that typically use reengineering in its most dramatic and radical sense are most likely to be in a market position where they have more to lose by not implementing dramatic change.

Capitation and managed care will force healthcare systems to scrutinize the likelihood that a disease care model will continue to generate massive amounts of revenue. Currently, several Midwestern hospitals are looking at reengineering how they manage their community's health and well-being. Through the use of health risk appraisals and supporting data collection, one Midwestern hospital hopes to manage the health of the entire population it serves by providing preventive services for identified community needs. By emphasizing a preventive line of products and services, the hospital has taken steps toward managing its population's health as opposed to just treating its diseases. If the market continues to move away from fee for service and toward capitation, other healthcare organizations are likely to follow.

Frequency of change

If an organization is reengineering the same process every two years, it is probably not reengineering. Whereas TQM and CQI are about continuous, ongoing, and sometimes simultaneous improvement across multiple processes, it is difficult to conceive of continuous large-scale innovation of 70 to 100 percent of the same process on a regular, ongoing basis. (It should be noted however, that continuous product innovation is possible and practiced in a variety of industries.) Although large-scale innovation is mainly a discrete initiative, the most successful organizations will combine their reengineering efforts with improvement programs. Even if a process is reengineered, a large number of opportunities to refine and improve that process will immediately arise.

Typical scope

Cross-functional teams have historically been a part of TQM and CQI. So how does the cross-functional approach of continuous improvement differ from the scope of a reengineering effort? Reengineering, although cross functional, is typically focused on the core processes of an organization. Considerable controversy has arisen over the number of core processes that can and do exist within an organization. The difficulty arises from the fact that processes are almost infinitely divisible; the activities in a patient visit, for example, can be viewed as one process or hundreds. The correct number of core processes has been identified as anywhere from 2 to more than 100 depending on the source of information. However, most companies currently undertaking reengineering have identified between 10 and 20 core processes (see Table 1).[11]

The number of core processes is less critical than understanding that if radical process change is desired, processes must be defined as broadly as possible. Many reengineering efforts fail because of lack of sufficient breadth when identifying processes to be reengineered. For example, a

TABLE 1
Example core processes

Market information capture	Customer engagement
Market selection	Inventory management and logistics
Inpatient services	Direct business
Outpatient services	Plan business
Customer fulfillment	Develop processes
Customer relationships	Manage process operation
Customer feedback	Provide personnel support
Marketing	Market products and services
Solution integration	Provide consultancy services
Financial analysis	Plan the network
Plan integration	Operate the network
Accounting	Provide support services
Human resources	Management information resources
IT infrastructure	Manage finance

European commercial bank decided to reengineer some of its back-office activities, expecting to reduce costs by 23 percent. The actual cost reduction was only 3 percent. The reason for such modest results was that the bank overlooked many back-office functions in planning the reengineering effort. Additionally, back-office costs represented only 40 percent of the bank's total costs. The breadth of the reengineering effort was too narrow to have a significant impact on the overall operating success of the bank.[12]

Risk of failure

If continuous improvement involves only incremental improvement, it also involves relatively little risk when compared to reengineering. With few exceptions, quality initiatives do not die highly visible and public deaths. Like old soldiers, they typically just fade away.

So why is the risk of failure so great when reengineering? Some of the most common factors include inappropriate use of information technology, lack of upper management understanding and support, and faulty process design and implementation. All can mean failure for any improvement or innovation effort. Thus, there are inherent risks within the approach of reengineering itself. Because reengineering initiatives require highly innovative and ambitious change efforts that rock the very foundation upon which an industry is built, the failure to meet these objectives is usually highly apparent. The level of change involved, the top-down approach, and the cross-functional nature of reengineering efforts greatly heighten the risk of failure. In addition, any initiative that threatens professionals with possible loss of power, positions, or resources is likely to meet strong resistance.

Key enabler

Unlike quality initiatives of the past in which statistical tools and controls were primary keys to success, reengineering makes use of information technology to make dramatic large-scale innovation possible. For years, organizations have tried automating processes by throwing computers at people in the hopes that automation would somehow change inefficient systems. Instead of analyzing activities and the way work was performed, healthcare organizations used computers to automate a number of processes in their current form. Thousands of hospitals spent millions of dollars automating their current processes to discover that automation made the process even more cumbersome and inefficient, in some cases creating the need to update both computer and hard copy versions of the same information. Healthcare, like many other organizations, forgot one of the golden rules of any redesign effort—"form follows function."

Its great potential notwithstanding, information technology cannot change processes by itself, nor is it an organization's only powerful resource. As healthcare systems continue to develop and implement reengineering initiatives it is critical to remember that the best way to perform work should be identified before the information technology is; otherwise an organization risks wasting an enormous amount of time, money, and resources to automate inefficient, redundant, or unneeded activities and work. Information technology counts, but no more than the human and organizational factors involved.

There are three basic building block technologies that are fundamental in the reengineering process: networking, databases, and desktop controls. To compete in the future, it is critical that healthcare systems pursue a network vision to connect all of their computers no matter where they are located. The large number of capitated lives with numerous geographical locations that a healthcare system will need to serve makes this technology much more critical to future success and customer satisfaction. Even if a healthcare system has a network architecture in place, it is wise to review the network's ability to assist an organization in remaining competitive in light of technology's expanded role in business. Will the network allow for centralized scheduling? A universal computerized medical record for each patient? Communications with customers and suppliers? These are just a few of the demands either currently in place or right around the corner for healthcare.

A database is the second technology critical to reengineering efforts, allowing the healthcare industry to store information in a more organized fashion; helping to break the ancient rule of the file folder and the medical record and allowing multiple people to access information at the same time. The airline industry is an example of how a shared database can help an industry meet the needs of its customers. The travel agent, the ticket agent, the gate agent—all can access or modify the traveler's record through a shared database. Without a shared database, it would be extremely difficult to move a large number of travelers to numerous destinations each year. For healthcare, database technology will do more to end sequential processing than any other technology.

The final technology is a set of technologies that cover the desktop interface. There are seven components to the basic tool set: a spreadsheet, word processor, presentation graphics, filing system (database or personal information manager), calendar, electronic messaging, and access to external data. One of the main advantages of this technology is that it allows people to switch quickly from one task to another. This ability to multitask allows people to have more than one application running at the same time. For example, a manager could be working on a spreadsheet and within an instant check the calendar, add an appointment, and then return to the spreadsheet. The older DOS-based application requires the user to save the spreadsheet, exit the program, load the calendar program, update the records, save the calendar file, exit the program, reload the spreadsheet program, and then bring up the worksheet. This represents time that could be better spent adding value to the process from a customer perspective.[13]

There is a broad array of communications, hardware, and software that healthcare has yet to fully explore including: client-server computing, interactive voice response, scanning, document imaging, rule-based routing, personal identification numbers, and multimedia and workforce automation software. Organizations such as Tufts Associated Health Plans have used software and scanners along with training to assist them to develop a paperless claims process for their customers, effectively cutting their claims processing time from 19 to 7 days. Tufts's ability to challenge the assumption of using paper as the key communicator of information in a claims process has reaped large dividends. Tufts currently has over 360,000 members, 165,000 of which have been gained since reengineering. Tufts's growth combined with its ability to adapt a process to meet the needs of its customers has eliminated the need for downsizing.

Organizational structure

Both continuous improvement and reengineering require cultural change. The necessary focus on operational results, measuring customer satisfaction, and empowering employees are all aspects of the changed culture within a successfully reengineered or continuously improved organization. While it is possible to implement a continuous improvement effort without making any major structural changes, large-scale innovation requires massive changes, not only in process flows and the culture surrounding them, but also in the distribution of power and control, management practices, reporting relationships, and organizational structure.

Elmhurst Memorial Hospital (EMH), a community-based hospital located in the western suburbs of Chicago, implemented this type of organizational structure where cross-disciplinary teams are just as important as traditional clinical support services. In a traditional healthcare model, up to 50 different clinical support services respond directly to independent physicians who order inpatient and outpatient services. By passing the responsibility of setting major operating parameters from technical experts in decentralized and independent clinical support services to permanent tasks forces oriented to specific clinical areas (e.g., oncology, behavioral health, or pediatrics), EMH is working to provide a framework that allows nonvalue-added work to be identified, reduced, and ultimately eliminated. Although restructuring or reorganizing an organization should never be confused with the actual reengineering, a restructured organization can provide a framework that assists a reengineering initiative. Reporting relationships are changed, power is redistributed, and the organization's structure is dramatically altered. These internal changes are often the most difficult part of any reengineering effort and at least partially account for the longer implementation time.

Marketplace

Even after the implementation of quality initiatives such as TQM and CQI, most healthcare systems remain highly bureaucratic. Departments act individually and pass along information, services, resources, and (most of all) problems to the next department. Different functions measure work and success in different ways and therefore have different goals. Because of these differences, barriers to overall business effectiveness are raised and turf is jealously guarded.

The ability to compete for a geographically limited number of capitated lives or potential customers is one of the driving forces behind reengineering. The number of capitated lives equals profit for a healthcare system if it can successfully manage risk and usage. This puts an interesting spin on a system that was originally built and designed to make money from people being sick.

Even though reengineering approaches may differ, at the heart of the concept is the idea of rethinking assumptions, whether implicit or explicit, about what work to do and the best way to do it. As customers needs change, the model that an organization uses for thinking about the products and services it provides, as well as how that work is performed, must also change. The problem for most organizations is not in challenging those basic assumptions but rather in dealing with the massive amount of change that breaking these assumptions requires of the supporting processes and systems. Few healthcare providers have identified and defunctionalized a major core process, challenged basic assumptions, and used information technology as a critical enabler to fundamentally restructure patient care delivery. More often than not, the majority of reengineering examples are more closely linked to methodologies such as continuous improvement or patient care redesign.

Does this mean reengineering in a healthcare environment is not possible? More likely, it reflects the opportunities that exist for growth and development as healthcare organizations struggle to discover which methodologies will serve it best in preparing for the future. The concept of challenging the basic assumptions within an industry and then using innovation combined with the appropriate information technology to strategically position an organization for the future is sound. The real challenge lies in discovering an approach to allow an organization to implement large-scale innovation within its existing system. For some healthcare professionals, reengineering may seem too risky a methodology to pursue. Others will proclaim that the potential payoffs of successful reengineering—for the individual healthcare system, for its patients and employees—are worth the risks.

NOTES

1. R. Wellins and J. Schulz Murphy, "Reengineering: Plug Into the Human Factor," *Training and Development* (January 1995): 33–37.

2. S. O'Connell, "Reengineering: Ways to Do It With Technology," *HR Magazine* (November 1994): 40–46.

3. G. Hall, J. Rosenthal, and J. Wade, "How to Make Reengineering Really Work," *Harvard Business Review* (November–December 1993): 119–131.

4. Wellins and Schulz Murphy, "Reengineering: Plug Into the Human Factor," 34.

5. O'Connell, "Reengineering: Ways to Do It With Technology," 42–43.

6. C. Currid, *Reengineering ToolKit: 15 Tools and Technologies for Reengineering Your Organization* (Rocklin, Calif.: Prima Publishing, 1994).

7. M. Hammer and J. Champy, *Reengineering the Corporation: A Manifesto for Business Revolution* (New York: Harper and Collins, 1993).

8. T. Davenport, *Process Innovation: Reengineering Work Through Information Technology* (Boston: Harvard Business School Press, 1993).

9. B. Filipczak, "Critical Mass: Putting Whole-Systems Thinking Into Practice," *Training* 32, no. 9 (September 1995): 33–41.

10. J. Flower, "Future Search: Power Tool For Building Healthier Communities," *Healthcare Forum Journal* (May–June 1995): 34–42.

11. Davenport, *Process Innovation.*

12. Hall, Rosenthal, and Wade, "How to Make Reengineering Really Work," 122.

13. Currid, *Reengineering ToolKit,* 60.

9

Aligning business goals and operations

Phil Nudelman, PhD
President and Chief Executive Officer

Linda Andrews, MFA
Assistant for CEO Communications
Group Health Cooperative of Puget Sound
Seattle, Washington

A T NEARLY 50 YEARS OF AGE, Group Health Cooperative of Puget Sound is the grande dame of managed care in
the Pacific Northwest. With 23 medical centers, 2 hospitals, and 3 specialty centers, the cooperative is stable and successful and serves one of
every eight residents in the five-county Puget Sound area. But by the
early 1990s, customers were saying premiums were too high, and Group
Health was beset by agile, well-financed competition that had never
been seen in this part of the country. The competition had studied
Group Health well and understood its ways of managing care. Group
Health, facing companies that were trying to emulate it, decided it did
not want to look like the rest of the world. One main challenge was to
become sleeker.

Like a house with many additions to accommodate a growing family,
Group Health's systems had become rather disjointed over the years.
The claims, patient accounting, and governance processes, for instance,
were a series of fragmented, specialized, and disassociated steps. Likewise, care was being delivered solely on an individualized basis, whereas
many health conditions, such as diabetes and heart disease, profit from

a population-based approach. As an integrated healthcare organization, Group Health encompasses all aspects of contracts, billing, insurance, benefit determination, and all levels of care delivery. The provision of so many different services to half a million customers made for intricate systems and daunting puzzles.

No off-the-shelf hardware or software could meet the needs of such a complex organization, and replacing one or two systems could not help either. A broader look at how it did business and delivered care made Group Health seem a perfect candidate for the reengineering of its business, clinical, and governance processes.

The prevailing wisdom is that it is almost impossible for a large, successful organization to change, especially when it is showing all the outward signs of success. Without the spur of crisis, most systems are incapable of well-worn habits. Group Health was not in crisis, but the selection of a new chief executive officer (CEO) in 1990 signaled that change had arrived. Group Health also faced intense legislative, competitive, and customer cost pressure, which challenged it to become more than a mature, well-established health plan. This chapter describes how Group Health altered its communication strategies and reengineered its business, clinical, and governance processes.

CEO communication

An organization faced with the reengineering of key business, clinical, and governance activities is asked to change some very basic levels of its operations. For Group Health staff to believe that change was necessary, they needed to hear it from the top.

A number of new communication tools let people know what kind of person now led the organization. The following tools showed that Group Health had to shake out its traditional ways of doing business.

- *CEO Week.* A weekly report from the CEO to the Board of Trustees discusses political changes affecting Group Health, market shifts, internal staff issues, healthcare reform, consumer satisfaction news, and CEO activities of the past week, including meetings with government officials or speaking engagements. The report is also sent to 300 managers, with the expectation that it be circulated to their staffs

- *FTEO* (For Trustees Eyes Only). An electronic memo sent only to the board of trustees contains information of a highly confidential nature. Topics might include early thoughts on expansion of service area, possible dues changes, or late-breaking news of community mergers or acquisitions. This memo is sent on an as-needed basis

- *Dear Colleague letters.* Staff is paid every two weeks. Included with their paychecks is a letter from the CEO, addressing a single issue of importance to Group Health. The range of topics—from the dangers of smoking to political initiatives to changing demographics—in these "Dear Colleague" letters spotlights Group Health as an employer, business, political force, and community member. The letters are philosophical and are accompanied by *Group Health News,* a just-the-facts staff newsletter

CEO communications, however, are not only written. There are also

- *Frontline meetings.* Several times each month, the CEO meets with groups of 10 to 15 frontline staff. No entourage accompanies these visits, no managers are present, and the agenda belongs to the staff

- *Group Health Visions.* This quarterly news video is shown at staff meetings throughout the organization. It looks very much like a news magazine-type show and is anchored by a staff member. Each video covers topics of late-breaking interest to Group Health and its staff, and each is shot on location at one or another of our medical centers

- *Leadership Conference.* This annual, day-long conference for all managers is designed for assessing of the past year and getting a look at what lies ahead

- *Leadership breakfasts.* Once or twice a month, the CEO has breakfast with a rotating group of regional midlevel managers and medical staff. With no more than 20 people present, it is an opportunity for conversation, questions, and consultation

- *Chatter walks.* Any staff members who would like to take an informal lunchtime walk with the CEO are welcome. These walks have proved to be a good way to informally discuss organizational and life issues—everything from enrollment growth and regional competition to career development and the importance of getting exercise to stay fit

For Group Health to succeed, the board of trustees and staff have to align their individual work with the goals and directions of the organization. In fact, the last staff survey showed that 81 percent were knowledgeable about Group Health's mission, goals, and vision. Keeping the vision alive takes relentless CEO communication; it is leadership's job to keep the goals always out in front of the organization. The English journalist G. K. Chesterton put it this way, "If you leave a thing alone, you leave it to a torrent of changes. If you leave a white post alone, it will soon be a black post. If you particularly want it to be white, you must be always be painting it again . . . Briefly, if you want the old white post, you must have a new white post."[1] Basic changes like business process reengineering require the same kind of constant, vocal commitment.

Business process reengineering

As Table 1 shows, not long ago Group Health was the only system providing comprehensive, prepaid healthcare. Now, it is one of many managed care providers, each with its own strength. One prime consequence

TABLE 1
Group Health's changing environment

	From	To
Market position	The only major managed care provider	One of many managed care providers
	Rapid enrollment growth	Slow to negative enrollment growth
Customers	Focus on individual members	Focus on multiple customers
	Comprehensiveness and quality as primary values	Price, quality, and choice are all important
Delivery model	Exclusively staff model	Mixed model with 700 provider contracts and 50 percent of providers in external delivery system—all to support
Products	Single product	Multiple products
	Product uniformity	Demand for flexibility and choice
Competition	Small, weak competitors	Strong, agile competitors
	Local plans with HMO options	National plans
Regulatory environment	Stable	Uncertain
	Few mandated benefits	Comprehensive mandated benefit package under health-care reform

of marketplace change was that Group Health had to be able to offer more new products or services, such as a point-of-service plan; tailored benefit packages; and creative payment and business arrangements, such as support for self-insured accounts, to accommodate its customers.

Group Health's distinctive strength has been its ability to manage healthcare. This core work implies strong interdependence of health plan and delivery system functions. In the changing marketplace, Group Health's ability to administer a variety of contracts, as well as collect and disseminate business and clinical information about its enrollee populations and purchasers' populations, became critical.

CASE FOR REENGINEERING

In response to its changing environment, Group Health refined its business strategy to focus on enrollment growth and rate competitiveness. In turn, enrollment growth depends on offering the products and benefits demanded by the market at competitive prices. And rate competitiveness depends on controlling costs in both the delivery system and health plan systems.

For instance, activities supporting the health plan—such as marketing, rating, and provider relations—were dispersed throughout the organization, scattering accountability and making it difficult to track and manage overall health plan costs. Also, while Group Health was successful in moving a growing number of its contracted providers from a charge-based payment system to risk-sharing arrangements that helped to control costs, most of the capitated, risk-sharing payment methods required expensive, time-consuming manual processing. While Group Health had been using quality improvement tools to solve the problems in existing systems, solutions were often constrained by departmental boundaries, lack of process ownership, and the limited capabilities of existing information systems.

Business process reengineering helped the organization look at the validity of the processes themselves, take them apart, and rebuild from the standpoint of customer requirements—whether those requirements were to reduce cost, ease information gathering, or streamline billing procedures. It was clear that to delay reengineering would ultimately prevent Group Health from achieving its strategic goals of enrollment growth and rate competitiveness.

A FEW EXAMPLES

Group Health has responded to purchaser demands for benefit flexibility by customizing the basic benefit plan offerings. Whereas it used to offer one basic set of benefits, today Group Health and Options, its point-of-service plan, together offer six basic benefit plans, with 55 categories of riders containing 507 variations.

Group Health's current computerized processes are unequal to the task of administering this degree of variety. This can result in lost revenue, manual work-arounds with resultant increased administrative costs, overpayment of benefits, poor customer service, reliance on expensive third-party claims administrators, and inconsistent application of benefits across the organization. These costly examples were the impetus for doing things differently.

REENGINEERING PHASES

Group Health business process reengineering consisted of three phases: the master plan, design, and implementation phases (see Table 2).

Master plan phase

The first step was to set up a work plan, with the goal of creating health plan systems to assist Group Health in achieving a sustainable competitive advantage. To that end, the aims were

- Responsive, easy-to-use, coordinated, and accurate administrative services

- Flexible and versatile personnel and information systems

- Reduced costs for administering all aspects of the plan

Achieving these aims would have significant impact on Group Health's administration of health benefits; business relationships with contracted providers, groups, and individuals; and the delivery and management of care.

Through the master planning phase, the decision was made to concentrate on the definition and implementation of benefits and products and on business relationships with contracted providers, groups, and individuals. These were the areas for which Group Health considered future scenarios, diagnosed root causes, and assessed the costs and

TABLE 2
Phases of business process reengineering

Phase one	Phase two	Phase three
Master plan	*Design*	*Implementation*
Define goal and objectives	Identify future process scenarios	Develop detailed project designs
Create core process model	Select a reengineering strategy	Develop and implement systems
Define project scope	Design processes and critical jobs	Train workforce
Develop design phase approach	Define information systems requirements	
Make the case for change	Develop change plan	

benefits of pursuing fundamental change. The approach consisted of fact-based, collaborative problem solving, with frequent decision points and an ongoing assessment of the information services marketplace for potential selection of a vendor.

Design phase

The design phase is organized into three work steps:

- Step one: This step includes developing alternative scenarios for the reengineered activities, evaluating and analyzing each alternative, conducting a preliminary cost/benefit analysis, selecting the desired scenario and deciding to proceed, and conducting an initial assessment of the information systems market. The focus of step 1 is on customers and providers

- Step two: This step includes redesigning the process, identifying early deployment opportunities, confirming the strategy, and updating the assessment of the information systems market. The focus of step two is on process

- Step three: This step includes refining the cost/benefit analysis. The focus of step three is on organizational priorities and resources

The design phase was completed in June 1995, with implementation of most recommendations scheduled to take place over the next four years.

Implementation phase

The implementation phase has just begun, but it holds the promise of vast improvements for Group Health's individual customers, employer purchasers, and contracted providers and partners. Through reengineering, the organization is aiming for these outcomes:

- Individuals will encounter reliable, trustworthy business systems, with convenient, speedy, and easy access to personalized customer service at any time from any place. They will be able to reliably determine the cost implications of their treatment plans as part of their healthcare decision making. And they will experience seamlessness between Group Health's delivery and insurance functions

- Purchasers will come to know Group Health by its flexibility of plan design, responsive purchaser account service, cost effectiveness, and its quality, access, and service in care delivery for enrollees

- Providers will confidently contract with Group Health because of its business competence, convenience, and respect for their ability to work in partnership with other providers and insurers to meet a population's health needs. Group Health's ability to work in alliance with other organizations will also be greatly enhanced

The organization's business process reengineering has been driven by critical assumptions, expectations, and business imperatives. Overall, the leadership of Group Health has sent a clear and consistent message that reengineering must not be constrained by current values, practices, or norms. It is meant to be a radical redesign of business and insurance systems for the purpose of decreasing costs and turning the currently jagged processes into one continuous flow in order to satisfy the customer.

The focus of the project is on creating solutions to enable Group Health to achieve a sustainable competitive advantage. Organizations that figure out how to smoothly integrate their health plan functions while delivering affordable, quality healthcare will be the winners in the competitive game.

Clinical Roadmap

Population-based care is similar to the three-dimensional picture in the Sunday comics. At first, the panel looks like a mass of brightly colored dots. But if one stares at it long enough, the thousands of individual points reorganize, and a picture appears. Likewise, population-based care also involves a new way of seeing the masses of individuals seeking healthcare. It is a way of looking at patients not just as individuals but as members of groups with shared healthcare needs. This approach does not detract from individuality but rather adds another dimension, as individuals benefit from the guidelines developed for the populations to which they belong.

Group Health's approach to putting population-based care into practice is called the Clinical Roadmap. It is a coordinated, multidisciplinary, data-driven approach to applying total quality management concepts and tools to clinical planning, measurement, and improvement activities at an organizationwide level. The mission of the Clinical Roadmap is to improve clinical processes and outcomes by focusing organizational attention and resources on a limited number of discrete clinical activities. These vital few clinical areas account for significant organizational, consumer, monetary, and human resources. For instance, 3 percent of enrollees on the typical physician panel have diabetes; however, these patients account for 12 to 13 percent of total costs. Similarly, although heart care patients comprise less than 4 percent of all enrollees, their care consumes nearly 14 percent of the budget.

To each of the vital few patient care areas, total quality management concepts and tools are applied, using Group Health's quality assessment and improvement methodology as a guide. The steps are to

- Understand customer needs and requirements

- Describe the existing process of care and assess the need for improvement

- Identify and convene the appropriate team(s) to lead the work in the specific patient care process area. Involve line owners of the care process, such as providers and managers

- Diagnose the problem, using data whenever possible

- Make improvements in the care process. When necessary, (re)design the process or system. Develop robust practice guidelines, as necessary, to support care processes

- Determine how improvements will be implemented, replicated, and maintained throughout Group Health

- Develop support activities and procedures, and clarify accountability to maintain the improvement

- Evaluate the effect on key processes and outcomes of care

AREAS OF FOCUS

At Group Health, the first four clinically significant areas chosen were diabetes, heart care, pregnancy care, and tobacco use cessation. Clinical Roadmap goals for 1995 through 1996 are

- *Tobacco cessation.* Reduce overall tobacco use by members from 17 to 15 percent; reduce use of tobacco by coronary disease patients from 13 to 8 percent; and reduce tobacco use by diabetics and pregnant women

- *Diabetes.* Reduce hospital admissions for ketoacidosis by 20 percent

- *Pregnancy care.* Reduce the cesarean section rate from 17 to 13.5 percent by the end of 1996

- *Heart care.* Reduce reinfarction and reduce the need for revascularization (i.e., coronary artery bypass graft)

Previously, Group Health had no overall guiding framework to coordinate and develop systemwide clinical assessment and improvement activities. In addition, there were multiple departments, work units, and committees independently setting priorities—with separate and significant effects on the delivery system. Through lack of coordination, the organization was losing the opportunity for synergy among these efforts, which impeded collective progress. The Clinical Roadmap strategy's two-pronged approach was designed to overcome these difficulties.

WORK IN PRACTICE

Group Health's Quality of Care Assessment department steers the development of practice guidelines in cross-functional clinical areas, while the delivery system deals with medical care team functioning to disseminate, implement, and evaluate the clinical guidelines. They also decide how to apply the guidelines for reorganizing their teams and their approach to patients. Both endeavors use a multidisciplinary approach, involving nursing, medical staff, and management, and seek input from customers.

Technology is also a factor. As Group Health revamps its approach to delivering care, it is investing $100 million in automation and clinical work stations over the next five years. These workstations will give physicians, nurses, and other clinical staff a powerful arsenal of tools for improving care and service. Group Health is building a total clinical environment oriented to population-based care, including wide-area and local-area computer networks, installation of several thousand clinical workstations, development of a central repository for clinical information, and software for easy retrieval of that information.

The computers will allow staff to

- View information from Group Health clinical systems such as pharmacy, lab, consulting nurses, and breast cancer screening

- Retrieve information about clinical guidelines

- Receive reminders of patients' preventive care appointment schedules

- Look up medical reference information

- Order lab work, prescriptions, and referrals

- Send and receive electronic mail

- Use the Internet to communicate with colleagues

- Link up with the appointment-registration-patient accounting system

One of the key characteristics of population-based managed care is the concept of planning for each patient's needs in order to keep that patient as healthy as possible for as long as possible. For instance, an enrollee may be an elderly female with diabetes who is also a smoker. People in each of these populations—elderly women, diabetics, and smokers—have distinct healthcare needs.

Using a systematic approach, the practice team will have identified this patient in terms of these three populations. Equipped with guidelines and effective patient education approaches, the healthcare team can pre-plan focused medical visits to address both the smoking issue and diabetes rather than wait for the patient to present with related symptoms. Computerized systems enable the team to track successive lab values and to provide reminders of future visits for eye and foot care. After evaluating the approach to care for the major populations in their practice, team members agree to take responsibility for the part of the visit or interaction that best fits each person's abilities. This may mean, for instance, that one member is primarily responsible for patient education, another does physical examinations and plans consultations, while another identifies members of the populations and tracks their outcomes.

CLINICAL ROADMAP GOALS

The goal of this system of managed care is to produce the best achievable health and satisfaction outcomes with the most effective use of resources for each patient served. Through the Clinical Roadmap, Group Health becomes a unified system where patient care is team based and integrated across providers, clinical services, facilities, and regions. Systematic assessment, measurement, and improvement of clinical processes and outcomes are features of this model.

The Clinical Roadmap aligns Group Health's direction and use of resources. It keeps leaders and providers going in the same direction toward high-quality care. It builds on the work of many individuals and groups, from preventive care and research to utilization management and the committee on emerging medical technologies. It also provides a focus for the clinical application of total quality management.

The Clinical Roadmap approach is deeply rooted in primary care and prevention—two things that Group Health was founded to promote. But this approach renews the organization's approach to prevention and makes care planning more aggressive.

Ideal process flow

In the 1980s, the board of trustees noted an apparent lack of connection between the nascent strategic planning efforts and the organization's historic budget-setting activities. There was no clear link between the organizational mission, emerging strategic objectives, and resource allocation. Efforts were then made to align the schedules for strategic planning and budgeting, in order to connect these two critical activities more logically. It became clear, though, that other important processes needed to be woven into an overall framework since a lack of coordination and systemic thinking had led, over time, to significant rework, a loss in efficiency, and ultimately higher costs.

DESIGN METHODOLOGY

Work on this issue began in earnest in 1991, when one of the CEO's goals called for the development of an organizational "master calendar" to tie together the key processes and decision-making events. A small group, whose members represented the suppliers and customers of the decision processes, were asked to create the design. Members came from the three spokes of Group Health leadership—management, medical staff, and consumers. Initial steps focused on evaluating the way decisions were traditionally made, as well as their underlying assumptions and structures. The areas examined included strategic planning, goal setting, budgeting, capital planning, and rate setting.

In the second stage of the group's work, the picture of the present flow was set aside in favor of creating a new, ideal picture. The group members examined which processes needed to be concurrent or sequential and which could be unrelated. For example, they noted that Group Health's rate-setting process took place between January and May each year, even though the organization could not have maximum information about competitors' plans this early for the following year. They saw that the process was being driven by at least one important internal structure—the need for revenue assumptions for the next year's budget preparation—and one critical external force—the need for rate proposals for both the federal and state employees' contracts. As they examined these conflicting needs, they repeatedly questioned why things were set up this way. By reviewing underlying assumptions and structures, constraints could be set aside to create something new. The group was free to propose new possibilities, rather than incremental change to what already existed.

The hoped for outcomes included increased alignment around organizational direction and priorities to achieve Group Health's mission and vision; increased meaning for staff's collective work through viewing the organization as an interconnected system; and greater flexibility. These outcomes became even more critical with the passage of healthcare reform legislation in the state of Washington. The time had come for consciously streamlining the way the organization did business to meet its own stated outcomes as well as its customers' expectations.

IDEAL FLOW OF ACTIVITIES

What had started as a quest for a master calendar became the ideal process flow (Figure 1). It is not a rigid calendar of decisions and events, but a logical flow of activities to support decision making. It reflects a fundamental commitment to articulating, integrating, and acting upon strategic priorities in all of the organization's work throughout the year. Ideally, it will result in more substantive progress toward the organization's vision, greater responsiveness to the environment, and enhanced opportunities for true collaboration among consumers, medical staff, and management.

The backbone of the entire design is a series of direct links, which drive all other processes in terms of sequencing and content. It includes

- Reaffirmed mission and key values

- Updated vision definition

- An environmental scan report, interpreting internal and external information related to Group Health's strategic priorities from the viewpoint of customer requirements

- Strategic scenarios used to test the impact of alternative futures

- A revised strategic plan

- Strategic priorities translated into rolling multiyear goals

FIGURE 1
Ideal flow of key Group Health processes

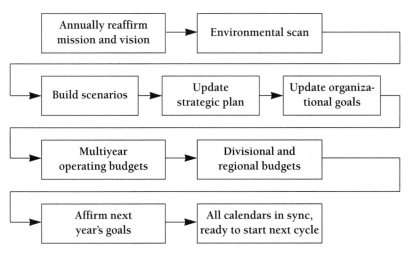

- Completed benefit design evaluation, rate setting, and negotiation of major labor contracts

- Systemwide operating budgets allocating resources to meet priorities, rather than allowing budgets to drive the goals

- Associated regional and divisional goals and budgets that show them in line with the organization's direction

- End-of-planning-cycle affirmation that Group Health's goals and budgets are in sync with each other and tested against the latest environmental information

IMPLEMENTATION

The closer alignment of planning and decision making required work to be done differently. Many of the changes brought about by the ideal process flow were straightforward, focusing on sequencing and greater attention to the linkages between processes. Some changes required the revision of board policy. Other changes, such as the timing of trustee elections and the annual meeting, required formal bylaw amendments, which were subject to membership approval. Full implementation of changes in governance and business processes associated with the flow took all of 1994 to complete.

Beyond the original flow implementation, the need for new components surfaced, including a global mission statement for Group Health and its affiliates, as well as a global strategic plan. Also considered were the impact of state and federal healthcare reform pressures, as they rose and fell in response to political changes. The ideal process flow concept is designed to support any future change in organizational structure, even if specific aspects of the flow have to be reconfigured to meet new needs of the organization.

Implementation required coordination and agreements among process owners, governance, and group leaders across many parts of the organization. Important by-products were the recognition and creation of genuine linkages throughout the organization's work and reduced cycle time for key processes. Further, creation of the ideal process flow helped to identify the structures and assumptions which sometimes invisibly shape the way business is done, thereby helping to create a more responsive, flexible organization.

Conclusion

Group Health's enrollment has been growing, as has its variety of benefit designs, financing arrangements, and affiliate organizations. Given the speed and flexibility of Group Health's competition, it was neither wise nor practical to accommodate these changes merely by adding new steps to traditional activities. What was needed, rather, was a shakedown of key business and clinical procedures through business process reengineering, Clinical Roadmap, and ideal process flow.

Success shows. By the beginning of 1996, Group Health had the enrollment of more than 630,000. A budget milestone of $1 billion in annual statewide revenue was also reached. The organization is optimistic that core values can be maintained, despite the marketplace maelstrom. The key is flexibility. Group Health is making good on its goal of not changing values in order to prove flexibility. Rather, it is acting flexibly in order to further the organization's values.

NOTES

1. G. Wills, *Certain Trumpets* (New York: Simon and Schuster, 1994), 143.

▦ 10

A strategic/tactical approach
to change

Anthony J. Kubica, MS, MBA
Executive Manager, Integrated Delivery Networks Practice
Superior Consultant Company
Farmington Hills, Michigan

REENGINEERING IS A POWERFUL TOOL for organizational change within healthcare delivery networks. It focuses on radically improving work processes across departmental boundaries to achieve significant operational improvements. It starts with a top-down vision followed by bottom-up implementation. The basic premise of reengineering is that current processes are either not working well or are not achieving the results required for the organization to be competitive in a rapidly changing healthcare marketplace. Incremental performance improvements (e.g., financial and operational) of 2 to 3 percent per year will no longer suffice. The marketplace is demanding more, and to be successful, healthcare delivery networks must deliver more.

Reengineering would appear to be the answer for organizations interested in improving their work and increasing their competitive edge. Yet the healthcare industry's success with reengineering is mixed. Thus, reengineering is at risk of becoming another management fad that passes away with time, only to be replaced by yet another management fad that also promises to be the answer to senior management's problem of improving organizational performance. Simply stated, there is no one answer to improve organizational performance. The power of reengineering is that it is not the answer but represents a way of thinking about how work gets done within an organization. It focuses on radically improving activities targeted to meet defined customer needs. It offers a dynamic approach to improving organizational performance, and it is supported by tools and techniques to help achieve desired results.

Senior management teams often argue: "Change takes time and we do not have the time. We need to create a sense of urgency, and we need action and results now."[1]

Change does take time, and it is critical that a sense of urgency be built into the change process. A bias for action is critical for success. Senior management must feel a sense of urgency and communicate it throughout the organization. Urgency without purpose is much like the irregular movement of molecules in a closed system, which, when heated, begin to move faster and bounce off the walls (of the closed system) at a higher velocity. There is motion—but no forward movement.

Organizational change and successful reengineering require both motion and forward movement, which can be created by a clearly defined purpose and a willingness to break down the barriers impeding change. This then is the challenge for all senior management if they are to position organizations for reengineering success.

Change management by event—Two case studies

When approached as an event, such as decreasing full-time equivalents (FTEs) per adjusted occupied bed or decreasing costs in a given department, achieving and sustaining success is difficult. FTEs per adjusted occupied bed may be decreased through downsizing, which is often mistaken for reengineering. Costs in a given department may be decreased by reducing overtime, not replacing vacant positions, renegotiating supply and service contracts, or through interdepartmental process improvement.

But the question is, will decreases be sustained? Invariably, the answer is no. Downsizing without interdepartmental process improvement results in fewer people performing the same amount of work the same way. An old adage states, "Insanity is doing the same thing the same way over and over again and expecting different results." After downsizing, productivity may improve temporarily. However, employees trying to cope with inefficient processes become frustrated and angry. Over time, staff size begins to approach predownsizing levels and may even exceed them. Disappointed with past downsizing and intradepartmental operational improvement efforts, organizations will be drawn to reengineering as a method to break the cycle of failed attempts to improve performance. Consider the following two case examples.

Hospital A was interested in reengineering based on a need to decrease operating costs. After 10 years of profits from operations, the hospital was facing a loss. A state law taxing healthcare providers, the introduction of managed care into the region (including Medicaid), and growing competition from other providers contributed to the downturn in financial performance. While reengineering appeared to be a reasonable approach to improve the hospital's financial performance, it represented the right solution at the wrong time. The need to improve financial and operational performance was no longer merely an interesting discussion at senior management meetings; it had become an imperative.

While the hospital was progressive in its market, this progressiveness represented incremental improvements in a stable marketplace with little competition. New programs representing new revenue streams were introduced, patient volume grew slightly each year, and competition among area providers was not an issue. Hospital A's business climate was similar to that facing U.S. industrial firms in the 1950s and 1960s. The oil embargo in the mid-1970s and the rise in global competition shocked U.S. industry out of its complacency in the same way that managed care and provider competition is shocking the hospital industry.

Hospital B was looking to reengineer its registration and scheduling function as it implemented a new registration and scheduling software package. These initiatives were performed independently of each other.

An interdisciplinary reengineering team composed of departmental members from registration, admitting, scheduling, and the business office was assembled to define a future vision and obtain consensus on it. The visioning process went well, the participants were enthusiastic, and creative ideas were generated on a desired future. However, senior management rejected the reengineering-visioning team's vision. They believed the vision was unrealistic, would cost more than was affordable, and was not consistent with the hospital's recent decision to purchase registration and scheduling software. The visioning team felt angry and betrayed. Rework is under way in an attempt to salvage the process and bring the software on-line.

Ideal conditions for success

When approached within the context of managing organizational change, the opportunity for reengineering success is great. Hospital A experienced market-based change and explored reengineering as a way to position the organization for success. Hospital B introduced reengineering into an environment that was poorly prepared to reengineer successfully. If Hospital A were to proceed with reengineering, its chance of success would be doubtful. Similarly, Hospital B's future reengineering efforts would most likely face strong resistance, as a result of the initial negative experience. Currently missing from both organizations is an understanding of the ideal conditions necessary for reengineering success:

- Clearly defined business purpose

- Top management support

- History of successful change management

- Commitment to follow through

- Open, timely, and candid communication

The ideal conditions for reengineering are like the organization's vision: they define direction and a desired future state. These conditions give the organization something to strive for, even if they may never be fully achieved. As the Cheshire Cat told Alice, if you do not care where you are going it really doesn't matter which direction you take. Knowing where to go is a prerequisite for successful change.

Positioning the organization

Before reengineering can be successful, senior management must prepare the organization for change. The process starts with understanding, accepting, and committing to the ideal conditions of reengineering success. These conditions must consist of internalized and deeply felt beliefs that senior management, as a team, believes are necessary for successful organizational change. Moving from intellectual acceptance to a deeply felt belief does not occur quickly or casually; rather it requires a defined process of change management.

An effective technique to position the organization for change and reengineering success is the strategic/tactical process. This requires

- Defining a strategic vision for the organization

- Identifying tactics to support the strategic vision

- Implementing these tactics

While this technique may sound simple, committing the entire senior management team to a strategic vision so that they work collaboratively on defining and implementing tactics is challenging. There is a danger that senior management teams will eschew this approach and move directly into a reengineering project. This is a mistake.

DEFINING THE VISION

The strategic/tactical process is shown in Figure 1. Defining the strategic vision provides organizational focus and direction. The vision need not be defined with pinpoint accuracy. What is required is to define a direction. For example, the hospital may decide to focus its efforts on building an integrated delivery network or expanding its ambulatory care program. It may decide that merging with another healthcare organization is critical for its long-term survival. By choosing a direction, senior management explicitly has decided not only where to focus its efforts but also where not to spend its time and resources. Knowing what not to pursue is as important as knowing what to pursue. Limited by

FIGURE 1
Strategic/tactical planning continuum

Strategic plan	Tactical plans
Define strategic initiatives	**Define tactics and begin**
Examples of strategic initiatives	**implementation**
Integrated delivery network formation	*Examples of tactics*
Financial stability plan	*Information system strategic plan*
Continuum of care model	*Open two satellite clinics*
	Medical staff development plan
	Reengineer results reporting

time and resources, a senior management team cannot successfully move in all directions at the same time.

As an example, Hospital A completed a strategic vision that focused on building physician relations and developing an integrated delivery network. Shortly after completing its vision and defining tactics, the hospital was offered an opportunity to manage and provide support services to a psychiatric facility in a neighboring town. Evaluating this opportunity against its strategic vision, it became apparent that entering into an agreement with the psychiatric facility was not consistent with the hospital's vision or tactical plans. Hospital A decided to pass on the opportunity. For another organization with a different vision, this may have been an excellent opportunity but for Hospital A, it would have been a distraction and an unnecessary use of scarce resources.

After the direction is chosen, the next step is to forge senior management commitment to the vision. This cannot be tacit commitment. To move the organization forward and overcome the barriers and challenges that will develop along the way requires total commitment to the vision. Committing to a common vision is a change step for the senior management team.

Senior managers must commit to the vision even if it means their turf will be adversely affected. Reengineering affects everyone involved in the process, and resistance to the change is a natural outcome. If the staff sees dissension in senior management's commitment to the organizational vision, they will have tangible evidence that not much is changing and reflect senior management's resistance. "Walking the talk" is a critical success factor in reengineering, and for senior management it starts with a commitment to the vision—regardless of its personal impact.

A technique a chief executive officer (CEO) can use to elicit support and commitment is a combination of consequence management and rewards. The CEO must clearly set the expectations for the senior management team. The expectations are that team members will participate in the process, voice their concerns and reservations, and, once a consensus is reached, support each other to achieve the vision. The CEO should reward those actively participating in the process through positive reinforcement, offering opportunities for future growth, challenging

assignments, and financial gains. Those who have chosen not to participate or to behave in a passive-aggressive manner should experience the
consequences of their behavior. The CEO will recognize passive-
aggressive behavior when a senior manager outwardly demonstrates support for the change process, readily agrees to commit the time and staff to
attain the stated outcome, but privately resists the effort by failing to meet
agreed-upon deadlines, not providing the best staff available for the projects assigned, and privately communicating (either through words or
behavior) that the change effort is not the senior manager's highest
priority.

The consequence of retaining a nonparticipating member on the team
is so dire it could result in failure of the change effort. When a nonparticipating individual is a member of the senior management team (or any
other change management team within the organization), the CEO or
the individual's supervisor should discuss the behavior with the individual, explain the behavior's damaging impact on the organization and
its change process, understand the reasons for the behavior, address the
reasons for nonparticipation (if possible), and request the team member's support and participation. If the team member still does not participate (either because he or she does not support the process or lacks the
skills to participate effectively), the CEO or supervisor should then
either help the team member acquire the necessary skills, transfer the
team member to a less critical position in the organization, or, as a last
resort, terminate the team member. Termination is an extreme measure
that should be used sparingly and only when the CEO or the supervisor
is convinced that it is the only viable alternative.

IDENTIFYING TACTICAL PLANS

When the strategic vision and senior management's commitment are
established, the next step is to identify the tactical plans that will move
the organization toward its vision. Successful tactical planning involves

- Selecting a manageable number of tactics

  The number of tactics considered manageable depends on the size
  of the management team and the resources available to commit to
  the tactical planning process

Each executive should be responsible for no more than two tactics when starting the tactical planning process

- Developing action plans for each tactic, which includes

  Description of the tactic

  Justification

  Resource requirements

  Cost/benefits assessment

  Work plan with time line for completing major steps in the plan

  Measurable key results anticipated and when they will be achieved

  Critical assumptions

- Defining and implementing foundation tactics

  Foundation tactics are those that must be accomplished first to provide the information or the infrastructure required to complete other tactics

- Allocating senior management time each month for updates and tactical planning progress reports

- Including tactical planning performance as a component of the senior management performance appraisal process

A number of benefits can be derived from the tactical planning process. Since tactical plans are often cross functional, executives must work cooperatively to successfully complete their tactics. This provides a common discipline and focus and builds a sense of team among senior managers. These characteristics are very important for the first reengineering project.

Moving from defining a strategic vision to identifying tactical plans can be an exciting and stimulating process. But so far, it is only a planning process. The arrow in Figure 1 demonstrates the work completed by defining a strategic vision and identifying tactical plans. Accomplishing these tasks only brings the team part way to its goal.

IMPLEMENTATION

Implementation is the third step in the strategic/tactical process, and it is the most difficult. Up to this point, senior management has been involved in a planning process. It has been essentially a paper process; the result consists of a written vision and well-defined tactics that support the vision. The true test of senior management's commitment comes with implementation.

Again, resistance will develop at this stage as it did during the visioning and tactical planning stages. It is critical to manage resistance at this stage because it will determine if the organization can move forward with change or will revert to past behaviors. A common concern voiced by senior managers at this stage of the process is, "We are so busy dealing with the daily issues of running this organization that we do not have time to add another project to our list of activities."

The reality is that the concern expressed by senior management is correct. Tactical plan implementation does impinge on their time to deal with the daily problems of running the organization, just as reengineering impinges on the staff's ability to run their departments on a daily basis during the reengineering process. This is one reason it is important to limit at the outset the number of tactics and the number of reengineering projects initiated. Both senior management and the staff need time to assimilate the changes under way.

An effective technique to maintain focus on tactical plan implementation is to schedule monthly meetings 12 months in advance. The senior managers should present a report that details progress on each tactic. The report should cover four areas:

- Progress on each tactic measured against the key results

- Verification of the implementation schedule

- Key results expected but not achieved

- Barriers encountered

If there is a deviation from the plan, it should be discussed. For example, if the implementation plan is not on schedule, the senior manager should discuss why and what is being done to bring it back on schedule.

If the key results expected have not been achieved, the senior manager should explain why and what corrective action is being taken. Finally, if barriers have been encountered, the nature of the barriers should be described and a plan presented to overcome them. The senior manager should also seek advice and assistance from other members of the management team in overcoming barriers.

Senior management also must present the strategic/tactical process to the board of directors to demonstrate how management is dealing with issues that affect the organization and its future. Semiannual progress reports should be presented to the board using a format similar to that used for the monthly meetings. In addition, the strategic/tactical process should be announced to the organization (including its physicians) with quarterly updates presented at management and physician meetings and through the organization's newsletter and other communication vehicles.

This level of communication is essential if the process is to take hold and become the organization's operating philosophy. It demonstrates to the board, physicians, and the hospital staff that senior management is committed to positive change and is taking a leadership role in the change process. It demonstrates leadership by example.

FIGURE 2
Tactical planning

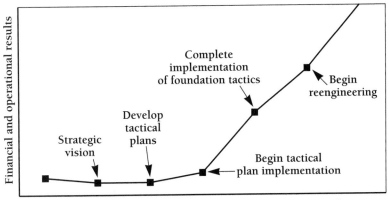

Note: The time (in months) is presented as a general rule. Each organization will vary in the time required to complete the objectives identified in the graph.

Figure 2 shows the relationship between time spent and results achieved in the strategic/tactical process. In the beginning it may seem that not much is happening. Time is spent defining a strategic vision and developing tactical plans, but there is nothing visible yet. Change at this point is a promise. As the tactical plans are implemented, progress becomes visible. When the foundation tactics are completed, new tactics are identified that build on the success of the previous tactics. Success builds on success until a momentum for positive organizational change begins to take hold.

For example, Hospital A spent a year defining and implementing its foundation tactics, which included creating a debt capacity study and a medical staff development plan, hiring a key executive, developing a business plan methodology for evaluating opportunities, completing a market assessment analysis to support its decision process, and initiating an assessment of the organization's culture. One year later, the positive experience gained from implementing these tactics served as a foundation to organize a working group of senior managers and physicians to define and pursue joint opportunities, incorporate the business development planning model into the budget process, and work with employees in a manner sensitive to the existing corporate culture. Hospital A is building the momentum necessary for successful change.

Alternatives to the strategic/tactical process

The strategic/tactical process provides focus for the senior management team, promotes team building, and achieves results. Two other management techniques (which can be described as "event management" techniques) are commonly used in many organizations today: crisis management and stop-start management.

CRISIS MANAGEMENT

In crisis management, small incremental improvements may occur over time. When the environment changes—such as with the introduction of managed care into the community, heightened competition from a neighboring hospital, or development of an integrated healthcare network in the area—a crisis develops. Senior management turns its attention to alleviating the crisis. Crisis intervention is not activated until there is a noticeable down-turn in operational or financial performance. In this reactive environment, emergency meetings are held, lists are developed, percentages of reductions in expenses and the workforce are announced, and partial action is taken. The situation may improve temporarily until the next crisis develops and the cycle begins again. Over time, only incremental improvements are realized as the organization moves from one crisis to another, with managers often surprised the last effort was not successful in achieving lasting results.

A crisis situation, however, can be an effective motivator for change. Crisis focuses the organization on a specific threat that must be addressed if the organization is to succeed. It grabs staff's attention and enables action. The challenge is to manage the crisis and not crisis manage. Managing the crisis results in using the crisis as a motivator to accept change; it requires action. Crisis management uses crisis as a disturbance, a surprise event requiring a reaction.

Under this latter mode of management, dramatic improvement does not occur. There is motion but little forward movement. The tragedy is that the same amount of time passes to achieve marginal results through crisis management as it does to achieve significant results through the strategic/tactical planning process. The constant is time, not results.

SAW TOOTH MANAGEMENT

Stop-start, or saw tooth, management is named for the distinctive configuration of lines on a graph, that depict a stop-start process. It represents managing independent events. In such a scenario, senior management, looking for the solution, decides to implement one of the latest management fads. They embrace the solution with vigor, hold retreats, voice commitment, create slogans, print and distribute buttons, coffee cups, and banners—and introduce the new idea organizationwide. When results do not occur quickly, interest begins to wane. Then another fad is discovered that promises to be the answer to their problems, and the process starts again. By the third iteration, the staff becomes cynical and positive results are more difficult to achieve. Often, the staff will posit: "Let's just wait this fad out and it will die just like the others."

The organization becomes acclimated to the start-and-stop change process and resistance becomes entrenched. The only solution for an organization in this cycle is to break it and begin a long-term effort of focused and sustained organizational improvement, as described in the strategic/tactical process.

Role of reengineering in the strategic/tactical process

Using the strategic/tactical process, senior management positions the organization for positive change, which includes reengineering. Reengineering is not the first tactic implemented but is introduced after the foundation tactics have been defined and implemented. In this sequence, senior management defines a strategic vision, develops tactical plans, implements the foundation tactics, and openly communicates the process that is built on a history of successful planned change. Equally important, senior managers, having experienced resistance to change themselves, will have learned how to overcome it to move the organization forward. Then, the organization is well positioned to introduce a reengineering project.

Reengineering projects must be defined, introduced, and managed with the same rigor and attention to detail used for the foundation tactics. The key to success is to treat reengineering as a component of the change process, not as an event. As momentum builds, results will become more dramatic and the organization will be on the path of active management to improve organizational performance.

Conclusion

The strategic/tactical process is planned change, and reengineering is a powerful tool for organizational change.

Organizations that have not had a successful history of implementing change should consider using the strategic/tactical process defined in this chapter. It is a positioning technique that provides a mechanism for senior management to define a vision for the organization and identify tactics required to move the organization in the direction of its vision. It also enables senior management to establish a history of successful change through implementing tactical plans. The work accomplished by senior management creates positive change in the organization that will carry over to the reengineering effort. Senior management teams having difficulty with the process should consider soliciting the support of an outside facilitator, which some organizations have found helpful in focusing the team's efforts.

The opportunity for reengineering success and improved organizational performance improves significantly when approached with purpose and commitment. There are no guarantees for success, and in a rapidly changing healthcare marketplace, surprises are common. Even though the senior management team will have gained experience managing within the context of the strategic/tactical process, surprises will still occur. The benefit, however, is that the team will expect surprises and will be prepared to deal with them effectively—they will no longer be surprised by the surprises.

NOTES

1. In this chapter, the senior management team is defined as the CEO, COO, CFO, staff, and operational vice presidents or assistant and associate administrators, and others who work directly with the CEO and are involved in the overall management of the organization. The senior management team may or may not include physicians, depending on the role of physicians in the overall management of the organization.

11

Balancing cost and quality through reengineering

Connie R. Curran, RN, EdD, FAAN
President
CurranCare
North Riverside, Illinois

MANAGED CARE IS A GREAT MOTIVATOR for many of the healthcare industry's reengineering programs. Hospitals are moving aggressively to significantly cut costs in anticipation of accelerating pressure from competition and local business coalitions of employers (Figure 1). Providers are looking to reengineering as an answer to achieve the costs results they need to remain competitive.

Reengineering is popular because it can attack the fundamental drivers of costs and streamline delivery while improving service to patients and the quality of outcomes. Most effectively, reengineering helps a hospital work on cost and service issues from two angles. The first is operational. Using work redesign and organizational restructuring techniques, hospitals can reduce the cost of a unit of care (e.g., days, tests, supplies) by increasing productivity, better leveraging highly skilled staff, and reconfiguring the organization to support core processes, such as ambulatory and surgical services. The second is clinical; hospitals can use clinical resource management techniques to reduce case costs (i.e., the number of units of care consumed per patient) by decreasing lengths of stay and resource utilization.

The combination of work redesign and clinical resource management reduces clinically unnecessary treatments and hospitalization while improving the service quality of those treatments, ambulatory encounters and units of hospitalization that are delivered. When these techniques are used concurrently, the medical, administrative, and nursing

182

FIGURE 1
Stages of managed care market evolution

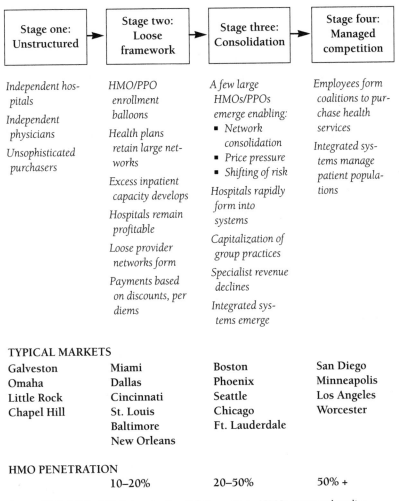

Stage one: Unstructured	Stage two: Loose framework	Stage three: Consolidation	Stage four: Managed competition
Independent hospitals *Independent physicians* *Unsophisticated purchasers*	*HMO/PPO enrollment balloons* *Health plans retain large networks* *Excess inpatient capacity develops* *Hospitals remain profitable* *Loose provider networks form* *Payments based on discounts, per diems*	*A few large HMOs/PPOs emerge enabling:* ■ *Network consolidation* ■ *Price pressure* ■ *Shifting of risk* *Hospitals rapidly form into systems* *Capitalization of group practices* *Specialist revenue declines* *Integrated systems emerge*	*Employees form coalitions to purchase health services* *Integrated systems manage patient populations*

TYPICAL MARKETS

Galveston	Miami	Boston	San Diego
Omaha	Dallas	Phoenix	Minneapolis
Little Rock	Cincinnati	Seattle	Los Angeles
Chapel Hill	St. Louis	Chicago	Worcester
	Baltimore	Ft. Lauderdale	
	New Orleans		

HMO PENETRATION

	10–20%	20–50%	50% +

Source: 1992, 1993, 1995 University Hospital Consortium–APM Incorporated studies.

staffs can work out agreements on clinical and administrative structures and procedures to ensure that the right amount of care is delivered at the right time and in the most cost-effective setting possible.

Undertaking a comprehensive reengineering effort can be like sending a management team on an Outward Bound wilderness survival experience. The team may call on guides or consultants who have led other groups through similar challenges to teach them which tools and techniques to use to overcome obstacles. In the end, however, the team has the responsibility to lead the organizational change effort and decide how to remove roadblocks to achieve consensus and major objectives. As in a wilderness survival experience, team members will have opportunities to learn about themselves, the organization, and how to work together. And, as in the Outward Bound experience, change comes from hard work.

Restructuring can succeed where strict cost cutting has failed in the past if it is sensitive to patient, staff, and organizational culture needs. In fact, to garner the financial results and quality outcomes that managed care demands, work restructuring must emphasize the human side of change management. All levels and disciplines of hospital and medical staff must be involved in decision making about changes that affect them. Thus, many hospitals must overcome "command and control" cultures that have stifled shared problem solving and innovation. Establishing a specific change management committee, in addition to human resources and communications, can smooth the transition to a more open culture that allows hospitalwide involvement and shared accountability for outcomes (Figure 2).

High levels of organizational commitment are required to manage organizational stress, which naturally accompanies a relatively short-term change process with lofty goals. A change management committee is instrumental in developing a plan to help staff understand what to expect during a time of transition, how to take best advantage of change, and how to deal with the emotional stress that accompanies rapid change. At the outset, the committee conducts an initial organizational readiness assessment and then periodically determines the impact of work restructuring on the organization, making recommendations for corrective or preventive actions.

The most important initial message to make clear to all constituents is that reengineering is neither a one-time project, a pick-and-choose approach, nor an exercise in slow, incremental change. It is a revolutionary change centered on the hospital's most important clinical, operational, and administrative activities. It must be comprehensive, viewed as a strategic realignment that requires total organizational commitment, and aimed at fundamental cultural change that will long outlive the current project's undertaking. Piecemeal approaches do not have a strong track record because they cannot effectively address any cross-departmental territorial issues that drive excess costs and limit service and quality.

Both the foundation and philosophy that underlie reengineering are

FIGURE 2
Managing change

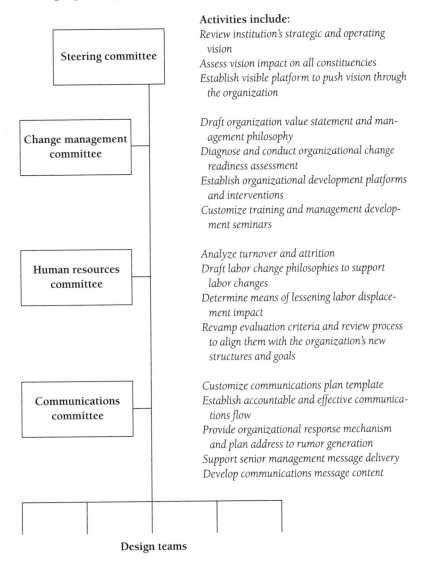

Activities include:

Review institution's strategic and operating vision
Assess vision impact on all constituencies
Establish visible platform to push vision through the organization

Draft organization value statement and management philosophy
Diagnose and conduct organizational change readiness assessment
Establish organizational development platforms and interventions
Customize training and management development seminars

Analyze turnover and attrition
Draft labor change philosophies to support labor changes
Determine means of lessening labor displacement impact
Revamp evaluation criteria and review process to align them with the organization's new structures and goals

Customize communications plan template
Establish accountable and effective communications flow
Provide organizational response mechanism and plan address to rumor generation
Support senior management message delivery
Develop communications message content

Steering committee

Change management committee

Human resources committee

Communications committee

Design teams

similar to that of most quality improvement programs: The work is performed by multidisciplinary teams charged by leadership to achieve positive changes. The teams, composed of the key stakeholders required to make the decisions, are given specific goals, defined time frames, and sufficient training to achieve the desired outcomes. Strong stakeholder involvement is critical to the success of such a change effort, which usually involves several hundred staff members from all parts of the organization working in 8 to 15 design teams.

Concrete goals and well-defined time frames provide the necessary degree of focus and discipline for the design teams. Example goals could include reducing the time spent in documentation of patient care by 35 percent, reducing turnaround time for operating rooms, or expediting patient rooms after discharge to speed the admission of new patients within a defined time window, especially those admitted from the emergency room.

The empowerment and support given to the team members by the organization's executives foster ownership, commitment, leadership, and enhanced capabilities. Acting as internal champions of change, the team members are key to successful implementation of the design because they can usually identify and overcome any internal impediments.

If outside consultants are involved, they should function as expert guides, providing training in analytical tools—such as work-flow analysis and staffing to demand—and change management techniques—such as group facilitation skills—to help team members carry out their assigned responsibilities. Hospital staff must be ready, willing, and able to promote the ideas they have decided to embrace organizationwide. The staff must direct the redesign efforts, lead all committees and design teams, and make all decisions, including those concerning the delivery of patient care, organizational design, and human resources issues.

Integrated approach

A large academic medical center (AMC) recently used the following integrated reengineering approach, which combined work redesign and organizational restructuring with clinical resource management.

An overall cost reduction target of 15 percent of annual operating expenses was set by hospital leadership. Under the direction of a steering committee composed of senior managers, clinical leadership, and departmental staff, 13 design teams were formed that included physicians, departmental managers, and staff from throughout the hospital. The teams were charged with developing recommendations to achieve the cost and quality targets set for each team by the steering committee.

The targets were based on a combination of strategic needs, comparative analysis, focused reviews, and a management assessment, all tempered by management judgment. A unique approach consisting of three major design teams was developed to address the resources and culture of the client.

The design teams fell into three categories:

- "Patient" design teams focused on opportunities to reduce the demand for clinical activities—i.e., reducing lengths of stay and ancillary resource use. These teams examined end-to-end clinical processes (e.g., from preadmission workups to postdischarge care) for patients with diagnoses that use similar care plans and resources. Team members were charged with developing "best practice" care maps and clinical practice guidelines, concentrating initially on high-volume case types or those where similar hospitals had better results or cost savings because different practices were used

- "Supplier" design teams focused on the providers, or suppliers, of care. They developed recommendations for redesigning jobs and interdepartmental working relationships and for revamping the activities that make up the major components of the continuum of care within the hospital, including the emergency room, operating room, diagnostics, inpatient unit care, and ambulatory care. These teams were charged with rethinking and integrating services used by the patient design teams

- "Service" design teams focused on redesigning the departmental organization and job functions that support the work of the supplier teams. These included patient services (e.g., environmental services, dietary, transport, materiel management, and pharmacy), corporate services (e.g., administration, finance, and medical records), and information management

Although these design teams undertook substantially different work and looked at the institution through different perspectives, each team was given the same generic reengineering principles to help identify opportunities for cost reduction and service improvements in a systematic and rigorous manner. Several key restructuring principles are critical to increasing the organization's resources used in direct patient care by reducing time spent in work that is duplicative or routine. The restructuring principles are

- Resize demand for clinical services by developing and implementing best practice care plans to manage clinical resources with reduced lengths of stay and ancillary resource utilization

- Group patients with similar resource needs in homogeneous clusters or clinical units or in ambulatory settings sized to operate at capacity (i.e., the number of beds filled or appointments scheduled) to meet the typical demand each unit has for patient care services. In addition, this should reduce the need for most patient transfers and unexpected staffing fluctuations

- Move services closer to the patients by decentralizing ancillary, support, and administrative services to the patient care unit. These shifts reduce costs (e.g., of "waiting around" and transport) while improving both quality of care and service and responsiveness to patients and physicians

- Delegate frequently performed, routine, manual tasks to the least expensive, appropriately trained workers. Simplifying, restructuring, and eliminating tasks will reduce unnecessary work. Remaining tasks can be better delegated, which lowers costs and increases the level of professional challenge for highly trained employees. They will now have more time, for example, to evaluate the effectiveness of interventions on the patient's condition

- Simplify and reduce the number of job categories by redesigning job responsibilities and cross-training workers to perform multiskilled functions, incorporating patient care assistive work and technical tasks such as venipuncture and electrocardiograms, and by eliminating excessive differentiation and specialization between departments and specialties

- Align authority, responsibility, and accountability for patient care outcomes by placing all unit-based clinical and support services under the direction of an operating unit manager, instead of having housekeeping and ancillary clinical staff assigned to units but still reporting to centralized departments

- Consolidate and centralize non-unit-based functions to improve economies of scale. Once patient care units have been reorganized, centralized services must meet the needs of the new units. There are significant opportunities in interdepartmental, rather than intradepartmental, consolidation. For example, bringing the laboratory subsections together under one management instead of having department walls between various subsections like pathology, histology, hematology, and blood bank

- Simplify, reduce, and eliminate complexities by redesigning patient care processes and using appropriate technology to free staff from routine, mechanical tasks. New technologies have improved performance in charting and patient management, pharmacy, and laboratory services. For example

    Charting technology capabilities maximized by the use of on-line (or even manual) flow charting with bedside access. Charting by exception and systems that incorporate record keeping with protocols and clinical pathway monitoring systems

    Patient management via predictable teaching-oriented protocols that involve the patient and family in many decisions and in accountability for outcomes. This occurs most commonly with protocols that help identify deviations from anticipated outcomes via clinical pathways

    In the pharmacy, technologies continue to improve that can provide timely staff access to regular and emergency medications via the use of automatic dispensing machines that function like automatic tellers

    Laboratory services can be greatly enhanced, especially in the emergency room or critical areas, with the installation of appropriately placed arterial blood gas analysis units that offer timely and accurate analysis of samples drawn by unit-based respiratory therapist (RT) or registered nurse (RN) staff members

- Flatten management structure to an optimum number of layers, usually no more than five from unit staff to CEO. Managerial titles and accountabilities as well as spans of control may vary widely from one institution to another. Substantial benefits include: improved communications, clearer identification with organizational goals, improved accountability for results, greater employee flexibility and adaptability, and greater professional satisfaction

Using the restructuring principles, the AMC then developed 15 guidelines grouped around the basic questions of what work should be done, when, how, and where it should be done, and who should do it. The 15 guidelines were

What and (how much) work should be done?

1. Define "best practice" care plans and guidelines to reduce costs while improving or at least maintaining quality of care. (This was a principal area of focus for the patient design teams.)

2. Reduce or eliminate nonessential activities, such as work done because of tradition instead of patient needs or gathering data that is no longer required, by considering ways to take advantage of streamlining opportunities:

   Eliminate tasks or activities—e.g., use charting by exception only

   Eliminate redundancies—e.g., develop an information system that integrates inpatient and outpatient care to avoid duplicated lab tests or x-rays done on an outpatient basis and then repeated during an inpatient stay

   Minimize communication and coordination needs—e.g., decentralize to the patient unit selected administrative, support, and clinical activities, such as admitting, housekeeping, and respiratory therapy

   Minimize duplicative control activities, such as requiring checklists to be reviewed three times

   Minimize patient and materiel transfers by bringing as many services as possible to the patient and keeping appropriate materiels on the unit instead of in a centralized department

3. Consider changing products or services to reduce costs while maintaining quality—e.g., look for sutures, prostheses, and scrubs

that can be used throughout the hospital, reserving specialized supplies for truly special purposes

When should the work be done?

4. Consider timeliness and urgency in terms of patients' needs. For example, make sure testing is "STAT" only when necessary

5. Consider the best time for performing activities from the patient's perspective. For example, have the room cleaned when the patient is not there or at least when the patient is awake

6. Keep patients' needs in mind, but consider opportunities to do the work during the daytime when it is least costly (striving to avoid premiums for evening, night, or weekend work or overtime expenditures, for example) and consider all opportunities to change staffing patterns to align them with predictable daily or weekly demand patterns

How should the work be done?

7. Standardize activities to minimize variation between caregivers performing the same clinical and nonclinical processes. This can be accomplished by grouping patients by their clinical support and equipment needs instead of by their diseases. For example, neurological and orthopedic patients could share a satellite physical therapy facility because they require the same type of rehabilitative clinical care

8. Streamline work processes

Minimize the number of steps currently involved in getting something accomplished by evaluating all activities to determine if they are really needed to achieve a given outcome

Minimize hand-offs of work from one person to another and, thereby, the number of people involved. Having the smallest number of appropriately prepared staff involved in a patient's care also minimizes the impersonality and fragmentation of care. For example, cross-trained x-ray technicians can draw time-sensitive labs and do EKGs for scheduled preoperative patients in the same or contiguous geographic space instead of having different people perform each test

Consider parallel rather than sequential processes to minimize turnaround times. For example, two teams with complementary responsibilities can get rooms ready for new patients

9. Use technology as a key enabler of reengineering. For example, developing hospital-clinic-physician information networks helps get the most out of reengineering ideas by linking the various sites that provide clinical services, requiring patients to give demographic and insurance information only once

Who should do the work?

10. Involve patients and other customers in work flows by considering, for example, if the clinic or physician's office staff or someone at the patient's home can do the work more cost-effectively and by considering if the patients and their families, with appropriate support and teaching, could do more to result in earlier discharges. For example, the clinic or physician's office could gather preadmission information, and timely preoperative training of the patient and family about postoperative self-care could speed discharge

11. Actively consider make-or-buy decisions for a wide range of products or services, such as dietary, environmental services, laundry, materiel management, and payroll. For example, consider the efficiencies as well as cost-savings potential in using the newer cook-chill-reheat technology in patient food service

12. Redefine jobs and accountabilities

Align responsibility and accountability and give appropriate individual authority over the resources necessary to get the job done. For example, getting a patient's room temperature adjusted or a light bulb changed should not require a work order and three days to accomplish

Reassign work to the least-expensive, appropriately trained—or cross-trainable—worker

Broaden job responsibilities to enhance worker flexibility (e.g., a unit assistant can help with patient room maintenance, admitting, and food delivery)

Use a team approach instead of a department-driven approach to delivering services

Where should the work be done?

13. Consider the best setting to deliver patient services, some of which might be better provided before or after a hospital stay, not necessarily during it. The service might happen at the physician's office or in a patient's home

14. Move resources as close as possible to patients and staff requiring these services. For example, a satellite physical therapy facility would benefit units with heavy physical therapy needs in terms of time saved and patient comfort

15. Identify relatively low-cost reconfigurations of physical facilities that could expedite work processes or enable consolidation of functions. For example, the satellite physical therapy facility would need only that equipment that pertains to the unit's patients' needs (as opposed to relocating expensive and less frequently used radiological equipment)

The AMC's design teams participated in classes in work flow analysis, Pareto analysis, staffing-to-demand, clinical protocol and outcomes assessment, brainstorming, task force management, and team facilitation skills with the leadership of the consultants. Team members then took the lead and

- Surveyed staff members on how they spend their time. (Usually, there is a significant gap between how staff members spend their time and how they would prefer to. Quantifying this gap helps to foster a patient-focused culture. Increased staff satisfaction is often linked to increased time spent in direct patient care.)

- Conducted productivity comparisons between internal departments and against departments in similar hospitals to establish cost and productivity "best practice" benchmarks

- Analyzed overall Medicare and non-Medicare ancillary resource consumption, length of stay, and cost per case compared to those of other, similar institutions

- Developed detailed utilization comparisons by diagnostic related group and by physician

- Analyzed and identified roadblocks to the efficient delivery of services (in part, from the patient's point of view)

- Drew the best ideas from the organization and introduced new methods and technologies on an as-needed basis

- Evaluated different options to determine the "best practices" for the hospital to pursue

- Developed service-by-service utilization reduction targets

- Reviewed pharmacy utilization analyses and hospital and physician reimbursement data analyses for cost and effectiveness as well as opportunities to use generic drugs in the hospital's standard formulary

- Worked through specific details of exactly how work will be redesigned and who will do what (which may be the most challenging aspect of this work for traditionalists of any discipline)

- Checked for potential operational impact of ideas developed by the task forces on service and quality of care by getting feedback from those who will be affected by the changes (including managers, physicians, and nurses)

- Quantified the impact of ideas using feedback from design team members, the finance department, steering committee members, and other managers

- Incorporated the feedback of users and key constituents and held ongoing discussions to make sure that they subscribe to each major idea of the redesign effort (with modifications) as well as to the final recommendations

- Developed detailed implementation plans of what, who, and when to expect to achieve results and designating one idea champion (or accountable person) to report back and maintain accountability

- Involved staff from throughout the hospital in multidisciplinary teams throughout the project, making sure they are focused on achieving the desired outcomes using internal communications vehicles to highlight positive experiences and bold leadership

- Transferred the aforementioned analytical, process, and computer database skills to the organization so staff members can continue to improve with confidence and a focus on quality outcomes

By charting operating work activity flows, conducting surveys, and performing external analyses, the design teams identified bottlenecks and then proposed restructured work processes to remove them. These included modifying the work steps, decreasing internal and external obstacles, or changing the way work is done in the current system. Sometimes this kind of scrutiny of previously accepted practice reveals illogical and quirky practices. The teams then identified the optimal mix of staff skills needed and the resulting cross-training required to support their newly developed processes. This would ensure that high-level skills and limited resources would be used most effectively. In addition, employees who were cross-trained in several less-skilled tasks, such as an x-ray technician who can also do EKGs and draw blood needed for necessary preoperative tests, will help reduce the amount of idle time in such areas as patient care operations, the laboratory, radiology, respiratory therapy, and the operating room.

As the teams discovered, restructured unit operations and new roles and responsibilities required new management models, particularly for the patient care units. The design teams looked for the most effective reporting relationships and distribution of management responsibilities. The objective was to increase the span of control and place decision-making responsibility at the lowest appropriate level. The teams evaluated alternative patient care models and philosophies of care for each unit's direct caregivers to determine how staff is assigned to patients and how to delegate accountability for patient care. Alternative RN-led patient care models include

- *Practice partners.* Here, one RN paired with a consistent assistive clinical care provider (licensed or unlicensed) is accountable for a designated group of patients for a specific time period

- *Clinical care triads.* The triads consist of at least one RN plus two others, who may be licensed or unlicensed, accountable for a designated group of patients for a given shift

- *Critical care teams.* These teams, which involve both the current RN and sometimes an RT in reformulated roles, share accountability for a variety of high-tech tasks for a small group of high-acuity, ventilator-dependent patients

- *Specialty-specific models.* These models are common to the emergency room or the labor, delivery, recovery, postpartum (LDRP) department. They add a unit-based support associate to the clinical care team on all appropriate shifts to take over the lower-tech jobs such as cleaning and stocking supplies. This permits a smaller number of RNs to delegate more of the routine tasks and take accountability for the patient's professional care needs

The practice partners model pairs an RN with another licensed or unlicensed caregiver on a regular shared schedule, instead of the less rigid practice of teaming RNs with other caregivers in ratios determined by the patients' clinical needs and the institution's specific local or regional labor supply conditions.

The number of people interested in and capable of filling entry-level and clinical technologist positions can be a problem and may require a significant investment in the screening, recruitment, and training of candidates. Some sensitivity is required because the local external pool of candidates may come from nearby long-term care facilities. One way to fill the void is to explore liaisons with nursing assistant training programs, offering ways to match the training of their students with the hospital's job requirements.

If either the internal or external environment of the institution is oriented toward collective bargaining responses, any changes are apt to be met with resistance. For example, one urban AMC went through leadership turnover after undergoing a large-scale reengineering project. The new leadership then faced strong challenges to many of the agreed-upon changes from the nurses' union representatives when their contract came up for review. The nurses were fearful that the expanded roles for nonlicensed assistive workers would ultimately cut the number of RN positions. Early in the reengineering process, preferably before it even begins, internal human resources or appropriate outside consultants should thoroughly evaluate the potential for organized resistance and develop strategies to counter it.

In developing any new patient care delivery model, the accountability for delegated activities must be clarified. The institution should develop new job descriptions and training programs that prepare the workers who will assist the RN in their expanded roles. As delegator to the assistive workers, the RN will need to know which coworkers have been trained and evaluated in each activity within a given job description. This underscores the importance of thorough training and explicit documentation of each individual's competencies in a user-friendly, computerized skills registry system.

Very few institutions are initially prepared for the challenges, which include

- The degree of personal and professional development needed for managers to be comfortable and perform well in the reengineered hospital

- The inherent distrust that department-based or unit-based personnel have for any changes that threaten their comfort with their current competencies or tacit "ownership" of particular clinical skills and tasks (specialization)

- An evolving realization that everyone's roles and responsibilities will be affected by this process and the concomitant waves of anxiety, which are expressed in a wide range of behaviors

To overcome employee fear of failure and skepticism, the hospital should commit to a serious, significant, and highly visible training and development program for all staff whose jobs have been redefined.

Another important consideration was the customer-supplier relationships between the patient units and the ancillary and support departments. For example, the design team determined that housekeeping staff should report to operating unit (nurse) managers but be trained through a central department. In this way, the units will have the authority to control resources allocated to their units and thus be able to establish and expect appropriate service levels.

At the end of the planning phase, the design teams recommended to the steering committee which ancillary, support, and administrative services should be decentralized to each unit. They showed exactly how services are to be provided, what equipment and staff should be relocated, how much training and certification is required, how reporting relationships are to be defined, and how current ways of doing things within and across departments are to be changed to support an integrated model of care delivery. They also included options for integrated computer applications or products such as drug dispensers. They also predicted the changes in work activities that would be affected by applying such technology on the units. All of the design team recommendations were synthesized into revised staffing plans with a detailed implementation plan for successfully rolling out the new model of care.

Value of incentives

Existing recognition and reward systems need to be evaluated during the restructuring process to make sure they promote the restructuring goals of lower costs and quality outcomes. A number of recognition and reward strategies can complement the leaner, flatter, more integrated organization. For example

- Send clear messages about the importance of multiskilling by compensating staff members for learning new skills. For example, a phlebotomist who is cross-trained to perform EKGs is paid more than someone who can do only one or the other task

- Relieve the stress that restructuring can bring by delivering positive messages aimed at staff retention. For example, semiannual surveys of employee satisfaction and priorities should be the norm so that benefits and rewards can be tailored to meet staff needs. This is often accomplished by offering a range of benefits pegged to age and life-stage priorities and then giving employees the flexibility to choose between them. Consideration also needs to be given to offering basic healthcare coverage (with higher copayments) for part-time staff

- Reward staff members' flexibility and development of multiple skills by establishing a prestigious, mobile, and highly skilled group of nurses and clinical assistive personnel (with their own designated leader) that can be dispatched to a number of clinical areas in response to unplanned census and acuity fluctuations[1]

- Reward managers who facilitate restructuring—even if it means their jobs might be reorganized or eliminated—by providing substantial career transition assistance and support. Some organizations have found it mutually beneficial for both the organization and affected staff to explore opportunities to enable inpatient managers to receive the necessary development in order to move into ambulatory and home care management roles within their own systems or in affiliated organizations[2]

- Reinforce the linkage between accountability and control by evaluating the potential for salaried staff of self-governed units to share the economic benefits from eliminating overtime and agency staff. This strategy works best with highly specialized, highly motivated staffs such as those responsible for a combined LDRP service

- Closely tie manager and executive rewards to outcomes in the areas for which they are accountable. Peer management input that reflects the level of collaboration among different areas and support for each other's goals can be formalized as part of the review process

One organization undergoing restructuring stepped up its efforts to foster behavior that furthers reengineering goals. They initiated a "You're a Star" nomination program to highlight collaboration. Formal "stroke notes" were forwarded to both the named individual and his or her manager and the nominations were cited in the organization's in-house newsletter.

It is also important to recognize managerial excellence that transcends narrow identification with a specific discipline. For example, one of the most successful reorganizations of a nursing department into a more inclusive patient care services team occurred largely because of the RN leader responsible for the new group. She looked beyond traditional nursing boundaries for her new directors of patient care services, choosing and supporting individuals with master's degrees from respiratory and physical therapy as well as nursing.[3]

Results

Well-run and realistic reengineering programs should generate substantial financial returns, which can range anywhere from a 5 to 21 percent decrease in operating costs within 12 to 18 months of implementation. The 500-bed Stanford University Medical Center, in Palo Alto, California, for example, began a multiyear "Operations Improvement" program in late 1989.[4] The goal was to decrease its $280 million operating budget by $26 million in the fiscal year beginning September 1, 1990, and by another $18 million in the following year. From the beginning of the project through August 1992, Stanford cut a total of $44 million in costs and enhanced revenues by another $10 million.[5]

The key was the involvement of people from every level of the organization, from housekeeping to nursing to finance. Using the top-down, bottom-up approach, Stanford established a steering committee composed of department heads, trustees, and administrators to set financial, service, and quality targets, but empowered employees and staff physicians working in task forces to figure out the specifics of how best to meet the targets.

In the first year, the targeted $10 million in nursing costs were eliminated, in part by changing skill-mix ratios and turning non-nursing activities over to nursing assistants, in the process eliminating costly overtime by registry nurses.[6] The targeted $7 million in ancillary services cost reductions was met in part by standardizing supplies so all staff could be cross-trained on a similar suture or catheter, for example. In addition, housekeeping (working on the same task forces) reduced its shifts to eliminate shift overlap.

During the second and third years, Stanford undertook major work redesign. Working closely with its internal nurses' union, Stanford restructured the work for its nursing and ancillary services, such as pharmacy, respiratory therapy, and laboratories.[7] Other innovations included

- Eliminating the hospitalwide transport service by assigning a designated and accountable transporter to one or two units. This eliminated waiting-around time by the more highly paid RNs, who often had transported patients themselves instead of waiting longer for a transporter from the centralized department

- Relieving RNs and housekeepers of delivery duties by purchasing three robotic carts to deliver meal trays, drugs, and other supplies

- Redesigning the cardiac monitoring system so it can be tapped into from any patient room, eliminating the need for RNs to watch a bank of cardiac monitors 24 hours a day. Eliminating these 13 positions saved $900,000 a year

- Eliminating overutilization of lab and x-ray services by implementing agreed-upon protocols that outline what tests a typical patient with a certain diagnosis would use

- Making the best use of high-level RN skills by making them "directors or coordinators of patient care," responsible for assessing the patient's condition and working with licensed vocational nurses and assistants (in nonintensive care units) to provide care, as well as the "overseer" of critical paths

- Using machine-based pharmacy delivery instead of a pharmacist on every floor

- Enhancing continuity of care by training 14 RNs to become service line case managers who oversee the patient from admission to discharge and follow-up by ambulatory and home health services

In most hospitals where reengineering has been successful, the process never stops. Stanford continues to implement new ways to provide care, while improving patient, employee, and physician satisfaction along the way.

Employee involvement was the key for the 275-bed St. Joseph's Hospital, Carondelet Health Care Services in Tucson, Arizona, which achieved $1.2 million in savings based on 1994 adjusted admissions.[8] The restructuring process, which reached the 18-month postimplementation mark in summer 1995, was led by direct caregivers. St. Joseph's selected a "unit-based care team" approach, in which teams are headed by a clinical manager, always an RN. The team also includes licensed practical nurses, patient care technicians (i.e., nursing assistants with some advanced training), and patient care associates, who handle the "hotel-management" functions that nurses clearly said they did not see as part of nursing. At least $400,000 of the $1.2 million savings in 1994 were attributed to the new care model.

According to the vice president for patient care services, St. Joseph's nurses learned that it was acceptable to delegate a few patient care tasks so that they could focus on the highly skilled services for which they were trained, such as evaluation of healthcare interventions. In the future, RNs will be the integrators and coordinators of care.

Lessons learned

While organizational cultures differ, the barriers to change are almost always the same. There is widespread disbelief of the need to change, at least on an unconscious level. Employees fear job loss or stressful role changes. Restructuring is a major time commitment for everyone. New, boundary-spanning working relationships are hard to create. Managers who have focused on maintaining the status quo find the process challenging. All of these barriers are exacerbated by the near-universal dependency needs of healthcare staffs and the paternalistic tendencies of administrators, which may conspire to stimulate a strong wish to return to old familiar and comfortable roles. Organizational development efforts can help employees understand that it is fine to wish for a return to yesterday while at the same time realizing that yesterday is gone. Focusing on the human side of change and developing ongoing, thoughtful communication about the need for change can overcome many of these barriers.

There are numerous factors that facilitate success in systemwide reengineering efforts which, if they are absent, require significant work before reengineering is launched. Among the positive predictors of success are

- A top leadership group absolutely convinced that significant, dramatic systemwide change is needed to assure viability and success in the future

- A leadership team that includes a vice president of patient care or director of nursing and clinical services who has both formal authority and internal professional credibility to drive changes in clinical care delivery

- A human resources department that anticipates and responds to the needs and expectations of management and staff

- Internal organizational development and training resources with the sophistication to lead two-way communication and training efforts or the readiness to bring in such culture-changing resources from outside the system

- A vigorous quality improvement effort with the requisite commitment and attention to quality and service outcomes among the staff

- Success in initiating case management or critical path guidelines with significant physician input and buy-in that include both clear clinical and fiscal outcome targets and accountabilities

- Movement toward a truly integrated healthcare delivery system that includes significant linkage and common goals with physicians, ambulatory, and home health services

- An accessible information system that effectively provides a computerized patient record and includes the ability to track fiscal, administrative, and outcomes data across all parts of the system

- A track record of having dealt fairly with employees in the past (without fostering a sense of paternalistic entitlement between the executive staff and employees)

- Participation or attendance at conferences where reengineering concepts and experiences are highlighted or in-depth research in the relevant literature

- The ability to examine all potential changes from the patient's point of view

- A thorough examination of alternatives, including visits to or interviews with key players in other similar institutions that have undertaken reengineering

- Selection of the most compatible and competent consultants to support the process and willingness to invest the management and staff time as well as significant fiscal resources to accomplish the project's goals

It is rare for any institution to have all of these assets in place at once. However, the most common problems are encountered when the system's leaders do not have an accurate perception of its assets and liabilities or when the leaders wish to use the process to help push out certain members of the leadership team. Problems also arise when a CEO suspects that a particular leader is not up to the challenges involved in a major change effort but is unwilling or unable to replace that individual with a more appropriate person before reengineering begins.

In conclusion, there are several major lessons including: getting leaders on board, setting a clear direction, agreeing on principles, creating support structures, preparing the organization for significant effort, picking a date, and beginning. The status quo is not an option, especially as managed care continues to push market evolution in healthcare delivery.

NOTES

1. S. Malone, "Developing a Mobile Nursing Unit: A Strategy to Handle Census Changes," *Recruitment, Retention & Restructuring Report* 8, no. 3 (March 1995).

2. S. H. Johnson, "Job Transition Assistance for Managers and Executives: Rekindling Entrepreneurial Spirit," *Recruitment, Retention & Restructuring Report* 8, no. 6 (June 1995).

3. B. Lockwood, "Developing the Role of Vice President of Patient Care Services: Pulling the Clinical Team Together," *Recruitment, Retention & Restructuring Report* 8, no. 7 (March 1995).

4. K. Southwick, "Multi-Year Restructuring Changes Stick at Stanford University Medical Center, Bringing Costs and Charges Down in a Managed Care Market," *Strategies for Healthcare Excellence* 6, no. 1 (January 1993): 2.

5. Ibid, 3.

6. Ibid, 4.

7. Ibid, 5.

8. C. R. Curran and D. K. Houghton, *Renewing the Catholic Healthcare Ministry, A Workbook on Redesigning Care: Become the Values-Driven, Low-Cost Provider* (St. Louis, Mo.: Catholic Health Association of the United States, 1995), 91.

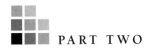 PART TWO

Systemwide transformation

12

Beyond traditional reengineering

Kurt Miller
Partner, Director of Care Delivery Solution Team
Andersen Consulting
Pittsburgh, Pennsylvania

P ROVIDERS, MANAGED CARE ORGANIZATIONS, and health insurance companies have undertaken a number of reengineering approaches during the past several years to reduce cost and improve quality. In some cases, these efforts have involved comprehensive, organizationwide reengineering of administrative, care management, and delivery processes; in other instances, more narrowly focused approaches have been taken.

To date, most initiatives have been first- and second-wave approaches. First-wave initiatives have targeted healthcare process improvements within discrete functional areas such as a laboratory or admissions in a provider setting or enrollment or claims in insurance or managed care settings. Second-wave initiatives—many of which are under way today— typically redesign organizationwide processes such as patient care delivery in a provider setting or customer service in an insurance or a managed care setting. Regardless of the scope, many of these efforts have succeeded, yielding quality improvements of up to 50 percent, cost reductions from 5 to 25 percent, and noticeable improvements in member, patient, and employee satisfaction.[1]

While providers and insurance companies have been reengineering operations, broader structural changes have been occurring industrywide. Merger and integration mania has swept the marketplace over the past several years, driven by organizations' desires to increase market share and decrease overall expenditures. To date, however, the cost advantages of these change initiatives have gone largely unrealized. This is partly the result of focusing on legal, governance, and organizational structure issues rather than on the operations aspect of these mergers, acquisitions, and alliances. In fact, in many cases these change efforts have added significant complexity to today's health services organization, often exacerbating any existing problems of fragmentation, specialization, and compartmentalization. This does not suggest that integration is an inappropriate strategy for a health services organization to pursue, rather it is a question to be examined and answered by each organization, based upon its strategic goals and objectives and specific marketplace dynamics.

However, the larger truth is that whether undertaking a merger, acquisition, or reengineering initiative, more fundamental change that is driven by comprehensive reengineering and transformation initiatives will be necessary to succeed in the future. As a result, a continuing emphasis on first- and second-wave reengineering initiatives will be necessary but not sufficient for health services organizations to transform themselves successfully to remain relevant in the future. Winning health enterprises of the future will also apply many of these concepts and principles across the entire administration, care management, and delivery continuum to achieve dramatic improvements in quality, customer service, and cost structure. These efforts will be recognized as third- and fourth-wave reengineering approaches.

Third-wave initiatives will focus on reengineering processes across horizontally integrated systems (e.g., care delivery, insurance, or managed care organizations). These initiatives are necessary because most new integrated systems (both provider- and insurance-based) still operate as fragmented, compartmentalized organizations. Within such a network, providers may be segmented into hospitals, physician practices, nursing homes, and others and within health plans into insurance and underwriting, member services, and others. For providers, third-wave efforts may encompass reengineering care delivery processes across an integrated delivery network (e.g., hospitals, clinics, and nonacute settings). In a managed care organization it may include reengineering enrollment and customer service processes across several recently merged health plans.

Fourth-wave initiatives, the most comprehensive, will take a very different view of process and organizational structure within an integrated health enterprise (IHE).[2] These initiatives will redefine the traditional boundaries between the two large industry silos, health plan administration (e.g., health plans and assumers of risk) and care delivery (e.g., hospitals and physician groups), to enable more fundamental organizational transformation.

In response to competitive pressures, many organizations have reengineered processes within these silos but have yet to bring the two together. Only recently have healthcare organizations begun to acknowledge that consumers are not interested in internal distinctions between health plan and provider. In fact, consumers increasingly want seamless service. This expectation should be viewed as a mandate for effective integration and coordination across the health services continuum, within existing integrated delivery networks (IDNs) as well as across "virtually" integrated systems. Fourth-wave initiatives will reengineer processes across these two large silos and achieve fundamental transformation of the organization.

Driving forces

To put the next waves of health service reengineering in perspective, it is important to understand the industry's evolution (Figures 1 through 3). These changes are occurring in numerous U.S. regions, as well as in Australia, Singapore, and several European countries. The broad evolutionary path is fairly consistent across most markets, although the pace and sequence of change varies dramatically. The changes are being seen in highly capitated markets where "tightly managed," or fourth-generation, managed care predominates.

In this environment, the distinction between provider, supplier, insurer, and even purchaser begins to blur (Figures 4 and 5). There are many examples: Delta Airlines and the John Deere Corporation have set up internal clinics to manage the health of employees, becoming both providers and insurers; Zeneca Pharmaceuticals purchased Salick, a chain of oncology centers, and entered the business of disease-state management; Merck acquired Medco Containment Services and added the role of benefits management. At Glaxo, another pharmaceutical giant, the chief executive officer stated that eventually "Glaxo will have to maneuver itself from drug firm to healthcare concern—from Glaxo to Glaxocare."

FIGURE 1
Traditional healthcare system

Historically, healthcare system participants have had segregated roles and positions in the care delivery paradigm.

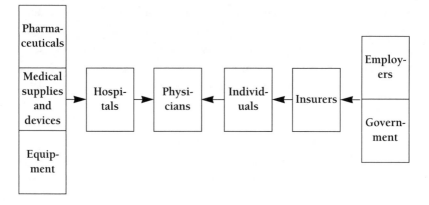

FIGURE 2
Managed care system

Managed care has brought together suppliers, selectors and payers or physicians, hospitals, and insurers. Most importantly, it has aligned hospital and physician incentives to reduce inpatient utilization, and therefore cost.

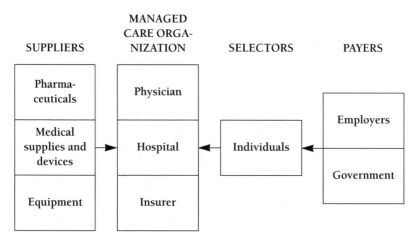

FIGURE 3
Future players

In the future, the individual will become an active participant in the healthcare delivery process and incentive structure.

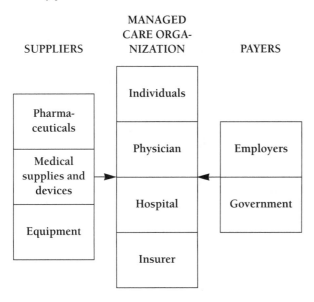

In addition to these developments, there is a stage beyond tightly managed care. This is the rapidly emerging world of virtual care, where time, space, and form are no longer barriers. In this world, health service organizations provide virtualized triage services via telephone and advanced database technologies, consumers are given on-line access to their medical records and extensive medical knowledge bases, and individuals with chronic diseases, forming virtual communities on the Internet, obtain advice from people with similar problems and in effect become their own primary care physicians and specialists. In such an environment, health organizations need to rethink their approaches to service and delivery and reexamine their value proposition.

This rapidly emerging environment provides important insights for third- and fourth-wave transformation initiatives. In addition to improving and reinventing processes, these initiatives must focus on building and enhancing capabilities in several areas: managing individual and

FIGURE 4
Future healthcare system

A cross-organizational view of the future healthcare system illustrates significantly different processes and players than currently exist.

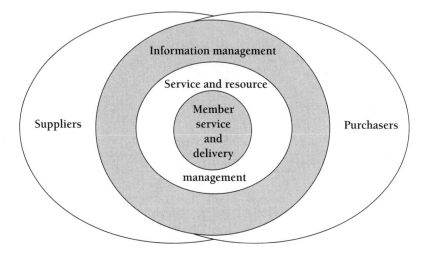

FIGURE 5
Supplier and purchaser relationships

An array of new suppliers and purchasers will emerge. The variety of arrangements between them and the products they offer will increase dramatically.

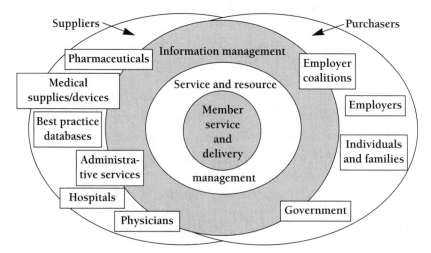

FIGURE 6
Philosophical shifts in care organization and delivery

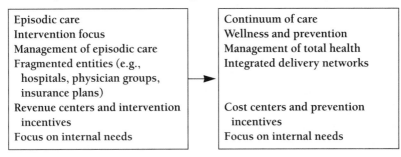

Episodic care	Continuum of care
Intervention focus	Wellness and prevention
Management of episodic care	Management of total health
Fragmented entities (e.g., hospitals, physician groups, insurance plans)	Integrated delivery networks
Revenue centers and intervention incentives	Cost centers and prevention incentives
Focus on internal needs	Focus on internal needs

population health, coordinating and delivering health services, building and managing relationships, and aligning services and resources. Information management plays an anchor role enabling all of the other competencies. The following section outlines the next waves of change and how these core capabilities contribute to organizational transformation and marketplace success.

The next waves

A number of philosophical shifts provide the foundation for third- and fourth-wave reengineering. These shifts influence how healthcare organizations organize and deliver a broad array of services to members. These shifts (Figure 6) drive corresponding changes in the way an IHE structures its processes, operations, and organization to move toward improved capabilities in the areas previously mentioned.

Managing individual and population health

How care is being managed at the individual member level is undergoing dramatic change. In many ways these changes reflect a departure from what Jeff Goldsmith has referred to as "the traditional 'diagnose-and-treat' paradigm of medicine to a rapidly evolving 'predict-and-manage' paradigm." Driven by the need for a new covenant between an IHE and its members, this concept is based on a two-way relationship—between a plan member and the IHE. Beginning at enrollment, the relationship focuses on wellness, prevention, and early identification of health risks. Through this process, members are encouraged to take a more active role in wellness and chronic disease management. This emphasis benefits members' well-being and reduces costs throughout the healthcare system.

The concept of managing individual and population health is an extension of the philosophies developed during early reengineering efforts such as patient-focused care and the Planetree model.[3] Bringing about such changes requires a radically different view of how processes are structured and organized. At the member level, the linkage between what traditionally has been viewed as separate processes for health plan administration and care delivery should be redefined. To provide more integrated, consistent, and seamless customer service, organizations need to bring together a number of traditionally administrative and care delivery processes.

Enrollment processing, for example, has historically been seen as an administrative task. It has focused on enrolling members in a health plan, establishing coverage categories, and defining copayment and deductible requirements. At one large managed care organization, however, this process is about to change dramatically:

- Individuals will be able to enroll from a variety of places, including home, workplace, or other locations

- They will enroll via technologies such as interactive television, personal computers, telephone, or free-standing kiosks

- If enrolling from the workplace, individuals will be able to access demographic information from the employer database, thereby simplifying the process

- Members will provide medical and clinical information (along with certain administrative data), including selected elements of their own medical history, family health history, lifestyle factors (e.g., use of tobacco, diet, and nutrition), and other clinically relevant information

- Using information entered by the enrollee, a preliminary health path will be established, and the enrollee will be prompted to select a primary care provider—that may or may not be a physician—and other team members (e.g., nutritionist, therapist). In the case of a young, healthy plan member, the member may elect to function as his or her own primary care provider and instead select a "relationship manager." The health path and primary care team will help the member maintain health and manage chronic illnesses. Information collected at this stage will also be used to identify educational, wellness, and membership materials that should be sent to the new plan member

- In addition to selecting a primary care provider, the enrollee will be asked to select one or more pharmacies to integrate the clinical aspect of pharmaceutical care, as well as streamline ordering, inventory management, and distribution

- An intelligent assist capability will be built into on-line member applications to facilitate selection of primary care providers, team members, and pharmacies. Knowledge bases containing extensive information and profiles—including location, languages spoken, experience, and credentials—will enable this capability

- The enrollment system will have intelligent capabilities for case management, thereby enabling immediate identification of high- and very high-risk members. In these cases, an initial appointment will be scheduled during enrollment

HEALTH PATHS

A key tool to manage individual health is the health path, a longitudinal map of all health-related events for an individual, including elements of preventive, chronic, and episodic care. The health path is a mechanism to maximize the probability of sustaining and improving individual health, as well as the length and quality of life. Plan and family members will work with the primary care team to update the health path with changes in status (e.g., an acute care episode), goals (e.g., weight loss), lifestyle choices (e.g., stop smoking), and best practices derived from an outcomes-based repository.

The health path identifies resources required by the member for care, treatment, and education. For an IHE, it models a process to forecast future demands (at both individual and overall system levels) as well as measure and improve outcomes. The health path also provides the basis for periodic assessments, thereby enabling both the individual plan member and IHE to target services to optimize the member's health.

Health paths are revolutionary because they represent the convergence and integration of three powerful forces for change within the healthcare industry by (1) redefining the relationship between the health plan and member from an acute, episode-driven focus to a long-term partnership based on member wellness; (2) using technology as an enabler of individualized service while coordinating utilization; (3) increasing the focus on health outcomes as a means of evaluating the effectiveness and efficiency of care delivery systems and suggesting improvements.

From a technical aspect, health paths are a set of data and a collection of tools to manipulate that data. These data and tool sets are used by providers, health plan staff, members, and other stakeholders to manage the long-term relationship between the members and their health plans and care delivery systems. In terms of their impact, and within the context of managing personal and population health, health paths are a powerful tool for providing substantive benefits to members, the IHE, and other stakeholders. Members will benefit from health paths as a straightforward and explicit way to understand the big picture of their health, as well as how to partner with their IHE to influence their quality of life over time. Health paths will also enable the member to simplify the relationship with the IHE by providing a planned schedule of activities for wellness and chronic disease management.

The individualized member care enabled by health paths will empower IHEs to build marketplace identity and establish their distinctive brand. Increased personalization is also intended to increase member satisfaction, which will strengthen the bonds between members and the health plan. Finally, increased individualization will enable better management of utilization due to the increased predictability and coordination of care.

PRIMARY CARE TEAM

In addition to the health path, the other fundamental element in this area is the primary care team, which is composed of physicians, nurses, pharmacists, dietitians, and others. This unit will take responsibility for working with the member to manage health and wellness as well as chronic illness. Composition of the team will be based on member and family health needs, as well as member preferences. In many cases, the team will be virtual and change over time as the members' health needs change.

At the population level, similar approaches will be taken to maximize the health of various member segments. Taking into account variables such as geographic location, ethnicity, and disease state, IHEs will identify and manage health risks for specific population segments (e.g., employer groups, the elderly). This broad scope of health management will also include standard items such as well-baby visits, routine mammograms, annual physicals, blood pressure screenings, and immunizations.

Coordinating and delivering health services

Coordinating and delivering health services will focus on planning, mobilizing, coordinating, and delivering services across the care continuum in a timely manner. Key concepts in this area will include triaging members to the most appropriate care setting and resources, scheduling appointments, longitudinal case coordination, and referral management and coordination. These concepts, which are closely linked and highly interdependent with practices for managing individual and population health, do not merely focus on the clinical aspects of coordination, they are used in both health plan administration and care delivery components of an IHE.

Excelling at coordinating and delivering health services will require fresh engineering, or building from ground zero, as well as creative reengineering of certain processes. It will also be important to integrate subprocesses that were previously considered either administrative (e.g., referral management from the perspective of an insurance company) or care-delivery oriented (e.g., case scheduling within a provider setting). The end result will seem similar to some of those achieved in the financial services industry. During a single transaction, for example, a banking customer might expect a service representative or automated teller to provide information about a savings account, loan application, and investment options.

Healthcare management and coordination are perhaps the most visible areas where the concepts of seamless customer service come into play, giving the IHE an opportunity to develop brand identity and build customer loyalty. Some of the key concepts include

- Proactive coordination of visits, tests, and procedures, which is driven by the member's overall health path as well as episodic care paths

- Proactive resource management through the extrapolation of historic data, knowledge of scheduled events, existing in-house demand, and appropriate look-ahead factors (e.g., membership growth). Not only does this enable better forecasting of demand at the macro level, but it allows this information to be mapped against event-driven care paths to forecast microlevel demand (e.g., care hours, office visits)[4]

- Exception-based care management that includes two primary components: care pathing (i.e., clinical guidelines and protocols) and documentation and work management. The anchor tools will be episodic, longitudinal, case-based care paths that include all required administrative and clinical interventions and expected outcomes on a daily basis (sometimes more frequently). Care paths will feature built-in quality indicators, referral guidelines, copayment and preauthorization requirements, and other administrative and clinical requirements

Care paths already developed for inpatient populations will continue to focus on effective management of patients through hospital episodes, taking into account both cost control and clinical outcomes. However, these paths should be viewed as components within longitudinal care paths that focus on the entire episode or event of care and ensure care is provided in the most appropriate manner. For example, while most hospitals try to continue to focus on reducing length of stay, there are certain cases in which it may be more cost effective, as well as clinically appropriate, to extend the inpatient stay rather than moving the patient to a skilled nursing facility or home-care setting. Similarly, longitudinal care paths will focus on minimizing the need for acute care services entirely through more aggressive health maintenance and improvement activities. These types of analyses, as well as various potential treatment and care-setting options, will be available through longitudinal care paths.

LONGITUDINAL CARE PATHS

In many cases, hospital inpatient care paths will be extended to include pre- and postacute activities. For example, care paths for joint replacement patients will begin with the initial exam in the surgeon's office and move through the operating room, inpatient unit, rehabilitation, home health, and back to the surgeon's office for follow-up visits and monitoring. The care paths essentially will become a comprehensive road map or work-management tool, guiding the activities required for a patient encounter.

These longitudinal care paths will include all appropriate clinical and administrative activities (e.g., precertification requests, and referral authorizations) and be based on both clinical guidelines and the member's health plan specifications. Consequently, many current administrative checks and authorizations will be handled on an exception-only basis, reducing nonvalue-added activities and enabling the identification of variations in treatment and administrative activities as they occur on a real-time basis. Care paths will also enable members and their families to take a more active role in managing their own care, as well as enabling associated network providers to play a more informed and integrated role.

SERVICE DEPLOYMENT

Effective care management will also require IHEs to rationalize programs across their delivery networks to reduce costs, enhance service, and improve clinical outcomes. At the IHE level, services will be distributed based on demographics and needs of the population in various service areas. The strategies may include establishing centers of excellence—particularly for technology-intensive services such as cardiac surgery and joint replacements—and consolidating administrative, clinical, and support services within the healthcare delivery system. Patient-focused, care-based reaggregation (i.e., grouping of like patients) will continue in both the inpatient setting and in other care delivery settings.

Similarly, IHEs will redeploy services at the broad system level to the most appropriate and cost-effective point along the care management and delivery continuum. This will mean reorganizing services and responsibilities within an existing IHE or actually building out the care management and delivery continuum (e.g., skilled nursing facilities or ambulatory surgery capabilities) in the case of single providers.

CHANGING ROLES

To support the reengineered processes described above, personnel roles will change dramatically. A number of the traditional responsibilities of physicians, such as assessing and triaging members to care settings, will be transferred in part to nurse practitioners and other clinical professionals. Additionally, as care delivery increasingly moves out of hospitals, the concept of bedside care will be broadened to patientside or memberside care. Such a shift will require adjustments in the skills included within cross-training, as well as how various care delivery teams are configured.

One such configuration is longitudinal, case-based teams that assume responsibility for the care management and delivery processes throughout a complete episodic event. For example, Grant Medical Center in Columbus, Ohio, has established longitudinal care teams for joint-replacement patients. The teams include personnel from the surgeon's office, operating room, inpatient care, and rehabilitation unit. These individuals are multiskilled across various care settings to function as an integrated team across the continuum.

Two other types of multiskilled teams will be developed in IHEs. Customer service teams are currently being developed at a large Blue Cross Blue Shield plan. These teams will be responsible for working with members to respond to a comprehensive set of member needs and inquiries, including enrollment, authorization and referral questions, claims, and other administrative items. Additionally, account teams are being developed to focus on meeting the complete service requirements of employer accounts and other purchasers—from product design through servicing and support requirements. These teams will be cross-trained to provide seamless customer service and integrated clinical and administrative support to plan members.

Another related organizational concept is the use of general (i.e., float) personnel resource pools. As with most of the other elements discussed in this chapter, this concept applies across most care settings. For example, within an inpatient setting, a pool of workers who are cross-trained and multifunctional—advanced nursing skills, electrocardiogram, phlebotomy, respiratory therapy, intravenous therapy—could provide support across patient-care centers and various central departments. Similarly, systemwide float personnel might be cross-trained to provide services in multiple settings, including inpatient hospitals, clinics, and home health.[5]

Information technology will play a vital role in developing this capability. Members of the primary care and episodic case-based teams, as well as members themselves, will need on-line access to schedules, member health paths, episodic care paths, and other pertinent clinical and administrative information in a real-time, user-friendly manner.

Building and managing relationships

Most organizations within the healthcare industry have not focused intently on maintaining long-term relationships with key customers and suppliers. Change is happening, however, in many ways. Leading-edge IHEs are beginning to develop ways of strengthening relationships with customers, key suppliers, and other partners.

RELATIONSHIPS WITH PURCHASERS
AND INDIVIDUAL MEMBERS

Establishing relationships with purchasers generally begins with the negotiation and product design processes and, for individual members, during enrollment and registration. In the coming years, IHEs will begin to actively manage the relationship with accounts much earlier in the process. This change will be enabled by developing purchaser-focused processes and teams that work with account representatives from initial product design and continue through enrollment, service delivery, claims, and customer service. These teams will be able to meet a wide array of purchaser needs through the application of mass-customization techniques being applied in other industries. Consequently, IHEs will offer a variety of both standard and customized products that can be configured on demand.

Delivering this capability will require a nimble organization. Enabling technologies will include object-oriented processes within the IHE, as well as a virtual delivery network (i.e., based on contracts and relationships with various providers rather than owning and operating all aspects of the delivery process). To meet demand-driven product specifications, a highly skilled and flexible workforce will also need to be assembled, disbanded, and reassembled in teams on a just-in-time basis.

Purchaser-focused teams will work with accounts to identify population health needs and risks and to develop programs and interventions to improve the overall health of the account population. Specific attention will be paid to improving performance in areas such as employee productivity (e.g., lost work days and return-to-work time lines following acute-care episodes). Enabling this capability will be account-based report cards to track cost, quality, and service. In many cases, IHE compensation will be driven, at least in part, by performance and value delivered to the purchaser.

A further illustration of this emerging partnership is that IHEs will work with accounts to reengineer claims and other nonvalue-added activities across both organizations to simplify operations and reduce costs within purchaser and IHE settings. An example of this trend will be "claimless" capabilities enabled by sophisticated information technologies to track utilization against forecast targets and settle accounts periodically, perhaps quarterly.

From an individual perspective, the IHE will view each member as unique and focus on maintaining lifelong relationships with individuals. The health path and primary care teams will be important elements to strengthen these relationships. The health path will provide an opportunity for the IHE to involve members in defining individual goals and expectations upon enrollment, creating an interactive process of collaboration between the member and IHE. The individual health path will also enable the member to work with the IHE to design a customized product that satisfies a member's needs.

This will be an ongoing process facilitated by the members' and their families' active involvement in care management and will enable the IHE to "touch" the member in a more proactive, meaningful, and continuous manner.[6] The heightened interaction will be driven by the health path and include items such as prompts and reminders (e.g., appointments), periodic report cards on health status, information delivered directly to the member based on interests and needs, and direct data entry by members in clinical and administrative (e.g., scheduling) areas.

Rather than functioning as a gatekeeper, the primary care team will act differently. These teams will focus on improving the overall health of the members by helping them achieve specific health goals and continually managing the customer relationship. In this capacity, team members will act as coordinators, putting a high value on education and communication and including members as important partners in health management and care delivery processes.

IHEs will also make accessing health services easier by using technology to enable members to receive services at a variety of locations. Examples will include interactive access via personal computers and interactive television, automated telephone access, and other distance medicine technologies. These points of access will be supported by a seamless presentation and one-stop-shopping for information across all

IHE contacts. For example, members will be able to ascertain various treatment options and associated deductible and copay requirements with a single contact. Additionally, IHEs will create consumer incentives to participate in these processes and supply the tools necessary to do so.

RELATIONSHIPS WITH SERVICE PARTNERS

Managing provider and supplier networks is challenging because of many factors (e.g., organizational and legal structures and various relationships between health plan, provider, and supplier networks). In general, IHEs will continue to own at least part of the delivery network and outsource other delivery system components. In some cases, ownership may be limited to selected clinicians, while in others it may span a broader range of settings. In either scenario, many of the issues will be similar—driven largely by customer-service demands and the need to reduce costs and improve operational efficiency.

Part of the challenge in an increasingly virtual world is to manage the many transactions among the health plan and various providers. These transactions include admissions, referral requests, and benefit inquiries from the provider network to the health plan as well as referral authorizations, case management activities, payments, claim inquiries and responses, and eligibility and benefit quotes from the health plan to providers. It also includes various reporting and feedback mechanisms (e.g., outcomes, guidelines). When done correctly, network providers obtain better information that drives a continuous quality improvement process.

IHEs will address these challenges in a number of ways. Multiskilled teams of service partners, for example, could manage the overall relationship with key network providers and suppliers. They would function in much the same manner as the purchaser-focused teams described above and would be supported by innovative processes already in place at the IHE.

From a provider perspective, examples of these techniques include

- Episodic, longitudinal care paths that include both clinical and administrative protocols (e.g., referral and authorization guidelines). This capability will enable most transactions between IHEs and network providers to take place without intervention and to be handled on an exception-only basis

- Best practices repositories with replicable procedures for bringing new network providers on-line quickly and inexpensively

- Enhanced ability to supply responsive customer service to network providers through capabilities such as voice response (e.g., for basic provider inquiries, extended hours), customer service databases (e.g., for contact monitoring and analysis, process feedback, and improvement), and customer service team representatives

From a supplier perspective, these techniques include

- Prepackaged kits for most care episodes. Such kits, including required items for a particular member episode, will be based on standard care paths and patient-specific adjustments. This approach is inspired by the mass-customization concept in manufacturing, whereby products such as cars and apparel are ideally tailored for a "market of one." In health management, the scheduling of an encounter will generate a patient- and event-specific care path that, in turn, will route a request to the health services vendor partners for a prepackaged kit. The supply kit and medication kit will be prepared and delivered on a just-in-time basis. With bar codes for scanning, tracking, and updating, these kits will serve as the charge mechanism for fee-for-service payers and for IHE resource utilization and cost-accounting purposes. A resource management and scheduling system will be an enabler of this vision, providing up-to-the-minute information, thereby allowing personnel to anticipate resources necessary to care for patients prior to arrival

- Ongoing performance feedback loops to monitor and reports the accuracy and timeliness of vendor deliveries

- Extensive standardization for vendor products (e.g., implants, catheters, food items). Integration with care-pathing processes will help monitor outcomes associated with vendor products

- New arrangements in which traditional suppliers share the risks and manage segments of patient care. Patient care outcomes will be measured by these organizations and guide product development and care standards

- Full-scale vertical integration, from manufacturer to supplier to delivery site. For example, one manufacturer of joint implants plans to establish and manage orthopedic centers of excellence. These centers will own the entire process, from initial screenings in a surgeon's office to implant production. The implant will be custom designed, manufactured, and delivered within 48 hours to the surgical suite. The process extends to the inpatient unit, rehabilitation facility, and home care, with each step referring to best practices and standard protocols. The entire process will be integrated via longitudinal care paths and care teams. An outcomes repository will be maintained to update best practices and demonstrate the value to purchasers. In this situation, the manufacturer essentially owns both risk and profit opportunities by contracting directly with purchasers on a capitated or other prospective-payment basis. The manufacturer assumes both operational and financial responsibility for providing comprehensive joint-replacement services

Aligning services and resources

Effectively aligning services and resources in the future will require very different capabilities than those of today's IHEs. Several components will be required to fulfill this capability: resource management, medical strategies management, and virtual enterprise components.

RESOURCE MANAGEMENT

More accurate demand forecasting is essential to align services, equipment, and personnel in the world of virtual care. Proactively addressing this need will require a combination of historic utilization data, scheduled inpatient and outpatient activities, and look-ahead factors such as projected member growth and population trends. This information can then be mapped against individual care paths to estimate demand for office visits, hospital care, and other services. This type of aggressive demand forecasting will allow IHEs to more effectively balance supply and demand at all levels.

A significant portion of this forecasting will be related to nonscheduled events such as last-minute clinic appointments and emergency room admissions, which typically account for 30 to 50 percent of inpatient hospital admissions. While difficult to predict at an individual level, unscheduled events are relatively predictable over a population of members and patients. They can therefore be incorporated into resource-planning processes. The opportunities enabled by sophisticated information technology are considerable and will allow supply and demand to be aligned more closely in both clinical and administrative settings. The following examples illustrate the potential:

- *Inpatient.* A rolling, four-week look-ahead schedule and rough-cut capacity plan (e.g., care team time, rooms and beds, operating room, other critical resources) reveals that the orthopedic care center may encounter care team capacity and room and bed problems in 23 to 25 days. Such forecasts are based on already scheduled surgeries, anticipated admissions to the emergency room, and care path information. With this information, calls for requested surgeries can be scheduled prior to, or following, this potentially problematic window

- *Clinic setting.* The schedule shows that clinic volume for selected services will be low the following month. Primary care teams can identify members scheduled for routine visits during the next two to three months, contact members, and, assuming it is clinically appropriate as well as convenient for the member, ask members to accelerate their appointments

Combined with a flexible, cross-trained workforce, resource management will provide the IHE with advance notice to manage demand and staffing with the most appropriate and cost-efficient personnel.

MEDICAL STRATEGIES MANAGEMENT

This concept is interrelated with individual and population health management, as well as delivery of health services. The primary goal is to optimize outcomes (e.g., cost, quality, and service) through development and use of specific clinical strategies, including pathways and guidelines, prevention techniques, and behavioral changes. The techniques include all types of care paths, referral guidelines, case management, demand management techniques, and various credentialing approaches.

This process targets the ongoing improvement of managed care programs and policies, clinical practice, and overall guidelines for care management. Included are care paths, high-volume routine programs (e.g., wellness), benefits policies and medical technology, and practice guidelines. The information that is used as input will include IHE clinical and outcomes data, medical literature and research, and benchmark data. Some examples include

- Case management performed across the continuum of care (e.g. episodic versus encounter focused), which implies greater involvement of case managers in settings outside of acute care

- A shift from managing the member's benefits to managing the case. Case managers, for example, would make exceptions to the member's benefits as appropriate. A five-day stay in a skilled nursing facility might be preferable to keeping the member in the hospital, even though skilled nursing facility benefits may not be included in the member's health plan coverage. Similarly, it might be better to keep a patient in the hospital for several extra days beyond authorized coverage limits if the costs and quality (risk) issues of home care would exceed those of additional hospital days

- Demand management via aggressive and safe self-care programs. IHEs will continue to move toward empowering members to self-diagnose and treat minor ailments and address other medical questions and concerns. This development will be enabled by a combination of individually customized life care paths, as well as advanced call centers and automated member records

VIRTUAL ENTERPRISE COMPONENTS AND RELATIONSHIPS

In the coming years, IHEs will align supply and demand through virtual service capabilities, enabled by shared incentive relationships with providers and suppliers. These relationships will enable delivery of services without necessitating ownership of physical assets. This approach will enable IHEs to focus on continuously improving core competencies to distinguish themselves in the market and outsource other processes.

Managing information

The ability to effectively manage information will be essential to building and strengthening the previously discussed capabilities. For example, to manage health effectively it will be necessary to obtain and analyze health risk factors, goals, and objectives at both the individual and population levels, as well as to link these needs to various outcome repositories.

Coordinating and delivering health services will require a seamless flow and exchange of clinical and administrative information across the health services continuum—both in vertically and virtually integrated systems. Additionally, information technology is the catalyst to virtualizing health services delivery. This innovation will offer the well-known "faster, better, cheaper" equation to an industry that increasingly demands ease of access, quality care delivery, and cost efficiency. Likewise, the ability to build and maintain relationships at the consumer and account levels will require a robust consumer database and customer information systems to enable a deep understanding of and the means to respond to customer needs. And at the supplier-partner level, the ability to support virtual integration through shared information and well-aligned performance incentives will be enabled largely by technology.

Similarly, aligning services and resources in a virtual world will require advanced information technology capabilities in order to mass-customize products and services, as well as to configure demand response on a just-in-time basis. Underlying all of these capabilities is the need for industry-level infrastructures that enable member health records to be shared across multiple independent organizations in a consistent, seamless, real-time manner.

Path to the future

Third- and fourth-wave initiatives will be substantial in both scope and ambition. Change of this magnitude will not be successfully accomplished through traditional reengineering approaches and techniques; IHEs will need to adopt a more comprehensive and holistic approach to change. They will need a model that moves them beyond reengineering processes to fundamentally transforming their organizations (see Figure 7).

Most healthcare reengineering efforts undertaken thus far have focused largely on improving processes. There has been limited emphasis on supporting infrastructures such as information system and human resource architectures and even less on reshaping culture and behaviors. Transformational change requires considerable emphasis in all these areas, as well as in reshaping the strategic intent of an organization.

A framework exists to understand transformational change. The building blocks include strategy, process, and behavior, as well as information system, organization, and human resources architectures. While still relatively new to healthcare, this framework outlines how businesses in other industries have successfully achieved transformational change. The key components of this framework are

- *Refocusing strategic intent and response.* Frequently the first step in the transformation initiative, this process begins by clarifying or redefining overall organizational vision and includes two major elements: strategic intent and strategic response. Strategic intent is driven by an understanding of various customer and stakeholder needs, as well as having industry foresight that anticipates future discontinuities. This combination of understanding enables an organization to redefine the value propositions that it will take to market and the core competencies and capabilities it will need to fulfill this proposition

- *Reinventing processes.* Processes are reexamined and modified to ensure alignment with the vision, elimination of nonvalue-added activities, and full leverage of core capabilities to provide unique and enduring value. Additionally, embedded information technology

FIGURE 7
Business integration model

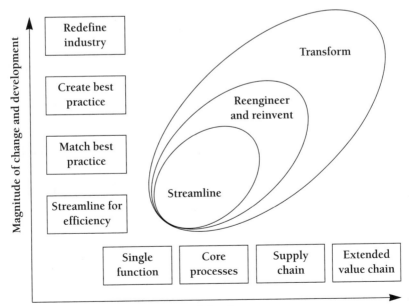

capabilities (e.g., exception-based processing) are defined and incorporated directly into process designs

- *Reshaping behavior.* Roles, responsibilities, jobs, and teams are designed and developed to support the vision and reinvented processes. Job and team design are performed in a manner that ensures alignment and consistency with core values and to support cross-team relationships

- *Rebuilding information architecture.* Two key elements are addressed: first, the application architecture, which includes all information systems and telecommunication applications, and end-user interfaces, as well as data, process, and user requirements; second, the technical architecture infrastructure, which acts as the glue bonding the telecommunication hardware, systems software, and computer networking hardware

- *Reconfiguring organization architecture.* The organization is designed and implemented to support reinvented processes and reshaped behaviors. Included are relationship maps, authority and decision-making structures, physical resources (including facility and equipment), communication channels, and business partnerships and alliances

- *Reorienting human resource management architecture.* This area is often neglected in major change initiatives. It includes recruiting and selection, training and development, performance measurement and appraisal, reward and recognition systems, and career pathing. It is highly related to the staying power of a transformation initiative and must reinforce desired behavioral changes

While each of these elements is discussed in discrete terms, they are highly related and interdependent. In fact, it is the dynamic and synergistic relationships between these various elements—when effectively aligned—that enable fundamental and sustainable transformation.

Conclusion

Organizations that already operate as IHEs—including providers, insurance companies, and managed care organizations—view cross-continuum reengineering and enterprise transformation as essential to maintaining marketplace success. Organizations, however, that are just beginning to establish networks and build their service continuum see these types of solutions as opportunities to leapfrog a generation of development and get it right the first time. In either scenario, health services industry leaders are beginning to recognize that transformational change is essential for success. They also know that change of this magnitude must be carefully orchestrated and include activities and interventions throughout all dimensions of the organization to be effective and enduring.

Rapid and pervasive change will continue to occur throughout the healthcare industry. The nature of this change is broad, transformational, and continuous, resulting in a radically altered landscape of the future—an environment where traditional boundaries and rules of engagement are no longer valid. These shifts are creating opportunities and challenges that will likely result in a new slate of winners and losers. But one certainty remains: by extending reengineering beyond the walls of an existing organization and across the entire health services continuum, IHEs will be better able to navigate the waves of change and emerge successfully in a transformed health industry.

NOTES

1. Based on the experience of Andersen Consulting's healthcare industry practice, such improvements have been seen across various reengineering measures, including inpatient base costs, ambulatory care costs, and various clinical quality indicators.

2. The term "integrated health enterprise (IHE)" refers to any organization that provides health services, whether those services include care delivery, health plan administration and insurance, or some combination.

3. This model was born in the Pacific Presbyterian Hospital in San Francisco.

4. The potential benefits in this area are discussed in greater detail in the service and resource management section that appears later in this chapter.

5. The float pool is an important input to the resource management processes described earlier.

6. Andersen Consulting's "Touch and Triage" refers to the ability to build and maintain relationships with individual members and guide them through a virtual system of health management and care delivery.

▚ 13

Applying Performance Engineering[SM] to medical care

Saad Allawi
Senior Principal
William M. Mercer Provider Consulting Practice
New York, New York

Brian Klapper
Principal
Mercer Management Consulting
New York, New York

Stephen Leichtman
Assistant Vice President, Organization Effectiveness
Tufts Health Plan
Waltham, Massachusetts

FOR THE PAST SEVERAL DECADES, healthcare providers have subscribed to the philosophy of providing "quality healthcare at any cost." But those days are now coming to an end. A growing industrywide trend toward managed care is forcing healthcare providers to reexamine their costs for the first time. Price discounting of 25 to 40 percent is now common nationwide. The average length of stay (LOS) in most hospitals is declining rapidly, and HMOs, formerly the bastions of moderately priced healthcare, are under considerable pressure to reduce their prices.

The gauntlet has been thrown down for healthcare providers: cut costs or suffer the fate of other consolidating U.S. industrial giants—bankruptcy, acquisition, or reduction of costs in an unplanned, haphazard fashion, resulting in significant layoffs and very low employee morale. Reducing costs is a daunting challenge to many healthcare providers, especially those whose markets require a substantial reduction in operating costs within the next three years.

This chapter on process redesign will serve as an operational road map for healthcare providers. As shown in Figure 1, process redesign is part of a broader performance engineering framework that allows companies to concurrently consider the scope of the project and its potential impact on the business. The scope of a performance engineering project varies greatly depending on the organization's requirements. Therefore, management must first determine the magnitude of the potential change. Performance engineering can be as focused as optimizing one process for a specific operation (e.g., treating the emergency room patients) or as broad as repositioning the entire enterprise to improve its competitive position (e.g., refocus hospital strategy to become the major outpatient surgery center for the region). This chapter details the methodology for process redesign for a moderate scope, moderate impact project that will reduce operating costs by 15 to 30 percent, maintain employee morale, and improve patient and stakeholder satisfaction.

FIGURE 1
Performance engineering framework

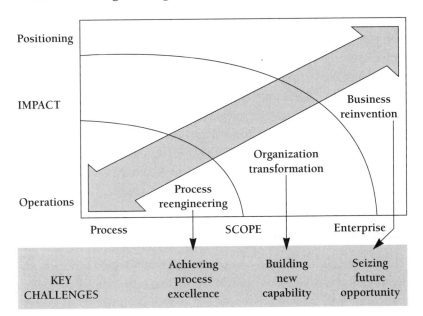

FIGURE 2
Framework for implementing process change

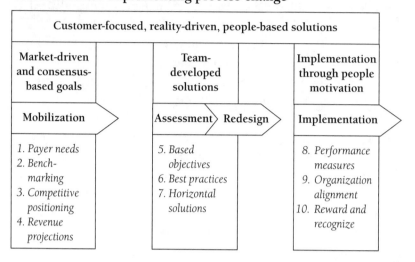

The process redesign methodology, as shown in Figure 2, can be conducted in four phases and is designed to achieve customer-focused solutions that are based on market requirements. The four phases—mobilization, assessment, redesign, and implementation—begin with a marketplace analysis to determine appropriate redesign goals. They end with a detailed step-by-step implementation plan that clearly defines activities, timing, and responsibilities. To ensure success, the organization establishes a transition team whose job is to manage the change process throughout the redesign effort.

The first step is to develop market-focused goals. These goals often include specific targets for cost reduction, cycle time improvement, LOS reduction, market share enhancement, and customer satisfaction improvement. While these goals are being developed, the transition team prepares the organization for the change. Throughout the process, the team works to focus the organization's talent to achieve the targeted operating improvements and to communicate the results.

Mobilization—setting the targets

The first stage of the process redesign effort is mobilization, which sets the overall objective and the pace at which the organization can achieve its goals. Here, a communication plan is developed to encourage employees to participate in the change process.

Initially, teams conduct extensive internal and external interviews to help the organization determine its internal customer requirements, payer demands, and competitive positioning. Within the hospitals, for example, internal interviews try to capture performance shortfalls and improvement ideas from all levels and departments. For the internal interviews, focus groups are used to facilitate the exchange of ideas. It is more effective to conduct individual sessions for different employee levels to promote a free exchange of views. This structure helps focus the participants to speak freely. The initial focus groups should concentrate on hospital staff most likely to make an impact, such as physicians, nurses, transportation, dietary, housekeeping, laboratory, pharmacy, and admissions.

While the redesign team and the transition teams are performing the internal interviews, the external team is assessing the local operating environment to determine current requirements, market status, and future trends. This includes payer mix projections, inpatient and outpatient trends, demographic trends, and competitive positioning. Interviews with local employers, physician groups, payers, and state governments also provide valuable insight into the changing nature of the healthcare market. The following case study from a large eastern academic medical center provides an example of some of the features of the mobilization phase.

During mobilization, joint medical center-consultant teams performed a comprehensive market diagnostic. One team performed a study that ranked 10 attributes viewed by the client as critical to success. These attributes were quality of care, patient satisfaction, type of hospital, price, hospital location, outpatient satellites, hospital-physician relationship, management information system (MIS) linkage, multihospital systems, and whether the hospital participated in risk sharing.

More than 50 interviews with payers across the country and in the local market enabled the medical center to conclude that quality of care, patient satisfaction, and price were the three most important features both across the country and in the local medical center's market. Paradoxically, although quality of care and patient satisfaction were critical features, they could not be quantified. Hence, price becomes the primary selection criterion on which payers base their affiliations.

Upon discovering that price was the payers' primary selection concern, the medical center administration needed to know how quickly it had to respond to the market's demand for lower price. The results of a

FIGURE 3
HMO penetration scenarios

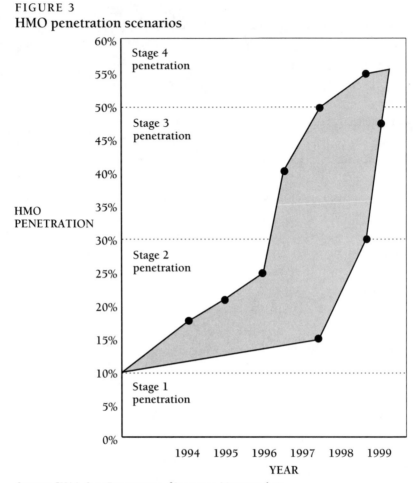

Sources: GHAA, State Departments of Insurance, Mercer analysis.

study projecting the speed with which managed care penetrates a local market is shown in Figure 3.

As the graph shows, there is a range of HMO penetration rates for a given market (represented by the shaded area). Each market has a different slope and thus a different managed care penetration rate. Table 1 shows the results of the case study whereby the mobilization team determined that its medical center was in an advanced stage of managed care penetration and that the market would have a 54 percent HMO penetration by 1999.

This analysis enabled the team to forecast the rate of penetration over the next five years. Once the team determined the rate of managed care penetration, it then performed a charge analysis that forecasted average

TABLE 1
Case study: Forecasted HMO penetration rate

Year	Projected HMO penetration
1994	17%
1995	22%
1996	27%
1997	41%
1998	50%
1999	54%

charges per adjusted discharge (as a proxy for cost) for different levels of HMO penetration. The team interviewed all payers (i.e., Medicare, Medicaid, commercial) from 12 managed care markets across the country and found startling declines in hospital charges as HMO penetration increased. Specifically, as HMO penetration increased from 15 to 25 percent, the average charge per adjusted discharge decreased from $12,000 to $5,000. The mandate for significant cost reduction was apparent.

A team then assessed the competitive positioning of the medical center relative to others in the area, analyzing average length of stay (ALOS) and cost projection. The analysis compared LOS for the medical center against two groups of local competitors for the medical center's top 10 diagnostic related groups (DRGs). The analysis enabled the team to determine whether the opportunity was driven by operating costs, treatment patterns, or both. Ultimately, the team found that for several highest-volume DRGs, there was a significant opportunity to reduce the length of stay by 20 to 40 percent.

The team then attempted to determine the interrelationships between the medical center's operational processes. The creation of an enterprise map for the entire hospital, as shown in Figure 4, enabled the teams to consider the hospital as a series of integrated processes that existed to support four "moments of truth." A moment of truth is any point where a customer (patient) has an interaction with a healthcare provider and comes away from that interaction with an impression about the quality and efficiency of the service provided. A "process" is a series of core activities that change inputs into outputs to meet customer needs. The processes classified as core (process categories into which all patients can be placed) include long-term acute care, short-term acute care, nonacute care, and academic support (e.g., education and training or research and development). Subprocesses, which transect the core processes, include patient transportation, billing and collection, dietary, housekeeping, and purchasing.

FIGURE 4
Hospital enterprise map

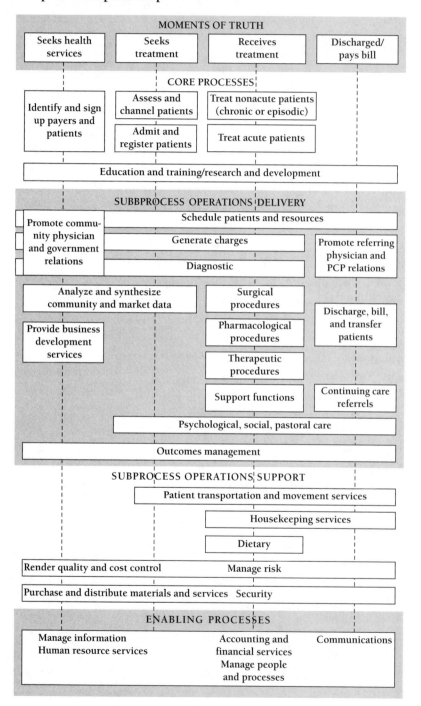

By viewing the hospital as a collection of processes, rather than as isolated departments, the team better identified processes for redesign that would have the greatest potential for overall cost reduction and quality improvement. Figure 5 shows an example of how the team allocated the labor resources to each of the core, sub-, and enabling processes to determine the extent of their operating resource consumption. The team worked closely with the controller's office to allocate departmental costs from the annual cost budget to the processes with which they were affiliated. The allocation enabled the medical center to view its costs as a set of processes, not departments, which more accurately reflected the ways in which costs behave. This allocation was then used as an input into the selection of the processes to be redesigned, with high-cost processes given a greater priority than low-cost processes.

Another tool that was used to help prioritize these processes was the importance/performance matrix shown in Figure 6. For a given process

FIGURE 5
Resource consumption (by thousands of dollars)

Subprocess	Allocated amount	Treat ambulatory patients	Treat emergency room patients	Treat inpatients	Percent of total
Perform diagnostic testing	$12,878	$2,833	$1,030	$9,014	7%
Perform surgical procedures	$2,493	$349	$0	$2,144	1%
Perform pharmacological procedures	$7,276	$1,746	$146	$5,385	4%
Perform therapeutic procedures	$7,780	$5,135	$0	$2,645	4%
Perform psychological, social service care	$840	$336	$84	$420	0%
Render clinical support	$6,955	$1,391	$696	$4,869	4%
Render patient transport	$1,477	$148	$175	$739	1%
Provide charging, billing, and collection services	$6,887	$827	$275	$4,408	4%
Render quality and cost control	$1,955	$293	$195	$1,271	1%
Assess and protect against financial and not-clinical risk	$148	$22	$22	$89	0%
Provide communication	$20,134	$3,020	$2,013	$13,087	12%
Provide accounting and financial services	$6,013	$902	$902	$3,608	3%
Coordinate processes and interfaces	$12,845	$1,927	$1,285	$8,350	7%

FIGURE 6
Importance/performance matrix (example)

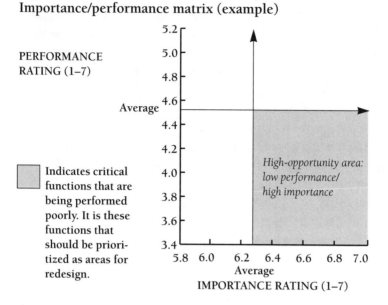

PERFORMANCE
RATING (1–7)

Indicates critical functions that are being performed poorly. It is these functions that should be prioritized as areas for redesign.

(e.g., diagnostics), the teams conducted interviews to determine how important each activity was to the overall process and how well the organization was performing that activity. Each process was given a score from one to seven; processes given scores of seven for both importance and performance indicated that the process was critical to the organization and that the organization was world class in its performance. This matrix enabled the team to visualize the entire process along these perceptual axes and ultimately focus its effort. For both the resource allocation and the importance/performance matrix, the team had to interview many people within the organization. It was therefore a critical step to educate the organization about the redesign effort and to allay employee fears regarding the impact of the potential change.

Throughout the mobilization phase, a transition team was dedicated to the process of change management. The case study team developed a plan to encourage all workers, managers, nurses, and physicians to become more involved with the effort. The transition team conducted more than 50 focus groups to measure the organization's attitudinal and cognitive readiness for change. The team also worked with the organization to develop a comprehensive communication strategy. The team found that most employees generally understood the concept of managed care and the need for change. Employees' fears focused on the potential impact on their careers and not on organizational change. In addition, the team found that most of the information circulated throughout the organization was done so by way of an informal grapevine. Most employees preferred that such critical news be communicated directly from senior management and be made available in print. This finding led the team to realize the importance of a communication strategy and the need to manage the informal communication process.

The communication strategy involved the creation of reengineering newsletters, an information hot line, suggestion boxes, informational videos, press releases, letters from management to the employees, and town meetings for the entire staff. Throughout the case study process, focus groups and employee questionnaires gauged the effectiveness of the strategy. The plan also included change management education for all levels of management. The education enabled management to assess organizational readiness for change, capacity to change, and the steps necessary to make the change happen smoothly.

The transition team's effort was vital to the project because it helped the organization generate ideas for improvement, provided a forum for discussion about change-related anxiety, strengthened the presence of senior managers as change leaders, kept employees feeling informed and involved, and created and maintained a feeling of openness. Transition management also mitigated the trauma associated with change, enabling the organization to view the change process in a positive, constructive manner.

After the case study mobilization, teams completed their analyses, one of the teams built an Interactive Strategy Model™ (ISM) to project future cost requirements based on the results of the interviews and analyses. The ISM is a computer-based forecasting tool that enabled management to enter their current cost structure and simulate various managed care scenarios. The ISM comprised many screens, each dedicated to one component of the business. Figure 7 shows some of the inputs to the model, including average length of stay, and departmental cost structures that build up to the inpatient costs. These inputs are then adjusted for projections in payer mix, charges by payer, patient volumes, LOS, price discounts, potential sources of revenue, and competitive positioning to yield revenue and expense forecasts. Management can then input required returns (e.g., return on sales) to determine what the revenue and cost structure must be to generate that return.

FIGURE 7
Sample Interactive Strategy Model output (by millions of dollars)

Inpatient costs			
	1993	1998	CAGR
Med	75.9	71.3	–1%
Surg	106.1	100.0	–1%
OB	24.5	23.0	–1%
Peds	31.8	29.6	–1%
Psy	15.9	14.8	–1%
Reh	8.9	8.4	–1%
Total	263.1	247.1	–1%

Return on sales

Variable cost				Variable costs				Fixed costs		
93	98	CAGR[1]		93	98	CAGR		93	98	CAGR
	By service				By service				By service	

Variable routine cost per day			Average length			Discharges			Variable annual cost per discharge		
93	98	CAGR	93	98	CAG	93	98	CAGR	93	98	CAGR
	By service			By service			By service			By service	

1. Compound annual growth rate.

During an off-site retreat, the project steering committee was able to work in real time to choose the most likely scenarios and project its required cost position. Management developed three future operating scenarios: a base-case scenario, which requires an annual cost reduction of 10 percent; an intermediate case, which requires a 20 percent annual cost reduction; and an aggressive case, which necessitates a 24 percent annual cost reduction. After extensive deliberation, the committee then chose the targets they wished to pursue. At the end of the session, the committee selected the intermediate scenario, and the cost reduction targets for the assessment phase were set.

Assessment—determining the opportunity

During the assessment phase, joint medical center-consultant teams worked to quantify the total potential cost reduction and service improvement opportunities by process. The following case study of work done with a 600-bed community hospital in the South will help illustrate the analysis performed during the assessment and redesign phases.

Initially, the teams created high-level process maps for each of the processes they were planning to redesign. The process maps included the department performing the activities on the left and the sequence of activities on the right. These process maps serve four primary purposes: definition of the process boundaries, determination of activities that constitute the process, assignment of customers (users) to the process, and allocation of costs to each of the activities within the process.

Interviews with the key customers of the process yielded additional insights into process problems. For example, in the diagnostic process map, the team identified four primary areas for further assessment, including order entry, patient tracking and scheduling, laboratory and radiology testing, and physician accessibility. Figure 8 highlights the measures used and priorities for these targeted diagnostic areas. To determine the potential gain from improving these areas, the teams conducted interviews, focus groups, and surveys to perform a gap analysis. As Figure 8 demonstrates, gap analysis is a comparison of customers' views of perceived performance compared to current actual performance and ultimately to customer requirements. Later in the assessment phase, after an extensive benchmarking exercise, the gap analysis was pushed a bit further to include best practice targets for all of the activities within the process map. This analysis led the team to develop "stretch" targets, pushing them to develop optimal processes.

Benchmarking is a critical component of process redesign. Typically, benchmarking includes extensive comparisons with other industries to help the team think "out of the box" and to learn how other businesses have dealt with similar issues. In the case study, the diagnostics team benchmarked its patient and specimen tracking and scheduling process against the package tracking and scheduling system of a world-class overnight package delivery company. The processes for the different industries were similar in that both are essentially highly complex, mass-volume delivery systems that require nearly error-free service. After the benchmarking, the team began to think about the applications for redesign, which included a zoning system for patient and specimen transportation and a computerized transportation tracking system that builds in accountability for each transportation event.

FIGURE 8

Performance measures and target diagnostic process

Priority level	Customer expectation	Performance measures
1	Good patient tracking and scheduling	Number of places that have to be called
2	Proper utilization of diagnostic tests and services	Standard performance (i.e., critical pathways, appropriateness standards)
3	Timely transportation	Delay time from request to patient arrival
4	Accurate orders	0% error rate
5	Quick STAT turnaround times	Average time in minutes until test result is received
6A	Accessibility to MD	Time in minutes to respond to page
7	Efficient MD interpretation of completed procedures	Daily interpretation of all completed procedures

After each process-design team completed its customer interviews, it assigned costs and times to the activities within the process, using an activity-based costing methodology. An organizational survey was then used to understand and analyze resource allocation by time spent per process step. This cost and time allocation enabled the team to begin quantifying the opportunities associated with improving or eliminating redundant and unnecessary activities. Assigning costs and times to activities also helped the team prioritize the areas on which it needed to focus in order to achieve maximum service improvement and cost reduction. Once costs were assigned to activities, the team performed a root-cause analysis to determine the origin of the problem. Root-cause analysis is complex and time-consuming but is essential to trace and understand the cause of the problem before it can be fixed. It is nearly impossible to redesign a process correctly without a complete and accurate understanding of all of the root causes that contribute to the process inefficiencies.

Throughout the assessment phase, the transition team continued to work with all organizational levels to help communicate some of the preliminary findings and to prepare the organization for future change. The team continued its focus groups to communicate the need for

Target performance	Perceived performance	Actual performance	Best practice	"Gap"
Single event (call or computer)	5–10 events	4 events	1 event	3 events
100% threshold	75% threshold	80%	100%	20%
15 minutes	30 minutes	20 minutes	10 minutes	>5 minutes
0% error rate	40% error rate	30%	<5%	25%
30 minutes	2 hours	41 minutes	20 minutes	>10 minutes
15 minutes	30 minutes	23 minutes	5 minutes	20 minutes
100%	75%	70%–80%	100%	25%

change in a managed care environment. All 3,000 hospital employees were told about the work taking place within the hospital and how it might affect them. These meetings occurred throughout the day—from early-morning physician advisory group meetings to midnight sessions with night-shift nurses, maintenance staff, and laboratory personnel.

The transition team also managed the shift in leadership responsibility from senior management to the department heads who participated in the reengineering training sessions. Separately, cross-functional teams developed "people strategies" to support the transition process. These strategies included career planning workshops, training sessions, and mentoring programs.

The final piece of the assessment phase was to develop a prioritized list of redesign opportunities and process targets as well as their potential impacts on the organization. Assessment, however, was only the beginning. For the targets to be attained, people within the organization were not expected to achieve performance improvement while operating within the old process. A new approach was established to reduce costs and improve service. Finally, all of the changes that were made during process redesign had to be consistent with the mission and the values of the organization.

Redesign—defining the solutions

In the redesign phase, the teams developed solutions to address the root-cause problems identified during assessment. The primary outputs from redesign were the new processes themselves, detailed cost/benefit analyses of the potential solutions, capital costs necessary for implementation, technology requirements, and finally organizational changes that must occur for the project to be successfully implemented.

Once the root-cause analysis was completed, the teams then delved deeper into the benchmarking module. During redesign, visits to other institutions (both within and outside of the healthcare industry) stimulated paradigm-breaking solutions. In one example, the team, exploring ways to improve bed turnaround time, visited a 10-minute automotive oil change service center. The team learned that the oil change shop's approach to cars was similar to the hospital emergency room's approach to patients. Since the oil change shop was measured on its ability to guarantee a quick turnaround time, it learned how to manage its labor force efficiently, move cars in and out of the shop, and document results. The visit gave the team readily implementable solutions to the hospital's problem of long waiting time, poor documentation, and substandard results.

In another example, a team analyzing the admission, discharge, and billing processes visited leading hotels and compared its processes to the registration, checkout, and billing system. The team learned how better to integrate reservations, room scheduling, billing, and discharge into one process by developing an improved preadmission process as well as an automated admission and discharge system connected to the billing system. Patients were then able to view their hospital bills from their rooms, sign the checkout form, and leave without going through the lengthy discharge process.

These visits generated ideas for significantly reducing patient waiting time, decreasing error rates, and lowering costs. Ideas for cross-training of staff came from visits to the baggage handlers at a major international airport. Baggage handlers are responsible for a variety of tasks including loading and unloading baggage, coordinating meal service, and performing a wide array of other duties. The team used the baggage handler training manual as a guide to create its own cross-training for hospital employees. Visits to best-in-class healthcare institutions were also used to find optimal solutions and help the buy-in process with employees.

Initial skepticism often yields to full support when teams can provide documentation of success in other institutions.

Benchmarking also helped to give credibility to some of the redesign solutions that the team had developed. In the case of the large community hospital, the teams identified $27 million in redesign opportunities, which represented approximately 30 percent of total operating costs. The following examples highlight some of the opportunities identified and approved by hospital management.

In a pharmacology process, the team reduced the number of process steps from 24 to 14, patient waiting time for medications by more than 50 percent, and cost by 14 percent. Some of the specific process improvements included: developing a unit-based pharmacist order-entry process, stocking required medications on the patient care unit, and achieving a more appropriate skill mix in the pharmacy by making better use of the pharmacy technician (see Table 2).

The diagnostic team identified cost-reduction opportunities of 30 percent and two hours per patient per day in cycle time improvement. Specific opportunities included implementing a centralized core lab concept that consolidated automated laboratory departments around machines and functions rather than around traditional laboratory departments; physical redesign of the diagnostic imaging space, catheterization lab, and gastrointestinal lab; streamlining diagnostic processes; implementing a one-call patient tracking and scheduling system to reduce the number of patient transfers per day by 50 percent; developing an automated

TABLE 2
Pharmacology process improvements

Eliminates need to tube MD order to pharmacy
Improves communication between pharmacist and nurses
Reduces physician callbacks
Eliminates 80% of unit dose medication process
Reduces drug credits by 80%
Eliminates daily narcotic counts
Reduces narcotic documentation time
Provides an up-to-date electronic medication profile
Reduces missing doses
Provides improved medication documentation and review
Eliminates the need for a floor stock cart and the associated maintenance
Provides immediate access to emergency drugs
Allows IV solutions to be maintained on the unit

order entry system; improved reporting of results; and using critical care pathways coupled with an expert diagnostic system to reduce diagnostic utilization.

The surgery team reduced cycle time by 130 minutes per patient per day and reduced cost by more than 17 percent. Specific changes included an improved surgery scheduling process, the development of preadmission testing, consolidation of surgical area entry points, improved use of operating room staff, and streamlined operating room processes.

The inpatient team identified a 32 percent cost reduction opportunity and significant opportunities for improved patient satisfaction. The improvements included developing a preadmission process; integrating discharge planning, case management review, utilization, and certification; reducing the number of steps in the admission process from 36 to 26; establishing a finance company to help reduce bad debt; reducing the number of days needed to issue a bill; streamlining the billing process (see Figure 9); decentralizing transportation department responsibilities, thereby improving efficiency; developing a patient-focused care delivery model; improving critical care bed utilization; and improving utilization of acute care days.

The information management team performed a comprehensive survey of the medical center's information systems capabilities, analyzing all hardware and software to determine its ability to meet the expanded requirements of the redesigned processes. The team found that the medical center had more than 1,000 databases, of which 75 percent were duplicative, and that these databases were largely unable to communicate with each other. Poor communication led to the inability to properly track patients throughout their stay; assign beds; schedule patients for tests, procedures, and, ultimately, discharges; and coordinate interdepartmental functions such as dietary, diagnostics, and billing. After completing the systems diagnostic, the team developed new systems that facilitated the changes to the pharmacological, diagnostic, surgical, and inpatient processes throughout the medical center. As a result, new systems were installed to link much of the hospital and enable the employees to adopt many of the changes recommended by the other process teams.

In addition to the process redesign, a restructuring team was engaged to manage a hospitalwide organizational restructuring effort. There were three primary objectives of the restructuring: align the organization structure to support its strategy, increase organizational effectiveness by determining optimal management processes and structures, and strengthen senior management leadership abilities.

The organizational alignment directly supported the hospital's ability to remain true to its mission statement, which was to provide the highest quality healthcare and be the first choice for patients and physicians in its region (see Table 3). The goal of the restructuring was to delineate operations instead of corporate structures and place responsibility and authority at the lowest appropriate employee levels. Increasing organizational effectiveness involved reducing or eliminating duplication of effort and standardizing the functional definition of managers, directors, and supervisors. This enabled the organization to arrive at the appropriate layers of management and spans of control (i.e., number of direct reports for a manager) and to ensure the organization developed sufficient support materials. Finally, senior management leadership had to be improved and the restructuring team needed to create a clear policy, easily understood and adaptable for future management staffing decisions. The team also had to develop and commit to an ongoing mechanism to establish accountability after these decisions were made.

TABLE 3
Structure should support strategy

Strategic initiatives	Structural components
• Provide ambulatory and outpatient care	• Become a lower-cost organization
• Provide emergency care services to the community	• Streamline decision making
• Be the first choice for both physicians and patients	• Ensure that information systems match strategic and operational needs
• Maintain or expand market share by ensuring that the hospital provides programs and services to meet patient needs in primary, secondary, and tertiary markets	• Provide a positive environment for physicians to work cooperatively with the hospital
	• Improve interdepartmental coordination
• Build upon hospital reputation while being sensitive to concerns about location	• Maintain effective leadership structure and communication mechanisms
	• Ensure that hospital resources align with changing patient needs and new payer programs

FIGURE 9
Billing process

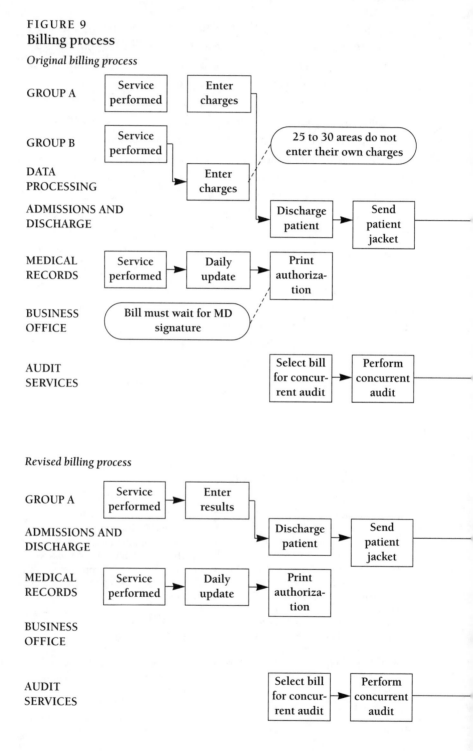

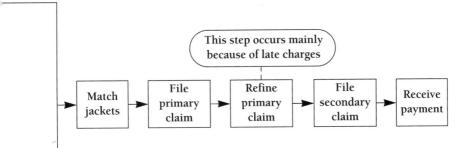

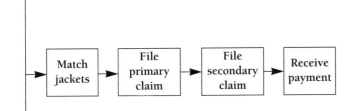

The specific structural objectives of the effort were to

- Develop consistent manager-employee ratios across the organization

- Determine the right number of employees to reduce unnecessary work and to ensure that jobs would be meaningful

- Eliminate or minimize duplication of effort

- Standardize functional definitions of managers, directors, and supervisors

- Develop appropriate levels of management based on organizational analysis

- Develop materials to support organizational redesign effort (e.g., education, training, and counseling services)

The restructuring team performed a comprehensive organizational survey completed by all employees. The survey focused primarily on how each employee spent the day and the structure of the employee's reporting relationships. Three primary measurements were calculated—the amount of time each person spent performing job tasks, the reporting relationships for each employee, and the types of tasks that they performed. The team then quantified the value of eliminating rework, reducing organizational layers, increasing the time that managers spent performing management tasks (in contrast to execution tasks), and increasing spans of control.

In one hospital, an organization team determined that more than $9 million (equivalent to 377 full-time employees) were being spent to do work that either was performed elsewhere in the organization or that had to be redone because it was not performed properly the first time. Of the $9 million, $4 million of rework was performed in the nursing department, $2 million in lab records and radiation, and $1.3 million in human resources. The team then performed an analysis on the level of job fragmentation in the hospital, defined as a job encompassing eight or more different activities, no two of which added up to 40 percent or more of a worker's time. Fragmented work is often unfocused and unsatisfying and should be kept to a minimum. In addition, if jobs are redefined and fragmentation is reduced, an organization can reduce staff without reducing productivity.

Table 4 shows the results of the job fragmentation analysis. The

TABLE 4
Fragmented jobs

	Department	Number of jobs	Number of fragmented jobs	Percentage of jobs fragmented
Manager profile	Nursing	62	21	34%
	Human resources, finance, executive	85	5	6%
	Other patient care	122	14	12%
	Total managers	*269*	*40*	*15%*
Worker profile	Nursing	1,290	419	33%
	Human resources, finance, executive	496	5	1%
	Other patient care	853	31	4%
	Total workers	*2,639*	*455*	*17%*
	Total company	*2,908*	*495*	*17%*

restructuring team calculated that 17 percent of all jobs were fragmented, a relatively high number for a typical organization. The team also found that the hospital had seven layers of management, which led to multiple meetings for even the smallest issues (e.g., 12 people were required to decide whether kale should be placed under the cake in the cafeteria). Employees at the lower levels of management were often frustrated by their lack of authority and the slow decision-making pace. One goal was to reduce management layers from seven to three or four.

The food and nutritional services department itself contained five management layers under the chief operating officer. Three directors, a manager, and a supervisor led the organization to low employee morale, high costs, and several management meetings to resolve even simple issues. As a result, the low- and mid-level managers did not have clear job definitions, which led to confusion and dissatisfaction. As a result, there was poor information transfer within the department, a lengthy decision-making process, poor customer service, and high costs.

When hospital managers were asked how much time they actually spent managing, defined as coaching, counseling, appraising, directing, training, measuring, and planning the work of the unit, they were startled to learn that only 41 percent of their time was spent performing management tasks, and of that 41 percent, 8 percent was spent performing support or indirect work. Of the 59 percent of the time not spent managing, 23 percent was spent performing secretarial and administrative tasks. Managers realized that they were not delegating responsibility sufficiently, a finding that was reinforced when the team analyzed spans of control. Spans of control are the number of direct reports each manager has. Appropriate spans of control indicate that the organization is appropriately delegating authority and empowering its lower levels of employees. In the case study, the organization team found that the average span of control was 7.3 and that if the medical center were to adapt its average span of control for all departments, which was 14.4, it could save over $4 million annually and create more rewarding jobs for both managers and employees. Finally, the restructuring team valued the potential savings from broadening the average span of control, eliminating rework, and eliminating job fragmentation. As Figure 10 shows, more than $15 million could be saved by focusing the workload and improving the organizational structure.

During the implementation phase, the restructuring team led senior management through a series of workshops to help them develop the optimal structure and realize the potential value.

Implementation—making it happen

In the implementation phase, the teams continued to work closely to ensure that the changes identified in the redesign phase occurred in an efficient, timely manner. During the initial phase of implementation, management assessed the organizational, financial, technological, process, and strategic impacts of the redesign recommendations. This assessment resulted in modified budgets, development of training programs, purchase of information systems and other new technology, and writing of job descriptions. The team also worked to develop appropriate management tools and systems to support the processes. Roles and responsibilities for departments and position categories were created, and compensation systems modified to align with the new tasks.

Finally, a detailed implementation plan and timetable were written that assigned responsibilities to specific individuals to ensure a timely completion. Figure 11 shows a time line of the rollout for all of the redesigned processes. In the implementation plan itself, several pages were dedicated for each activity that listed the activity, tasks required, timing, expense, capital required, expected annual savings, performance measures, and roles and responsibilities of those expected to execute the changes.

Redesigning healthcare processes

The process redesign techniques outlined above are an effective means to improve the efficiency and effectiveness of marketing, administrative, and back-office functions of healthcare providers or payers and to improve the direct delivery of healthcare services to the patient. As healthcare providers and payers come to the realization that they must improve their performance and processes—or else risk being outdistanced by their competitors—they are searching for ways to streamline and redesign activities throughout the organization.

FIGURE 10
Potential cost savings from focused work and improved organization structure

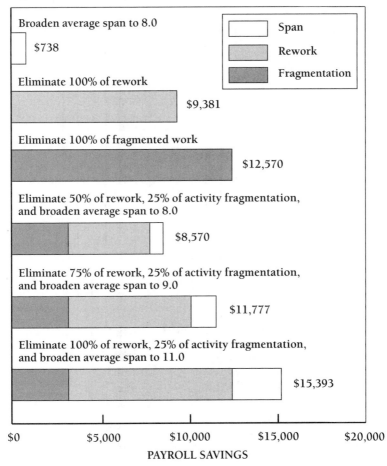

FIGURE 11
Implementation time line

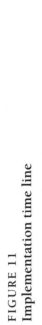

For example, a fast-growing family of managed care companies (including an HMO and a point-of-service plan) with more than 500,000 members, more than 1,000 employees, and annual revenues exceeding $500 million reengineered its claims, customer service, case (new or renewing group) installation, and provider development, installation, and servicing processes. The HMO's approach originally involved a survey of customers to determine which process changes or improvements they valued most highly. An enterprise map of all the organization's core processes was then created, resulting in a prioritization of processes for reengineering.

The goal for claims processing was to reduce costs and enhance turnaround time. Some of the problems identified included multiple access points for customer inquiries, resource-intensive claims processing, and lengthy processing and payment cycles. Work began on this project with the formation of cross-functional teams (mobilization) and proceeded through a process mapping stage. The mapping typically included determining the process participants and steps, calculating the cost and time to perform each activity, and calculating the total cost and time for the entire process. The team assessed the data collected during that stage and recommended a set of redesign efforts to address the functional inefficiencies it discovered. Through these efforts, the HMO was able to redeploy 27 percent of its data entry staff and 17 percent of its claims examination staff. It also found a way to discontinue the use of a data-entry service bureau, which eliminated a major source of handoffs and rework.

Just as important, turnaround time was greatly accelerated. The percentage of claims entered within seven days of receipt grew from 65 percent in 1993 to almost 100 percent the following year, thereby allowing the percentage of claims paid within 21 days of receipt to increase from 60 percent in 1993 to 96 percent by 1994. Additional reductions in cost and turnaround time were anticipated as a new imaging system was brought fully on-line—another critical recommendation of the reengineering team.

The goal of the customer service portion of this reengineering was to provide one-stop-shopping for customers by setting up a single customer service telephone number, eliminating the need for call transfers and improving response time. This redesign relied heavily on benchmarking work to locate and define best practices, a determination of what the ideal organization structure would be, a review of telephone and related information systems, the evaluation and planning of human resources issues, and, finally, implementation. One of the outcomes was to consolidate member relations, claims, and enrollment customer service functions into a single unit. As a result, response time was improved by nearly 50 percent and the abandonment rate (i.e., caller disconnects prior to answer) was reduced from 10 percent to 4 percent within two years.

Case installation, which encompasses everything that occurs from the point of employer group sale to the newly enrolled members' receipt of their identification cards and benefit information, was a poorly performed function that required performance improvement. The goal of this project was to identify all systems required to provide new and existing members with correct information on their specific plan procedures and benefits in the most efficient and effective manner.

A redesign team, consisting of members from all departments involved, assessed existing performance and developed redesign recommendations. The team was guided by a steering committee of senior management, whose role was to provide overall guidance and give approval of the team's recommendations. Other process participants provided specific expertise as required. The reengineering approach was to map all major processes, develop cost and time cycle data, identify gaps between customer needs and current performance levels, use team and subteam meetings to identify quick fixes and long-term recommendations, benchmark other HMOs, set design goals, and define requirements for the major systems enhancements and development.

Three primary themes emerged when all of the activities were mapped. First, the processes were far too complicated, which added to cycle time, costs, and employee dissatisfaction. Second, the teams seldom found an individual or team that was accountable for a process from beginning to end, which hampered the organization's ability to focus on the customer. And third, simplifying steps and clarifying responsibilities increased the organization's ability to meet the needs of its customers. As a result of its work, the HMO has been able to outline its ideal process and has developed a comprehensive implementation plan. Elements of this plan included an electronic communication system to eliminate paper forms, decrease cycle times, and improve internal distribution. The plan also included a centralized management, production, and distribution system that improved the quality and utility of the information provided to customers.

Conclusion

There are countless methods an organization can select to institute a change process. However, a few basic rules must be followed to ensure organizational success. Employee involvement must be active throughout the process. Change cannot be done to an organization; it must be done by the organization. When reengineering engagements fail, it is usually because employee support was never established. The best method to obtain employee support is open, honest, and frequent involvement and communication. Even though the employee grapevine will continue to function, formal communication is needed to provide not only answers, but also to establish the right context to many employee questions and concerns. This communication must come from top management; the employees going through the change must believe that management fully supports their efforts.

Finally, leadership and vision are required to gather and maintain support for the change process. The process is long and it can be tiring. However, if senior management empowers its employees, it will be rewarded by the tremendous growth of its people and the quality of their work. As one chief operating officer said following a redesign engagement, "I no longer have employees, I have marines. I never realized how much latent talent we had in this hospital. My job now is to continually find problems for them to solve."

Redefining the work of healthcare organizations

Tim Coan
President
Aslex, Inc.
Denver, Colorado

T HE CASE FOR ACTION no longer needs to be made. Dramatic change in how healthcare entities approach their work is a prerequisite for survival. The questions now being asked in every quadrant of the industry are "What should be done?" and "How should it be accomplished?" Many have realized that incremental improvement programs, even those that are successful, cannot keep up with the scope of marketplace demands. Now healthcare executives, previously rewarded for cautious management approaches, are looking to reengineering as a way to respond to these relentless market demands. Yet streamlining processes, enhancing efficiency, and developing cost-cutting strategies alone are not enough. Customers, redefining what they expect from the healthcare industry, are forcing industry leaders, and even survivors, to rebuild their operations to deliver new value, not just improve past practices and update old strategies.

This chapter outlines a methodology to transform an organization, offering specific steps along with lessons learned from applying this methodology in healthcare organizations. This approach incorporates three foundational aspects of transformation:

- Strategically rethinking the value delivered by the entire business

- Reengineering critical business processes to change how the work is performed and managed

- Changing the management context and the organizational culture to reinforce and sustain the change

Many in the industry, cognizant of the positive results of reengineering, question if this concept truly can be applied to healthcare. Others view reengineering as a pure negative and want no part of it. Unfortunately, the concept and label of reengineering have been thrown around loosely, often misused by consultants, organizations, journals, and the popular media. In spite of how the label is frequently applied, reengineering is "the fundamental rethinking and radical redesign of business processes to achieve dramatic improvements in critical, contemporary measures of performance, such as cost, quality, service, and speed."[1] Four phrases in this definition capture its essence:

- Fundamental rethinking is the start-from-scratch aspect of reengineering. The success starts with rethinking both the overall value the organization delivers to customers and the specific processes to be reengineered

- Radical redesign implies creative and possibly unorthodox ways of executing work, but more important is the connotation of radical that means "core" or "foundational." The redesign aspect of reengineering goes beyond surface changes and examines why the process exists, what it is expected to produce, and entirely new ways of delivering the outcome

- Business processes are collections of activities that, when taken together, produce a meaningful outcome, usually for an external customer. In reengineering, business processes are driven by the strategy and they in turn drive everything else about the organization

- Dramatic results are more than a hoped for outcome. Those who are serious about reengineering know that while many projects fail, it is impossible to produce dramatic results with a limited and safe scope. Large and significant pieces of the business are the focus and the goals are bold and ambitious

Case example: Catherine McAuley Health System

A discussion of the recent reengineering experience at Catherine McAuley Health System (CMHS), Ann Arbor, Michigan, will be used as an example in parallel to the in-depth discussion of the methodology.

CMHS is a large community healthcare system owned by the Sisters of Mercy Healthcare System in Farmington Hills, Michigan. CMHS consists of 1 large regional tertiary hospital, 2 community hospitals, and more than 12 outpatient facilities. CMHS is a $400 million system with almost 1,000 licensed beds, 200,000 inpatient days, 635,000 outpatient visits per year, and more than 4,600 employees. During its reengineering effort, CMHS signed a joint operating agreement with Providence Hospital in Southfield, Michigan, a 459-bed facility owned by the Daughters of Charity National Health System in St. Louis, Missouri.

Reengineering facades

Before exploring the steps involved in transformation, it is helpful to sift through the myriad of approaches currently running under the reengineering banner, but which are clearly something else (Table 1).

First, due to the frenzy associated with reengineering, many old methods have been repackaged as reengineering for marketing purposes. Executives want to buy it, boards want to support it, and consultants want to sell it. Yet program after program, now labeled as "reengineering," is nothing more than downsizing or team building or information systems development or simple basic management decision making. Many organizations say that they have been doing reengineering for years, yet very few have taken a start-from-scratch, process-oriented look at their business. While there is no one standard definition, care should be taken that reengineering-level outcomes are not expected from an "old wolf masquerading in sheep's clothing."

Often, selected aspects of reengineering are used, producing meaningful but limited results. A frequent example in healthcare is staff cross-training. Building broader jobs that take on more responsibility is often part of a reengineering solution. Yet to simply train employees to do

TABLE 1
Masquerading as reengineering

- Old ideas with new label
- Selected aspects of larger concept
- Streamlining and process redesign
- Process change without culture change
- Redesign without fundamental rethinking

another job with no change to the fundamental design of the larger process is not reengineering. Again, there are benefits to be gained, but they are usually not significant.

Many organizations view reengineering as nothing more than a better version of the cost-cutting mousetrap. Existing activities can be redesigned and streamlined for efficiency. Though many organizations have learned firsthand that redesigned work usually operates at a lower cost, the essence of the value delivered to customers remains unchanged. Such a narrow approach leaves behind the major benefits that come from completely rethinking the business.

Another common flaw occurs when redesigning work is done without addressing the surrounding organizational culture. Process changes alone result in temporary improvement spikes, but the organization quickly migrates back to the old status quo. Conversely, isolated attempts to change an organization's culture, either through empowerment programs or team-building efforts, fail to produce business results because nothing is changed about how work activities are done.

The major problem with many so-called reengineering efforts is that redesign is completed without the fundamental rethinking upfront. Where there is any rethinking, it is limited to the confines of the activities being redesigned, not the broader issue of how to deliver more value to the customer. Consequently, many organizations end up with an improvement, but something that delivers much less than dramatic results. For example, many hospitals have been involved in implementing the patient-focused model of care. While this has produced many innovative ideas and challenged longstanding conventional wisdom, most efforts have been limited to delivering nursing and ancillary care on an inpatient unit. Thus, this model does little to prepare the organization for the continuing decline in hospital utilization, much less build new capabilities required for an integrated health system.

Principles of transformation

The methodology outlined here is built the following principles (Table 2) that represent critical factors for successful transformation.

TRANSFORMATION IS A HIGHLY STRATEGIC EFFORT AND THEREFORE MUST BE ACTIVELY DRIVEN FROM THE TOP. As with every other important change effort, transformation requires top management support. The difference

TABLE 2
Principles of transformation

- Strategic effort driven from top
- Bold effort, not reswizzling of status quo
- Strategy drives processess that drive everything else
- More than restructuring or streamlining
- Combination of innovation and change management
- Changes to strategic framework, system of work, and culture
- Effort requires disciplined approach
- Cannot be done by an outsider

with transformation is that support alone is not enough. If this is about recreating the organization, senior leaders should be actively involved throughout the process.

The CMHS project had extensive executive involvement throughout all stages. In the beginning, the chief executive officer, the presidents of the three hospitals, the vice president for patient care and human resources, and the chief financial officer spent several day-long work sessions framing the effort. The executives wanted to make sure this effort was aligned with other initiatives such as hospital-physician integration and community health programs that were part of the transition to an integrated system. A vice president, who is also a physician, was taken off-line for two years to lead the effort on a daily basis. Senior executives from Mercy's corporate office were involved all along the way as were executives from the medical staff. Throughout the project it was clear that management not only endorsed the project but also was involved in the design, decision making, communication, and rollout.

In the beginning, new strategic directions will be defined. As the effort progresses, the entire equation to deliver value to customers will be recreated. Finally, massive change will be implemented, causing disruption for employees and customers. Unless a leadership team is willing to devote a significant amount of time to the effort from beginning to end, transformation will not occur and should not be started.

TRANSFORMATION IS A BOLD EFFORT, NOT A "RESWIZZLING" OF THE STATUS QUO. What begins as transformation often drifts back to incremental improvement. Immediate operating pressures reduce the vision of the transformation in search of short-term gains. Political hurdles can cause management to back off of innovative ideas that will upset existing power bases, either around clinical disciplines such as nursing or a section of the medical staff or a department head who controls critical resources. Other initiatives compete for the time and attention of senior management causing the transformation to shrink by default. If transformation is to succeed, there must be a deeply held belief that the current system of work, while successful in the past, will not work in the future. The extent to which the organization bets its future on the transformation greatly influences the boldness of the stretch.

Given its intent to build a broad-based community health system, CMHS decided that how clinical information was managed across the entire system was going to be a critical success factor. The intent behind the first project was to fundamentally change the way care was delivered to patients by changing the way information was used, both between caregiver and patient as well as from caregiver to caregiver. In fact, many people in the organization would now argue that managing clinical information is now a primary business of the institution, not just a support activity.

TRANSFORMATION STARTS WITH THE BUSINESS STRATEGY THAT DRIVES BUSINESS PROCESSES THAT DRIVE EVERYTHING ELSE. Many approaches to change work on a discrete area such as the organizational structure, marketing approach, cost accounting system, performance evaluation system, or customer relations. Transformation begins with a view of how the organization will compete in the future environment. Once a strategic direction is established, the activities necessary to execute that strategy can be defined and built. Only then can everything else in the organization be put in place. With this thinking, the organization is rebuilt with a zero-based mind-set, evaluating decisions against the test of whether it adds value to the customers.

For CMHS, its decision in the mid-1980s to move from a stand-alone hospital to a vertically integrated community health system was the driving force behind all reengineering discussions. Clinical information management was seen as the process that united hospitals, physicians, health plans, acute care facilities, preventive care programs, and all other aspects of the system.

TRANSFORMATION IS DIFFERENT FROM RESTRUCTURING, REORGANIZING, DOWNSIZING, AUTOMATION, OR STREAMLINING. As reengineering has become a popular concept, loose use of the term has caused confusion about what is actually involved. While many existing concepts are incorporated into reengineering and transformation, there is a difference. Rather than attempting to somehow improve the existing system of work by changing some part, transformation puts everything on the table in light of the coming demands on the organization. Organizational changes, new information systems, and new policies should be driven by the new business requirements, not ends unto themselves.

From the beginning, there was an expectation at CMHS that some elements of restructuring, reorganizing, downsizing, automation, and streamlining would all occur. However, specifics in these areas were not discussed until the design of the work processes began to take shape. Unlike most reengineering efforts, the information technologists did not directly participate at CMHS until a conceptual process design was developed by clinically oriented personnel. In the final design, there were many types of change, but each was positioned as part of the larger transformation.

TRANSFORMATION REQUIRES THE UNIQUE COMBINATION OF INNOVATION AND CHANGE MANAGEMENT. Two apparently conflicting ideas have to be managed for a successful transformation. First, innovative ideas generally come from a relatively small group of people working in a politically protected environment. New ideas represent changes to organizational power bases because roles are redefined and control of resources shifts. New roles, especially those that put people in charge of entire processes such as patient access or clinical information management, instead of functional departments, such as admitting or medical records, require new and generally broader management competencies. With these changes, the very definition of organizational and personal success is turned on end. Thus, if the creation of a new system of work is the responsibility of the entire organization, incremental improvement, not innovation, is most often the result. As has been said, "change has no constituency." On the other hand, for such a change to be implemented successfully, a critical mass of the organization must embrace and support the change. This is best done by allowing staff from all levels in the organization to participate in the process and the conflict. In addition to a methodology designed to bring these ideas together, strong and active leadership involvement is required to manage the conflict or the balance will tip too far one way or the other. A highly innovative design that is not accepted, or an incremental design that is accepted, produce the same marginal results.

In the first half of the CMHS project, direct staff participation was limited as senior executives rethought the business and the reengineering team developed a new vision for the work processes and infrastructure related to clinical information management. In the second half, many staff members from across the organization were involved to work out the details of the vision and implement the changes. Leaders of the transformation must be able to make the shift from one context to the next.

TRANSFORMATION COMES FROM CHANGING THE STRATEGIC FRAMEWORK FOR THE FUTURE, THE SYSTEM OF WORK, AND THE SURROUNDING CULTURE OF THE ORGANIZATION. Many approaches to transformation tend to focus on either strategy (e.g., markets served, competitive positioning, resource allocation, and strategic alliances), hard issues (e.g., organizational restructuring, work flow, and information systems), or soft issues (e.g., team building, empowerment, compensation programs, and communication), often to the detriment of each other. For genuine transformation all three must come together, although there is an appropriate way to approach the integration.

The new strategic framework must lead because it establishes how the organization defines itself and the surrounding industry. From that new framework, the system of work (i.e., how work activities flow, how information is moved and used, how organizational boundaries are defined) is next because it is this system that delivers value to customers—the reason a business organization exists. Then the management context and organizational culture can be built to support and facilitate the new strategic framework and system of work. While the system of work creates value for the customer, the way an organization is managed and the resulting culture delivers much of the value to employees. Though there is a hierarchy in terms of which components drive the transformation, all are equally important. Unless they are aligned, changes will not last.

TRANSFORMATION IS A COMPLEX EFFORT THAT REQUIRES A DISCIPLINED APPROACH. While there are a variety of approaches to large-scale change, to undertake such an effort without a clear plan of action can mean failure.

Too many companies launch early activities without full consideration of all of the steps required. To be unclear about how the new world will be created and how the transition will be managed is impulsive.

The CMHS leadership team spent a good deal of time studying the approach to be used and the commitments that would be required of the organization. Because of the demands of other challenges already under way, the reengineering project was not launched for six months after the initial strategic work was completed. This allowed the organization to "clear its plate" so that the project could receive the care and attention required for success.

TRANSFORMATION IS ABOUT CREATING THE FUTURE AND CANNOT BE OUT-SOURCED OR DONE BY AN OUTSIDER. Real transformation means redefining the rules of the organization and potentially the industry. It is more than a program or a plan. The vision for the future has to be developed and implemented by the organization. An outside partner can provide guidance through the process, offer a structured approach, teach and coach new skills, provide objective feedback, develop ideas for consideration, and challenge the status quo. However, an outside partner cannot and should not drive the process, impose their ideas, or make key decisions along the way. A corollary to this principle is that the role of a consultant should be carefully defined. Many successful organizations advise against undertaking such an effort without an outside partner. Each of the functions listed above is necessary for success and it is as difficult for an organization to do it alone as it is for a physician to provide their own personal care.

CMHS made all of the decisions at every phase of the project, and all work that will be described below has been completed by CMHS personnel. Consultant support was limited to one person on-site only a few days per month. The consultant provided only the support listed above to executive management and the reengineering teams.

Transformation methodology overview

This approach to transformation integrates three complementary ideas: development of a new strategic framework, reengineering key processes to change the system of work, and rebuilding the management context and organizational culture to support the other two. Though there are certain steps and activities that clearly relate to one of the three ideas, the intent of the methodology is to intertwine all three, forming a multidisciplinary platform for transformation.

The strategic framework articulates the organization's basic assumptions about the industry's future and how it expects to compete in the coming years. At the heart of the framework is where and how the organization is going to add value for its customers.

Once a new strategic framework is developed, the system of work itself can be reengineered. This involves the redesign of many things: how the work flows, how activities are executed, who does what, the information that is used along the way, the organization's structure, the skills of employees, and even the layout of the physical infrastructure.

There are several ways to approach changing the context within which the work is performed. First, simply recrafting the strategic framework changes the rules of engagement for employees. With the shift to community-based care comes the rise of primary care providers in a world long dominated by specialists. Investments that traditionally went to high-cost equipment now go to buying or growing primary care practices. The management of chronic conditions becomes as important as heroic episodes of acute care. New careers develop, such as case managers, while others diminish.

Second, a new strategy and system of work demand a new way of managing the business. Work groups, traditionally organized around functional disciplines such as nursing or finance, are built around broader processes and result in staff with diverse backgrounds working together on the same team. Jobs become broader as employees perform tasks that were formerly spread across many people. Human resource practices are changed to reward new behaviors. Instead of just building deep technical skills, training aims to create an understanding of how the entire system works together. Costs and revenues are tracked and reported by process instead of by old cost centers. What is measured, discussed, evaluated, and rewarded all changes.

Third, it is impossible to truly reengineer a major business process without changing the culture. A major feature in the CMHS design is a single integrated patient chart in lieu of the professional segmentations in the existing chart. This was not approached as a ploy to change the culture but was determined to be the right thing to do. Such a process change will not only require a major culture change, it will also create it.

FIGURE 1
Transformation methodology

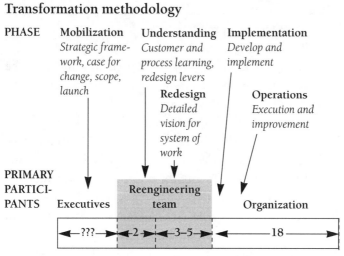

Time frame (months)

The methodology is broken into five major phases (Figure 1):

- Mobilization

- Understanding

- Redesign

- Implementation

- Operations

Each phase represents key milestones in the transformation process, and each operates with a noticeably different set of dynamics and issues. All three components of transformation are embedded along the way as appropriate.

Mobilization phase

The first phase of a transformation effort involves mobilizing the key leaders of the organization for change. This phase is the least structured of the five due to the nature of building commitment to a new but ambiguous venture in their minds. The end result of the mobilization phase is a fully launched transformation (Table 3).

TABLE 3
Mobilization phase: Key steps

- Begin transformation education
- Develop new strategic framework
- Develop enterprise process map
- Define reengineering project scope
- Develop synchronization plan
- Establish commitment to transformation
- Create case for change
- Finalize transformation staffing
- Launch project

While the results of each step are designed to build upon one another, organizations work through this phase in a variety of fashions. Often it is difficult to pinpoint when this phase actually begins because many individuals may be sensing the need for dramatic change, although a coherent idea of what should be done has not yet developed. Transformation rarely starts in a completely clean and deliberate manner but rather takes hold when disparate pieces of information and thoughts about where to go in the future begin to coalesce. At some point, a critical mass of leaders, usually executives but occasionally middle managers, share the belief that something needs to be done, even if they are not sure what it is.

The duration of this phase varies from several weeks to many months. How quickly an organization launches an effort depends on a variety of factors. The style of leadership and decision making, the degree to which there is a broad base of executive talent and not just a few carrying the load, and other strategic initiatives that are already under way all contribute to determining the pace of the mobilization phase. However, a collective sense of urgency seems to be the most important determinant. As expected, companies facing severe operating problems or pending strategic changes tend to move faster. On the other hand, those which are strong in terms of market position, operations, and financial performance usually move slower. This is largely due to the difficulty of coming to grips with the idea of abandoning what is working, and working very well, to build a new system that will work under tomorrow's rules. This psychological feat, as proven by IBM, Sears, and the big three automakers, is not easy for those who are currently enjoying success.

In spite of the popular trend toward innovation, many executives and managers still believe, whether publicly stated or privately held, that there is truth in the old adage "if it ain't broke, don't fix it." This is the first of many pitfalls since transformation requires just the opposite—a willingness to deliberately and intentionally dismantle systems while they are still working.

BEGIN TRANSFORMATION EDUCATION

A basic understanding of transformation and what is required is necessary before leaders can decide if it is the best course of action for their organization. Organizations should not go too far down this road without a grasp of the effort, difficulty, risks, costs, and steps involved.

Throughout the mobilization phase at CMHS, work sessions were interlaced with "just-in-time" education concerning the issues that would be faced (e.g., political resistance, synchronizing multiple efforts, managing the implementation), the amount of executive time required, the skills needed for various roles (e.g., creative design, business case development, project management), potential risks, and projected implementation costs.

DEVELOP NEW STRATEGIC FRAMEWORK

Meaningful transformation requires a new conceptualization of how the organization will provide value to its customers. Many organizations take the process redesign aspect of reengineering without the fundamental rethinking of what must precede it. There are many examples where companies are realizing "eye-popping" performance improvements. Process costs can be cut in half and cycle times can be reduced by 90 percent. Quality can be improved by an order of magnitude. But for all intents and purposes, the company is serving the same customers and meeting the same set of needs. Such improvements in performance are positive and can often be used as a basis to attract additional market share, but only for a time. These types of changes are the ones most easily replicated by competitors, making the competitive advantage transitory. On the other hand, companies that dominate over time are continually redefining the value that gets delivered to customers, reshaping the boundaries between their organizations and the customer, and rethinking their entire ways of working. These changes to the total relationship between the company and the customer are the kind that can set new minimum performance requirements for an entire industry.

For example, one health system reworked the admitting process at the hospital, reducing patient wait time by 75 percent and eliminating 50 percent of the forms to be signed. By contrast, another organization took a broader view of how patients access the entire system and eliminated asking patients for information previously gathered by employers, health plans, or physicians. The little remaining portion of admitting activities was performed in the physician's office or at the bedside. Not only was wait time and paperwork reduced even more than the first example, but a new value was also delivered. Before hospital-based care even began, the fact that no one asked the same questions over and over again signals to the patient that staff were working together—evidence of a coordinated health system that goes deeper than its marketing brochures. Changing the strategic framework completely reframes the reengineering effort from one aimed solely at gains on key operating measures (e.g., the time required to admit a patient) to one of creating new forms of value (e.g., giving the patient a seamless experience across multiple providers).

A new framework for the business is developed by examining changes in the environment that will require the organization to deliver different value in different ways. This step requires a series of concentrated discussions with the senior executives and other leaders who influence the organization. Changes to customer needs, competitor responses, new regulations, emerging technology, and new competitors must all be considered. The very basic assumptions about the business must be examined. A new view of how the organization will compete and add value will emerge from these dialogues. This vision will be expanded and fleshed out throughout the transformation as the organization develops a deeper understanding of what will be required in the future. Ten years ago, CMHS, long recognized as a premier provider of high-end tertiary care, shifted to a position that it would add value by improving the overall health status of the community. This new framework required a redirection of decisions, investments, and resources. Many people participated in the initial development of the new framework. At the beginning of this project, the top six executives of the system worked through the steps of the mobilization phase to identify potential reengineering projects. Additional people were brought in to help finalize the initial scope, staff the project, and get it launched. By way of contrast, other organizations have included as many as 40 to 60 people in this phase of the approach. Generally speaking, small groups move faster while large groups build a larger base of consensus around the new framework.

DEVELOP ENTERPRISE PROCESS MAP

Reengineering, as an approach to transformation, works with core business processes as the fundamental building blocks of the organization. It is through work activities, not organizational structures or information systems, that value is delivered to customers. To properly frame potential transformation projects, a map of the major processes that cut across the enterprise and their relationship to one another is developed. The map developed by CMHS has six major processes (Figure 2):

- Patient/member acquisition

- Health maintenance

- Health restoration

- Governance

- Resource management

- Continual learning

By way of example, CMHS defined patient/member acquisition to include activities such as managed care contracting and marketing since they each worked to influence the number of patient/members cared for

FIGURE 2
CMHS Enterprise process map

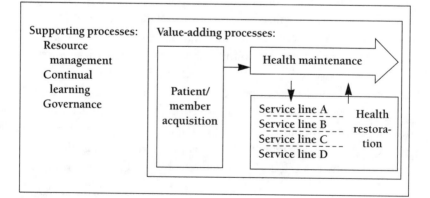

by the health system. Under their old functional-based organizational structure, each resided as distinct departments with distinct reporting relationships rather than under a single process owner.

To ensure clarity of the concepts portrayed in the first-level map for the team, each component shown is broken down into second-level maps. These maps reflect what is required to operationalize the vision of a vertically integrated system, not work as it currently exists. For CMHS, many of the processes existed in some form, though the performance might not be acceptable in the future environment or may not be geared to support a vertically structured healthcare system. Others, such as health maintenance, had limited activities operating in isolation, but nothing on the scale required for the future.

Processes come in three types (Table 4):

- Value-adding

- Support

- Asset building

Value-adding processes deliver an outcome that meets a need of an external customer. Counter to the movement that classifies everyone as a customer, that designation is reserved for those who consume or pay for the products or services of the organization. For example, activities that are directly related to a patient receiving treatment are value-adding, but verifying insurance and authorizing treatment is not.

Support processes do not add value directly but are necessary for operation of the business. Some are prerequisites for value-adding work in that they produce an outcome used in value-adding activities. For example, admitting falls within CMHS's health restoration as a sub-process. Patients do not come to a health system just to be admitted, so

TABLE 4
Process types

Type	Definition
Value-adding	Outcome directly satisfies a need of an external customer
Support	Outcome necessary but not valued by an external customer
Asset building	Outcome builds future capability:
	• Prerequisite for value-adding process
	• Required by an external stakeholder
	• Business prudence

there is no value added. However, the admitting steps produce outcomes required for direct patient care. Other support processes are required by external stakeholders such as regulators or reimbursement intermediaries. An example is the classification and coding of work done for billing purposes. Finally, processes like budgeting or maintenance are not required by value-adding steps or external stakeholders but are supportive because of the dictates of simple business prudence.

The final category of processes is asset building, such as continual learning in the CMHS model. These produce outcomes that will be used in the future as opposed to executing current operations. All of the things that work together to develop employees, from recruiting to training to coaching and feedback to career planning, are building a future asset—the competent workforce.

Processes in all three categories can take on one of two natures. Some are relatively linear in that they move from a logical beginning to end. Linear work flows are the easiest to recognize. Integrating processes, by contrast, are more ambiguous in that they usually cross several linear processes and synthesizes multiple outcomes.

While there are no rules for the number of processes that should be on an enterprise map, a few guidelines are helpful. First, all activities in the future organization should be able to be placed on the map. The map should be inclusive of everything the organization will do. Second, having too many processes at the first level creates confusion. More than 20 is difficult to handle. The number depicted on the first-level map should be limited and the second-level maps should be relied on to provide clarity.

DEFINE REENGINEERING PROJECT SCOPE

Determining the initial transformation scope is a tricky step. Too large a scope is difficult to manage; yet for this type of transformation, it is more risky to take an effort that is too small. If the scope is too narrow, the potential for radical change is limited. Breakthrough opportunities come by changing large processes that cut across the enterprise. Even a dramatic redesign of a small process is consumed and assimilated by the status quo resulting in little real change. At CMHS, some people wanted to restrict the scope to the specific activities related to the patient's medical record. However, by taking the broader view of all work related to clinical information, the team was able to address issues such as narrow organizational boundaries that resulted in duplicate work and, thus, duplicate documentation. In several cases, the fragmented patient care drove the need to write down more and more information in an attempt to keep the care coordinated.

Another common temptation when scoping the initial effort is to start with a safe process that allows the organization to start reengineering with minimal risk. By definition, there is no such thing as a safe transformation effort. If the scope is in fact safe, it is either too small to produce meaningful results or so unrelated to the heart of the business that is does not really matter. If the organization is in need of something as risky as transformation, will there be time for two cycles, first through the safe process and then through the core business? Usually the environment requires a faster solution.

Scoping the initial transformation project involves bringing together all of the work completed to date. It is not a straightforward decision, but one that must balance many disparate and often contradictory factors. First, and most important, is the consideration of the new strategic framework. What capabilities does the organization need to have to be able to realize the new direction? What has to be changed to increase the value delivered to customers? Unfortunately, many of the reengineering case studies that are found in the literature fail to consider these questions. All scoping decisions are made based on potential cost reductions and current performance improvement opportunities. Unless a significant portion of the initial effort goes toward building new value, the strategic framework will never materialize.

Thus, existing operations should not be ignored. The current position is the starting point that impacts the end point. It should be evaluated, but consider that this does not become a license for one of management's greatest stalling techniques: endless analysis. The question, far more basic than what is implied in a three-inch-thick situation assessment, is "Where is the organization bleeding?" Transformation is too risky an approach if the current performance simply needs to be fixed. If performance is creating or will create a strategic disadvantage, then complete reengineering should be considered.

With this comes the question of cost reduction. As demands continue to escalate throughout the industry for price cuts, organizations will have to look for ways to reduce costs. Often, all of the easy cuts are made and the market still requires more. Given a choice between slashing services or sacrificing quality, many are hoping to garner big financial gains through reengineering. When Willie Sutton, the infamous bank robber, was asked why he robbed banks, he declared: That is where the money is! Thus, if financial returns are a primary consideration, the scope should target the processes that contain the most cost. In healthcare, the cost is in people. If significant cost reductions are required, it has to come from a reduction in people, and that is neither safe nor risk free.

If the transformation effort serves only to catch up to the state of market competitors, no advantage is gained. The organization might live to fight another day, but the battle is far from over. During the effort, others have moved ahead, raising the bar once again. There is also a false belief that cost reduction alone is the key to survival during this industrywide feeding frenzy. Clearly, high-cost players are in trouble. However, it is impossible to shrink to a position of future strength. If competitive realities dictate an initial project aimed at reducing significant costs, it should be balanced with another effort geared toward building for a new future. For example, a hospital-based health system facing cost pressure might opt to reengineer processes related to inpatient nursing and diagnostic testing because those processes drive most of the current cost structure. However, to not simultaneously begin to reengineer processes that help build a truly integrated system (e.g., chronic disease management, outcomes management, patient routing and scheduling) poses a risk of having a cost-effective but empty, 1980s-type hospital.

Finally, these considerations must be balanced against the resource constraints of the organization. While everyone needs to reduce costs, they should be moving to a new strategic position that necessitates creating entirely new processes or at least the complete reengineering of existing ones. Now, all activities have become a top priority. Here the executive team must step up to one of the hardest responsibilities of management and reject important initiatives. History is replete with examples of organizations that were spread too thin, aiming for everything and hitting nothing. This chronic problem becomes acute when transformation is being considered because of the size of the effort. Significant resources are required, including things such as operating expenses, capital, management time and attention, staff that will work directly on the project, support from key areas such as human resources and information systems, and employee time during the implementation. Here it is better to scale back a bit than to "underfund" an effort.

The scoping decision is strategic because it identifies the key critical success factors and leverage points for the organization in the future. But executives must also be comfortable leaving some wiggle room in the project scope. Once into the details, it is inevitable that the reengineering team will find opportunities and dependencies that were not visible before. The CMHS project provides an excellent example.

After exploring several potential projects, the executive team selected the clinical information management process for its first project. The scope of this project included the complete redesign of the manner in which individual patient-specific health information was collected, input, integrated with other applications, and stored in the CMHS universal database. All individuals coming in contact with the CMHS system or its affiliated physicians were included. This integrating support process, far more than an information systems initiative, was viewed as the lifeblood that tied the entire system together. Furthermore, the project offered a return on all three scoping considerations: it addressed the frustrating operational problem of moving clinical information between caregivers, the cost of the process was huge and could provide substantial savings, and the way clinical information was handled would have to change dramatically to accommodate a vertically integrated health system. With these considerations, the executive team intentionally left a wide berth as evidenced by the scope statement. Yet even with this level of ambiguity, the reengineering team pushed the boundaries even further as they found seemingly unrelated issues that impacted how clinical information was managed.

DEVELOP SYNCHRONIZATION PLAN

Any project of significant scope will invariably have overlap or conflict with other work already under way. For CMHS, the joint operating agreement with Providence Hospital, the continuing rollout of a clinical information system, and a large-scale construction project at one of the hospitals were just some of the issues to be synchronized. In the beginning, management can identify the obvious issues. While the project progresses, the reengineering team will uncover other initiatives that need to be coordinated. A resolution process should be established to keep the various projects from getting crosswise with one another. Resolution can involve changing scope to remove the overlap, rolling one project into the other, stopping one and letting the other continue, or letting a short-term effort play out knowing that a solution will be temporary until the larger transformation is in place.

ESTABLISH COMMITMENT TO TRANSFORMATION

Before transformation can be launched, it is important that the organization's leadership is fully committed. Transformation is a difficult undertaking, and in fact, most organizations are not successful. One of the most damaging types of failure is to begin and not finish. Not only are valuable resources wasted, but the capability to change is weakened by yet another grand plan that fails to materialize. Employee skepticism is deepened, making the next change effort even more difficult.

Before going too far, a realistic assessment of the organization's ability to complete this is necessary. Leaders should consider the other initiatives under way, the level of personnel that can be committed to the effort, the financial position of the organization, and the depth of belief between the members of the leadership team in the approach to be used. An overly optimistic assessment confuses supportive leaders for those who are committed. While there are many ventures that can succeed with only support from the top, transformation is not one. In fact, the extent to which leaders bet the organization's and their own future on the transformation is a good indicator of the level of commitment. If this is one of many strategic initiatives, chances are that the distractions will prevent the requisite level of support.

CREATE CASE FOR CHANGE

No organization in the healthcare industry needs to discuss the general case for change. Surprisingly enough, all of the turmoil about the future of the industry does not translate to a workforce motivated to change. In fact, many, especially successful organizations, will quote the apocalyptic industry projections while simultaneously rationalizing how those forecasts do not apply to them. Even where everyone in the organization accepts the need for change, full-blown transformation is not often what they have in mind. It is too alarming to think about walking away from what is working today in exchange for a very difficult process that will produce a strange future that might not even work.

Consequently, executives must construct a highly compelling story that explains why this specific organization must transform, not just improve, and transform now. The litmus test for the case for change is whether it delivers a compelling reason to justify the pain and effort that will be required. If not, employees will not muster the energy to give it a try. Moreover, they do not believe executives will stay on course without a strong business reason to do so. CEOs come and go, operational crises create distractions, a new concept comes along, or another consultant pitches another plan. Ironically, the first question of employees is not "What does this mean to me?" but "Why are we doing this?" If the answer is not strong enough, why worry about what it means personally? It will pass.

Once the case for change is developed, it must be communicated often throughout the organization. Before the launch, a top-down communication should be completed at least through the middle management ranks. Many organizations kick off this communication with a formal meeting or management retreat. General industry forecasts are used to set the stage, then a detailed look into the organization's future is presented. Market share and competitor strategies are discussed. Financial projections are shared along with critical assumptions about the future and the related impact. Customer research is analyzed. The current operating model is reviewed in light of future demands with emphasis given to those things that have worked in the past but will not in the future. The objective is to move people to the point where they personally believe that significant change is required.

However, the complex idea of changing almost everything about the organization cannot be communicated in a one-time meeting. The case for change must be reinforced throughout the transformation effort. Department meetings, budget reviews, the employee newsletter, and even board meetings should continually refer to the need for change. Even if people accept the message, there are many reasons to settle back and just try to fix the status quo. The case for transformation must overcome this inertia.

Care should be taken to not assume that the same message rings true for multiple audiences. A common trap is to frame the message in a way that reaches the board of directors and then expect that same story to excite and motivate middle managers. The CMHS board was most interested in how reengineering the clinical information management processes would help make the vision of a seamless community health system an operational reality. For people who provided daily patient care, the case for change was less about the overarching vision and more about problems the current processes presented to caregivers and patients. For all audiences, a portion of the message dealt with the coming financial pressures that CMHS would face. Frontline employees and middle managers who knew that cost cuts would be required preferred to reengineer out those activities that did not contribute to patient care rather than live with the typical across-the-board cost cuts.

FINALIZE TRANSFORMATION STAFFING

Once the initial work is scoped, the next challenge is to staff the effort. This is where the organization puts its money where its mouth is. Though there are many different methods for reengineering, one common success factor that cuts across them all is a full-time, off-line team of people. This particular approach usually calls for 6 to 10 people for a period of 12 to 18 months. This model for approaching a transformation project usually prompts protests, objections, and descriptions about how lean the staffing is already. The consternation goes up even higher with the realization that it is not just any 6 to 10 people but top performers. It only makes sense that the project to recreate the organization's future should be staffed by "first string" employees. Further, these employees are already busy, usually carrying more than their share of the load, especially in times of tight staffing.

Without question, this is one of the first hurdles to successful transformation. Many companies do not succeed here. Some believe they can run against established wisdom and work with a part-time team. However, it does not work. Often, the team is pulled in many directions and never gives transformation the effort required. Other organizations sign up for the full-time team, but staff it with the wrong people. Top performers not only create more innovative designs, but they are also crucial to selling the change to the organization. Employees know "who's who" in the organization and do not believe a transformation project is the most important priority if it is staffed with people having little else to do.

The most important position on the team is that of team leader. Early impressions about the seriousness of management regarding transformation will be formed based on the stature of that of team leader. With a substantial scope and a true strategic shift, it is reasonable for the team leader to be at the vice president level. As with the notion of a full-time team, many organizations resist the prospect of committing an executive to a single project for more than a year. In part, this is a reflection of the lack of bench strength one level down in the organization. While this concept may be foreign in healthcare, organizations that understand what is required for transformation quickly see the need for extensive senior leadership and find a way to make it happen. The CMHS team was lead by the vice president of medical services, a physician who had moved into hospital administration three years earlier. Management responsibility for his departments was spread among the other vice presidents. The best operational managers are not necessarily the best suited to lead a multifunctional team through a process of creating an innovative future for the organization. It is more important that the leader be able to lead in an unstructured and ambiguous environment.

There are several factors to consider, other than performance, when selecting team members. A cross-section of perspectives and skill sets enhances the quality of the result. Most team members should come from areas directly impacted by the scope of the project, although a few should come from somewhere else in the organization. These team members, those outside of the process, provide fresh insights and ask good questions. There are particular characteristics (Table 5) that relate to transformation. As with the team leader, all top performers are not suited for this type of work. Many employees who are solid day-to-day contributors do so within a well-defined role. Their tasks are completed, deadlines are met, follow-through is consistent, and customer service is superb. However, these same people can sometimes find the loose nature of redesigning and the related change process unnerving.

In addition to the team leader, the CMHS team had seven other full-time members: two clinical nurse managers, a research coordinator, the director of clinical information services, an associate director of the emergency room, an industrial engineer, and a recently retired family practice physician. Through this staffing, all three hospital locations were represented on the team.

LAUNCH PROJECT

Once planned and staffed, the transformation effort is launched to the entire organization. This includes communicating the case for change, the vision for the future, the project scope and expected outcomes, the approach to be used, key milestones, which people have been staffed to

TABLE 5
Reengineering team skills

Organizational characteristics	Interpersonal traits	Cognitive abilities	Management skills
Recognized leader	Commitment to ideas and ideals	Creative thinker	Group facilitation
Top-level performer	Empathetic, helps people with change	Open to new, unconventional ideas	Project planning and control
Long-term potential above current position	Resilient in face of setbacks	Comfortable with ambiguity	Knowledge of organizational resources
Department head level or above	Enlistment mentality	Intuitive, able to extend from one idea to another	
Line operations background	Strong communications	Analytical, able to synthesize diverse data and draw conclusions	
Inside or outside process	Willing to compromise on details to get to the desired end		

the team, and what employees will be able to expect along the way. Team members are removed from their current positions and assigned to the transformation project.

Understanding phase

For most people in the organization, the understanding phase is the beginning of the transformation effort for it is the first visible activity (Table 6).

The objective of this phase is to create learning across the organization in two ways. First, it is a prerequisite to develop the new design. It is said that when scientists ask new questions, they are then able to find new solutions; the same is true for transformation. Until the team sees the situation in a different light, the tendency is to produce the same answers as in the past. Second, it furthers the case for change by helping people continue to understand why a complete rethinking of the business is required. The reengineering team works along two tracks, customer and process, while other parallel activities go on in other parts of the organization.

TABLE 6
Understanding phase: Key steps

- Finalize process definition
- Create process view
- Document customer values and requirements
- Document stakeholder constraints
- Complete process valuation
- Identify redesign levers
- Establish redesign targets
- Assess key supporting infrastructure
- Launch communication campaign

This phase should take about two months to complete. Although this is longer than may be desired, many factors contribute to the time frame. First, members of the team are learning to work together in a true project environment, which is something new to most people. Second, the work of this phase, while sometimes tedious, clearly orients the thinking of the team along process lines. Third, team members individually go through the change process that allows them to be more innovative designers. It is the hope that all team members are forward thinking and open-minded, yet they too have been immersed in the current world and must work through old ideas and beliefs. Periodically throughout the phase, the team will meet with executives to share their findings. There are not a great number of decisions to be made during the understanding phase, but frequent communication between these two groups helps keep everyone on the same page going into redesign.

FINALIZE PROCESS DEFINITION
Once in place, the first task of the team is to take the project scope provided by the executives and break it into the various subprocesses that are involved. This will serve as the basis for the work during the understanding phase. Since clinical information management is an integrating process, the CMHS team took two cuts at the process definition. One perspective identified the subprocesses that are involved to manage information, such as gathering data and abstracting, codifying, storing, and delivering information.

The other perspective viewed clinical information management as a process that is intertwined with operational activities. Information and the information management processes run in parallel to those functions that provide patient care. While the first perspective helped to understand what must occur to fully manage clinical information, the team opted to let the second perspective guide its work. The rationale for this decision was that the processes to manage information should be driven by the delivery of patient care. Therefore, the process definition identified the patient-oriented activities that created or used clinical information. A partial list of these includes emergency services, admission from emergency services, physician office visits, presurgical testing, inpatient care, and scheduled diagnostic testing.

The result of this step is a shared understanding between team members and the executive team of what is in the scope to be addressed. It also serves to provide a good education for the team to identify and understand processes.

CREATE PROCESS VIEW

Once the scope is understood, the team begins research on the current operation. This starts with the creation of process maps (flowcharts) that depict how the process currently operates. It is important to remember that these processes are going to be reengineered so this activity does not require the same level of detail that would be suitable for a continuous improvement effort. Instead, the team seeks to identify the fundamental weaknesses in the current design, the key dynamics that drive the performance of the process, and potential ideas for redesign. Rather than a detailed portrayal of every task and activity, the intent is to focus on instances where information or responsibility transfers between people and departments, activities are duplicated, or work adds no direct value to customers. Further, the team must understand when information flow is required in order for the process to be completed.

As the maps are developed and validated by others who work in the process, the team begins to collect process performance information. Again, this can become a bottomless pit of interesting but meaningless analysis. The information should concentrate on the results delivered by the process (quality and volume), the execution of the process (cycle time, potential variations, and bottlenecks), and the cost of the process (payroll and nonpayroll). The potential data to be collected should be tested by asking what will be done with the information (i.e., does it contribute to building the case for change for people? Will it help the team make design decisions in the next phase?).

The risk of overanalyzing the data cannot be overemphasized. The activities in this step are comfortable and familiar. Team members feel capable examining existing processes. Substantial insights, be they new or simply a confirmation of what has been suspected all along, are stimulating. Those who continue to push for more detailed analysis are generally using the information as a sophisticated stall tactic and may not be as committed as they publicly profess.

DOCUMENT CUSTOMER VALUES AND REQUIREMENTS

Feedback from external customers is crucial to orient the work of the redesign phase. This step is geared toward gathering information about customer needs relative to the specific activities inside the scope of the project. To begin, the team will identify external customers for each subprocess. Some subprocesses may be supportive by nature and have no external customers, while others may serve multiple customer groups.

When customers are identified, the team develops a strategy to obtain feedback. Interviews, focus groups, surveys, and literature reviews are common tools. Another powerful way to learn about customer needs is through direct observation. Team members, as unobtrusively as possible, watch the process in progress to find things that either enhance or frustrate the customer's experience. By videotaping customers standing in line, one bank received better information on the tolerance of wait times than was provided through interviews or surveys. Observation also provides additional insight into the performance of the process itself as it makes the problems identified in the previous step real. As with the process view, it is easy to spend too much time at this step. The research should be sharp and clearly focused.

Knowledge gleaned from this step will be documented and translated into customer values and requirements. Values are general statements of customer needs (e.g., timeliness and being treated with respect by staff). Requirements are specific expressions of a particular value. As part of timeliness, for example, customers may expect that call lights be answered in less than 2 minutes, bills be processed in less than 3 days, or a physician's office wait be less than 10 minutes. Requirements can be measured, where values are more amorphous and general. During the research, some feedback from customers will come in the form of value statements with no specific requirements attached (e.g., "I want to be treated like a human being"). Other findings are more similar to requirements (e.g., "I want to be called by my name").

It is the team's job to sift through the feedback and identify values and the related requirements. As a rule of thumb, no more than seven total values should be identified. In the end, requirements may be more powerful because of their specific and measurable nature, although values provide a powerful platform to redesign and find additional ways of satisfying customers. Once the values are understood, the new design can enhance those values in areas that customers have not even considered.

Though these steps are presented here as clean and sequential, there is much iteration. For example, once the customer values and requirements are documented, the team should refer back to the process performance measures to see how they align with customer requirements. It may make sense to measure the key customer requirements to see how the organization is stacking up.

DOCUMENT STAKEHOLDER CONSTRAINTS

This step seeks to document the constraints, restrictions, and minimum performance requirements placed on the process by stakeholders. Stakeholders are broken into two groups: external and internal. External stakeholders are those outside the process that can impose parameters on how the process is executed. For CMHS, external stakeholders included regulatory and review agencies, insurance companies, defense attorneys, and CMHS billing and finance needs. Each of these groups either used some output from the clinical information management processes or stipulated minimum standards. Internal stakeholders are those who participate in executing the processes and have specific needs as well. Physicians and their staff, nursing staff, ancillary providers, medical records, admitting, utilization review, and quality assurance personnel are all internal CMHS stakeholders. A clear understanding of the stakeholder issues that must be considered when redesigning the process should be the result of this step.

As with the customer groups, research must be conducted to identify stakeholder constraints on the process. Most constraints look like requirements in that they tend to be specific. However, one major problem with many current processes is that a general stakeholder constraint is interpreted too specifically and the collective organization may believe the process cannot be designed any other way. For example, CMHS, like other healthcare organizations, believed that malpractice cases require as much medical record documentation as possible to substantiate a position in the event of a legal challenge. After clarifying these assumptions, the team concluded that what was needed was a single complete story of what happened to the patient and why. In fact, during chart review, there were numerous examples of contradictory information, inevitably occurring with volumes of paper in a six-inch-thick chart. It is important, therefore, that work teams drive to the factual external stakeholder constraints, not the collective historical interpretation.

In the hierarchy of all groups, internal stakeholders come last. The process must satisfy customer values and function inside the boundaries established by external stakeholders. Needs of internal stakeholders cannot stand in the way of accomplishing the best results for customers. If necessary, the organization has the power to change internal stakeholder needs. Too often, great ideas never get past this point because the design is overly accommodating to internal needs. While those internal to the process should not be ignored, the aim should be to find ways to design the work more effectively, not simply gear it to the personal comfort zone of those who work in it. Ironically, examples repeatedly show that a process designed to maximize the value for customers is actually a better work situation for employees. Fragmented processes frustrate customers by requiring them to navigate a byzantine collection of many people in many places operating under a variety of, and often contradictory, policies and procedures. Working in that type of situation frustrates employees as well. Choosing between the needs of customers and employees is generally not the painful tradeoff that it appears to be.

COMPLETE PROCESS VALUATION

The customer and process view will be brought together in a valuation exercise. By comparing the work that is being done to customer values and requirements, the team can determine which activities add value for customers and which do not. This step can be both emotionally difficult and very positive for the team as well as the broader organization. Regardless of industry or organization, a relatively small percentage of the work directly contributes to satisfying customer values.

To complete this step, the team will classify each activity in the process maps into one of three categories:

- Value-adding activities are those that provide a result that directly meets a customer value or requirement. For example, patient education, a subprocess within clinical information management, directly contributes to the patient value of maintaining as much control as possible while receiving care. The value of personal control is enhanced when caregivers provide the patient with information regarding the assessment and diagnosis, treatment options, the plan of care, expected outcomes and risks, and key milestones. The activities that directly communicate this to the patient are value adding

- Support activities such as support processes, are necessary in that they enable a value-adding activity or satisfy a stakeholder requirement. To continue the patient education example, the work of the caregivers to develop a specific plan of care is a support activity. Though critically important, developing a plan of care in and of itself does not add value to the patient. Only when the plan is communicated (value of personal control) or enacted (value of receiving treatment) is value actually added for the customer

- Waste activities are, by definition, any activity that does not add value to a customer or satisfy a necessary constraint. An example of a waste activity would be a nurse copying every aspect of a standardized plan of care into a patient's chart. It is not helpful for communicating to the patient and not required by the caregivers to execute because they can work from the standardized plan, noting only the exceptions

Presenting this fact in a graphic way is how the case for change finally hits home for many people. The team walks through the maps, placing colored dots on each activity according to its classification. It is difficult for people to accept that only a small number of activities are value-adding. In clinical information management, which is a support process, value-adding activities are few and far between. This is not to say that these activities are not important. Yet if the organization wants to start with a clean slate, it is critical that the entire system be stripped down to what the customer truly values. Everything else adds cost, time, and potential complications—but not value. The experience can be sobering.

There are two cautions at this step: First is the battle between the reengineering team, now oriented to customer needs and processes that cross organizational boundaries, and those people who work in the current system. The team will be more aggressive in labeling activities as something other than value-adding and this will create conflict. This is a reflection of where team members are in the change process vis-à-vis the rest of the organization. When the CMHS team decided that diagnostic testing is not a value-adding process but a support activity for treatment, which is what patients come for, their conclusion was not warmly received by everyone in the organization. Their point, however, was accurate; customers do not come to be tested, they come to have their health improved.

The second caution relates to the activities labeled as waste. Some people will erroneously assume that the waste activities can be immediately discontinued. That would be a recipe for disaster because most waste activities work around inefficiencies in the system and hold the current process together. Without the duplication, double checking, and logging, the work could not get done. This points to the heart of redesign. Nonvalue-added work is marbled into the system and cannot easily be removed. The process has to be redesigned to eliminate those activities.

IDENTIFY REDESIGN LEVERS

As a summary of the understanding phase, the team will identify the redesign levers, those key things that must be changed to successfully reengineer the processes. Identifying levers enables the team to sort through its learning in this phase and reduce it down to no more than 12 statements that will serve as guideposts during redesign.

One type of lever is a customer lever. Customer levers highlight opportunities to add extra value for customers' met and unmet requirements or to potentially expand the business by targeting unserved market segments. An important customer lever for CMHS was the elimination of duplicate questioning of patients. In the existing system, patients were repeatedly asked the same questions, and for some, providing five or more complete medical histories was not uncommon. Given patient values of timeliness and confidence in the caregivers, taking five histories is not a good thing. Other examples of customer levers include

- *Determine patient's desired level of information.* Some patients want a lot of clinical details, while others do not. To best serve people with different needs, the new design should require a mechanism to allow for tailoring

- *Design working documents so they can be used to communicate with patients.* The team opted to use the fact that urgent tasks generally override important tasks in the design rather than fight years of history. Instead of separate documentation for communicating with patients, which would have increased the work, the principle was to design forms for the chart that could also be used directly with patients

- *Reduce the number of people who interact with the patient.* Care delivery is highly fragmented with many people contributing a small part to the total picture. Such narrow job responsibilities not only increase the amount of time spent coordinating and communicating among staff members but heighten the confusion for the patient. An endless stream of people going in and out of the patient's room is not comforting

Process levers, by contrast, indicate changes that will improve process cost, quality, or cycle time. To the surprise of the CMHS team, much of the work in the clinical information management processes had nothing to do with communication between caregivers about the patient. Instead, there was a sophisticated employee management system lurking. Patient care plans, which require extensive amounts of nursing time, were more a tool for nurse managers to evaluate their staff than they were for patient care. In another example, the operating room staff had created a "face sheet" for each patient coming to surgery. The stated purpose of the face sheet was to capture summary information on the front of the chart so it would be easily accessible during surgery. Nursing staff spent time extracting lab values, patient allergies, and other types of information from within the chart to the face sheet, but operating room personnel still went into the chart to check the information themselves. When this was highlighted, the true reason for the face sheets became clear. Operating room personnel felt that nursing unit personnel were not doing the necessary things to prepare a patient for surgery, so the face sheet was developed. In short, a simple "to do" list became a part of the patient's permanent medical record. Another example of process levers includes collecting only relevant information. In many activities, employees are collecting more information than is actually used. Over time, questions had been added to forms and assessment protocols that were no longer relevant. For example, one physician had a standard block of questions asked of every patient that was challenged by the team. The physician admitted that regardless of the patient's answer to a particular set of questions, the plan of care would not change.

Another process lever was the decision to move only the patient information that is needed. Several problems arose from the fact that when patients left the nursing floor for tests and treatments, their charts went with them. Consequently, nurses charted in a "shadow" system and later transferred the information when the chart returned. Physicians would arrive for rounds and would not be able to review the chart and test results would arrive on the floor with no place to go since the chart was missing. Most people accepted this as a fact of life, cured only by an electronic medical record. The team found that personnel in the ancillary departments did not need the entire chart, only selected pieces of information such as patient allergies and resuscitation directives, information that was relatively stable over time. Through a minor modification to an existing system, all of the information that needed to travel with the patient was printed once and placed at the bedside. The single sheet of paper went with the patient, allowing the chart to remain on the nursing unit.

ESTABLISH REDESIGN TARGETS

To conclude this phase the reengineering team and the executives will establish a limited number of outcome targets for the new design. Outcome targets can be set for any performance measure that is important to the process being reengineered. Some targets are cost based, others measure process cycle time, and others examine customer satisfaction with the postreengineered process. Some redesign targets for the clinical information management process include

- *No duplicate documentation.* At times, multiple caregivers need to repeat assessments due to professional discipline or level of skill. Once the first assessment was documented, the goal was for subsequent caregivers to simply note points of agreement and only document discrepancies or new information

- *Seventy percent reduction in the size of the chart.* The average inpatient chart for a four-day length of stay was 140 pages. The goal was to reduce that to less than 45 pages

- *Fifty percent reduction in nurse documentation time.* Approximately 20 percent of the typical nurse's time was spent charting. The goal was to reduce that to less than 10 percent

Whatever the arena, the targets play an important psychological role in the redesign. If the targets require only a minor improvement over current performance, it is unlikely that the redesign will be highly innovative. Instead the team will solve a few problems in the existing processes and determine they are done. Targets should be set high enough to cause the team and the organization to realize that the current model will never get there, no matter how finely tuned through improvement efforts. Only then will people be pushed to the creativity required for innovation. Besides, if significant targets are not required, odds are that transformation is not either.

Setting targets should incorporate the learning gained from the understanding phase. By knowing how much of a process is waste, for example, an estimate can be developed for how much of that waste can be eliminated through reengineering. This is also a place to insert benchmarking data into reengineering. Comparing current performance to best practice organizations is another way to help executives and the team arrive at targets that are a stretch yet achievable. If targets are set appropriately high, there is not a problem if the redesign and implementation fails to reach them. What organization would be disappointed with an effort that aimed for a 50 percent cost reduction in a process but delivered only 40 percent?

ASSESS KEY SUPPORTING INFRASTRUCTURE

A parallel activity that should occur during the understanding phase is a high-level assessment of the key infrastructure components required to support the new design. This includes areas such as human resources, information technology, physical space, and the information used to run the business. From the new strategic framework, it is possible to begin to project what will be required of those areas in the future. Of course, until the new design begins to take shape, specific requirements will not be known.

During the understanding phase, executives and managers responsible for those areas can begin the task of evaluating existing capabilities. Emphasis should be given to the strength of support organizations such as management information systems, finance, and human resources. Do current policies, systems, and employee competencies support the new strategic framework, or will extensive changes be required? How flexible and adaptable are the support areas? How strong is the leadership in key areas? Will they be able to maintain daily operations while also implementing major changes?

This will not only help those areas prepare, but it will also serve as important information for the reengineering team during the redesign phase. When the team develops the business case for the proposed changes, they need to know where capabilities stand and, thus, what will be required to move to the new design.

LAUNCH COMMUNICATION CAMPAIGN

Throughout the transformation, communication with the organization is vital. During the understanding phase, the focus is to reinforce the case for change and facilitate ongoing discussions around the new strategic framework.

While the reengineering team is completing its portion of the understanding phase, the discussions that began in the mobilization phase about the case for change and the new strategic framework should continue throughout the organization. Before the details of a new design can be accepted by people in the organization, they must buy into the new strategic direction and understand why it is the right change. When executives frame a new way of thinking about the business, it takes a while for that to go deep enough to provide a foundation. It must go deep enough within the executives that they instinctively make decisions based on the new framework instead of the old.

The consensus reached in a few working sessions during the mobilization phase should not be mistaken for the depth of understanding needed to lead the organization toward the future. New concepts need subsequent conversations as executives grapple with the full implications of such a shift. The framework also needs to go deeper into the organization. Managers and frontline employees need to hear about the new framework, have an opportunity to react and ask questions, and even be able to refine it. Getting a deep level of understanding around the new framework facilitates acceptance of the redesign that will be built to help realize it. This also lays the groundwork for the changes to the culture. As people throughout the organization come to understand the new direction, they begin to see things that may have worked in the past but will not work in the future.

These conversations should be driven by members of the executive team. A list of people to participate in these discussions should be developed and a plan for meaningful dialogue established. How the discussions are structured depends on the style of each organization. Some opt for large gatherings and others prefer several smaller discussions. Either way, the objective is to share the new strategic framework and prepare those who are critical in implementing it so that they personally understand and are committed to the direction.

Overcommunication about the design itself at this point can be frustrating to both the reengineering team and the organization. Many people want details that are still several months away. This phase can be used to get the communication process itself running smoothly. Target groups should be identified as well as the best mechanisms with which to reach them. Expectations should be established about the candor which the organization can expect along the way. Additionally, there should be an explanation of the steps of the transformation effort, who is involved, and key milestones coming in the future.

Redesign phase

In the redesign phase, a detailed vision is developed for everything within the scope of the project. This includes new process designs, organizational and job changes, information flows, specifications for information systems, infrastructure changes, and policy revisions. The design will address the changes required to fully implement a new system of work (Table 7).

A significant shift occurs when the team moves into the redesign phase, which is highly creative and far less structured than the understanding phase. Rather than analyze, the team must start putting a stake in the ground about what the solution will be. The redesign targets become very real as potential solutions are evaluated against projected outcomes. As specific ideas begin to emerge, political resistance surfaces. Most of the steps discussed below are iterative, with many in progress at

TABLE 7
Redesign phase: Key steps

- Create ideal design
- Design work processes
- Design process management system
- Define implementation projects
- Develop business case
- Approve implementation
- Conduct change management education
- Continue communication campaign

the same time, which requires a different operating style compared to the generally linear nature of the work in the understanding phase. The difficulty of the team's tasks goes up substantially.

This phase should take between three and five months to complete. Where the understanding phase can be limited to work that can be done in two months, the redesign should be complete before implementation begins. Factors that influence the length of this phase include the complexity of the project scope and the proposed solution, the political hurdles regarding the design that must be overcome, the number of people who have power over design decisions, and the organization's speed in making decisions. While it is important that redesign be given enough time to address the relevant issues, it is equally important that the organization keep moving toward implementation. No benefits are realized until the design is implemented. Momentum, which is the critical issue during implementation, begins to build during redesign.

Executives, with a minor role during the understanding phase, must now become more active. Key decisions regarding process flow, organizational structure, operating policies, and priorities must be made. Change management begins to require more time and attention as middle managers begin to see how the new design will affect them and individuals who report to them. Additional resources are now needed as personnel from human resources, finance, and information systems work to help the team flesh out specific ideas.

CREATE IDEAL DESIGN

To start this phase, the team will spend a short time, about a week, documenting ideas for the absolutely ideal design of the processes. The team will work from the perspective of the ideal to unleash the greatest creativity possible.

This step usually looks like a science fiction exercise because all constraints, be they technological, financial, or political, are removed. The question is, "What is the very best that can be imagined?" Many other programs begin with organizational "givens" and work to find improvements within those constraints. Such an approach tends to result in incremental, not innovative, gains.

This produces some interesting ideas. Part of the information used in caring for patients is demographic data. In this step, the CMHS team took the position that demographic information has already been collected many times. Why not get this from sources such as the local utility or telephone company? Nightly updates to the health system computers would mean that 98 percent of the patients who walk in the door would already be in the database. Though there are several practical reasons why this is not part of the design, the discussion did point the team toward other sources of information such as physician offices, health plans, and employers. By skipping over the optimal and starting with the ideal, the creativity of the team is greatly enhanced.

There are a variety of ways to complete this step. Some teams take each process and brainstorm ideal possibilities. Others create new process maps of the ideal flow. These tend to be very short because all of the waste steps are gone and most of the necessary steps are fully automated, occurring instantaneously. A third approach is to have team members write stories about a customer's ideal experience. Most of these tend to take the form of an ecstatic patient writing a letter to the CEO. Regardless of technique, two things are important. First is the stimulation of the team's thinking. Such innovative creativity is not natural for most people. Second, the team should tease out the underlying ideas that need to be carried forward in the design process. By articulating why it would be better for patients to be educated through their interactive television rather than by a caregiver upon discharge, the team can look for more practical ways to accomplish all or part of the same benefit.

DESIGN WORK PROCESSES

This step begins the basic work to create the solution to be implemented. This is a highly iterative process concerning not only the activities described in this step but the work in the next several steps as well.

The transition from ideal to optimal design is accomplished by introducing constraints one at a time. After a couple of days with literally no limits, a technological constraint is imposed. Money is still no object and all political barriers can magically be overcome, but the team is told their solution must be supported by technology that is currently on the market. Later the financial constraints are added and eventually other constraints that will confine the design. One constraint that has proven to be helpful is the time frame for implementation. By limiting the team to a design that can be fully implemented in 18 months, for example, the scope of the change can be managed. The longer the period required for implementation, the less likely the design will ever be put into play.

Drawing new process maps has proven to be one of the most effective ways to capture the optimal design on paper. Using the same technique as in the understanding phase, the team begins to lay out the process as it should operate in the future. An advantage of optimal process maps is that the team can sit down with people throughout the organization and review the maps, getting feedback on what will work and what will not. The maps can also be compared to those developed earlier to make sure problem areas and waste activities are being addressed.

As the new work flow begins to take shape, the team starts to work on surrounding issues. This includes how information will be used, the skills that employees will need, the technology that will be required to support the work, changes that will need to be made to physical space, and performance metrics that will be used to evaluate performance. This points out why design is so iterative. An initial process flow may be developed only to find that the skill-building effort required to do it that way is too costly. Ultimately, the team is responsible for putting together a complete design that works for customers and does so within the constraints of realities such as investment limitations, the capability of the existing workforce, or the physical assets of the organization.

The team begins to involve more people during this step. Selected managers and employees provide critical review and feedback. Other specialists help work out portions of the solution. Executives provide direction about how emerging ideas fit into the bigger picture. This is the beginning of resolving the conflict between innovation (small group of people developing ideas) and change management (broad participation to achieve buy-in). Be careful not to swing too quickly to broad participation. The team must still own the design decisions or the effort runs the risk of backing off from innovative ideas. Not everyone will initially like new ideas. If too many people are given veto power, the ideas will die.

The purpose of the CMHS example is to help illustrate the transformation process, not provide a detailed case study. However, a few highlights from that design show the scope of reengineering. A partial list of features from the final design includes

- Multidisciplinary (e.g., doctor, nurse, therapists, and diagnosticians) patient management plans that address practice guidelines, treatment protocols, critical pathways, and clinical algorithms

- Charting by exception in an integrated medical record

- On-line information system that supports patient management plans, charting by exception, and an integrated medical record

- On-line access by all caregivers

- On-line order entry by those who generate patient orders

- Point-of-care registration

- Relocation of patient-based business services (e.g., insurance verification, coding, and billing) to point of care

- Changes to role definitions for all clinical personnel

- Elimination of presurgical testing

- Change from two stages of recovery for ambulatory surgery patients to one stage

Many of these features are in place in other organizations. The key point is that the design addressed all aspects of the way clinical information is managed. It is the way the design is put together, not the individual components, that provides the power for change.

DESIGN PROCESS MANAGEMENT SYSTEM

The design itself has two major portions. Detailed process design, the step above, is about the direct work activities. Process management design is focused on changes to the surrounding organization that will be required to not only manage the new process, but also to sustain the change. A lack of sustainability is a common problem with change efforts. The problem is usually not with the process design itself, but the fact that the surrounding context was not changed as well.

The new management system is bigger than the process being reengineered for it affects the entire enterprise. Included are matters such as

- *Organization design.* Given this new approach to work, how should work groups be organized?

- *Reward and incentive programs.* How should employees be incented to reinforce the process orientation?

- *Career paths.* How do career options change for employees in a process organization?

- *Performance tracking and reporting.* What type of information should be looked at on a regular basis?

- *Management development.* What new skills and abilities do managers and executives need to lead a process-oriented organization?

- *Continual improvement.* How does the approach to ongoing improvement change in a process world?

- *Technical architecture.* How does the approach to information systems need to change to support this orientation?

- *Space utilization.* How does the use of physical space need to change?

Designing a new process management system presents several unique challenges. On one hand, the issues being addressed are larger than the process being reengineered. This prompts some organizations to separate design of these areas from the design of the process itself, giving responsibility to the appropriate functional disciplines. Yet that violates the premise that the business processes that deliver the value should drive the design of everything else about the organization. Furthermore, functional experts from areas such as finance and human resources who have not been participating in the project are not likely to design the innovative solutions required to support the new process. The very act of working through the detail of designing processes from scratch brings a new perspective to functional support areas. While not perfect, it seems that leaving responsibility for the complete design with the reengineering team is the best answer. Again, the team should have responsibility to deliver a complete and integrated design that encompasses the surrounding management practices as well as the direct work activities.

However, the team will have to collaborate extensively with both functional experts and executives on issues impacting how the organization will be managed. By understanding how management practices need to change to support the new process design, the team can develop ideas for how the management system should be changed overall. If the organization is committed to moving from a profession-based functional orientation to a process orientation, changes to budgeting and finance, human resources, information systems, and performance reporting are all required. The reengineering team is best suited to understanding what changes are needed because they have been immersed in a process mind-set.

On the other hand, these changes go well beyond the scope of the project, so executives and managers responsible for those support systems must be involved in finalizing the design. This tension can stimulate creativity, but it also may cause a battle. The reengineering team, which wants to push for the ideal, may believe that the functional managers are protecting turf and are stuck in their old ways of thinking. Functional managers and many executives think the reengineering team consists of a bunch of loose cannons spouting theoretical ideas without considering the practical implications. Here, extensive management time is required to work through what it means to be a process-based organization. Resolving policy issues, handling personnel transitions, and teaching new ways of thinking are time-consuming efforts. How the management practices are changed has much to do with the long-term results that are realized.

Many people at CMHS believed the project was focused on automating the medical record, yet the team spent much time redesigning the overall management system. The final design included radical changes to the organizational structure, the medical staff organization, and even the structure of the budget. The variety of role changes driven by process changes will require extensive alteration to human resource practices such as job definitions, performance evaluations, recruiting, and compensation.

DEFINE IMPLEMENTATION PROJECTS

The optimal design, both the work processes and the management systems, are converted to a series of implementation projects. Each project represents a specific and discrete piece of the overall design to be implemented. CMHS had 22 implementation projects ranging from development of the integrated record to installation of wireless computer terminals.

Breaking the design into projects accomplishes several things. First, the business case for implementation is more easily developed on a project by project basis. Second, multiple implementation projects support the change management principle of broad participation. In the implementation phase, many people will become involved through staffing on the implementation projects. Third, projects break the design down into more manageable pieces. Fourth, implementation teams will have responsibility for all details required to see a project through to completion. From this point forward, the design will be viewed and managed as a series of projects rather than a collection of ideas.

DEVELOP BUSINESS CASE

The team will develop a business case that covers both the one-time implementation and the ongoing operation for each project (Table 8).

In developing the one-time portion of the business case, the team will address all costs related to getting the project fully implemented. Possible cost categories include the following: time for a detailed design, information systems development and installation, changes to physical space, specialty consulting services related to the project, unproductive employee time for communication meetings and training, redeployment and severance, and lost revenue during the implementation.

Each organization handles implementation costs differently. Some count everything while others only want to know about actual cash that will be expended, exempting payroll costs that would be incurred anyway. When dealing with payroll costs for training and other types of downtime, some count it at straight time and others use time-and-a-half. Depending on the features of the design, some dollars that will be used for the implementation have been already budgeted somewhere else and management may only want to count the incremental spending. At the beginning of the business case development, the reengineering team and executives need to agree on the assumptions and rules that will be used to count costs.

TABLE 8
Business case

Implementation costs:
- Implementation team time
- Employee training and communication time
- Capital (i.e., technology, equipment, physical infrastructure)
- Severance and outplacement
- Consulting services
- Lost revenue during implementation

Impact on operating results:
- Personnel
- Supplies and equipment
- Maintenance

Payback:
- Implementation costs ÷ (impact on operating results ÷ 12 months)

Though most of the one-time portion of the business case deals with the financial cost, the team should also document other issues that should be considered when each implementation project is evaluated. Interdependencies with other projects, political risks, and confidence in the technological portions of the project are examples of nonfinancial issues that could be part of the business case.

The ongoing operations portion of the business case is more difficult to develop. Here, projections about staffing levels after implementation usually present the greatest sticking point. Care must be taken to only count productivity gains in the design that can be translated into realizable benefits. In many cases, a few minutes saved here and there do not result in the ability to reduce personnel. As a general rule, benefits from staffing changes occur when an entire person can be reassigned. If a whole person cannot be taken out of the process, the benefits become more elusive.

There are financial benefits that come from nonpayroll areas such as materials and supplies, but again, caution should be used to not overstate what can be realized. It is also important to make sure that new costs related to managing and maintaining the process be included in the going-forward projection. As with the one-time portion of the business case, nonfinancial costs and benefits should also be noted here.

A common temptation of reengineering teams trying to justify a business case is to project increases in volume due to improved performance. While some design changes can be linked to direct volume or price increases, most are second- or third-level effects. An example is the reasoning, "With these changes, the process will be faster and more customer-friendly, which will make more patients want to come here, which will translate into more business." Though there is no disagreement with the thinking behind the argument, the effect is usually too spurious to be built into a business case.

To provide a business case summary, the one-time implementation costs are compared to the annual impact on operating results to calculate a time for payback. Some projects will never show a payback and should not be expected to do so. They represent foundational pieces required to support the entire design or added costs that create even more value for customers. Bringing physician offices on-line is such a project for CMHS. Paybacks longer than two years (the positive impact on annual operating results is less than half of the one-time implementation costs) begin to be suspect for projects being evaluated primarily on financial grounds. Too many things can happen to derail the economics of the design if the time frame is too long (e.g., new strategic alliance, changes to technology, or preemptive action by competitors). The most important payback number is not the one for any particular implementation project but the overall solution. A design that meets other expectations and offers a payback of less than two years is a good candidate for receiving management approval.

APPROVE FOR IMPLEMENTATION

An organization has a major investment in transformation at this stage. Yet it is relatively minor compared to the costs and risks incurred during implementation. By developing a fully integrated design and a detailed business case, management can take another hard look before going forward. This step should not be handled as a big event presentation by the reengineering team to executive management at the end of the redesign phase. If the team has lost its focus, a lot of time and energy has been wasted. Instead, executives should be actively involved throughout the phase, looking at both the design and the business case as they are being developed. If things are done right, the official approval to move into implementation should be easy.

CONDUCT CHANGE MANAGEMENT EDUCATION

As the reengineering team develops the new design, a broad educational campaign should be rolled out to help prepare people in the organization for the change. Since the details of the design will not be finalized, the education will deal more generally with how the future will be different from the past. What does it mean to manage a process organization rather than a functional department? What new skills will be required? What norms and barriers will have to be removed? What new norms and expectations will have to be built to fill that void?

There are many general education programs related to change management. These should be supplemented with specific ideas that begin to develop during the design process to make the education more relevant. Middle managers as a group may be the most important target constituency at this point. After the new design is in place, the jobs of executives and frontline employees will change, probably a great deal, but the nature of their roles will be roughly the same. Executives will still lead and frontline employees will still execute. Middle management jobs, on the other hand, are defined by and exist because of the functional work groups they lead. If the new design fundamentally changes the model of work, then the very basis for middle management jobs will be different. Add to the formula the expectation that middle managers help employees work through their personal concerns caused by the change and a potentially volatile situation is created. It is more than the shrinking of middle management ranks. The switch from boss to coach, from an owner of many employees to the owner of a process using someone else's employees, from a supervisor to a doer, and from a position of control to a position of service makes this change traumatic.

CONTINUE COMMUNICATION CAMPAIGN

The communication campaign that started in the understanding phase will continue in redesign. Three specific topics related to communicating during a transformation effort are discussed below.

First, the assumption that the team should tell everyone everything is erroneous and dangerous. During redesign, a whole host of ideas will be considered and discarded. If every crazy concept that floats through the team is publicly spread to the organization, many people will fight battles over things that may never materialize. In one instance, the CMHS team was contemplating a radical change that would dramatically alter the practice patterns of one physician specialty, and thus negatively impact physician income. Eventually the idea was dropped from the final design. If this discussion had been communicated too soon, the CEO would have spent much time on a problem that never occurred. There will be enough other challenges without sending the organization on unnecessary emotional roller-coaster rides. This is not to imply organizations should go to the other extreme and withhold information. Instead, the ground rule should be, "We will tell anything we know when we know it for sure."

The second topic is about rumors. As various people participate on the fringes of the design process, rumors will begin to grow like a wild vine. Managers have somehow convinced themselves that it is their job to eliminate all rumors. One might well try to hold back the sea. Rumors exist during a time of change because traditional norms and expectations are removed. Norms and expectations are a valuable, though unspoken, form of information. Communication fills this void until new norms and expectations are established. Rumors are a form of communication, and in a large organization they are unpreventable. They should be rectified when appropriate, but an organization should not spend too much time or energy trying to eliminate or prevent all rumors.

Last is the issue of employee discomfort during the change process. Again, many have been deluded into believing that enough communication can remove employee discomfort. In fact, a common way to camouflage resistance to change is to couch objections under the mantle of worry about the employees' level of comfort. Change, if it is meaningful, creates pain and discomfort. It is not and should not be the goal of management or the reengineering team to remove employee discomfort. Rather, the focus should be on employee productivity. During design and implementation, as well as after the change, the role of management should be to move employees to a point where they can operate at their maximum productivity. Only where rumors or discomfort begin to hinder productivity is action required. In many cases, the discomfort should be recognized as part of meaningful change and be allowed to play out in a supportive environment.

Implementation phase

This phase is where changes become an operational reality (Table 9). Ideas and concepts leave the flipchart pages and begin to affect the way work is done. Compared with the redesign phase, the challenges are different and in many ways more difficult. Every detail has to be addressed and loose ends must be tied up. Problems and mistakes are not theoretical but are made in the presence of customers. Many organizations develop impressive designs and plans, but few follow through with implementation. At this point, momentum and perseverance are more important than a brilliant design.

Success factors in this phase are like those found in any major implementation. Good planning, the ability to make decisions that keep things moving forward, clear responsibilities and accountabilities, effective communication mechanisms, and well-conceived roll out plans are all important. For transformation, the added challenges come from the scope of the change and the fact that it represents significant role adjustments for so many people. Executives must become more involved, not less—as tends to happen with many initiatives—as the transformation moves along.

TABLE 9
Implementation phase: Key steps

- Develop implementation plan
- Develop redeployment plan
- Establish program management approach
- Launch implementation teams
- Develop and test changes
- Implement changes
- Transition to operations
- Measure and evaluate
- Continue communication campaign

The reengineering team itself goes through an interesting transition as it begins to release control of the project to other people throughout the organization. Like any creator, team members face intellectual struggles when their ideas are not implemented exactly as designed. Executives switch from guiding a handful of people to the more amorphous task of leading the entire organization through the change. Yet these transitions are necessary for the new vision to take root and grow. Employees and managers need to feel significant ownership within the framework of the design to make the changes stick.

DEVELOP IMPLEMENTATION PLAN

Once the design is approved, the team develops a comprehensive implementation plan. This plan defines when each implementation project starts and ends, the resources needed to implement the project, and key dependencies with other projects or initiatives.

Timing is the biggest issue in implementation planning. The following factors must be considered as the plan is developed:

- *Pace of implementation.* No benefits are realized until the changes are implemented. Long implementation plans mean delayed results

- *Benefits realization.* Depending on the needs of the organization, implementation projects that deliver tangible results may need to be scheduled earlier. Many organizations use such an approach to help fund subsequent capital investments in the transformation

- *Resource levels.* The amount of resources, whether time, energy, operating expense, capital, or political chits, that can be committed to the transformation is limited. Implementation plans must be constrained by what is available

- *Dependencies.* Some implementation projects need to finish and be rolled out at the same time. In other cases, one project must finish before another one can begin, while still others have long lead times. The implementation plan must incorporate these dependencies or the program will face difficulty in the roll out

- *Impact of changes.* In most cases, a particular work group will be impacted by multiple implementation projects. The plan needs to anticipate where downtime for training or postinstallation adjustment periods will negatively impact a work group. It may make sense to spread changes out over time or synchronize them so change will be felt only once

CMHS spent six weeks finalizing the implementation plan. The complexity of the various projects required the synthesis of the different planning perspectives cited above. Several functional experts were brought in to help the team work through issues such as information technology dependencies and the amount of time required for training on activities such as charting by exception.

DEVELOP REDEPLOYMENT PLAN

Any design of significance will result in job changes. Unless the organization can realize new growth, major productivity gains mean that fewer jobs are required. Even if staffing reductions are not necessary, employee skills may not match the new jobs. It is safe to assume that redeployment will be a major issue during implementation.

Many decisions about redeployment must be made in the mobilization phase. As soon as a reengineering project is announced, the question about layoffs will be raised by employees. Once the project scope is determined, management can anticipate which groups of employees could be impacted. Some foresight in hiring and staffing during the project can minimize the number of employees affected later. Freezing hiring in the affected areas and using temporary staff is one common tactic to reduce the number of employees to be redeployed.

Each organization must make its own decisions about retraining, layoffs, transfers, and staffing decisions. Rather than manage redeployment decisions on a project by project basis, an organization-wide approach is more appropriate. The redeployment plan should specify how decisions about personnel will be made, the commitments that will be made to employees, and the tactical procedures that will be followed. If this aspect of the transformation does not run smoothly and fairly, many problems are created.

When the redeployment plan is developed, consideration must be given not only to the changes driven by the initial reengineering project, but also to the larger policy issues involved. What criteria will be used to decide which employees are affected? How much severance and out-placement support will be provided? How will entirely new positions be staffed? Decisions made as part of the first project tend to be viewed by employees as ground rules that apply to all subsequent projects.

The amount of support given to affected employees remains the purview of each organization, but a strong case can be made to provide more support than would be normally considered. An effective and humane redeployment plan includes details such as retraining, extended severance packages, and outplacement counseling. These factors are tangible and so are the costs, but the costs of not taking care of people are hidden and thus often ignored. Though it is more difficult to calculate the specific costs of unproductivity due to survivors' remorse, confusion, anger, and sabotage, it is significant in large-scale change projects. The best antidote is a demonstration that the organization is bending over backward to help employees, both those with jobs and those without, through the transition. After all, most employees have worked hard for the organization in the past. It is not their fault that the environment changed to the point of requiring a radical transformation. The aim of management should be to return to maximum employee productivity. Investments to help people through the transition can pay off by restoring the productivity of remaining employees more quickly as well as reducing the risk of legal action and associated costs from outplaced employees.

ESTABLISH PROGRAM MANAGEMENT APPROACH

During the understanding and redesign phases, the work of transformation is completed primarily by two groups—executive management and the reengineering team. During implementation, the effort has a different mode of operation. With many implementation teams operating in parallel (simultaneous multiple projects), an overall program management approach is required.

Program management has responsibility for six functions: coordinating the work of the various implementation teams, resolving issues that span across teams, protecting the integrity of the design by keeping implementation teams from straying too far from the original concept, facilitating communication across teams and the organization, tracking and reporting progress, and managing the general momentum of the effort.

This approach is meant to give implementation teams as much freedom as possible, thereby letting people closest to the work have significant influence on the details of how new processes will operate. However, there are a few things that should be tracked and reported by program management. These are also the areas that senior management should pay attention to during the implementation phase:

- *Design integrity.* Have the implementation teams discovered something about the original design that cannot or should not be implemented? Such decisions to change the design cannot be made unilaterally for there are often implications that affect other implementation teams

- *Projected benefits.* As the details are worked out, do projected benefits change, either positively or negatively? Management must be kept aware of benefit changes because the business case is also altered

- *Schedule.* Is the project on track to be implemented in the planned time frame? Delays affect other projects and push the realization of benefits farther out

- *Budget.* Is the cost of implementation within the established budget? Budget overruns require even higher gains to deliver the expected return on investment

- *Decisions.* Are there decisions that must be made by management in order for the implementation team to move forward? A common problem is projects that stall due to slow decision making

- *Change management issues.* Is political resistance inhibiting the progress of the team? Management cannot help resolve objections or deal with obstructionists unless those issues are surfaced

- *Realized benefits.* As portions of the design are put into operations, what benefits have been realized? Management needs to know to make sure the design is working and performance gains are actually being realized. Employees need to know so they may see their efforts are paying off

The program management function is usually filled by the reengineering team. Depending on the size and scope of the implementation, either all or a portion of the team members are required. For the CMHS project, the entire reengineering team remained in place to work with the implementation teams.

LAUNCH IMPLEMENTATION TEAMS

Each implementation project will be staffed by an implementation team with a team leader and team members with the skills necessary to completely implement the changes. Most implementation teams will work on a part-time basis with team members continuing with their other responsibilities. For certain projects, it may make sense to use a full-time team and shorten the time frame for the project.

Once the implementation teams are in place, responsibility for the transformation begins to shift. The reengineering team, in its program management role, depends on implementation teams to flesh out remaining details, develop training material, establish necessary policies and procedures, and roll out the changes. Almost 200 people at CMHS, from all sites and all levels and many professional backgrounds, staffed the various implementation teams.

The teams receive an orientation to the design and a detailed explanation of their specific project. Reengineering team members support the implementation teams by providing background information and consultative support.

DEVELOP AND TEST CHANGES

Implementation teams flesh out all the details required to fully implement the projects. Working from the vision developed in the redesign phase, each team has responsibility for all aspects of the implementation, all the way through the complete rollout and evaluation.

Where at all possible, changes should be pilot tested during this development step. Before going through the effort of rolling changes out to the entire organization, the solution should be tested in a limited situation. In some cases this can be done in one department. Other changes such as a new compensation program or new methods of contracting with health plans require crossing the entire organization, but can be tested with a limited group of customers (e.g., patients from one set of physicians, patients from one or two employers, or only patients requiring a specific type of service) or employees (e.g., one department, one physical site, or one or two job classes).

IMPLEMENT CHANGES

Once developed, the changes will be rolled out to the organization. The roll out approach should consider the downtime related to installing the changes, the learning period required for employees to reach a minimum level of competency, other initiatives affecting the work group such as regulatory reviews or busy seasons, and the postinstallation support that is needed.

TRANSITION TO OPERATIONS

Since reengineering is an off-line development effort, the transition of control from the teams back to operational managers is critical. From the beginning of the implementation phase, thought should be given to making this transition as smooth as possible. As soon as new management-level staffing decisions are made, those people can become directly involved with the implementation. Regardless of how involvement is accomplished, it is important that implementation teams understand that the operational managers must eventually take ownership of the new work processes and the surrounding management practices.

MEASURE AND EVALUATE

Each implementation team is responsible to measure and evaluate the specific changes it implements while program management measures and evaluates the transformation as a whole. This includes financial scorekeeping and tracking performance against the redesign targets and the business case. In addition to being reported to executive management, these results should be shared with managers and employees. Many people sacrifice to get the design in, whether working directly on a team or carrying an extra load to cover for a colleague who is, and they need feedback that indicates the effort is paying off.

CONTINUE COMMUNICATION CAMPAIGN

The communication campaign continues in the implementation phase, but the emphasis shifts again. Detailed information begins to become available and many specific questions can now be answered. Employees care less about the big picture and begin asking for information that is relevant to the changes that will affect them directly. Communication tactics may need to be modified to deliver specific information to targeted audiences rather than general information to the entire organization.

Nuts and bolts information is the heart of implementation phase communication, but the most important outcome is establishing new norms and expectations. Fortunately, much of this is done with very specific facts. The point is to make sure the underlying principles are not lost in the tactical details. As new norms and expectations are formed, the amount of communication required begins to decrease.

Operations phase

The final phase of the methodology is really not a phase at all, but the continuing realization of the vision developed during redesign (Table 10).

As the off-line portion of the effort comes to a close, the pursuit switches to operations-oriented activities. The intent of these steps is to make sure the gains from transformation are protected and enhanced.

TRANSITION TO PROCESS MANAGEMENT

Transition from traditional management approaches to a process management system is not easy. People must adjust to new roles and responsibilities. Managers and employees must learn how to operate with a process orientation. Process performance data, such as total process cycle time, require different analyses and interpretations than data geared to running a single department. Executives, who are also learning to live inside the new model, should provide support and continuing dialogue for employees and managers until process management becomes as natural as the old functional management.

IMPROVE PERFORMANCE

Ongoing improvement is important in any system of work. This is especially so, however, for recently reengineered activities. If the redesign is

TABLE 10
Operations phase: Key steps

- Transition to process management
- Improve performance
- Document lessons learned

appropriately aggressive, it is unlikely that the full vision will be realized during the implementation phase. Managers should be held accountable for improvements in the key operating measures as well as for design elements that were not part of implementation.

DOCUMENT LESSONS LEARNED

At some point, it is important to declare the end of the initial project. Since the transition from off-line development to on-line operations is gradual, one way to do this is to stop and document collective lessons learned regarding transformation. It is also a good idea to host a big party to celebrate the successes. Closure is important for all of the people who have been involved in the effort.

Conclusion

Organizational transformation is a very difficult venture and should not be undertaken lightly. Many efforts fail or fall short of expectations. The approach described above is designed to help an organization improve its odds. Yet on paper, things always appear cleaner and easier than they actually are. Transformation truly tests the resolve and commitment of the organization. No methodology can replace the leadership required for success.

In spite of the many pitfalls along the way, many organizations are willing to undertake a transformation for a simple reason—those who succeed reap tremendous rewards.

NOTES

1. M. Hammer and J. Champy, *Reengineering the Corporation: A Manifesto for Business Revolution* (New York: HarperCollins, 1993).

▝▘ 15

Implementation strategy issues and options

John J. Skalko
Assistant Vice President, Operations Improvement
Lee Memorial Health System
Fort Myers, Florida

WHEN EMBARKING ON REENGINEERING as an organizational initiative, a major decision is to select the most appropriate implementation strategy. The primary methods are vertical, horizontal, and blended strategies. Each approach has specific advantages and disadvantages and requires varying degrees of capital, operating, and management resources. Reengineering is a major initiative that requires significant management energy for success. The implementation strategy selected has a direct impact on the resource requirements for full implementation. The common denominators of time, money, and corporate culture are all decision criteria in an organization's selection of the most appropriate implementation strategy.

Defining the approaches and how they are applied during implementation will serve as a point of reference throughout this chapter.

Vertical strategy

In the vertical strategy, a particular patient population (unit or units) is selected for reengineering. The patient groups are usually centered around clinical product lines (e.g., cardiology) or resource consumption of the patient types (e.g., orthopedics, neurology). In this approach, the redesigned care delivery model is defined and implemented to match the clinical and operational requirements of the selected patient popula-

FIGURE 1
Vertical strategy

Design and fully implement a comprehensive, reengineered care model in a defined patient specialty care area.

| | Care center #1 | Care center #2 | Care center #3 |

Electrocardiography
Phlebotomy
Intravenous therapy
Respiratory therapy
Charting by exception
Bedside computers
Laboratory
Radiology

Source: Health Care Resource Group, Fort Myers, Florida.

tion. Once fully implemented, a second patient center is selected for redesign and implementation. This process continues until all patient care areas are fully redesigned and implemented. (See Figure 1.)

The vertical approach, which uses the input of a design team and a project team, was adopted by the pioneer hospitals that pursued reengineering. A guiding principle of the pioneer architects was that aggregating patients in terms of common resource consumption would enhance economies of scale and lead to increased synergy among the nurses and other bedside caregivers. It was under this premise that early reengineered care delivery models were developed.

Horizontal strategy

In the horizontal approach, a commitment is made to redesign care delivery across the organization, but a fully developed model is not implemented in a single patient-specific unit. Instead, reengineered components of the redesigned delivery model are sequentially implemented, across (horizontally) all care areas. One important feature of this approach is the evaluation of each component for clinical, operational, and financial feasibility within the defined patient unit. However, not all redesigned work flows and work methods lend value in all patient units. Components are implemented simultaneously in multiple units. Although this approach was not readily used by hospitals that pioneered reengineering, today it is a more common and readily accepted practice. (See Figure 2.)

FIGURE 2
Horizontal strategy

Design and fully implement redesigned work methods across broad range of care areas.

	Care center #1	Care center #2	Care center #3
Electrocardiography	————————————————————————▶		
Phlebotomy	————————————————————————▶		
Intravenous therapy	————————————————————————▶		
Respiratory therapy	————————————————————————▶		
Charting by exception	————————————————————————▶		
Bedside computers	————————————————————————▶		
Laboratory	————————————————————————▶		
Radiology	————————————————————————▶		

Source: Health Care Resource Group, Fort Myers, Florida.

Blended strategy

A blended strategy uses a combination of both vertical and horizontal approaches. Some hospitals decided to focus on a few specific patient units to create centers of excellence to leverage the reengineering benefits, to differentiate clinical services, and to provide a competitive advantage in their market. To accomplish this, hospitals concentrated their redesign efforts in the strategic areas, such as orthopedics, to develop and implement fully the reengineered care model. As various redesigned components were developed and implemented in the centers of excellence, they were selectively chosen for integration into the other care areas of the hospital. The blended strategy tries to balance effectively the clinical, operational, and financial benefits of a comprehensive model to enhance a care center while selectively deriving implementation benefits of components in other care areas. (See Figure 3.)

Prior to selecting any of these strategies, it is important to understand the advantages and disadvantages of each approach so the selected strategy will fit the organization's fiscal, operational, and clinical requirements. This is critical, since incongruence can effectively derail a reengineering initiative.

Vertical strategy advantages

Reengineering has been referred to by many experts as the "radical redesign of processes" and its implementation can be akin to "managing

FIGURE 3
Blended strategy

Design and fully implement a comprehensive reengineered care model in a designated care areas while concurrently implementing selected redesigned work flows and work methods across a broad range of care areas.

	Care center #1	Care center #2	Care center #3

Electrocardiography
Phlebotomy
Intravenous therapy
Respiratory therapy
Charting by exception
Bedside computers
Laboratory
Radiology

Source: Health Care Resource Group, Fort Myers, Florida.

chaos." From a change management and organizational development perspective, a vertical strategy is favorable. By concentrating the reengineering initiative in a specific unit, the activities are localized, allowing the organization to pay special attention to the change process. Education programs can be provided for the management and staff dealing with change, team building, self-directed work teams, and governance. It is important to recognize that redesigning processes and providing technical skill training is easier than transitioning through the change process and cultural shift needed. Thus, localization allows programs to be customized to meet the unique needs of the staff. It also creates more opportunity for the staff to give ongoing assessment and feedback to the reengineering effort. This two-way communication is invaluable in problem solving and refining the redesigned model.

A way to understand a reengineered care model is to visualize a collection of integrated work flows and work methods that have been redesigned to eliminate structural inefficiencies and activities that do not add patient care value. In most models, this may involve multiskilling bedside caregivers (e.g. phlebotomy, EKGs, and noncomplex respiratory) or work simplification (e.g., charting by exception, streamlined charge capture, and standardized protocols). Implementing a single area allows an organization to develop a model and use the process to determine which redesigned work flows and methods have significant clinical, operational, and financial benefits. It is through this validation process that organizations can define the reengineered care model that best meets their needs. In addition, by approaching implementation in this manner, the education programs and support tools can be developed that provide a strong foundation for broader implementation activities in other units. The organization can gain valuable insight to help establish realistic implementation schedules and budgets.

By understanding the concepts of reengineering, an organization can apply the techniques and approaches that work best in a particular setting. Organizations should not be wed to a single redesigned model that has been implemented in another hospital setting—that model may not benefit a different hospital situation. In other words, one size does not fit all. It is through this validation of components that organizations can define the reengineered care model to best meet their needs.

Another advantage to the vertical implementation process is that it allows the systematic reengineering of all care areas. By approaching each patient area individually, implementation schedules and training requirements can be adapted to the particular unit to ensure that the complete model is in place and fully operational before moving to another unit. This allows an organization to build on its success and gain operational momentum. In some situations, the vertical strategy may provide the most significant opportunities for improved performance. This is based on the fact that some reengineered components not implemented in an initial horizontal approach may never be implemented due to loss of organizational momentum and focus. This point, however, is only valid if the omitted redesigned work flow components have real value. If no significant value was originally identified, the cost/benefit will probably not warrant later implementation.

Vertical strategy disadvantages

One of the most frequently cited disadvantages of a vertical strategy is that implementing one unit at a time protracts the overall implementation time frame; some of the operational, clinical, and fiscal benefits will not be realized quickly. If an organization is faced with competitive pressures to reduce costs, timing is a major consideration. Organizations have various time opportunities depending on their financial stability and the impacts of managed care pricing in their specific market. A central question becomes, "Does the organization have the luxury of not realizing tangible benefits in the short term?" A vertical strategy can take as much as two to three times the duration of a horizontal implementation schedule.

The second drawback of a vertical strategy is that implementation is generally more expensive from an operational and capital cost standpoint. Another model implemented in the various patient care areas may contain reengineered components that require substantial capital but offer no significant value to the delivery of care or performance improvement in that patient unit. For example, installing a x-ray unit in a patient care unit that does not have high imaging needs for clinical care will result in underutilization of the equipment and increased costs because of the low volumes. With a vertical approach, staff training generally is concurrent with the daily operations of the care unit. This is very costly if all caregiver hours for patient care need to be replaced during staff training. If time savings gained through work simplification are not used to offset training time requirements, training hours and expense become additive. Regardless of which approach is used, training requirements should not be compromised and adequate resources should be committed on the front end of the implementation process. Failure to do this may end up costing more time, money, and management energy than if it is done well the first time.

Another disadvantage of the vertical strategy is the requirement to run dual care delivery systems through an extended implementation period. This tends to create operational problems as ancillary departments or units become impacted by the redesigned care model. For example, if a simplified charting system is part of the reengineering initiative, the unit will chart differently than the rest of the traditional care areas. This can create confusion in medical records and utilization review departments and create staffing inflexibility since employees may not have the knowledge or skills to float to the reengineered unit. These are the types of operational issues to be dealt with throughout the implementation phase. As implementation is occurring, there is also a tendency for staff to see a disparity between the redesigned units and those maintaining a business-as-usual environment. This can create employee relation conflicts and tensions for managers and staff during the implementation phase.

Horizontal strategy advantages

Reengineering involves redesigning work flows and work methods (components) into streamlined processes. The horizontal strategy deals with the implementation of various reengineered components sequentially across a broad range of care areas. In contrast to a vertical strategy, a selected redesigned work flow and method is implemented in patient units. Once in place, another component is implemented and so on until all selected components are fully operational within the areas. The intent is to build progressively on each redesigned work flow method implemented. Some of the advantages of this approach are as follows: this strategy tends to have a much more rapid implementation period. Since components can be implemented sequentially and concurrently in several areas, the overall schedule can be condensed. Accomplishing implementation in a shorter period of time will allow faster realization of the clinical, financial, and operational benefits. By approaching the reengineering process on a component-by-component basis, a broader range of concurrent activity is achieved. In some organizations where one unit at a time (vertical) has been implemented, the effort is initially viewed by staff as a trial that may or may not impact them in the long run. With multiple units undergoing redesign activities, there is little chance the initiative will be viewed as anything but a new way of doing business.

Second, implementation is less resource intensive from a capital and operational perspective. For example, resource intensity increases if capital dollars are spent on equipment, facilities, or system modifications in areas where tangible performance gains will not be realized. In many vertical approaches, this occurs because the reengineered model is not generally adapted to the unit. In a horizontal approach, there is more of an opportunity to evaluate each work flow and method's impact on a unit. This can prevent spending capital where it offers little clinical, operational, or financial benefit to the organization.

For operational resources (expenses), a horizontal approach allows an organization to blend redesigned work flows and methods that have direct impact on freeing up or taking additional staff time. For example, if one of the redesigned work methods is charting by exception, a simplified patient charting process, this component can have a tremendous positive impact on reducing the amount of charting time required by caregivers. Actual time savings vary by organization depending on its current documentation system, but reductions in charting time of 30 to 60 percent is not unusual. By isolating charting by exception in a horizontal approach, a hospital can use the time savings for training, rather than pay for additional training hours. Also, by freeing up caregivers' time, a hospital can integrate other bedside clinical activities that historically are performed by central departments (e.g., phlebotomy). The end result is greater efficiency and patient care continuity. The blending of work flows and methods that are "time-givers" and "time-takers" is a distinct characteristic of the horizontal approach.

A faster implementation used in a horizontal strategy will allow a hospital to realize the benefits of reengineering more quickly. This is particularly important if the financial or market conditions warrant speed. Speed can minimize the operational problems and confusion normally encountered with running a reengineered and traditional care delivery model concurrently.

Horizontal strategy disadvantages

The horizontal strategy implements reengineered work flows and work methods in multiple care areas concurrently within an organization. The sheer magnitude of the change process requires a higher level of management involvement. As multiple patient units undergo change, it is critical that the process be well managed. It is essential that the managers be available to support effectively their staff through this intense change. Staff must be prepared to let go of tradition to accept a reengineered care delivery model. Simply stated, redesigned work flow and methods inherently changes staffs' jobs and roles. The management team must be prepared and capable to provide leadership in this process.

The change can have an adverse impact on job satisfaction and morale, particularly if the organization's culture does not readily accept change. A commitment to organizational development should be sufficient to prepare the management and staff to support the cultural shift. Managers cannot be effective role models if they do not "walk the talk." Obviously, involvement of managers, supervisors, and staff in the implementation process is a prerequisite to help the staff understand and gain ownership of the redesigned care model.

The second disadvantage of this approach is the impact on the organization's human resource policies. As part of a broad-based redesign effort, it invariably affects inplacement and outplacement strategies, job descriptions, performance appraisals, and compensation. Because of the speed of implementation, it is critical to have well-developed human resource policies as a foundation for the change management process. For instance, if during the redesign process an individual learns and assumes additional clinical responsibility (e.g., a nurse performing phlebotomy), what will be the additional compensation for the function, if any? Such significant policy decisions will need to be made during a reengineering initiative. Generally, organizations are slow to develop and adopt new personnel policies that reflect new ways of doing business. Therefore, the rapidity of a horizontal implementation could force an organization to develop and adopt policies and procedures in an unusually short time frame, thus causing additional stress. There is no reasonable alternative than to create an effective human resource strategy and structure to support successful implementation.

Blended strategy advantages

The advantages of a blended strategy echo the positive factors that apply to vertical and horizontal approaches. Integrated redesign efforts can be contained in a few units, which allows for development of education and implementation. Because of the localization in the units, change and cultural shift can be better managed in the designated care areas where full redesign is slated.

With a blended approach, an organization can concentrate on a few strategic service lines with total redesign, while implementing some of the reengineered work flows and methods in other care areas. This allows gaining the full range of benefits in those strategic units while selectively implementing components that have the greatest value in a broad-based fashion. The end result can be significant performance improvement and competitive advantage in key areas coupled with incremental gains in the others. As for duration of the implementation schedule, the time required is between that of a vertical and a horizontal approach. With all approaches, once the implementation plan is in place, the duration of implementation depends on resource commitment and the organization's willingness to embrace fundamental change.

Blended strategy disadvantages

The disadvantages of this strategy are a combination of some of the weaknesses outlined in the other approaches. However, the dynamics of the change process are significant. Because there are major reengineering efforts in one or more care areas, and component implementation in several patient units, the change process becomes complex. Having to develop change management programs to deal with the various degrees of redesign becomes an organizational development challenge. Ultimately, a full range of educational needs must be provided for all areas, but the level and intensity varies by redesign scope and implementation schedule of the units.

Another disadvantage of the blended strategy is the concurrent redesign of total units and individual components. If an implementation team is established to support the transition of fully redesigned units, there are limits on how many units can be adequately supported. If the implementation team becomes consumed with the fully redesigned units, what additional levels of support will be required for the rest of the units undergoing component level reengineering? Running dual tracts complicates the implementation process, and more support may be required to complete the project. The level of support will be determined by the scope of redesign and the pace of schedule implementation.

Conclusion

Reengineering is a major strategic initiative that can effectively position an organization for the future. However there is no universal best strategy for implementation. Many of the implementation approaches must be considered to determine which one best meets the organization's needs and circumstances. Based on this inventory of factors, an administrative steering committee for the reengineering initiative should decide the specific strategy and approach. To validate the ownership of this important strategic initiative, this decision must represent active executive support and involvement.

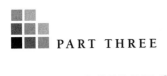

PART THREE

BUSINESS
PROCESS
REDESIGN
TECHNIQUES

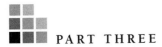

PART THREE

Healthcare industry

case studies

▚ 16

Catholic HealthCare West: Documenting operational improvement

Roger Hite, PhD
Executive Vice President and Chief Operating Officer
Dominican Santa Cruz Hospital
Santa Cruz, California

FOUR YEARS AGO, the president and CEO of Catholic HealthCare West (CHW), a multihospital healthcare system, brought together senior management from each of its hospitals and challenged them to understand and apply total quality management (TQM) principles and philosophies to their operations. To help the hospitals survive and prosper in a turbulent reform environment, they needed to reengineer many arcane hospital processes and develop methods to continually improve productivity and quality outcomes produced by the reengineered processes.

Members of CHW senior management were asked to look at their organization through the eyes of its external customers—patients and third-party payers. Hospitals had to stop looking at quality as something that was assumed by patients and asserted by administrators; CHW demanded more from hospitals and medical staffs. Quality had to be demonstrated with data that measured both clinical outcomes and service excellence. Old methods of patient care needed to be reengineered into integrated healthcare delivery systems designed to effectively use resources. And, as leaders of Dominican Santa Cruz Hospital soon realized, the true challenge was to reengineer the culture so that there was support for and buy-in to redesigning key interdepartmental patient care activities and to committing staff to constantly improve the quality of care as perceived by the patients.

331

Dominican Santa Cruz Hospital took this opportunity seriously. Within weeks, Dominican's senior management team was searching for a TQM approach compatible with the hospital's culture. After interviewing a number of consulting firms, Dominican selected an external process consultant and adapted AT&T's customer/supplier model, where quality is defined from the perception of the customer. Although senior managers did not realize it at the time, the hospital was not introducing TQM or reengineering; it was initiating a complete and irreversible cultural transformation—one that continues to grow three years later.

It was not easy to convince a traditional hospital organization to view itself from the patient's (customer's) perspective. There continues to be sincere objection to the notion that a patient who comes to a hospital is a customer, but as the cultural transformation matures at Dominican, even the most ardent opponents of the term "patient/customer" realize that there is an intertwined and inseparable relationship between clinical and service excellence. Anyone who has lost baggage when traveling on an airplane knows how technical excellence of a service process is inseparable from service excellence. Hospital organizations are just beginning to understand this.

Dominican's "quality journey" is founded on a basic principle of quality management—to learn how to see the services of a hospital from the patient's perspective and learn how to measure and monitor how well the hospital meets and exceeds the expectation of its customer patients.

The purpose of this chapter is to describe the significant systems and process redesigning necessary to transform the culture of a hospital into one that is truly customer driven.

The patient as "customer"

When Dominican's senior management began learning about the principles of TQM there was significant resistance to view the patient as a customer. The rationale was simple: healthcare creates a special relationship between the caregiver and the patient that does not exist in the traditional business transaction between customer and merchant. Patients, it was argued, rely upon the caregivers to tell them what they need to purchase. A healthcare provider is an expert who has a different responsibility than a merchant who is trying to sell something to a customer. This environment creates a higher ethical responsibility on the part of the caregiver—an ethical dimension that is missing in the general business marketplace where suppliers sell a product or service to customers who are presumed to know what they need and how to evaluate the purchase of goods and services.

The resistance to seeing the patient as a customer turned out to be one of the significant clues to transforming the traditional hospital organization. Virtually all of the operational systems and management systems, from admitting through discharge and continuing on through billing and collection, were designed to accommodate the needs of internal customers. Little attention was paid to how patient/customers might perceive what was happening as they moved through the care and treatment activities in the hospital. Each hospital department had its own policies and procedures, which made perfect sense when taken in isolation, but few departments spent much time working to improve interdepartmental communications. Nowhere was there an assessment on how well the cross-departmental activities were integrated to satisfy the patient/customer needs and expectations.

Senior management was asked to consider the macrostructure of the hospital organization from this customer/supplier perspective. The following key processes were identified and categorized into three distinct areas: (1) direct service processes experienced by patients (e.g., admitting, patient care units, and food service), (2) indirect service processes supportive of direct services (e.g., laboratory and radiology), and (3) administrative functions (e.g., accounting, human resources, administration, and safety/security). When viewed from the customer perspective, each process has cycle times and adverse indicators that can be defined, measured, and improved.

Senior management first learned in its weekly continuous process improvement (CPI) meetings that its organizational chart was a great barrier toward cultural transformation. It did not reflect the patient's perspective.

Organizational process reorientation

The hospital organizational chart illustrated that the status of internal customers took priority over the status and importance of the patient/customer. In fact, there was no mention of the patient/customer on the traditional organizational chart. Instead, it showed the hierarchy and status of departments and division. The president's box resided below the board at the top of the chart, directly below the president was the COO, below the COO were the vice presidents and the departments contained in their divisions.

As senior management defined and managed key processes of the organization, it became clear that a new picture was needed to describe the new process improvement culture. Dominican's new organizational chart now identifies 30 key processes. More importantly, the customer is now placed at the top of the organizational chart.

Process improvement council

Central to the reengineering effort at Dominican is the Process Improvement Council (PIC), which consists of officers, vice presidents, and three key managers. The PIC initially was created as an educational forum for senior and middle managers responsible for large multiple-cost center departments. During the first six months of the PIC, weekly hour-and-a-half sessions were conducted by a process consultant. The focus of each session was to teach senior management the fundamentals of CPI. Management learned to view the organization as a system of intertwined key processes. Each process was viewed from the perspective of the patient/customer. At the conclusion of the formal training process, the PIC developed a curriculum to introduce management and first-line supervisors to CPI concepts and philosophies.

Instead of relying on the external process consultant, members of PIC accepted the responsibility of being faculty/coaches/mentors to instruct the rest of the management team. This required that the hospital's management development program be converted to a new curriculum centered on TQM philosophy, and the customer/supplier approach to process definition and management. The first quarterly training session was highly rated in postseminar evaluations, with comments made about the importance of seeing senior management in educational leadership roles.

In addition to its teaching and mentoring role, the PIC also was responsible for systematically initiating all key process improvement teams. A priority selection criteria was developed to guide the PIC to determine which of its more than 30 interdisciplinary teams should be launched first. Priority was assigned based upon such factors as number of customers served, number of transactions, process cost per year, upstream relation to key process, and importance to external and internal customers. Furthermore, the PIC validated the use of a six-level process qualification criteria system used by teams to measure progress, from having no definition of process to meeting world-class quality standards.

The following presents the most recent statement of goals and objectives for the PIC:

1. Organizational quality assessment

    a. Maintain the assessment of process qualification levels for all key hospital processes and work with process improvement team (PIT) leaders to establish goals to continuously improve process quality

        - Choose at least one key quality measure for each process or department for which a service target will be established, measured, and improved

        - Publish a summary grid that tracks each chosen quality measure, its measurement value, and its target for improvement

    b. Benchmark at least half of the key defined processes of the hospital with at least one outside organization

    c. Use the Malcolm Baldrige National Quality Award (MBNQA) criteria as a rigorous method to measure and plan quality improvement activities

        - Complete and submit the application

        - Educate the full management team in the applicability and use of the MBNQA criteria, score current processes, and set improvement goals in light of the results of this self-assessment and the feedback from the Malcolm Baldrige reviewers

2. Process improvement team development

    a. Refine and standardize documentation formats to be followed by all PITs (e.g., issues and action items, process qualification criteria, and minutes)

    b. Schedule the start-up of uninitiated key PITs, including

        - Billing, charging, and collecting

- Mental health

- Rehabilitation

- Scheduling patients

- Patient record management

- Community health and outreach

- Others to be determined

c. Develop and implement recognition methods for team accomplishments

d. Increase, by at least 10 percent, the number of direct service delivery staff participating on process improvement teams

e. Recruit at least 10 percent more physicians and their office staffs to participate on PITs

3. Process improvement education

a. Continue regular training programs (at least two sessions) for appropriate CPI topics

b. Continue the PIT STOP (Process Improvement Team, Strategic Tips on Process) meetings as a method of interteam collaboration and learning

c. Ensure the organization's ability to support teams with new or replacement facilitators, as well as the materials for team start-up and ongoing team management

Complaint process management

The first PIT initiated at Dominican was the Complaint Process Team. Initially, there was resistance to starting with complaints because it was perceived as a negative approach to process improvement. However, senior management began to look at complaints as a way to obtain useful feedback from customers that could be used to improve processes and increase customer satisfaction. Complaints were viewed as valuable to provide information about customer perceptions and satisfaction.

Since only one person out of eight will make the effort to make a formal complaint, the comments came from individuals who genuinely wanted the hospital to change and be successful. Complaints provided the lowest-cost, most accurate information about what needed improvement in the organization.

One of the basic principles of TQM is, "If you can't measure it, you can't manage it." Unfortunately, some organization leaders rush headlong into reengineering departments and processes without first questioning if they can measure and quantify what isn't currently working. If they cannot measure, how can they detect if the reengineered process or procedure is superior to the old? Once reengineered, the organization must be brought under some structure of process management if it is to enjoy the full benefit of CPI. Dominican's leadership realized that having a better system to capture and record complaints—those that are resolved and those that remain unresolved—was an essential process.

The previous complaint resolution process could be described as follows: A complaint was received by anyone—physician, patient representative, board member, employee, or volunteer. If the complaint could not be resolved on the spot, it was forwarded to the patient relations department. The complaint was investigated and resolved, often with little involvement from others. No database existed and little information was shared about trends and results. The process ended after the complaint was received by the patient relations department.

The problem with this traditional model for handling customer complaints was that it missed an opportunity to learn from errors or to see the "bigger picture" issues that are imbedded in isolated, individual complaints. The most management could hope to achieve with this method of handling complaints was to resolve each complaint to the customer's satisfaction. CPI, however, demands more.

The reengineered complaint process created a different perspective. It was designed to ensure that Dominican was collecting 100 percent of customer complaints in a timely fashion and that the process enabled the organization to sort, analyze, and discuss changes needed in patient care processes to prevent the same type of complaints from recurring. Collecting and acting on patient feedback is the essence of patient-focused care.

The new process created by the complaint PIT was designed to fulfill the following mission statement: "To provide a system for the timely and satisfactory resolution of complaints, and to efficiently provide managers and staff with the information to support the implementation of process changes that address complaints and improve customer satisfaction."

The complaint PIT determined that the "process owner" of the complaint process should ultimately receive all complaints and should be committed to immediate contact with the person issuing the complaint. The CEO and COO were selected for such ownership.

The team identified three cycle time measures for the complaint process: (1) initial response time—how long did it take before the customer received acknowledgment that the complaint was heard by the organization? (2) resolution time—how long did it actually take to resolve the complaint? (3) follow-up time—how long did it take until the source of the complaint (patient, physician, staff) received follow-up communication that the complaint was resolved?

Once the complaint process team was launched, it quickly adopted a positive attitude toward complaints. Buttons were produced that read, "Every complaint is an opportunity to improve quality." Once the complaint process was reengineered, the complaint PIT developed a training module used to educate all employees in the hospital regarding the importance of complaint management and how the new process was designed to work.

Using the creative energy of team members, a video script was developed that described the methods and process to resolve customer complaints and record the data for process improvement purposes. The cohost of *Good Morning America* provided an introduction and conclusion to the videotape. The tape has become a part of the materials that Dominican shares with other hospitals across the country who are interested in reengineering and continuously improving a new approach to customer satisfaction.

The total reengineering of the traditional patient relations department was key to successful complaint management. It was redesigned so that complaint management was not the sole responsibility of the patient relations coordinator. Instead, under the reengineered process, complaint management engaged the attention and actions of all staff, especially those working at the bedside. The complaint process was redesigned so that a more systematic method was used to collect, evaluate, and use customer data obtained in the complaint process. A computer software program to allow complaints to be recorded and entered into a matrix to assist other process teams focus on root causes of recurring complaints was developed by the complaint PIT. All complaints received from staff during a patient's stay in the hospital were recorded on a short blue form collected daily and brought to the COO's desk. The goal of staff was to address and mitigate the sources of complaints at the point of customer dissatisfaction. All complaints were recorded on the short blue form, whether or not they had been resolved. After COO review, the documents were sent to the Patient Relations Department where they were tabulated into the database and distributed to the appropriate parties for future follow-up.

To assist staff in making immediate amends for actions that caused patient dissatisfaction, the complaint PIT developed a tool called "DominiScrip," a pad of $5 scrip available to any hospital staff. Each department developed criteria and reasons to use the scrip to deal with customer dissatisfaction with service in a particular department. A recent customer survey and focus group results indicate that the DominiScrip program is highly successful.

Complaints received in letter form or by telephone after the patient/customer's discharge were recorded by the staff person who received the complaint and recorded it on a "long form" (the complaint form used when investigation and follow-up is required). One of the measures of the success of the complaint process team is the cycle time required to respond formally to the dissatisfied customer. The team also measured the cycle time required to complete the investigation, make adjustments, and achieve customer satisfaction. A control chart was used to communicate to all management staff that the process was under statistical process control.

In addition to managing the complaint process and improving the cycle times of response and resolution, the complaint PIT regularly analyzed the database that captures and classifies the areas of the hospitals where various types of complaints were received. The data was distributed to the full management team and used by key process teams as a source to focus on recurring problems creating dissatisfaction. A Pareto chart was distributed monthly to all managers. The types and frequency of complaints were displayed, and the data was used by departments and PITs to analyze root causes.

Part of the ongoing activities of the complaint process team is to analyze complaints to determine if root causes of complaints can be determined and engineered out of the current processes. Frequently, case studies are developed and presented to process teams for discussion purposes. The following two case studies illustrate how complaints have been used to improve operations.

CASE STUDY ONE—COMPLAINT: BROKEN EQUIPMENT

A 70-year-old man was brought to the emergency department after an automobile accident. The treating physician wanted to check for cracked ribs and abdominal trauma and several x-rays were ordered: a chest plate, a side view of his chest cavity, a back view, and a semisitting posture view.

The technician handling his case repeated four of the eight x-rays and told the patient that the equipment was not functioning properly. It took several retakes to finally fulfill the physician's x-ray order.

The patient later sought out the COO to complain about his experience. "I am an old man, and I don't worry any more about cancer," he said. "But you shouldn't be exposing patients to unnecessary radiation. Get your equipment fixed!"

The patient was assured that the clinical treatment he received was well within the guidelines for x-ray exposure, and he was informed that the failing equipment was already scheduled for replacement. The feedback of the complaint to the radiology department manager provided an example to explore with his staff. How can reasonable expectations be better communicated to the customer? Should equipment malfunction procedures be clarified? The complaint also served as a catalyst for a broader range of questions: (1) What was the real cause of the patient's dissatisfaction? (2) Did he get an appropriate clinical diagnosis? (3) If the technician had not said anything about the equipment, would the patient have been dissatisfied? (4) What is appropriate for technicians to tell patients when equipment is the cause of retakes? (5) At what point is equipment removed when retakes are required? (6) If a retake is necessary because of legitimate equipment failures, should it be included in the patient's bill? (7) How much of redone medical treatment is related to the reasonable variation associated with the application of technology for performing diagnostic procedures?

Obviously, these questions cut across the organizational chart and involve many different departments and personnel. They are important questions to ask and to answer, but would they have been so thoughtfully considered without the customer complaint?

CASE STUDY TWO: COMPLAINT—INACCURATE DIAGNOSIS.

A 59-year-old male came to the hospital's emergency room and complained of severe stomach pains (he previously had been treated for a heart attack.) The examining physician gave him a nitroglycerin tablet and ordered several tests to rule out heart attack or other critical conditions that could cause the pain. When the test results came back negative, the patient was given a prescription to aid one of the several conditions that could have caused his stomach cramps and was sent home after four hours.

The pain persisted for another two days, and the frustrated patient turned to the phone book to find an internist who could give him an appointment that same afternoon. This physician diagnosed a classic case of a parasite infection, which the patient probably contracted on a recent camping trip. In 30 minutes, he had a different prescription, which brought him relief from the pain. The patient's complaint was that he did not receive an accurate diagnosis in the emergency department.

Under Dominican's reengineered complaint process, the complaint was noted and acted upon immediately. The original message the patient left on the hospital president's phone mail on a Wednesday evening triggered the initiation of a customer complaint form. The form was forwarded to the manager of the emergency department, who then contacted the treating physician and the patient by late Thursday. The COO (the process owner) contacted the customer on Friday to reassure him that the hospital was taking his comments very seriously.

The process provided a completed complaint form that was entered into the database for trending and tracking purposes. It was determined that the patient received clinically correct care. Ruling out a heart attack was a service consistent with the customer's condition upon arrival to the emergency department. The real complaint was that the hospital failed to meet the patient's expectations. He expected to get his pain fixed, and the hospital did a poor job of communicating with him about his condition and the care he received.

The following critical questions were posed at the weekly meeting of the PIC as a result of this customer's complaint: (1) Is it possible the customer received "appropriate medical treatment" but was still dissatisfied? (2) What prompted the customer to visit the emergency department? Was it to rule out heart attack or find a cure for the stomach problem? (3) Why did the customer not complain about the length of time in the emergency department? Why was that not a priority for him? (4) What does this episode tell about the role of "customer expectations"? (5) Why did the customer go to the phone book to find a physician? (6) Is there anything that could be done to improve the connection to follow-up care? (7) Is there any way the care provided by the follow-up physician could have been better coordinated with the care given in the emergency department? (8) Should the customer's bill be adjusted? If yes, what should be the rationale? (9) What reasonable actions should be taken to follow up on this customer's complaint?

One of the major outcomes of analyzing this emergency department complaint was the initiation of a volunteer working with staff to help ensure that important arrival and departure communication takes place and that customer expectations are addressed at the time of service.

How PITs operate

There are currently 22 PITs operating across the hospital. A PIT team is formally launched by the PIC. Initial membership is determined by the PIC and is usually based upon discussion regarding which departments and key staff are currently engaged in work that is related to the key process. Additional members can be added at the discretion of the team once it is formed and operational. Most teams have membership that does not exceed 10 to 12 members. A team is formally launched by the COO and coached by at least one of the VPs. General orientation to the "rules" for participating on the team and guidelines for how to effectively work as a team are presented in the initial PIT meeting. Meetings are scheduled, usually once per week, not to exceed an hour and a half. The process owner and facilitator plan the agenda in advance of the meeting. Each PIT has a facilitator, often someone not working on the daily activities of the work process.

The first activity of the process improvement team is to validate the preliminary customer/supplier model developed by the PIC, which requires that the process be viewed from the eyes of the patient/customer. The team is asked to use nominal group process (a discussion method) to maximize input of members and to keep one person from dominating discussion. The initial activities are done when the team completes the following tasks: (1) agreement on a statement that describes the object of the process, (2) consensus on when the process begins and when it ends, (3) a clear understanding of who the suppliers are of the resources needed for the process to work, (4) a clear statement of what the expectations are of the customer regarding outcomes, (5) an identification of at least three quality indicators from the customer's perspective, (6) listing key adverse indicators of the process, and (7) key process cycle times that can be measured and improved upon.

Another important PIT activity is the early generation of an issue list. The list is a result of allowing all members to identify what they hear, think, or feel about what is not working well in the way the process serves the needs of the patient/customer. These lists help the PIT focus on where problems can be resolved within the PIT and where to focus on areas for true process improvement.

To make sure PIT teams are making progress to improve the way the key process meets customer needs, each PIT is required to make a semi-annual progress report to the PIC. These formal presentations are highly structured and usually rehearsed prior to the presentation. There is a great deal of team bonding and pride generated in these reports. Ordinarily, the reporting of results is shared by most members of the team. For some, it is one of the few opportunities they have for formal business speaking and an opportunity to improve their own presentation skills.

Each formal review allows the team to assess and demonstrate its progress, to gain additional insights into the team's accomplishments and goals, and to provide recognition of the team members.

Process qualification levels: What do they mean?

CPI is an active endeavor that goes beyond simple problem solving. At the heart of the activity is an effort to constantly view the services delivered from the customer's perspective. With this focus, the PITs look for ways to improve the service level beyond its current level.

Process qualification, a methodology taken from the experiences of other industries such as manufacturing, formally evaluates and ranks the level of performance for the key processes at Dominican. It consists of specific, verifiable activities that PITs target. Once certain targeted activities are completed or are in place, the process is considered to have reached a certain level of performance.

Increasingly demanding efforts make up the criteria for higher levels of performance. Listed below is a description of the six-level process qualification system in use at Dominican.

LEVEL SIX: UNKNOWN STATUS

This is the initial status of a process, until a PIT has been formed and the customer/supplier model has been developed.

LEVEL FIVE: DEFINED STATUS

Processes performed at this level are documented by the PIT. A customer/supplier model is validated, and the requirements of the process (outputs and inputs) are understood. Performance of the process is beginning to be measured from the customer's perspective, and minimum operational requirements are being met. The team has targeted improvement objectives for the customer's three most important quality measures.

LEVEL FOUR: EFFECTIVE STATUS

The process meets all of the requirements of the previous level. The process is fully described through a flowchart depicting the customer's point of view. The process is being improved, based upon the knowledge of the PIT members and data gathered about the process, while the measures taken help identify areas where streamlining efforts should be made. The primary customer expectations are being met. The team is tracking customer complaints as an approach to understanding the areas to make improvement changes.

LEVEL THREE: EFFICIENT STATUS

The process meets all of the requirements of the previous levels. It is being streamlined to reduce cycle times (the elapsed time to deliver a certain service to the customer) as well as to reduce adverse indicators (e.g., the number of times the customer was inconvenienced in some way with the delivery of the service). Process defects and costs are being reduced, and the PIT is actively benchmarking the process with other hospitals and other industries (e.g., hotels).

LEVEL TWO: ERROR-FREE STATUS

The process meets all of the requirements of the previous levels. Process deliverables (outputs) have been error free for more than six months.

Schedules are consistently met and worker stress levels are lower because the PIT functions in a mode of "fire prevention" rather than "fire fighting." All performance measurements show improvement from the previous six months.

LEVEL ONE: WORLD-CLASS STATUS

The process meets all of the requirements of all previous levels. The process is rated among the top 10 percent of its kind. Other organizations, from various industries, are frequently benchmarking with Dominican to learn about its experiences and approaches.

One of the things Dominican learned about using process qualification criteria is how useful the criteria are to help teams keep focused on process improvement, rather than simply problem solving. Initially, the criteria were only reviewed prior to the six-month reviews so the team could stake its claim regarding level. Now the levels are reviewed frequently at PIT meetings to keep focus on process. The other thing Dominican learned is that the criteria are difficult to meet and require extensive systematic design and redesign so that data can be collected and quantified. Most teams are still working to achieve level-four status. The complaint process team is the most advanced, having met much of the criteria for level three and some criteria in level two.

All of the teams are cautioned that it may not make economic sense to move all processes beyond level three (efficient). There is a cost-benefit test to apply before one sets the goal of creating a world-class process. But all teams are encouraged to work toward level three status.

Manage patient care PITs

One of the important design elements of Dominican's process improvement culture is the integration of clinical and service processes. The organizational chart indicated the center of all hospital processes are the managed patient care activities. The chief medical officer (CMO) is responsible for coordinating and coaching the activities that occur in each of these teams. To date, the following managed patient care PIT teams have been launched: oncology, maternal and child health, medical and surgical, and cardiothoracic services.

The managed patient care teams are dynamic because they involve physician support and bring together physicians, nurses, and support staff to discuss patient care processes. The managed care teams are used to develop the clinical pathways and care plans. Perhaps the most important aspect of the teams is that they use the same process language to talk about care activities as other support and service process teams use. This common language spoken by all caregivers and support staff goes a long way toward dissolving old culture problems that plagued medical organizations.

To bring physicians into the CPI culture, the CMO conducted special management training and orientation for medical staff leadership. All key medical staff leadership participated in the seminar. In addition, the CMO is responsible for the Support Physician Services PIT, which provides all physicians and staff with the clinical database and resource utilization data. The data helps patient care teams understand the economic and clinical outcomes data as decisions are made to improve patient care.

Departmental service standards

As Dominican's CPI effort continues to mature, it is important to show that progress is being made from the customer's point of view. What are the critical points of service most important to the patient? Establishing service standards means setting improvement of performance targets using quality measures. There is a progression of steps involved in setting service standards: (1) select areas to measure improvement based on criteria using patient expectations, (2) identify key requirements from the patient's point of view, (3) establish key quality measures for these requirements, (4) determine improvement targets and, (5) implement a tracking system to indicate continuous improvement.

Some of Dominican's service standards are set by the organization as a whole (e.g., noise reduction and improvement in parking accommodations are areas that patients and families say Dominican needs to improve). They also are set by hospital departments, units, or process improvement teams. It is important to follow the steps involved to select and measure areas for improvements as indicated above. Cycle times, number of retests, or errors are often selected by departments or teams because these are high-priority expectations on the part of patients.

The ultimate purpose of setting and measuring standards is to decrease the gap between Dominican's service delivery and its customers' expectations and requirements. A recent management training seminar was devoted to a curriculum designed to assist each manager and supervisor to develop measurable service standard targets for all areas of the hospital. All departments have a wall-mounted document that identifies the service standard for all hospital departments. Annually, Dominican will use the matrix of standards to report on how well processes and departments have met targets. The document will be used to continually set higher targets of service standards.

Malcolm Baldrige criteria

One of the important tools being used by the Dominican PIC is the Malcolm Baldrige Quality Award criteria. For the past year and a half, the PIC has studied the criteria used by the Baldrige Award to define how its organization pursues quality. The Baldrige criteria comprise seven broad categories, including leadership, information and analysis, strategic quality planning, human resources development and management, management of process quality, quality and operational results, and customer focus and satisfaction. There are 28 examination items, each focusing on a major management requirement. Each criterion has a point system that allows an organization to quantify its overall progress in achieving excellence. Improvement in year-to-year totals is Dominican senior management's goal. Winning an award is secondary to the value the criteria hold in providing a paradigm for evaluating and monitoring organizational excellence against standards held in high esteem in American manufacturing and business sectors.

Dominican is preparing an application for the Baldrige Award and has been using the criteria to organize senior management's plans for total organizational improvement. The value of the Baldrige criteria lies in the discipline it requires of management to systematically evaluate key organizational functions and to develop methods to measure and quantify.

Productivity management

Concurrent with Dominican's focus on CPI is its senior management's concern for effective productivity management. Like hospitals across the country, Dominican faced the challenge of adapting to reduced revenues and reduced patient days. Dominican found it necessary to "rightsize."

Productivity management is an ongoing and concurrent responsibility of a hospital's leadership that is engaged in process improvement and reengineering its culture. All divisions at Catholic HealthCare West real-ized that the system fell far short of adjusting expenses to changes in rev-enues, resulting in a significant shortfall from budgeted expectations. Each division took steps to better manage productivity and to cut expenses this last fiscal year, so CHW returned to the level of success it enjoyed the previous years.

Leadership at various divisions took different approaches to produc-tivity management and organizational downsizing. The following des-cribes Dominican's approach to reduce the number of full-time equivilents (FTEs) in light of declining patient days and describes the lessons learned about attrition analysis, reengineering, management restructuring, early retirement, layoffs and outplacements, and ongoing productivity management.

Dominican's statistics

Dominican's challenge to restructure, reengineer, and downsize started with two distinct advantages: It had one of the best productivity levels in the CHW system, whether measured in terms of FTEs per adjusted occupied bed or adjusted admission. Secondly, with the acquisition of a nearby community hospital, Dominican gained substantial efficiencies, thus avoiding layoffs for Dominican employees. When operations of the two facilities were consolidated, the number of FTEs was reduced by more than 125.

With the consolidation and the introduction of a productivity moni-toring system, Dominican was able to eliminate the increase in FTEs that occurred prior to 1990.

The problem Dominican faced in 1993, however, was that recent staffing did not adjust to declines in volume. Dominican saw the inex-orable decline of a few adjusted occupied beds every year since 1990, while hospital staffing stayed the same. Therefore, FTEs per adjusted occupied bed that used to be 4.83 in 1992 now approached 5.20.

When the performance of individual departments was examined, they were performing effectively relative to their standards. The major problems were twofold: more ancillary services were being provided in a patient day than historic norms, and more patient days were taking place on the critical care units. This would not be a problem if revenue adjusted to the increased intensity of service. However, Dominican's case mix index did not increase, and per diem contracts did not reflect the intensity of services.

As Dominican looked at fiscal year 1995's budget, the combination of not meeting the standard in fiscal year 1994 and the budgeted decline in census of fiscal year 1996 required a reduction of at least 40 FTEs. Unlike previous years, Dominican recognized that actual hours would need to be eliminated. Otherwise, Dominican would be in the red by $2.4 million.

The challenge: Develop an alternative approach

Like many CHW divisions, Dominican's senior management holds a weekly administrative meeting to communicate important management information among senior staff.

One important dimension of this meeting is the routine analysis of productivity and why certain variances occur. Dominican identifies the "hot spots" where variance seems to be consistently below budget standard, and the VP for the area works with the manager to further evaluate why variance is occurring and what can be done to meet the standard.

While this analysis is important to reinforce the need to constantly monitor and investigate productivity variance, it did not help Dominican reduce FTEs. Dominican recognized, though, that if certain key areas such as intensive care units (ICU), telemetry care units (TCU), medical and surgical units, mental health units, and laboratories could meet current productivity standards, Dominican would minimize the need for layoffs.

When senior management acknowledged the need to downsize, and when it calculated that the reduction amounted to 40 FTEs, it was evident that Dominican needed to refocus its efforts. The first step to create this focus was to put management restructuring and downsizing on the agenda for the annual senior management planning retreat.

At the previous year's annual senior management planning retreat, Dominican's management talked about how it could restructure middle management and how senior management's role would change as a result of management restructuring. This year, Dominican's leadership talked candidly about another CHW hospital's approach of eliminating vice president (VP) roles and whether Dominican could justify all of its VP roles since department managers had been combined into "megamanager" roles. Some VPs felt uncomfortable having so few direct reports. The planning retreat produced a rough cut that represented senior management's perspective on how Dominican could achieve savings in middle-management expenses by combining middle manager's roles into fewer megamanager roles.

When senior management returned from the retreat, it realized that it needed to involve middle managers in testing the assumptions senior management made in designing cuts within departments. Dominican leadership invited each department manager in areas it had targeted for reduction to meet with senior management and work out a specific plan for reengineering and redesigning work. Dominican developed a matrix to allow it to track which departments were redesigning and eliminating work and positions. The final task was to identify the people who would be affected by either early retirement, reengineering, management restructuring, or layoff. Dominican wanted to make sure it was not just pushing numbers and was truly effecting a reduction in workforce.

Benchmarking productivity management: St. Mary's and Santa Rosa Memorial

One of the things Dominican did early in its downsizing activity was to find other hospitals that were effectively managing productivity or that successfully engaged in reengineering and downsizing. Dominican met with senior management staff from St. Mary's Hospital in San Francisco and talked about how they reengineered. Dominican adopted the concept of making all departments variable and it adopted St. Mary's approach to attrition management.

Dominican also met with a senior vice president at St. Joseph's of Orange Health System to talk about his experience in managing the remarkable turnaround of the operations at Santa Rosa Memorial Hospital, a division of St. Joseph's, which went from an $8 million loss to a $10 million profit in one year. While Dominican leadership was proud of its operational productivity levels, Santa Rosa, which is identical in size to Dominican, employs 100 fewer FTEs. Several of Dominican's department managers made contact with Santa Rosa counterparts and benchmarked their programs.

In analyzing data from Santa Rosa, Dominican leadership noted four important contrasts: (1) the difference in staffing between Santa Rosa and Dominican was not in nursing, but rather in the support and ancillary departments. Even though some of Dominican's best departments ranked favorably relative to other CHW hospitals and state data, Santa Rosa exceeded Dominican's performance by 30 percent in certain large departments; (2) relative to inpatient volume, Santa Rosa had much lower utilization of ancillary services than Dominican; (3) Santa Rosa faced a "near death" experience. It is much more difficult to make productivity improvements at institutions with excess operational revenue of $6 million a year, like Dominican, than at one losing $8 million; and (4) the circumstances at Santa Rosa in the late 1980s and Dominican in 1994 were different. Patient volume at Santa Rosa was increasing. Santa Rosa's success related to not adding staff when volume increased; for example, the ancillary departments did not have variable standards. Dominican's challenge was to modify staffing levels to lower volume. Nevertheless, this benchmarking experience was helpful.

Attrition analysis process

One of the lessons Dominican learned from St. Mary's and applied to the Dominican management process was the implementation of "attrition analysis." St. Mary's told Dominican senior management that they had long since passed the point where net productivity gain could be achieved by not replacing people when they left. While they no longer have attrition, they scrutinize the neccessity of each position before it is posted for new hiring.

Dominican still had a number of people vacating positions across the hospital. Instead of allowing the manager to get a VP's approval to post vacant positions, Dominican decided that no vacated or new job could be posted until the manager completed an "attrition analysis" form. The form asks a series of questions designed to assist the manager in considering less costly alternatives to replacing the position in total or in part. The VPs bring this attrition analysis to the weekly administrative meetings, and Dominican's senior management team "gently" debates if vacant positions should be posted.

There are several lessons Dominican has learned from this process. First, savings have been gained because some managers are simply reluctant to go through the grilling associated with justifying refilling the position. The process has lead to the policy of posting most positions for internal applicants only, or has caused departments to share employees. For example a nurse's aide may spend two days a week on a medical surgical unit and three days at the skilled nursing facility. Further, it has reduced the number of 0.5 FTE and 0.6 FTE positions. With the cost of health benefits, these are by far the most expensive positions in the organization. Instead, managers are asked to see if the work can be reengineered into other staff positions or if the position can be posted at an unbenefited 0.4 FTE position. Finally, Dominican also learned that over the years it had abused the practice of hiring per diem employees. Dominican's management team and employees thought of per diem as though it were a job classification rather than a pay category. As a result, Dominican hired regularly scheduled, nonbenefited per diem staff who work more than 0.5 FTE. This was a way for managers to get around hiring benefited staff, even though it often proved to be more expensive.

To address these issues, the following solutions were introduced: (1) instead of hiring per diem, Dominican hired unbenefited, part-time staff but made sure they worked no more than a 0.5 position; (2) for all current per diem staff, they assigned a specific FTE status so that 0.2 staff were not routinely worked 0.4, thus contributing to FTE creep; (3) in cases where a 0.4 or less position was vacated, Dominican looked to see if staff working 0.5 or 0.6 could absorb hours. This was more cost effective because a full benefit package was available to people working 0.5 and more.

The net effect of not replacing vacated positions in a four-month period resulted in a savings of 23 FTEs.

Redefining the core (regularly scheduled staff)

Some departments have had greater reductions in volume than others. The difficulty is that even with calling off staff during low census periods, more employees are often used instead of reducing the core staff and providing more consistent work schedules for the fewer numbers of staff. Thus, when volume increases, there is a challenge to increase the number of staff. This concept certainly has more applicability in nursing departments than in other departments. Dominican was able to reduce the core staff on the mental health unit, intensive care, and emergency room through the use of attrition and reducing per diem hours as well as decreasing the number of charge nurses in critical care. These actions mean that departments that used to be averaging 93 percent productivity are now at 100 percent performance as measured by Mecon's OPTI-MIS productivity system.

Reengineering targeted areas

One of the lessons Dominican learned about reengineering was from Care 2000 at Mercy San Diego Hospital (a CHW division). Dominican initiated "care partners" in Dominican's Telemetry Care Unit (TCU). A care partner is an upgraded nursing assistance position that enabled Dominican to cost effectively provide services previously done by respiratory therapists and laboratory technicians. Unlike Mercy San Diego, Dominican has not decentralized the radiology, pharmacy, and admitting functions because of the capital costs, limited opportunities for cost savings, and major architectural and staffing issues that precluded decentralization in a cost-effective way.

While it is still very much in its infancy, Dominican expects that major reengineering will occur in the respiratory and laboratory departments as this concept spreads to the remaining nursing units. Dominican has already seen some reductions in its laboratory and respiratory FTEs.

Dominican's great challenge is to make the "care pods" (nursing unit) work effectively in a unit where there is significant fluctuation in patient census. It is far easier to adjust staffing with a staffing grid based on going from 26 to 24 patients than a care pod when census goes from 4 patients to 3.

Management restructuring

Management restructuring began at the senior management level. When Dominican's VP for physician relations resigned, Dominican reassigned his responsibilities partly to the CMO and partly to one of Dominican's remaining vice presidents. Dominican also reduced one other VP title by downgrading the position's responsibilities and salary and having that individual focus on developing and implementing Dominican's new outreach care programs for the poor.

While Dominican did not significantly reduce senior management, it did make major changes in middle management. Dominican attempted to establish some common criteria to use to determine if a person could be a manager, a director, a megamanager (someone who manages multiple departments), or a program coordinator. Dominican's goal was to alter titles that had become important status elements in its organizational culture. After creating a special ad hoc group of managers to assist in the development of the criteria, Dominican gave up on the idea of tampering with titles at this time because it discovered how sacred titles are in the traditional hospital paradigm. Dominican expects that as its CPI culture takes hold, traditional titles will naturally fade away as it develops new titles related to functional roles of intradepartmental process teams.

Dominican's plan for middle management reengineering finally resulted in the combination of a few departments into megamanager roles and the elimination of the several assistant department manager roles. This net effect was that Dominican reduced middle management by eight people and 5.5 FTEs. Most managers now have multiple departments or are responsible for at least 60 FTEs.

Dominican leadership recognizes that management restructuring is not complete and that further restructuring is necessary. Not all of Dominican's process improvement teams are up and running, and Dominican does not have many self-directed work groups in place yet. Once Dominican has more work groups experienced in self-direction, it will be easier to transition away from the traditional command and control management and further reduce middle-management roles.

Early retirement

Other CHW divisions have used early retirement programs as a method to reduce workforce and redesign departments. Dominican learned from the experiences of other CHW divisions, gleaning the following: (1) early retirement must be implemented as part of a broader staff reduction program. It was made quite clear to managers and staff that if savings were not achieved in this area, then the number of staff being laid off would increase; (2) management at Mercy Hospital in Redding, California, told their counterparts at Dominican to target only positions that would not require replacement. No nurses who would have to be replaced were offered early retirement; (3) given Dominican's limited pension plan benefits, what most staff members want in their retirement is health coverage. Dominican provided the cash equivalent for employees to purchase health coverage on their own until eligible for Medicare. Dominican made it explicit that it was not setting the precedent of offering retiree health benefits.

Dominican's early retirement plan was offered to 35 people. Dominican thought that about 8 to10 FTEs would be gained through this plan. It also estimated that the cost would be a one-time expense of $200,000. Dominican's leadership was surprised that 18 people, representing 14 FTEs, or half of those offered early retirement, accepted. Therefore the cost of the program was closer to $400,000. Given the cost, the payback period would be one year. The cost also forced senior management to make sure that the positions were not filled.

Taking advantages of opportunities

There are certain support services where savings could be gained through outsourcing. Along with St. Luke's Hospital in San Francisco, Dominican was one of the last hospitals in northern California that still operated an in-house laundry. Previously, Dominican had studied the situation and knew that substantial savings could be gained from closing the laundry; however, it chose not to eliminate laundry workers' positions at that time.

In early May, 1994, Dominican had an electrical fire in the laundry that put it out of service for at least two months. Dominican decided to close the laundry, but the staff was given four months' notice. Dominican was also able to place all but two employees in other vacancies at the hospital; some staff members were retrained for positions in dietary, housekeeping, transportation, and medical records.

Dominican remained consistent with its mission and its values and treated the displaced employees with dignity, yet at the same time was able to gain savings of at least $150,000.

Layoffs and outplacement

Dominican was not able to target the number of FTEs it would have to lay off until the early retirement candidates declared their intentions.

When the final plan was put in place, Dominican had to lay off 17 people, which translated into 10 FTEs. The layoffs took place on all levels of the organization, including registered nurses (RNs).

All of the affected people were provided severance pay in accordance with hospital policy and all were given the opportunity to work with an outplacement counseling firm.

Dominican also established, through its employee assistance program, a series of debriefing sessions for staff who found it difficult to work in an environment where coworkers had been laid off. Interestingly, relatively few people participated in sessions. One speculation was that the actual number was small compared to what people read about elsewhere and what they expected. Also, Dominican communicated early on that it was developing a plan designed to have the least possible impact on the organization. Restructuring management and announcing it a few months earlier, as well as instituting an early retirement program, created the climate that the hospital "did it the right way."

However, one of the issues Dominican wrestled with was a conventional wisdom that suggests if an organization is going to put staff through the agony and disruption of a layoff, it should be as big as possible so operations are not disrupted again in the near future. This conventional wisdom does not seem to apply in healthcare. There are seasonal spikes in census, and it makes little sense to lay off people and hire them back a few months later.

Dominican recognized that the key to successful rightsizing was to establish a communication system to allow all employees to know where the hospital stands in relation to budget assumptions that drive the operational plan for each fiscal year. The long-range trend that will drive the size of the labor budget each year is the average of occupied beds. For every one-day decline in the adjusted occupied beds, Dominican will have to reduce the equivalent of 5.5 FTEs.

Summary of savings

Dominican has exceeded the 40 FTE target and may reach a reduction of 60 FTEs. This is due to a combination of layoffs and particular departments meeting their productivity standards. However, since the census decline is a little greater than budget, Dominican appears to be on the right course for its current fiscal year.

Next steps

Dominican has communicated to staff that while these reductions should be sufficient for the remainder of the fiscal year, staffing reductions are not a one-time event. There will be further declines in census, which will require additional reductions in staffing. The decline in census will be due to two factors, the first of which is the tendancy of Medicare and Medi-Cal programs to shift patients into managed care. Medicare HMO enrollment will cannibalize existing Medicare fee-for-service activity (e.g., if 4,000 enrollees sign up and days per 1,000 decline from 1,700 to 1,000, there will be a decline in census of 9 patients). Second, the opening of a new maternity and short-stay surgery center by a competitor in early 1996 will reduce Dominican's acute volume by about 10 patient days.

While Dominican has designed a series of strategies to compete effectively with the new facility, Dominican has stressed to the staff that it must implement improvements in service quality so that patients and physicians will prefer Dominican. Dominican is stressing how important it is to have a physical plant that looks first-rate and a staff that meets or exceeds the needs of patient/customers. Dominican's philosophy is that "the only true job security anybody has is having patients at our front door (or in our affiliated health plans for capitated activity)." If Dominican does things to drive patients to a competitor, all employees' job security is impacted.

Given the anticipated volume reductions, over the next year Dominican will need to continuously reduce staffing in the organization. Some of its strategies include

1. *Changes in resource consumption.* The long-term strategy to reduce staffing in the ancillary departments is to reduce ancillary utilization. Like other CHW hospitals, Dominican is aggressively developing critical pathways as part of business improvement. It is also designing the risk pools for managed care contracts so that there are withhold incentives for physicians that reward cost-conscious behavior by the medical staff. Two of the more successful operational changes are related to the appropriate use of the critical care unit. A cardiac intervention unit was established, and certain cath laboratory therapeutic procedures patients are now recovered on a unit with staffing equal to that on the TCU, not the ICU. Dominican has also implemented the Apache

Information System, which assists physicians and staff in determining on a concurrent basis the appropriateness of a patient for critical care

2. *Census tracking.* Dominican wants all employees to be sensitive to how changes in census impact staffing levels. It prepares a daily flash report that goes out on the e-mail system. Rather than just listing the midnight census, Dominican also shows a census thermometer. Volume has been divided in to nine zones, and each department will design staffing levels based on these zones

3. *Cross-training.* The most effective way to eliminate departmental barriers is to have staff float across units. Dominican has placed the management of medical records, admitting, emergency department registration, and patient accounting under one manager. One job classification was developed—patient services representative. Staff will float across all of these departments based on changes in workload. A savings of at least four to five FTEs is anticipated.

   Like many other CHW divisions that have limited cardiac volume, Dominican spends a huge amount on standby pay in both the cath lab and operating room, even though the frequency of staff callback is low. Dominican is in the process of training staff to work in both the cath lab and critical care and also reducing the number of employees on standby in surgery by one FTE

4. *Eliminating pay premiums.* Some staff are working 12-hour shifts in the ICU, the nurseries, and to a limited extent, the emergency department. They receive an 11 percent pay premium. Under its union contract with the California Nurses Association, Dominican has the right to eliminate 12-hour shifts. This issue will be addressed with the union because of ongoing pressure to further reduce expenses.

   Dominican also changed some if its pay policies. It has a large number of part-time benefited employees. When employees worked greater than their status, paid time off (PTO) was accrued on the hours worked. However, a peculiar policy is that when fewer hours are worked, PTO is still accrued based on the employee's status. This policy is being changed to make the PTO accrual rate a function of actual hours worked. This will save $200,000 dollars annually

5. *Outsourcing.* At the time of a nursing shortage, Dominican started an offcampus childcare program to encourage nursing recruitment and

retention. It was heavily subsidized because of the staffing levels and the level of flexibility provided for parents who had varying work schedules. Dominican eliminated this service and received the expected criticism from participating parents who had to make other childcare arrangements. However, at a time when cutbacks were being made elsewhere throughout the hospital, this level of subsidy for a small number of employees could no longer be justified

Ongoing productivity management: Customer focus

Dominican recognizes that it must keep a close eye on how well its productivity standards are met. Dominican continues to stress with all hospital staff that it is not changing the standards for nursing hours per patient day for nursing units. Dominican currently has standards that are at or slightly better than industry norms. Like many hospitals, Dominican has some poorly designed care systems that are inefficient and serve as barriers to optimum productivity. Some of the systems problems are procedural, others are related to core staffing, and still others are related to not aggressively calling off staff (e.g., sending some people home when there are fewer patients to care for than the budget projected).

Dominican recognizes, though, that productivity management is not directly connected to the way patient/customers perceive Dominican's services. This is where Dominican's customer-driven CPI activities fit into the management vision.

Dominican now has more than 20 teams involving 200 employees and 15 physicians working to improve cycle times, reduce and eliminate rework, and measure improvements in key process indicators. The new organizational chart describes how Dominican's leadership is rethinking the organizational structure so there is more emphasis on how processes, not departments or divisions, allow staff, physicians, and volunteers meet customer/patient needs

Dominican's most recent CPI activity is the education of managers and first-line supervisors on how to establish and maintain service standards for all departments and services. Each department now has a service standard (e.g., "We answer all call bells within ____ minutes," and "We have a waiting time in our emergency department of less than ____ minutes before a nonemergency patient is seen by a caregiver.")

Conclusion: Developing leadership vision and cultural transformation

Reengineering is more than blowing up an existing department and process and starting over. It is more than reallocating resources to perform the same amount of work with less staff, and it is more than a faddish buzzword defining the most vogue techniques of management. Reengineering is most effective when it focuses on an organization's culture. Changing how people think about the whole fabric of an organization is the greatest challenge to hospital management.

When Dominican began its CPI journey more than three years ago, it had little idea about how integral CPI would be to productivity management and organizational downsizing. CPI provides Dominican's staff with a common language to talk about the behaviors and processes used in the hospital to meet or exceed the expectations of customers. This new language allows everyone, whether they are working in the business office, the food services department, the admitting area, or a patient care unit, to have a common language to talk about how clinical processes of care and nonclinical service or support processes meet customer needs. It takes staff beyond productivity statistics and links all staff through a common language. In addition to monitoring whether or not the hospital is on budget, Dominican staff now also ask questions about whether resources are being used to reinforce the customer's perception of quality.

▤ 17

Marion Merrell Dow: Reengineering to meet customer needs

John L. Aitken, PhD
Principal
Ernst & Young, LLP
Kansas City, Missouri

THE FORMATION OF MARION MERRELL DOW (MMD) in 1989 through the consolidation of Dow Chemical's Merrell Dow Pharmaceuticals unit with independent Marion Laboratories is an example of the mergers that have occurred within the industry over the past 10 years. In general, such consolidations have been interpreted by industry analysts as a requirement to afford the costs of basic research, product development, and regulatory approval. More recently, however, it has become clear that consolidations will continue—perhaps at an even faster pace—as a response to fundamental structural changes, such as the emergence of very large healthcare providing organizations, taking place within the broader setting of healthcare.

Healthcare—the actual delivery of treatment for illness—has been and continues to be in a process of industrialization. The traditional patient-selected, fee-for-service physician mode of delivery is rapidly being replaced by a model whereby payer-selected healthcare providers not only treat illness but also engage in disease management, healthcare maintenance, and illness-prevention interventions. At the root of this transformation is the introduction of economics as a factor of equal importance to the traditional concerns of safety and efficacy. MMD launched a major reengineering of its U.S. commercial business in early 1992 in response to these far-reaching changes.

Unlike many projects started to restore economic health to badly deteriorated businesses, MMD's reengineering activities began in a period of exceptional financial success. The project, named USBR (U.S. Business Reengineering), was seen as a strategically focused initiative designed to develop and implement business processes to successfully meet the changing needs of U.S. customers. The business case for the project involved a strategic recasting of the company's approach to conducting business based on changes that had occurred or were expected to occur in its marketplace.

The emergence of myriad forms of organized healthcare in the United States has had the following specific implications for pharmaceutical suppliers:

Creation of formularies. To manage drug costs, many organized healthcare providers have adopted formularies—lists of recommended or approved drugs—to prescribe and dispense to patients. Typically, drugs are selected for inclusion on formularies by panels consisting of both healthcare professionals and business administrators. In these deliberations price is viewed as a criterion of equal importance to safety and efficacy. Although healthcare providers vary in the vigor with which they insist on physician compliance with formularies, it is clearly better for pharmaceutical manufacturers to have their products included on formularies than not.

Negotiated price. A direct offshoot of the increased use of formularies is the movement toward contractual relationships between healthcare providers and pharmaceutical suppliers wherein drug companies provide rebates to healthcare providers upon demonstrated performance (i.e., quantities of drugs prescribed or dispensed). The quantities of drugs actually prescribed within any specific managed care organization reflect the degree of physician compliance the organization is able to achieve. Absent a contractual relationship, the manufacturer is likely to sell less.

Curtailment of promotional practices. Organized healthcare providers increasingly recognize that representatives deployed by pharmaceutical suppliers to sell to healthcare professionals are effective and persuasive. There is little doubt that the frequency of contact between pharmaceutical representatives and physicians correlates with the number of prescriptions written. Since this is seen as inimical to healthcare providers' economic interests, these organizations increasingly are barring access of pharmaceutical representatives to healthcare professionals. This clearly threatens the use of products produced by firms that have representatives who are denied access. On the other hand, it can lead to a reduction of promotional expense as a result of diminishing the number of representatives who can be productively employed. Reduced expense can, in turn, allow suppliers to make more competitive contractual proposals to providers.

Disease state management. As healthcare provider organizations gain in economic sophistication and organizational complexity, they also are becoming more aware of the need to look at economic issues on a broader base. A lower-cost drug that leads to longer hospital stays may be of less value to a provider who covers drug costs and hospitalization than a more expensive drug that produces therapeutic improvement more rapidly, resulting in shorter hospital stays. Likewise, in some cases, an over-the-counter drug may be as effective in providing symptomatic relief as a more expensive prescribed product.

In dealing with these complex issues healthcare providers are finding it useful to develop disease state management guidelines that, like formularies, set forth practitioner directions based on economic as well as ethical and safety considerations. These guidelines or treatment protocols call for the lowest-cost treatment based on all elements of the treatment process as well as all available products. They also call for well-documented outcomes analyses concerning these products. Pharmaceutical companies having products that provide genuine value based on total healthcare costs as well as those capable of providing a wide range of over-the-counter, generic, and prescription products will prosper while those whose products are without demonstrable economic benefit—even though therapeutically competitive—will suffer. This chapter discusses the reengineering of MMD to accommodate these changing circumstances.

Project development

Marion Merrell Dow's USBR project was initially broached by the company's chairman and CEO in a meeting in December 1991. From then until the official launch date in April 1992, a number of critical pieces of infrastructure were developed. A high-level project steering committee

consisting of the president of the U.S. business as well as the heads of all
the major functions in the company (i.e., sales and marketing, manufacturing, product development, finance, and human resources) was
formed to provide cross-functional support and "political coverage" for
what would be a project demanding behavioral change at many levels
and functions of the business. A project leader and facilitator were identified, and they, in turn, created an eight-person project team to lead the
project through its initial stages. Those named to the team were selected
primarily on the basis of their individual capabilities and performance
rather than to represent one or another of the company's functions. Also
during the start-up phase, and after a period of careful study, an outside
consulting firm was chosen as reengineering consultants.[2] Finally, to
gather information on current and projected customer needs, an outside
marketing research firm was selected to conduct "customer-based customer research."[3] The project was organized into six distinct phases: current state analysis, benchmarking, visioning, future state design,
implementation, and continuous improvement.

Current state analysis

An initial task of the project team was to create a process model of the
business. This proved to be more difficult than expected as the concept of
process in an organizational setting was unfamiliar to most members
of the team who were much more oriented to a functional model of organizational design. In retrospect, the "process" model originally developed
turned out to be little more than a "functional" model turned on its side.
It proved adequate, however, to enable the current state analysis
to go forward. More than 90 associates were organized into nine current
state analysis teams built around the processes identified in the model.
Each team was asked to put down on paper, in considerable detail, precisely how their assigned process was currently being handled in MMD.
To enable the activity, each team was assigned a trained facilitator and
given forms to record inputs, transforming activities, outputs, systems
support, and personnel support. The current state analysis occurred over
a six-week period and resulted in a substantial accumulation of documentation. The project team then used this material, as well as information derived from the customer-based research, to diagnose the
organization's effectiveness to meet the customer needs.

A significant number of "disconnects" were identified by the team. These disconnects included the discovery that sometimes work performed by one group of well-intentioned and well-trained associates in one part of the company was not, in fact, of much value to another group of associates who were its intended users. Other disconnects involved duplication of effort in several organizational entities as well as procedures that added time and cost but no value to the final output. Likewise, systems inadequacies and human performance factors (e.g., inadequate training) sometimes resulted in excessive costs, unacceptably long cycle times, and work products of unsatisfactory quality. These improvement opportunities were compared with a ranked ordering of customer needs (identified by customer research). A list of processes for improvement most likely to be of value to customers was then developed.

Benchmarking

The second stage of the USBR project took place between September and November 1992 and began with secondary research—the electronic scanning of networks of published information using key words associated with the process to be improved. The good news for MMD was that no other pharmaceutical company emerged as having established "world-class" proficiency in the subject processes. However, a number of well-known firms in other industries were found to have more effective or less costly business procedures that paralleled those of interest to MMD. The project team reviewed these results and identified target companies for on-site visits. Using networking techniques, such as relationships built through participation in professional associations, arrangements were made to visit these companies. The project team then prepared detailed questionnaires and organized site visits so as to maximize the learning and value of each trip. Companies visited included Hewlett-Packard, Wal-Mart, USAA, Federal Express, and General Electric.

During the benchmarking stage of the USBR project, the project team was also exposed to several days of expert testimony, where subject matter experts from both inside and outside the company gave members of the team an in-depth and future-oriented understanding of the dynamics affecting MMD's marketplace. Topics included prospective healthcare legislation, health economics, future technologies, industry dynamics, and competitor activities.

Visioning

With the background of the customer needs analysis, the current state analysis, the findings obtained from benchmarking, and the knowledge and perceptions of leading thinkers in the future of healthcare, the project team went off-site in December 1992 for a one-week visioning process. The output of this activity consisted of developing

- A theme—a customer-oriented company

- A new conceptual model of the organization described through a series of six statements contrasting the present with the proposed future state

- A new process model of the business identifying "megaprocesses" that incorporated the customer-centered ideology

- A recommended organizational structure

  A summary of the vision is shown in Table 1.

  The project team presented the vision, the process model, and the proposed organizational structure to the steering committee in January 1993 and asked and received approval to proceed to the future state design.

Future state design

In some sense—but with an important difference—the future state design phase of the project was reminiscent of the current state analysis. Using the new process model discussed below, multifunctional teams of knowledgeable associates were assigned to develop a very detailed description of the new processes, the systems necessary to support or enable these activities, and the training and structural support necessary to implement the new activities from a behavioral and organizational viewpoint. Thirteen teams of between 8 and 12 dedicated members each (plus ad hoc participants) worked on future state 60 percent of their time over a four-month period. As with all teams involved in the project, facilitators were provided for each team. A description of each megaprocess (the highest-level process developed in the model) as well as the thrust of the improvement initiative is provided below.

TABLE 1
Summary of vision statement
Marion Merrell Dow—A customer-centered company

Marion Merrell Dow will so effectively satisfy the needs of its customers that all patients will have access to its products.

As a customer-centered company we will transform ourselves from a company in which associates have been focused internally to a company in which each associate knows and understands each customer, is dedicated to meeting their needs, and is motivated and rewarded on the basis of achieving customer satisfaction.

As a customer-centered company we will transform ourselves from a company organized around traditional management functions to a company organized flexibly around the geography and processes necessary to satisfy the needs of each customer.

As a customer-centered company we will transform ourselves from a products-oriented company to a company driven by the desire to provide the best value to each customer through outstanding products tied to the most customer-valued support services in our industry.

As a customer-centered company we will transform ourselves from a company too often limited by our own perceptions and resources to a company whose products and services are developed, manufactured, and offered in partnership with customers and suppliers.

As a customer-centered company we will transform ourselves from a company in which information has been viewed mainly as a vehicle for administration and control to a company whose culture encourages the use of unbiased information and treats it as a highly valued and deeply embedded source of associate empowerment and customer enablement.

As a customer-centered company we will transform ourselves from a company which has presented itself to its customers with many unconnected faces to a company that provides each customer on every transaction with only one point of contact, backed up by process support teams and by the spirit of customer-centeredness that permeates the entire organization.

As a customer-centered company we will transform ourselves from a company whose image with customers has not been well established to a company whose image is firmly associated with leadership in our industry, with a commitment to continuous improvement in all that we do, and with a total dedication to being "customer centered."

CUSTOMER INTERFACE

This process involves any interaction of any sort between any MMD associate and any customer. Most of the company's interactions with customers are carried out by field representatives; however, for the purpose of the new process model, this process also includes phone and written interaction between MMD and its customers. The primary highlights of the process changes that were developed to support this megaprocess consisited of

- Systems enablement of the representatives to assist them in providing information needed to manage their customer interactions as a small business

- The introduction of account management teams that link together the representatives who call on physicians affiliated with the same managed care organization. These teams are under the strategic direction of an account manager who has responsibility for overseeing MMD's relationship with that account

- The development of a 24-hour per day, 365-day per year customer service center staffed with administrative associates and staff personnel who can respond to technical and scientific questions

- The development of a single system to enter all data obtained from all sources of customer contact

DISCOVERING AND ANALYZING CUSTOMER NEEDS

The second megaprocess involves understanding the information received from customers. In the classic representative-physician interchange, it occurs just seconds after the representative has heard whatever it is the doctor has to say (the first megaprocess). The transformation of information into understanding is the heart of this process—whether it occurs through conversation or in writing. It is through this process that customers—and potential customers—are identified. It is also through this process that MMD develops an appreciation for customer needs. Highlights of the changes being developed to support this megaprocess include

- The creation of an "intelligent" system to collect, analyze, and interpret data on customer needs that is accumulated and entered on a routine basis from all customer contact (most commonly from field-based associates)

- The use of micromarketing data to improve the effectiveness of each representative's call—both through increasing the percentage of calls made on more rigorously "qualified" customers and through more focused, customer-tailored call plans

- The institutionalization of customer-based customer research to maintain a continuous assessment of MMD's performance in understanding and meeting customer needs

PLANNING AND ALLOCATING RESOURCES

Traditionally MMD's planning process has been product-centered and top-down driven. At its core has been a process involving the creation of a plan of action to generate appealing financial results from an investor viewpoint. In the reengineered planning process, these elements were not eliminated, but they were complemented by the introduction of a customer-centered, bottom-up planning process which fed off of the second analytical process. The new planning process initiates planning at the account level using the new account management team structure. This leads in part to field-inspired proposals for marketing support materials that are discussed across the four business regions in the field to determine if materials can be developed nationally based on common customer needs. These customer-centered proposals are then debated and reviewed within the context of similar proposals (i.e., those that traditionally have held sway over the available marketing budget) advocated by product-centered managers. Account-centered planning is now used also to develop service programs and educational presentations which, in the past, were often developed with minimal customer input as to relevancy and content.

DEVELOPING AND PRODUCING PRODUCTS AND SERVICES TO MEET CUSTOMER NEEDS

Of the megaprocesses depicted in the new process model, this process is the most complex and absorbs the most resources. Since it includes all research and development, manufacturing, marketing, and certain elements of the administrative functions (e.g., accounts receivable), more of the company's associates are employed in this process than elsewhere. Although these are the processes most often targeted for improvement by an organization's management (presumably because they frequently absorb the bulk of the organization's people), many of them are invisible to customers and, consequently, generate little customer interest. Indirectly, however, the customer is impacted significantly by these processes since the process outcomes—the product or services produced, the information communicated, and the accounting statements issued—are all of great interest to the customer. Thus, unless process improvements in these areas make a difference to the process outcomes, little gain in customer acceptance will be realized.

Given this perspective it is perhaps surprising that so many of the improvements initiated in the USBR project—focused on meeting customer needs—were located within this internally centered process. Part of the explanation undoubtedly stems from the aforementioned proclivity of management to push for change it can appreciate (e.g., improving productivity, reducing cycle times, and reducing costs). To the extent these process improvements lead to reduced expense and, ultimately, to lower prices, the changes can be said to be customer focused.

Some of the major initiatives in this area are described below:

- Reconfiguration of the planning process to develop informational materials, sales aids, and brochures beginning in the field at the representative level, based on customer input. Previously this process was initiated in headquarters

- Allocation to field-based associates of budgets that will be used to order support materials from headquarters coupled with a field-based process for ordering such materials from an electronic catalogue. This process replaces traditional bulk distribution of these materials to all field-based personnel. (This process change is estimated to result in millions of dollars of savings over a five-year period. By itself this change will pay for more than 50 percent of the cost of the reengineering project.)

- The use of cross-functional teams to plan and develop support materials. Virtually all of the content of the materials used by MMD to communicate about its products and services is regulated by the Food and Drug Administration. To ensure compliance with regulatory guidelines, a group of associates with legal and regulatory expertise traditionally have approved or disapproved such materials following their creation. In many cases, disapproval meant substantial rework. By using cross-functional teams in the creation process, including regulatory personnel, compliance will be built in to the initial cycle, thus reducing rework

- Enabling field-based associates to engage in contract negotiations with accounts with electronic support from the headquarters-based contracting department. In the past, field-based associates essentially gathered information for forwarding to contracting departments, which developed draft contracts for review and negotiation with the account. All issues resolved at the customer contact level required approval from headquarters. The contracting process often took weeks—sometimes months—to complete. The new process calls for contracting to establish negotiating parameters and boilerplate language to be electronically available to the field so on-the-spot negotiations can be conducted within a few days. The new process also provides for contracting across the company's product line instead of on a product-by-product basis

- The development of a reward system that, in addition to the conventional link between sales success and bonus payout, ties bonuses to meeting customer needs as well as other changes coming out of this project

CUSTOMER FULFILLMENT

This process contains those activities that move products, materials, services, information, billing statements, and all other forms of response from MMD to the customer. At the moment the customer receives the response, the customer fulfillment process is completed, and the customer interface process is again in play. Highlights of the process improvements made in this area include "one order, one shipment, one invoice"; automatic replenishment of warehoused inventories; better management of inventories in general; and accommodation of customer desires for specific customer fulfillment processes (e.g., through a distributor or directly from MMD).

The future state design was presented to the company's management committee and board of directors and was approved for implementation in August 1993.

Implementation

The implementation phase of the USBR project was managed primarily through cross-functional teams aided by facilitators. In the case of the implementation teams, many of the participants were those who would ultimately be involved on a daily basis in using the new processes and systems. In addition, two enablement teams—a systems enablement team and a training enablement team made up of professional employees in these respective functions—were established. Members from these two teams were assigned to participate on each of the implementation teams. This made it possible for the two enablement teams to influence the implementation plans as well as gain a direct and clear understanding of the requirements of each of the process implementation teams. Coordination between the implementation teams was also critical. While each process could be conceptualized separately, the processes were closely linked to each other and each team needed to take into account decisions and actions being taken by the other teams. Weekly team leader meetings were scheduled during this period to facilitate communications and to resolve conflicts.

The structural recommendations were the first elements of the new future state to be implemented. These changes, among others things, involved the creation of four regional organizations to manage MMD's commercial business. The regions replaced one national business unit and were announced by the North American MMD president at the outset of the implementation process. The four new regional general managers were then added to the USBR steering committee and became active in shaping the implementation of the new processes and systems.

Two decisions made early in the implementation process turned out to be critical. The first involved the creation of a user advisory group to support the creation of new systems. The new systems required more sophisticated hardware, as well as more and more complex software, than many associates had previously experienced, particularly those in the field. Many good suggestions that made the new systems more user-friendly were received through this activity.

A second decision was that all training would be conducted through the management hierarchy. Again this proved to be an important and constructive decision. The magnitude of the training task was substantial and alternative approaches to training would have required either significant investments in outside resources or stretched the implementation process out over a prolonged time period. This latter consideration brought with it the specter of a headquarters organization having to maintain the capability of dealing with two distinct and unconnected systems over many months. By using line management for training, the transition process occurred over six to eight weeks. Headquarters staff were trained first, followed by senior field managers who trained their staffs. Training then cascaded throughout the organization.

In an earlier unrelated rollout of a new system, the company had elected to go directly to the frontline field organization—the field representatives—with new equipment and a new system, bypassing intermediate line management. This was a mistake since field managers were unable to assist representatives in the new system and were themselves at a disadvantage in not having access to information as it became available to representatives. In the USBR project, using managers as trainers ensured their understanding and familiarity with both the mechanics and the uses of the new capabilities.

Continuous improvement

This final phase of the USBR project consisted of recognizing that marketplace changes, which prompted the formation of the project in 1992, are far from over. The adaptation of MMD to these changes cannot, therefore, be a one-time event. It was recognized early on that decisions on process and systems design would be time-limited by marketplace events. Therefore the concept of a process champion—an individual with ongoing responsibility to the activity for its viability and effectiveness—was built in to the latter phases of implementation and considered the chief element of the continuous improvement stage. The process champion, typically with management responsibility at a level that provides a broad overview of the commercial organization, is authorized to initiate action to convene new cross-functional teams as necessary to modify or even radically redesign the processes. In looking back at the overall project, the following emerge as critical success factors.

COMPELLING BUSINESS CASE

The axiom that change is resisted is as true in business as in other arenas of life. The marketplace served by MMD is in a state of dramatic change. This fact was made clear by virtually every edition of every newspaper and television news reports on the dramatic changes occurring in healthcare across America. To MMD associates, living through these times without seeing any reaction or response from their employer would have been more upsetting than seeing the company undertake a change process of this magnitude. Change simply for the sake of change would be a difficult business case to sustain within an organization, but change to accommodate new circumstance and conditions was a persuasive and compelling rationale for MMD's associates and aided in their personal readiness to adjust the ways in which they performed their work.

CUSTOMER-BASED FOUNDATION

The use of customer-based customer research as a foundation for understanding customer requirements was important to USBR. In other reengineering projects, a database predicated on the experiences and observations and conclusions of management was used as a foundation for analysis and priority setting. While there may be considerable overlap between what management thinks are the needs of the customers and what customers actually think, the availability of independent data provided a solid basis for refuting or supporting internal opinions.

INVOLVEMENT

The magnitude of change involved in a true reengineering project is akin to the magnitude of a merger or acquisition. Unlike those events in which legal restraints and negotiations strategies get in the way of massive participation and involvement until after the fact, the reengineering process lends itself to getting many people involved from the beginning. The sense of ownership that easily develops if people are involved in substantive ways in change design activities greatly facilitates implementation and acceptance.

MANAGEMENT SUPPORT

Virtually every article or textbook refers to the importance of top management leadership for a massive reengineering project and certainly USBR benefited from that kind of support. At the same time, however, the support of middle management proved to be critical to USBR—particularly during the implementation stage of the project. Middle management is in an ideal position to bury unwanted changes in bureaucratic minutia and procedural obfuscation even in the face of top management endorsement. More positively, middle management can also provide the hands-on leadership for inculcating new ideas and new approaches to work that makes it possible to get things done more rapidly and more easily.

PURSUING AN ESTABLISHED METHODOLOGY

The use of external consultants on the reengineering process itself provided MMD with a known road map. At each stage it was possible to articulate with reasonable clarity what was being done and why it was being done. The linkage to what had gone before and what would follow was also easily understood as a result of following an established reengineering process. This understanding made it possible for the MMD people to focus on content and to avoid endless debate on how things should be done.

QUALITY OF PEOPLE

The leadership, the facilitators, and the participants were among the best and brightest in MMD's associate pool. When this pattern was established with the appointment of the very first project team (which took the process through visioning), it became apparent to many in the organization this was a good project with which to be associated. The reengineering project manager was often in the enviable position of being able to choose from several well-qualified candidates. There is little doubt the quality of the outcomes of USBR directly reflected on the quality of the people performing the work.

COMMUNICATIONS

This project was moved forward—particularly subsequent to the rollout of the vision—in an atmosphere of openness and transparency. Although this might have been assured simply by virtue of the number of people involved, the various teams went to considerable lengths to communicate about what they were doing, what they were thinking about doing, and what they were hoping to achieve. The company's communications department routinely carried stories about the project and the progress being made. Team leaders made frequent presentations at department staff meetings and to small groups of associates that would be affected by the changes being made.

LUCK

It is perhaps not surprising that in a project of this scope that luck would emerge as a critical factor. USBR was launched during a period of prosperity. In 1993, however, the company experienced a downturn in sales as a result of the introduction of generic competition for one of its major products. The need to adjust expense to match falling income led to downsizing activities in 1993 and 1994. These reductions were attributed, correctly, to business circumstances. However, it is likely the USBR project eventually would have led to reduced personnel levels. In reports of other reengineering projects, dealing with downsizing has sometimes prevented organizations from truly reaping the full value of their reengineering effort.

As indicated earlier, the USBR project is a story of one company's response to dramatically changing market conditions; changes that are, in fact, ongoing. Thus while the project is now completed, the spirit that gave it birth must be maintained. The continued responsiveness of MMD to the further evolution of the U.S. healthcare market will be essential to its survival and success. USBR enabled MMD to be positioned effectively to meet this challenge.

NOTES

1. Prior to his retirement in December 1994, Dr. Aitken was vice president, quality performance, for Marion Merrell Dow. He became a principal with the consulting firm of Ernst & Young LLP in January 1995. In May 1995, Hoechst (the German chemical and pharmaceutical company) announced the acquisition of Marion Merrell Dow and the formation of Hoechst Marion Roussel, which will be the world's third-largest pharmaceutical company.

2. Ernst & Young LLP served as reengineering consultant for this project.

3. Customer-based customer research was provided by Anjoy Consulting of Ann Arbor, Michigan.

18

CAPP CARE: Reengineering utilization management

Mark Kimmel, PhD
Principal
Kimmel and Associates
Berkeley, California

Michael Henry
President and Chief Executive Officer
CAPP CARE
Newport Beach, California

MANAGED HEALTHCARE ORGANIZATIONS control costs either by reducing inappropriate units of service (volume) or by negotiating preferred rates in return for channeling business to selected providers. Healthcare management (HCM) focuses on the appropriateness of services, thereby reducing service volume or intensity. This article chronicles how CAPP CARE, a national managed healthcare company, redesigned its services and operations based on healthcare management principles.

The context and time frame into which these reengineering efforts fit are important and instructive. CAPP CARE is a national managed healthcare company with networks of 110,000 providers and 4,300 facilities serving 4 million members in 41 states. Its principle product line is its national provider network. However, it also provides healthcare management services such as utilization review (UR) and case management to many of its customers.

As the market demands have changed, (diminished returns, changes in providers' behavior, customer demands, advances in technologies, and practice management techniques), so has CAPP CARE's HCM product design. This product evolution and resulting reengineering of operations is ongoing at CAPP CARE, incorporating products such as practice guidelines, outcomes information, and physician empowerment tools.

CAPP CARE's long-term view of HCM expands on the traditional concept of healthcare management. This vision is based on CAPP CARE's strategic belief and commitment to the concept that success in managed care is built on the breadth, depth, and effectiveness of its network providers. Accordingly, CAPP CARE is focusing on positioning itself as a network-based company, providing HCM services in sophisticated and innovative ways.

The company's strategic vision involves the full use of cutting edge technology to select providers and, most importantly, equip them with innovative tools to achieve a best practices approach to patient care. The company is developing powerful handheld, pen-based computers housing multifunctional software applications. These include algorithmic clinical practice guidelines, point-of-service precertification of care, specialist referrals, formulary-based prescription ordering, disease management, and outcomes management. Each uses the "information super-highway" to process information. Such technology is intended to differentiate CAPP CARE from its competitors by achieving HMO-like results through broader and more accessible provider networks.

The notion of a managed care company as a knowledge-creating organization provides the proper context for healthcare in the twenty-first century. As healthcare services become increasingly information-based, there are opportunities for various stakeholders to harness information to create knowledge. Learning at the individual and organizational levels must be valued in order to create knowledge. It is important to note that each stakeholder requires different kinds of information and has different objectives in using information. For physicians, practice guidelines and other specialized clinical information augment existing knowledge about how to treat medical conditions. Given the uncertainty of medical outcomes for certain conditions and the explosion of clinical information, there are opportunities for physicians to combine their experience and judgment to produce better results. The availability of clinical data and other tools will enable physicians to provide better care with greater control and autonomy. Through the appropriate use of information technology (IT) many of the administrative hurdles that now exist in most "gatekeeper" point-of-service plans can be avoided.

Similarly, patients will have greater access to various information channels that can assist them in managing their health and treating a wide variety of common medical problems that do not require professional intervention. Clinical information has been provided in medical self-help books, videos, and advice nurse services, but in the near future on-line services will offer a broader range of services. As the baby boomers age, self-care will become a cornerstone in managing utilization. In order to manage chronic illnesses people will have to become more knowledgeable about various medical conditions and treatment alternatives.

Employers are also key players in using information to create knowledge. There are enormous costs associated with disability that require employers to understand the medical and psychosocial root causes of illness and injuries. Information about the causes of disability can lead to carefully tailored illness prevention and wellness programs. When individuals are injured, clinical tracking combined with management involvement can facilitate an early return to work. Employers can use IT to track outcomes and integrate healthcare management and quality management.

A truly knowledge-based healthcare management system requires more sophisticated business processes and information systems (IS) as well as different employee skills. In addition to computer literacy, business is likely to be conducted in project-oriented and team-based environments. There will be a requirement for managed care professionals to understand the workplace and to be able to partner with employers. For example, there are many opportunities to improve health in the workplace, through health and safety programs, prevention, and disability management programs. These health strategies suggest a different organizational capability than found in acute care hospital settings and the competencies of health professionals need to be refocused to provide a different but equally valuable set of services. Rethinking organizational capability and competency is at the heart of reengineering.

Historically, HCM has consisted of a few labor-intensive and tedious UR strategies such as precertification, which requires physicians to receive approval prior to providing care; concurrent review, where nurses or other staff follow the episode of care to determine the appropriateness, level, and placement of care; second opinions, where other physicians are used to confirm or reject the recommendations of the treating physician; and retrospective review, where the cost and quality of care is analyzed after it has been provided. These administrative procedures often cause physicians to feel micromanaged and unsupported by managed care companies, creating animosity and conflict. While a basic level of accountability has been established through a "sentinel effect" (essentially watching physician behavior), the larger and more important goal of improving quality is addressed only tangentially. In response to UR procedures, physician behavior has changed over time, yielding diminishing returns for ongoing reliance for these procedures. Thus, savvy managed care companies are beginning to realize their unique role, to improve care through outcome management strategies.

CAPP CARE's redesign of healthcare management services illustrates how innovation can be conceived and implemented in a rapidly changing industry. Over the course of a three-year period, 1993 to 1995, HCM services were reengineered using a variety of tools borrowed from four disciplines; these included quality improvement, project management, operations research, and IT. At the heart of any reengineering project is a transformational strategy that integrates work flow and appropriately skilled employees through advanced information technology. From this perspective, reengineering is a strategic means to redraw the boundaries and change the rules of engagement between CAPP CARE, providers, and payers.

This strategy must be implemented in an evolutionary manner for three reasons. First, many payers, providers, hospitals, and insurers are just beginning to acquire the requisite IT to collect and distribute data. Secondly, the handheld devices and other information intensive transmission tools are only now being fabricated. Moreover, health data standards and computer-related functionality are just emerging. Finally, new healthcare products are being integrated into CAPP CARE's healthcare management program, causing a continuous shift in the skills and organization design required to deliver services.

Reengineering of healthcare management services is being conducted at three levels: business reengineering, business process reengineering, and business process improvement.

- Business reengineering at the strategic level is the planning and adoption of enterprisewide strategies and initiatives to establish its business drivers and framework. These initiatives define CAPP CARE's vision and mission and determine the basic scope of products and services offered. It is essential to establish the business architecture prior to reengineering organizational processes. Isolated process improvements without a strategic context (e.g., customer focus, competitive practice, and patient well-being) may cause operational efficiencies without impacting customer satisfaction and overall value

- Business process reengineering, the architectural level, is the radical redesign of existing business processes and establishment of appropriate organizational architecture to achieve dramatic improvements in critical measures of performance. In most cases, the organizational architecture is supported by advanced information technology

- Business process improvement, the operational level, is the ongoing refinement of existing business processes focused at improving the manner in which things are accomplished. This approach uses quality improvement and process redesign methodologies and is geared to make incremental changes

Reengineering phases

Reengineering requires a structured and disciplined methodology to coordinate planning and problem solving. A phased-in approach provides order and coherence to innovation activities (Table 1).

PHASE ONE: ORGANIZE FOR IMPROVEMENT

1. Defining reengineering leadership and committee structures

CAPP CARE senior managers created a committee to focus on improvements in core business processes and provide leadership as reengineering projects were identified and undertaken. The committee, named the business process improvement committee (BPIC), included senior managers. It began its work by analyzing core business processes to prioritize necessary changes. A change agenda was developed to provide direction and coherence and help sequence redesign efforts. The objective was to focus on a few core processes (e.g., those with central activities

TABLE 1
Phase-in methodology

This framework will be used to describe each phase of HCM reengineering with illustrations of key activities, tasks, and results.

1. Organize for improvement
2. Strategic planning
3. Understand the process
4. Redesign the process
5. Implementation
6. Continuous improvement

and functions) essential for current customer satisfaction and future competitiveness.

The BPIC identified and prioritized core activities in terms of value to customers as well as revenue and profitability. The first process to be reengineered was customer implementation due to the influx of new business and the importance of accurately understanding the needs and preferences of customers at the beginning of the relationship. The second reengineering project was HCM.

At the outset of the reengineering effort, an infrastructure was created to support the HCM project. The elements of the infrastructure included the BPIC, a cross-functional HCM redesign team, an IT committee, and a customer service group (see Figure 1).

The director of review operations, an experienced clinical and UR nurse, was selected as the HCM redesign project director. She was responsible to the BPIC for coordinating redesign tasks, acquiring necessary resources, and reporting to the BPIC. The membership of the HCM redesign team included the head of case management, CAPP CARE's medical director, the director of network development, the director of budget and analysis, and two business analysts with IS and project management backgrounds. The rationale for including IS staff was the recognition that IT support would be needed.

Since HCM, customer service, and IS were identified as the business units that would be most affected by the redesign changes, nonmanagement representatives were selected from these areas to participate on the redesign team. Department managers in each area needed to be involved to support recommended changes and accelerate implementation. These department managers were consulted regularly to provide necessary information for analysis and to solicit their suggestions for change.

FIGURE 1
Organization

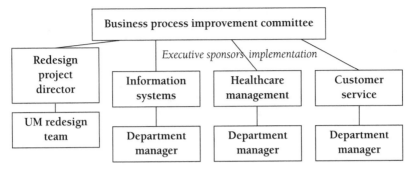

The HCM reengineering project demanded leadership to link the company's strategic choices with operational effectiveness and efficiency. The reengineering infrastructure was designed to facilitate coordination and communication between organizational functions and levels. In addition, five critical factors were identified for project success: effective project member behavior, clearly defined roles and responsibilities, project scope definition, effective problem solving and teamwork, and appropriate use of IT.

PHASE TWO: STRATEGIC PLANNING AND PROCESS ALIGNMENT

Strategic planning for HCM was initiated by gathering information from various sources: an internal assessment by managers and staff regarding current and future products and services, customer satisfaction research, and interviews with industry leaders regarding healthcare management trends.

The information gathering provided confirmation of the vision and strategic direction described in this section. CAPP CARE has been working to integrate IT, practice guidelines, and outcomes management to form a new basis for HCM. As this new model of HCM is evolving, physicians' offices are becoming computerized, purchasers of healthcare are demanding information about quality, and there is a growing consensus on best clinical practices. These developments suggest that HCM will be practiced in significantly different ways in the future.

Because these industry changes will occur over time, there is a need to maintain existing products (e.g., traditional precertification and UR

TABLE 2
The evolution of healthcare management

Current	Future
Screen cases	Health information and education
Approval of low-cost, low-risk cases (sentinel effect)	Demand management
	Early detection
Case management of potentially high-cost cases	Case screening and management
	Disease management
Treatment plans	Outcomes measurement
Centers of excellence	

services) while investing in new ones (e.g., practice guidelines and enhanced IT). This stretch in strategy was jokingly expressed by one manager's statement, "when we reached a fork in the road, we took it." The discontinuity between current HCM approaches and those being designed requires a company to leverage existing resources. This includes developing or acquiring core competencies (e.g., advanced case management skills), partnering with other firms with complementary competencies (e.g., IT and practice guidelines), and developing a migration plan from the review (i.e., precertification and UR) approach to an outcomes strategy. This transition must be actively managed to build the competencies required for the future.

As outlined above, the transition from traditional modes of HCM to the new IT model requires substantially different core competencies. Core competencies are the essential or distinguishing bundle of skills and technologies that make a disproportionate contribution to customer value, differentiates a business from its competitors, and provides a pathway to future markets. To develop these skills and technologies, a targeted set of skill development activities is being instituted. All too often, reengineering strategies are based on reducing staff to enhance productivity. What is frequently ignored is the constituent skills that must be assembled to compete in the future.

An employee development program was also instituted at CAPP CARE as a set of activities parallel to the reengineering effort. The objective was to define and develop critical skills and competencies needed to fulfill the vision. As part of this program, greater emphasis was placed on project management, software development, IT, and team problem solving. The employee development program helped to define these skills as core competencies and then provided training and, in some cases, placed skilled employees in different functional areas. For example, nurse reviewers who previously had focused solely on precertification were trained, using case management tools and practice guidelines, to provide mini-case management, thereby upgrading their skills and enabling them to provide greater value to customers. IS staff were used as internal consultants on a variety of projects, such as the practice guidelines effort to disseminate knowledge. Technology paths must be managed so the migration paths of employee skills are defined and upgraded to support the business strategy.

An important issue related to the migration of HCM is its pace and time frames for proposed changes. Some managers believed that utilization review and precertification will be eliminated in the near future and that redesign may be a waste of time. Others thought the time horizon for such changes were far enough away to warrant incremental improvement of existing HCM services. Proponents of this position argued that outcomes management and practice guidelines require all providers to have computers to utilize available databases efficiently and that this development was far enough in the future to warrant a major overhaul of the current HCM process. There was also a belief that the marketplace was becoming sophisticated enough to use products such as practice guidelines and outcomes management and that resources should be reallocated to these strategic products as well. While there was disagreement about time frames, consensus developed about the increased emphasis on practice guidelines and outcomes management through electronically coordinating care. IT provided the tools to streamline transactions by electronically linking patient, provider, and payers to reduce inefficiencies. But the midterm reengineering effort was to focus on shifting the HCM emphasis so that cases needing individual attention would receive case management services to ensure quality and cost-effective treatment interventions.

CAPP CARE views itself as a network-based organization where value to customers is based on the quality and accessibility of contracted physicians and hospitals. Accordingly, emphasis is placed on recruiting and credentialing outstanding providers. Once providers are accepted into the network, a sophisticated outcomes-oriented strategy for supporting and managing them is needed. By maintaining this network focus, CAPP CARE has been able to frame the HCM reengineering work to empower physicians. Not surprisingly, CAPP CARE's healthcare IS is named physician empowerment technology (PET). PET will reduce administrative overhead; provide for easy information exchange between providers, CAPP CARE, and the payer; and enhance physicians' time caring for patients. More importantly, PET contains a combination of performance support services embedded in the software package, such as practice, referral, and formulary guidelines. These services function as both comprehensive references and advisors to the physician, and they help, but are not substitutes for, clinical decision making. Through the use of these guidelines, practice variation is expected to decrease and yield improved outcomes.

Electronic data interchange, such as PET, is made possible through the use of sophisticated technology such as mobile, wireless computing and sophisticated software. Given the enormous resources required, strategic partnerships with leading technology companies and alliances with various medical societies promulgating practice guidelines are being formed. This enables CAPP CARE to focus on its core competencies (clinical decision making and HCM) and leverage the expertise of related industry leaders. The components of the PET system are being currently defined and developed, and decisions are being made regarding which ones CAPP CARE should make or buy. There will undoubtably be opportunities in the future to integrate a PET system with a computerized patient record to provide a truly comprehensive outcomes management system. These product development considerations are in the near-term future while the current HCM system is entering the last phase of its life cycle.

PHASE THREE: UNDERSTAND THE PROCESS—HEALTHCARE MANAGEMENT REDESIGN TEAMWORK

The BPIC authorized the redesign team to assess and recommend changes for the utilization management process (UM), a major component of CAPP CARE's core business. The objective of the review was to simultaneously improve the level of quality care to customers while increasing productivity.

Team formation, structure, and approach

The HCM redesign team began its work by discussing team characteristics that would enhance discussions and decision making. This was particularly important since they were a cross-functional team with different perspectives and skills. Team members did not initially perceive interpersonal obstacles and underestimated the potential for conflicts due to their focus on tasks rather than relationships. Team members were asked to talk to other teams about what worked and what factors they thought were responsible for good and bad teamwork. Issues such as openness, respect for different perspectives, and a willingness to suspend judgment were noted as essential for problem solving and brainstorming.

The team then discussed goals to redesign the UM process, although there was enough vagueness in the project definition that the redesign team had the discretion of considering a wide variety of options. The performance goals for the redesigned UM processes included increased customer responsiveness, improved clinical outcomes, reduced company costs, improved quality of data, and faster cycle times. The UM process goals were to be operationalized in the near term without the benefit of advanced technology and, thus, a plan for incremental improvements and partial solutions was accepted in the interim. Redesign team representatives had meetings with senior managers to discuss ideas and align emerging process redesign concepts with the long-term strategy.

Team members initially approached discussions from the perspective of their functional area (e.g., customer service), but over time they made comments and observations that displayed a more sophisticated understanding of the overall system. This sharing of perspectives surfaced uncovered knowledge in individuals and various business areas. As these perspectives were discussed and made explicit, a shared understanding emerged of UM processes and critical concepts that provided a foundation for the teams' analytic work.

The redesign team met for a half day twice each month for three months. At the end of each session, assignments were made to conduct interviews, collect data, or assess the functioning of a subprocess that had been discussed in the session. Work outside the regularly scheduled meeting created a sense of continuity and enabled the team to make rapid progress through analysis of subprocesses. The redesign team used a structured project management task time line to ensure efficiency and adherence to timelines. Although participants had competing time demands with their primary jobs, they believed the team could move quickly if it worked efficiently.

A number of different methods were used to gather information about the UM process. A walk-through process provided a descriptive model of the UM work flows by examining each process flowchart. At each step in the flowchart examination, the team was informed about key process characteristics, including the triggers for an activity, organization and current technology being used, the outputs, and performance levels.

The walk-through familiarized all team members with each of the process steps and associated tasks; more importantly, it facilitated a dialogue essential to the problem-solving effort. As each process step was scrutinized by the team, the central assumptions, implicit process rules, and pertinent thoughts were recorded on a chart pad. When an issue was deemed to be outside the boundary of the UM process discussion, a separate chart pad was used for "parking lot issues." Thoughts and assumptions were recorded, as were process steps and tasks. In many instances further analysis was required to determine accurately how an activity worked. For instance, team members were assigned to observe UM nurses making and taking phone calls, several managers were interviewed, and numerous queries were run to analyze UM data.

Once the UM data were collected from various sources regarding anticipated competencies, process specifications and desired outputs, discussions were held to combine and convert data into concepts and a prototype model. These concepts were developed through collective reflection in which redesign team members used metaphor and analogies to broaden their thinking. Analogies were drawn from different industries such as financial services organizations that were also involved in complicated transactions. The multidisciplinary composition of the redesign team provided a unique perspective that challenged the group to think about HCM in different ways. For example, one redesign team member wondered why a CAPP CARE card could not be used to store and transfer information. Many creative ideas surfaced and were recorded for consideration at a later date.

The UM application on the AS/400 has been developed and progressively enhanced over the past nine years. Observations of its use and questions about its functionality (to all levels of staff) confirm that it supports the current process effectively, with a few minor exceptions.

Assessment findings

The redesign team categorized UM processes to better allocate labor. The team analyzed the skill sets of CAPP CARE staff to determine where additional training was needed and where staff could assume additional responsibility. The appropriateness of documentation was reviewed to determine whether excessive or unnecessary data was being collected. The redesign team analyzed call management procedures to determine if CAPP CARE could initially segregate calls to connect the caller to appropriate staff in order to improve customer service and satisfaction. The redesign team also identified manual activities that could be automated to increase efficiencies and work product quality. In the course of the reengineering project, the analysis of tasks and handoffs identified opportunities for increasing quality of outputs that had a positive effect on service levels.

As a result of automating some reviews and eliminating bottlenecks in work flows, the number of preadmission reviews taken per full-time equivalent (FTE) each day averaged 12 during the first quarter of 1995 (FTEs include only nurses and processors). This number indicates a significant improvement compared to the 6.5 average in 1993. There is still room for further gains.

In summary, the review of HCM labor costs and financial returns for customers for prospective, concurrent, retrospective review, and case management suggested significant progress with additional opportunities for improvement. Some routine medical reviews were automated, freeing labor to provide support for complex or problematic medical procedures. This analysis also revealed business process bottlenecks and skill deficiencies. The review suggested a number of recommendations, which are discussed in the following section.

PHASE FOUR: REDESIGN RECOMMENDATIONS

Based on the above findings, a number of conclusions were reached and the following recommendations were made:

- Identify data requirements to streamline UM notes

- Look for further opportunities to automate reviews and referrals to internal physician staff based on analysis of impacts on review automation (e.g., costs and clinical outcomes)

- Identify UM activities that can be more effectively handled by case managers and activities that are managed by case management that can be more effectively done by UM

- Redefine reviewers' roles to promote an increased scope of responsibility, thereby eliminating unnecessary handoffs and labor costs

PHASE FIVE: IMPLEMENTATION AND
CONTINUOUS IMPROVEMENT

These recommendations formed the basis for a work plan that served as a source document to monitor progress. Recommendations were translated into business objectives with specific outcomes and time frames. Examples include

1. Objective: Improve and maintain systems and processes that result in efficient handling and tracking of UM activities
   Outcome: Graduated increase in UM productivity throughout 1995 to achieve 50 percent greater than baseline by year-end

2. Objective: Dedicate staff and resources to facilitate the evolution of the UM process into a mini-case management approach
   Outcome: 25 percent of preauthorization reviews (or diagnoses) will be managed using mini-case management principles

3. Objective: Expand the current training and professional development program and tailor it to meet the changing department service and productivity requirements as well as the evolutionary needs of the managed care industry
   Outcome: Retention of qualified staff who service customers at levels identified in service goals

4. Objective: Revise and implement a metric system to document UM quality improvement
   Outcome: The cost of the UM process will decrease by 50 percent within one year

During the 18-month reengineering period many substantive changes were made, resulting in increased work efficiencies, decreased lengths of stay, significant financial savings to customers, and intensified focus on quality improvement through case management and practice guidelines.

Concluding remarks

HCM is being transformed by advances in IT, practice guidelines, and an increased emphasis on treatment outcomes with the objectives of reducing cost and improving clinical quality. The underlying principle of knowledge creation is driving advanced managed care companies to creatively redefine HCM, through the use of easy-to-use handheld computers, practice guidelines, and outcomes measures embedded in expert systems. The result will be the ability to manage care less intrusively and at a fraction of the cost.

The evolution of HCM is gradually replacing inspection methods, leading to an increased emphasis on knowledge-based strategies. For CAPP CARE, this requires creativity in managing the migration from old to new HCM methods while maintaining customer satisfaction. New approaches to HCM require different core competencies (e.g., employee skills, IT, and clinical database applications) efficiently linking providers, patients, payers, and managed care companies. The acquisition and integration of these competencies requires an organizational development blueprint that includes a strategic human resource program to build desired employee competencies, software and technology development initiatives, and business process management. To develop this blueprint, it is essential to consider time horizons of proposed changes, the potential benefits and costs of new technology, and the changes required of internal and external customers.

The HCM reengineering project illustrates some practical realities. Reengineering is a time-consuming activity that competes with other organizational priorities. It must be identified as a strategic priority and receive ongoing support and attention from senior managers during all phases of the project. At CAPP CARE, the reengineering project was temporarily displaced by an acquisition but regained priority status because of its critical importance to the organization's survival. The benefits of reengineering are compromised when proposed changes are not adequately managed. Frequently, this becomes apparent in poor communication and coordination or inadequate resources and organizational commitment. A key factor that helped get the HCM reengineering project back on track was senior management's ability to talk about conflicting strategic and organizational issues. Management was able to consider the important issues in real time and maintain a strategic focus.

As HCM evolves, new organizational forms and technological tools will be developed to create and share knowledge. These will offer opportunities for patients, healthcare professionals, and payers to improve health outcomes. The challenge for advanced managed care companies is to engage consumers in the knowledge creation cycle.

19

Department of Veterans Affairs: Redesigning cost recovery programs

Walter J. Besecker
Director, Medical Care Cost Recovery
Department of Veterans Affairs
Washington, DC

Carol A. Craft
Program Director, St. Louis Continuing Education Center

Melissa McCanna
Assistant Director, National Media Development Center
Department of Veterans Affairs
St. Louis, Missouri

IN 1993, THE MEDICAL CARE COST RECOVERY (MCCR) Program of the Department of Veterans Affairs initiated a major effort to examine its mission and rethink its process. Static budgets, flat recoveries, and challenges from management to enhance revenue recovery and reduce operating costs motivated this effort. The goal was to improve recoveries, and create measurable improvements for customers, management, and employees. The MCCR effort involved redesigning the business process, standardizing operating procedures, automating as much of the process as possible, and developing training tools to sustain the changes.

The lessons learned from this effort provide practical insights for management and project team members considering large- or small-scale process redesign. Business reengineering need not be traumatic or threatening and can result in positive outcomes for the organization, its participants, and its customers.

This chapter presents the four major phases of the MCCR project and discusses the steps, issues, and critical factors associated within each phase.

The mission of the MCCR program is to maximize the recovery of costs incurred by the Department of Veterans Affairs (VA) in providing medical care to veteran patients and other users of the VA system. The source of recoveries includes third-party insurance and copayments.

The VA is unlike private healthcare providers in a number of ways. Its size alone separates it from most private sector healthcare corporations. The VA operates one of the largest healthcare systems in the country, 173 medical centers, 209 independent, satellite, and community-based outpatient clinics, 131 nursing home care units, and 39 domiciliary care units. This large infrastructure generates staggering statistics. In fiscal year 1994, the VA provided care to more than one million inpatients and recorded more than 25 million outpatient visits.

Unlike private healthcare providers, VA depends on annual congressional appropriations to fund the operation of its healthcare delivery network. It has limited authority to recover any share of its cost from patients and other users of the system. All revenues recovered by medical centers are deposited directly into the federal treasury. In essence, the VA may not retain any revenue it collects through the MCCR effort.

Complicating the recovery process are the facts that fewer than 20 percent of VA patients have commercial health insurance and that patients with insurance using the VA system have few incentives to disclose their coverage. Unlike a private or other public healthcare provider, the VA may not bill or impose charges (other than minimal copayments) for healthcare services. And, unlike private facilities, the VA may not bill patients for the insurance deductibles or for any care provided but not reimbursed by the insurer.

The cost recovery process developed independently within the 173 VA medical centers. Hospitals were free to create organizations and operating procedures to identify veterans with insurance and to collect on that insurance to the fullest extent possible. As a result, there was little standardization and no clearly defined or uniform cost recovery process in the early days of MCCR.

Legislation in 1990 changed how the recovery effort was funded, created the MCCR program office, and also redefined some of the care for which claims could be established. During the first year of operation, the MCCR office defined its mission and introduced a number of major initiatives directed toward rethinking the VA's recovery effort. Task groups, made up of medical center staff, assessed, recommended, and implemented a variety of specialized programs, methods, and activities. These initiatives established

- A comprehensive training and education program for frontline staff and midlevel managers

- Automation of significant portions of the recovery effort

- An extensive awards and recognition program

- New technologies for data capture and claims processing

- A variety of communication pathways within the organization

- Sophisticated goal setting and resource allocation models

- A national database and performance measurement process

- A competitive and entrepreneurial spirit among facilities

Based on this new foundation, the program realized some degree of success between 1991 and 1994, growing in recoveries by approximately $300 million. While these statistics on nationwide recoveries appeared solid, facility data indicated that there were variances in recovery performance among medical centers in five key areas: identifying the insured population, the cost to recover a dollar, the number of staff required to generate claims, the management of aging receivables, and the numbers and reasons for rejected claims. The data also indicated that substantial growth in recoveries was still possible. The situation was ripe for a serious look at process redesign and standardization.

Reengineering experience

The MCCR program office called together a group of field and headquarters staff in early 1993 and asked them to respond to four objectives designed to achieve the goal of improving total recoveries while limiting costs. The four objectives were to

- Streamline the entire cost recovery process

- Automate as much of the streamlined process as possible

- Develop standardized procedures for each operation in the MCCR process

- Develop a comprehensive training program for frontline staff and managers

A project coordinator was needed for this effort. The MCCR program office had established a working relationship with the St. Louis Continuing Education Center (CEC), part of the educational network within the Veterans Health Administration (a part of the Department of Veterans Affairs), and the principal internal unit developing MCCR's educational programs. In accepting the request for participation in reengineering, the CEC stepped beyond its traditional role of content planning and delivery, evolving from training coordinator and planner to project coordinator and internal consultant for the entire reengineering project.

Components of reengineering

There were four phases identified in the cost recovery reengineering project: process flow analysis, process redesign, preparation for implementation, and pilot site testing (Table 1).

PROCESS FLOW ANALYSIS

Before MCCR could improve the cost recovery process, it had to understand the details of its current recovery effort. Process flow analysis offered an approach to this understanding, beginning by identifying all the detailed steps of a process through the visual schema of a flowchart. The completion of a process analysis involved several steps.

Steps

Involving a consultant. A reengineering consultant joined the VA project to offer content and process expertise. The consultant served as faculty for quality improvement principles and practices, reengineering approaches, and facilitator skills. The consultant also worked with the program office and CEC to develop the overall approach to process analysis, process redesign, and pilot site testing.

TABLE 1
Phases of reengineering

Process flow analysis—10 months:
    Involving a consultant
    Involving initial process owners
    Creating macrolevel flows
    Training facilitators
    Creating microlevel flows
    Coordinating logistics

Process redesign—9 months:
    Listing process breakdowns and recommendations
    Involving other process owners
    Visiting private sector hospitals
    Peer review
    Completing ideal process

Preparation for implementation—13 months:
    Planning for pilot test
    Requesting proposals
    Reviewing proposals
    Selecting sites
    Training
    Organizing at pilot sites

Pilot site testing—18–24 months:
    Distributing work plan tasks and schedules
    Establishing communication mechanisms
    Developing a reporting structure
    Determining needed resources

Involving initial process owners. A small group of MCCR employees representing medical administration, fiscal, pharmacy, utilization review, outpatient clinics, MCCR units, and the MCCR program office initiated the process flow analysis.

Creating macrolevel flows. Over several days, 16 to 20 major steps of the process were identified in "macrolevel" form, which captured activities at a general or overview level. An example of macro-level flow for the data capture and validation process is displayed in Figure 1.

Training facilitators. The next step was to prepare facilitators to lead small groups to expand the development of the process flow. Facilitators were educated in the concepts of quality improvement, flowcharting, benchmarking, and performance measurement during a week-long course. Through practice teaching sessions and small group discussions, they developed their skills in team leading, negotiating, and creating flowcharts of the MCCR process at macro- and microlevel detail.

FIGURE 1
Macrolevel of data capture and validation

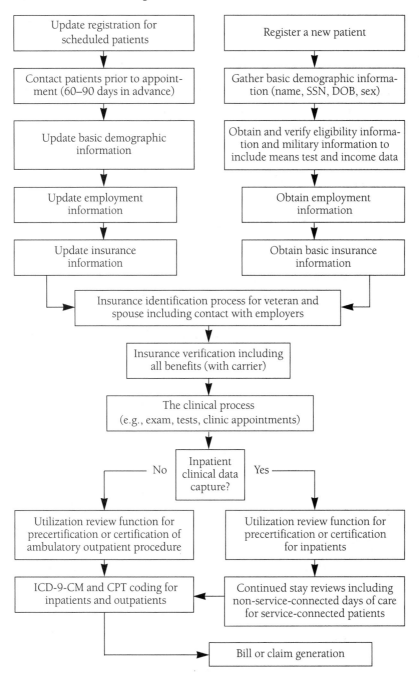

Creating microlevel flows. The program office solicited volunteers from the system of 173 VA medical centers to continue the process flow activity, but at a very detailed level. Microlevel flows expand the macrolevel by articulating all of the detailed steps and decision points associated with those steps. Such detail was required in order to analyze and evaluate the process for rework loops, redundancies, and inefficiencies. More than 100 employees, representing a variety of functions within MCCR, initiated the task. They began with one intense week-long workshop, and continued with conference calls, homework assignments, and validation of the resulting flowcharts with peers back home. This effort yielded a first draft of microlevel detail on 16 major components of the MCCR process.

It became clear that the work of completing and then analyzing the flowcharts would require considerable time and personnel investment. It was not feasible for the original group of 100 employees to continue with this task. Twenty facilitators assumed responsibility for this task, meeting monthly to continue the microflow and identify major breakdowns and inefficiencies. Ongoing education was provided to this group, focusing on methods for data collection and analytic skills. These skills proved valuable to critique the existing MCCR process for its effectiveness and value.

Coordinating logistics. Work accomplished by the MCCR process flow groups was coordinated by CEC staff. A flowchart software program was used to capture the numerous paper versions of the flowcharts. CEC maintained ongoing correspondence, arranged conference calls, and directed the travel plans and meeting arrangements for all those involved in the project. The CEC also served as a clearinghouse for process improvement and reengineering-related literature and documented the "story" of the project.

Issues of process flow analysis

The process flow analysis phase spanned 10 months, during which time two major issues surfaced.

Lack of MCCR standardization. It was difficult to determine whose version of the current process most accurately represented reality. This issue was significant because the current flow was to be the structure from which the ideal flow would be created. Process flow groups addressed this issue in one of two ways: either they created a "generic" model that represented the majority of what each medical center did, or they allowed a medical center that seemed to have a well-defined process to offer its flow as a representation of current reality.

The difficulty and tedium of the process. People working on the flowcharts often felt their way was best. They also had a tendency to spend excessive amounts of time on minute levels of flowchart detail. By so doing, they frequently lost sight of the overall purpose of this activity, which was to establish a base of current practice and then, most importantly, create an ideal process. Sometimes this flowchart development was inefficient and oftentimes frustrating.

Critical factors of process flow analysis
Three factors seemed critical to the success of process flow analysis.

Ownership. Many frontline and first-level supervisory staff throughout the VA system were involved. Most of the employees chosen to participate clearly bought in to the task. They took ownership of the flowcharts they were creating. This sense of ownership was sustained throughout the course of the analysis and process redesign stage.

Varied background skills. Employees who represented varied functional tasks and medical centers were key to success. No one individual knew enough about all the MCCR process details, so representatives from multiple services were needed. The variety of medical centers that these employees represented offered a broad range of experiences and processes. They were from large and small, urban, rural, and suburban facilities from all areas of the country.

Use of facilitators. Facilitators, also drawn from multidisciplinary backgrounds, were chosen based on several criteria: demonstrated ability to work effectively with groups; strong belief in the value of the project; willingness to commit time and talent for an unknown period; adequate content knowledge of some portion of the MCCR process; and ability to increase the scope and depth of that knowledge. Some facilitators were picked prior to this phase, while others emerged as leaders out of the initial process flow groups.

PROCESS REDESIGN

The outcomes of the process flow analysis phase initiated a nine-month period of redesign to create an ideal process flow. This process redesign involved various elements.

Steps

Listing process breakdowns and recommendations. This activity began during the preceding stage of process analysis but received more attention during process redesign. As the current flow was analyzed and inefficiencies and breakdowns identified, solutions surfaced. The list of breakdowns and recommendations became the foundation for the redesign process. An example of the major breakdowns and recommendations for the data capture and validation process is contained in Table 2.

The recommended changes prompted an environment of creativity. "What if . . . ?" and, "Why can't we . . . ?" were frequently heard throughout this stage. Many changes proposed were so radical that "reengineering" became a part of the group's vocabulary.

Involving other process owners. Some of the MCCR process lies outside its direct control. Any success in reengineering is clearly dependent upon getting other departments that hold some control to cooperate. Dialogue began at a national level with key departments within VA and external agencies (e.g., the Treasury Department). Initial communication was informational, but these groups quickly were asked to become involved in a collaborative manner. As a result of this ongoing dialogue, several major new efforts were initiated, designed to positively affect the VA system as a whole. One such effort was the creation of a multidisciplinary work group charged with overhauling the entire VA patient registration process. Another effort targeted systemwide automation of patient accounting functions, benefiting both MCCR and financial management activities.

Visiting private sector hospitals. During this stage of the project, facilitators visited model private sector hospitals to examine their cost recovery processes. These visits confirmed that the components of the ideal VA process being developed were consistent with the private sector, which is more experienced in efficient billing and collection.

Peer review. Midway through the process redesign stage, the original 100 members of the microflow process were invited to meet to critique

TABLE 2

Data capture and validation: Major breakdowns and recommendation

Major breakdowns	Recommendations
1. Incomplete and inaccurate registration data ■ Special consents ■ Lack of specificity of service-connected disabilities ■ Lack of patient privacy ■ Notification that means test is due	■ Preregistration of patients with scheduled appointments to update any and all information in decentralized hospital computer program (DHCP) ■ Potential automation of eligibility and military information through automated medical information exchange (AMIE) system and hook-up with Department of Defense (DoD) computer system ■ Electronic simplification of certain datafield entries (e.g., county, city, and state automatically stuffed based on street address and zip code) ■ Enhanced patient data card compatible with interactive computer capabilities
2. Verification of coverage, lack of monitors to identify date of latest verification ■ Problem with the insurance list ■ Inability to create HCFA 1500	■ Enhanced insurance software package in integrated billing (IB) package 2.0
3. General breakdowns ■ Cooperation from physicians ■ Lack of information resources management (IRM) support ■ Lack of medical record availability ■ Delay in patient treatment file (PTF) coding ■ Incomplete information on fee patients	■ Pursue use of electronic form that ties into the eligibility fields of the patient information management system (PIMS) package that lists service-connected and non-service-connected conditions and also ties into the integrated billing (IB) package for automatic generation of a claim ■ Enhancement to future packages (PIMS, IB, accounts receivable) will hopefully include automated record request functionality. In the future, an electronic medical record will completely eliminate this problem ■ Enhancement in the future should provide for an automatic generation of a bill once patient treatment file (PTF) is closed ■ Once closed, the PTF information will be electronically transmitted to the UB-92. Fee and other ancillary services will need to be included in future versions of software packages

what had been created by the facilitators. Frontline staff looked at the flowcharts with a fresh view and judged their value and feasibility. Participants offered suggestions, raised questions, and confirmed the direction of the process. This session also identified additional content experts who were needed by the facilitators to help with selected portions of the process redesign. These individuals served in an ad hoc fashion for the remainder of this phase.

Completing an ideal process. While process redesign can be a never-ending effort, human and material resources usually do end. Several months after peer review, the facilitator group determined the ideal process was ready for testing. This signaled the end of the process redesign phase. As a result of this redesign, the steps in the MCCR process were reduced from 781 to 400 and the ideal flowchart depicted a smoothly functioning, well-detailed, and highly automated process.

Issues of process redesign
Three major issues surfaced during this phase of the project.

The extent of the ideal created. The sophistication of what had been proposed as the ideal began to clash with the reality of what could be created before the pilot began. Many of the projected changes for the ideal process involved technology development and its acquisition, which were outside the project group's control. For example, the ideal process included a magnetic data card that patients would use to easily and quickly update their demographic and insurance information. This technology was not in place within VA, and a department other than MCCR was responsible for all patient databases. Yet the accuracy of the database was critical to MCCR to establish a potential billing case. Achieving the ideal process was further complicated by the acknowledgement that reengineering was only one of many initiatives occurring in MCCR, several of which impacted a total process redesign.

Process versus technology. Which should be the leader? Process redesign groups were attempting to create the ideal MCCR process, but their vision frequently was constrained by the available technology and reengineering project time lines. This precipitated a roller-coaster phenomenon in the group's cognitive and emotional approach to redesign. When the group perceived that technology was a possibility to enhance or accomplish a task, they were enthusiastic and creative in considering possible ways the process could work. When the constraints of technology proved a deterrent to the ideal process, however, they were discouraged about their redesign efforts and reluctant to alter their vision to fit the available technology. The multiple versions of the redesigned flowcharts were among the tangible effects of this conflict between the driv-ing forces of process versus technology.

Territorial prerogatives. Many organizational units at the national level had ownership of processes and technology that affected MCCR's process redesign. From the outset of the project, the MCCR director recognized the importance these units played in the project. In exchange for their participation, MCCR offered these units one of their desired outcomes or the resources to accomplish those outcomes. Informational sessions, formal meetings, and identification of collaborative projects were the mechanisms used to solicit their involvement.

Critical factors of process redesign
During this segment of the project, several critical factors were evident.

Balancing the ideal and the real. Those engaged in process redesign needed frequent encouragement to think beyond the available technology; those creating the new technology, such as software developers, needed ongoing feedback and information from the group about the ideal process flow so that the software could be developed accordingly.

Collaboration with groups external to MCCR. The redesigned process had extended MCCR's crossing of traditional functional lines. For reengineering to succeed, MCCR had to increasingly solicit these groups for their buy-in, support, and collaboration.

Continued involvement of individuals initially invested in process flow analysis. Engaging the original process owners to critique the ideal process fostered ongoing owners' support for the project and MCCR as a whole. Their expertise from the frontline perspective helped to clarify the practicality and efficiency of the ideal process.

PREPARATION FOR IMPLEMENTATION

Thirteen months prior to the implementation of the ideal process, preparation for the pilot test began. Several steps were necessary to complete this phase.

Steps

Planning the pilot test. MCCR was committed to pilot testing the reengineered, or ideal, process. The anticipated scope of pilot testing and subsequent implementation of MCCR reengineering across the VA system required a larger and more diverse planning group. It was reasonable to look to the existing facilitators as a core planning group. They represented varied expertise, had a strong background in the project, and had a substantial investment and interest in seeing reengineering succeed. The core planning group developed a request for proposals, began designing the logistics and time lines for implementation, and identified the approach needed to meet the training needs of the pilot sites.

Requesting proposals. The request for proposals was distributed to all VA healthcare facilities. Its key features are outlined in Table 3. Seventy-nine letters of intent, with 56 subsequent proposals, representing almost one-third of VA healthcare facilities, spoke strongly to the interest and excitement that medical centers had for the potential of this project.

Reviewing proposals. Members of the proposal review group included the core planning group, selected MCCR program office staff, and other key process owners such as representatives from information resources management. A three-member team reviewed and independently scored each proposal. One member of each team served as lead reviewer whose responsibility was to summarize individual scores and present the proposal at the review meeting. Criteria supporting the recommendation of a site included strong commitment and tangible support by both top administration and MCCR-related department heads, effective leadership displayed by the pilot's team leader, willingness to commit staff time for a period of 16 to 24 months, and previous experience and commitment to total quality improvement. Recommendations from the proposal review group were sent to the MCCR director, who made the final selections.

TABLE 3
Key features of the request for proposals

- Reasons for submission
- Past successes within MCCR
- Effectiveness of MCCR unit
- Administrative and clinical commitment
- Support services commitment
- Experience with total quality improvement

Selecting sites. Ten VA medical centers were selected as pilot sites, with four additional sites chosen as alternates. These sites represented different patient populations and organizational structures and varying levels of success in achieving previous MCCR collection goals. Once sites confirmed their willingness to participate, they assembled a pilot team leader, team members, and identified other content experts, such as pharmacists and prosthetic representatives, to be used as ad hoc resources to the pilot team. Each site was assigned an advisor from the core planning group to serve as a resource, advocate, and program office liaison to assist the pilot in a successful implementation.

Training. Top management, team members, and the pilot site advisors needed information prior to the pilot's initiation. To achieve this training

- A one-day informational session was held to provide a project overview for top management, key department heads, and the pilot's team leader

- A five-day session was conducted with medical center teams. Learning activities were conducted in small group settings, with a heavy concentration on team building, process flow and analysis, and implementation guidelines for the process redesign. Teams received a comprehensive manual containing information that was key to the site's success, such as team concepts, flowcharting, data gathering, and analysis. A second manual presented the entire microflowed MCCR process, with reference notes

- Pilot site advisors received additional training for their role, particularly in reengineering, data-collection tools, coaching and mentoring

Organizing at pilot sites. In addition to the educational preparation, participants at pilot sites were asked to complete several surveys intended to establish a baseline of performance and resource needs. Site team leaders began marketing the project to an expanded group of key personnel within the facility, including local unions.

Issues of implementation preparation

As in the other phases of reengineering several new issues emerged.

Increased demands on the core planning group. The core planning group's role in the project had evolved from facilitation to project planning to pilot site advising. The group had committed to week-long meetings each month for a year; however, planning and implementing the pilot would demand continued monthly or bimonthly meetings for the life of the pilot. Individuals in the core planning group held full-time positions within VA, and the reengineering project duties were assumed as additional responsibilities. In some instances, medical center directors were unable to allow their employees to continue in the project because of the time commitments. New planners and advisors had to be identified, recruited, and prepared for their roles.

Baseline performance measurement. A survey was created to identify a baseline of performance in the pilot sites. Several problems existed with this initial measurement: some data were unknown or very labor-intensive to obtain, and some were inconsistent because of ambiguous terminology. Much of the data were based on "guesstimates." This issue was readdressed later in the project by the core planning group. It decided to track a very limited number of MCCR general performance indicators specific to each medical center that were known to be valid (Table 4).

Additionally the group intended to track a number of measures associated with the major categories of the ideal process. An example of performance indicators for the preregistration process is listed in Table 5.

Critical factors of implementation preparation

Two critical factors emerged during the phase of preparing for implementation.

Detailed planning. A work plan, with tasks and time lines, was created for the pilots. An example of the tasks and time lines developed for

TABLE 4
Baseline performance indicators

General measures
Operating cost ratio to dollars collected
Collections to full-time equivalent (FTE)
Percentage increase in collections fiscal year 1993 to 1994
Percentage of insured inpatient stays billed
Percentage of insured outpatient visits billed
Average claims generated by FTE for insured outpatient visits billed
Average claims for insured outpatient visits billed
Average age of insurance claims outstanding

Organizational measures
Position within MCCR
Functions within MCCR

TABLE 5
Performance indicators for preregistration

Specific subprocess measures
Preregistration (monthly):
    Number of calls attempted
    Number of calls connected
    Number of demographic changes
    Number of next-of-kin changes
    Number of employment changes
    Number of insurances identified or changed
    Number of billable insurances of total identified
    Dollar amount billed: inpatient
    Dollar amount billed: outpatient
    Dollar amount collected: inpatient
    Dollar amount collected: outpatient

preregistration is provided in Table 6. The core planning group created its own work plan for orchestrating the implementation and also developed performance measures and a reporting structure for the pilots.

Educational preparation. Education was targeted to all the initial groups invested in the pilot: top management, key department heads, the pilot sites team leaders, team members, and the advisors. It was important for the advisors to participate in these training sessions, both as teachers and as learners. Their faculty role helped them establish credibility as advisors with pilot site representatives, and their student role ensured that they had maximum opportunity to develop their own knowledge base in the reengineering of VA's cost recovery effort.

TABLE 6
Work plan for preregistration

Activity

	Oct	Nov	Dec	Jan	Feb	Mar	Apr	May
Preregistration in place								
• Evaluate and modify position description (PD)				1/13				
• Classify PD	10/1							
• Develop performance standards								
• Determine orientation and training needs for new and existing FTEs								
• Determine orientation and training needs for other individuals involved in preregistration (e.g., MDs, all clerks)								
• Evaluate and modify preregistration template								
• Evaluate and modify protocol for phone interview								
• Determine equipment needs to do job								
• Install equipment								
• Receive allocation of FTEs		11/22						
• Hire or reassign FTEs								
• Orient and train FTEs								
• Initiate preregistration process								
• Monitor preregistration process and make changes as appropriate								
• Final flow of process								

5/13

PILOT SITE TESTING

Testing of the redesigned MCCR process began in October 1994. The intent was to see if the perceived ideal MCCR process would stand the test of implementation. To the extent that it did, the pilots' experience would be the guide for subsequent systemwide implementation. Several elements of the pilot testing phase warrant discussion.

Steps

Distributing work plan tasks and schedules. A six-month work plan was developed by the core planners as a guide for the pilots. It stipulated the tasks and measures that would be used to indicate successful accomplishment and delineated the expected dates of completion.

Establishing communication mechanisms. Project communication was designed to flow in a two-way fashion. Pilot team leaders' first level of contact was the advisors. The advisors' principal contact was the project coordinator in CEC, who in turn communicated with the director of MCCR. The advisors began working with the teams at the time of the first team training, then continued with conference calls and site visits. Electronic mail groups and quarterly meetings also were established for team leaders and advisors.

Developing a reporting structure. The guiding principle in creating the report structure was to gather meaningful information about the progress of the pilot in as simple a fashion as possible. A one-page monthly report, tailored to capture the implementation of the work plan tasks, including copies of meeting minutes and process measures was submitted by the sites. A quarterly report represented a narrative account of milestones, barriers, and schedule and job function changes (Table 7).

Determining needed resources. No additional staffing or technology was immediately available to the pilot sites. However, within the first four months of the project, the MCCR program office was able to provide some limited contract and salary funds. These monies were dedicated to the preregistration process. Sites were assessed for their hardware and software needs, both for the pilot test and as potential test sites for new software and hardware. Within the first eight months of the pilot, electronic scanning technology was installed in the pilot sites and used for patient data capture.

Issues of pilot site testing
A number of important issues emerged during the first year of the pilot program.

Dual roles of team leaders and advisors. Team leaders at three of the pilot sites also served as their site's advisor because they had been members of the core planning group. As the pilot began, they had some concern about their ability to fulfill both roles as well as continue to serve on the core planning group. They also were concerned that within their own facility they would not have the same credibility as an outside advisor. As the pilot progressed, the duality of roles became more of an asset than a concern. There were two benefits to having some team

410 REDESIGNING HEALTHCARE DELIVERY

TABLE 7
Pilot site quarterly report

MEDICAL CARE COST RECOVERY (MCCR) PILOT INITIATIVE
QUARTERLY PROGRESS REPORT

VAMC:_____

REPORTING PERIOD (month/year): _____

1. *Milestones/achievements*

   A summary statement of accomplishments and impact MCCR change has had on other services, areas, functions

   _____
   _____

2. *Project schedule*

   Major changes to implementation schedule and rationale

   _____
   _____

3. *Issue or barrier encountered*

   A. Explanation of the issue or barrier (who, what, where, when, why)

   _____

   B. Effect on the overall pilot

   _____

   C. Strategies or action proposed to resolve

   _____

4. *Changes in working conditions, job activities, and function*

   _____
   _____

5. *Miscellaneous comments and questions*

   _____
   _____

leader/advisor positions: the core planning group received very detailed information about the pilot's progress in those sites, and those individuals with dual roles have enhanced the communication between team leaders and advisors in other medical centers.

Loss of consultant. Unexpectedly, the consultant left the project, creating a void in the project's management and a sense of uncertainty within the project's core planning group. This group had not yet acknowledged to itself that it possessed the knowledge, skills, and judgment to steer the project in the right direction without outside assistance. The CEC, previously responsible for the educational aspects of the project, assumed direct project management responsibility and coached the advisor group to see itself as empowered to effectively direct the reengineering project.

Critical factors of pilot testing

At the current stage of pilot testing, several factors seem critical.

Detailed implementation schedule. This document offered significant guidance with concrete tasks to accomplish according to stipulated dates. The timetable was not perfect and in some cases had to be revised, but it offered pilot sites a clear sense of direction and progress. It also offered to the core planning group a method of tracking each site's success in implementation.

A formal plan for communication. Written reports, informal dialogue with advisors, and regular meetings of the advisory/team leader group were essential to track the progress of the project and to direct attention to future planning elements. Sustained communication within the medical centers also was needed. The most successful pilots worked hard to inform other employees and veteran patients what the pilot was attempting to accomplish and what benefits it would yield.

Lessons learned

To date, MCCR's experience supports the impression that actually doing reengineering demands courage, considerable patience, and a tolerance for uncertainty in moving through uncharted territory. Several lessons were learned.

Confusion in terminology exists in the literature on process improvement and reengineering. Key words, such as "reengineering," are not defined consistently. Clarity and consensus on the meaning of concepts is particularly important as groups struggle to apply those concepts. Groups involved in process improvement and reengineering efforts will need to agree on definitions of concepts they will use.

Despite the current surge of writing on reengineering, few materials have touched the surface of how to do it. Many questions about the concept itself arise as implementation occurs. How radical and revolutionary is reengineering in its implementation? Are the terms "radical" and "revolutionary" even appropriate to apply to human processes? Or are they best applied to industrial processes? Can a process be revolutionary in its redesign, yet evolutionary in its implementation? Is reengineering just a gradient of a process improvement approach? Answers to these questions will be forthcoming only when groups involved in reengineering document, analyze, and report their experiences.

A shared vision and project ownership is critical for successful reengineering. This project benefited from having a leader with a clear vision of MCCR's reengineered future that he shared with others. Added to the shared vision was a sense of ownership by all involved. Ownership was actively solicited, then nourished throughout the project's duration by the MCCR director and the core planning group. As a result, the pilot teams were very committed to the project and the implementation of an ideal MCCR process.

The process of reengineering is even more complex, lengthy, and detailed than is anticipated at a project's beginning. Reengineering is further complicated when organizational functions cross traditional lines of responsibility and authority, as MCCR does, and when operations are significantly affected by external agencies, such as Congress, as is the case for VA.

It was invaluable for the MCCR project to use a core group in planning, advisory, and implementation capacities. These individuals represented a variety of skills, ideas, and approaches, and convening them as a core ensured commitment and continuity for the duration of the project. Unfortunately, not enough individuals were prepared in this role from the beginning. Resignations from the group for reasons of time and relocation necessitated replacements. These replacements needed orientation and preparation for their roles, a task that would have been more efficient to accomplish at the project's beginning. Another critical human resource was a capable project coordinator.

Performance measurement is important, but it demands considerable planning to be effective. Questions that should be asked include: How important to the project are the indicators to be measured? How valid are existing data about the indicators? How easy are they to obtain? Does every site gather the same data, and in the same way? MCCR resisted the temptation to develop an abundance of performance measures to track the project's success; rather, it selected a few based on the questions posed above.

Communication about the pilot is a never-ending activity and needs to occur within two separate environments, the medical center and the VA organization. Informing the involved parties prior to the project was only the beginning. As the pilot progressed, the teams wanted feedback on how they were doing. Medical center administration wanted their own pilot results and comparisons with other pilot sites. Other medical center employees wanted to learn what reengineering was. MCCR needed to update representatives of the larger VA organization on the technology and process changes to foster the continued support of the project.

Early outcomes of reengineering

Four features of the reengineering pilot have achieved early success: walk-throughs, preregistration, technology enhancements, and paperless processing. Each is discussed below.

WALK-THROUGHS

Walk-throughs were an effective mechanism for understanding process details. With flowcharts in hand, pilot teams walked through every MCCR process step to see if tasks were done as represented by the flowchart. The pilot sites discovered efficiencies and inefficiencies, rework, and too much paperwork. Benefits of the walk-throughs included an immediate improvement in communication because staff from varied functional areas had a clearer understanding of every MCCR activity. Internal processes that could be changed immediately were targeted and other tasks that could be improved by implementing the reengineered ideal process were clearly identified.

PREREGISTRATION

Preregistration of a veteran prior to an outpatient visit had not been a uniform practice within VA. Pilot sites received funding to add temporary staff to assume this function. The goal was to clean up the database, identify new cases of billable insurance, and ultimately increase collections. In the first two weeks of operation, staff at one VA medical center identified 120 veterans with new addresses, new spouses, or employer changes. In the first six months, another VA medical center identified more than 1,000 new billable insurances, which generated more than $8 million.

TECHNOLOGY ENHANCEMENTS

Improvements due to technology enhancements have occurred many ways. Computer-based templates have been developed to facilitate the preregistration process. One of these allows data gathered through phone calls to be entered on 3 screens, instead of the 14 screens contained in the normal registration process. These data are then automatically updated in the computer database. A major enhancement was the implementation of technology and processes to capture patient diagnostic and treatment data via scannable encounter forms.

PAPERLESS PROCESSING

Paperless processing has been a goal espoused throughout reengineering. Its early success is seen in the growing electronic interface between the medical center and regional counsel, the legal arm of the medical center. It is the referral avenue for billable cases that requires formal negotiation or legal action. Prior to reengineering, the medical center and regional counsel had separate computer systems and different ways to track referred cases. Transactions between the two parties occurred at the paper level only, however, a template has been developed to standardize data entry and regional counsels have been given access to the hospital's computer system. Ultimately, complete electronic transfer of cases will occur.

Summary

The final outcomes of the MCCR reengineering project are unknown at this point. The objectives of the project have not been fully realized, but progress on the first two, namely streamlining and automation, is substantial. Changes are occurring, consistent with the redesigned process and according to the project timetable. The data, which will allow a thorough and objective evaluation of these changes, are beginning to appear on the monthly reports. The implementation of technology and the remaining ideal processes, the pilot evaluation, and subsequent national implementation and training are being planned.

The core planning team identified four elements of the MCCR reengineering project that provided the unique and necessary combination of ingredients for its early and continuing success. These were

- The cross-functional scope of the project

- The effort to cultivate participant ownership of the process

- The careful planning and execution of the project redesign steps

- Management's commitment and ongoing support

Broadly defining the nature and scope of the project was critical. MCCR bears the direct responsibility for collections, but must rely on the work of people beyond its organization. Similarly, the products it generates have value to others outside MCCR. Based on these organizational realities, the scope of the reengineering effort was intentionally designed to bridge organizational lines and to be cross-functional rather than department specific. This meant including those organizations and individuals outside of MCCR in the reengineering process. Coupled with this broad scope was developing a "win-win" strategy to provide incentives for every organization involved in the reengineering process to participate fully.

For this cross-functional effort to succeed, a strategy was developed to involve and obtain the buy-in, commitment, and contributions of all staff, supervisors, and other MCCR customers. The involvement of these individuals from all levels of the organization created a sense of ownership, pride, and clear commitment to succeed.

The third element involved the careful planning and execution of every step of the project. Flowcharting, work plans, performance measures, data collection, and analysis were just a few of the tools employed. One measure of the importance of the planning stage is that most of the issues discussed were raised or anticipated. Although the extent of their impact could not be accurately predicted, strategies for dealing with them could be outlined and ready. Planning is a continuous activity in reengineering.

Management support of the reengineering effort and long-term commitment to the project's success are essential. Support begins with management's ability to create and clearly communicate the organization's vision, where it is going, and the role it will play. Management must

- Envision and communicate the full scope and the challenges of the reengineering effort without overtly prescribing solutions

- Gain and retain the support of employees, supervisors, customers (e.g., patients and physicians), and other stakeholders critical to sustain the total vision over the life of the project

- Be involved with the team in planning the critical steps of the reengineering effort and in establishing the project's major objectives

- Support the effort within the bureaucracy by providing necessary resources, empowering its participants, and facilitating the evaluation and implementation of the process redesign

MCCR employees already are benefiting. Those involved in the pilot project are growing in their ability to function effectively in teams and are broadening their expertise and expanding their roles in the cost recovery effort. Above all, they are growing in their commitment to continuous improvement and the belief that they have a significant influence over the course that improvement takes. This makes them an important resource to the MCCR program both at their own medical center and nationally.

In addition, MCCR better understands how its organization functions at each medical center in the country. It also has acquired a better ability to manage a complex project and integrate implementation strategies, education, analysis, and evaluation.

Reengineering is a test for any corporation, but for a government organization with 173 medical centers across the country, it proved, and continues to prove, particularly challenging. The stereotype of a government organization constrained by bureaucratic inertia, rules, regulations, and territorialism was soundly dismissed during this project. Old stereotypes did not affect the enthusiasm and actions of VA management and employees dedicated to reinventing their department. While MCCR is only in the middle of its reengineering efforts, it already has achieved success in many ways important to cost recovery and the Department of Veterans Affairs as a whole. Reengineering can be frustrating for any organization, but with patience, an understanding of the issues, a commitment to the amount of time required, and careful planning, it can be a successful experience.

20

Penrose–St. Francis Health System: Redirecting service mix

Donna L. Bertram
Senior Vice President and Chief Operating Officer

Sharon Roggy
Vice President, Strategic Planning and Business Development
Penrose–St. Francis Health System
Colorado Springs, Colorado

IN THE 1990S, THE OPERATIVE WORD in the healthcare industry is "change." Incremental change, however, often fails by using quick fixes or decisions based only on today's challenges. Rather than significantly reducing expenses, the healthcare industry is rushing to restructure and reengineer, taking zero-based approaches to operations management. Positioning a healthcare system to accept risk for its populations through contracts with managed care organizations requires much change. Executives must consider closing existing beds, converting high-cost, low-volume services to wellness and prevention programs, consolidating hospital units, and shifting high-technology inpatient services to outpatient services.

This chapter identifies the steps necessary to eliminate unnecessary duplication among services offered by the hospitals in a large healthcare delivery system. This framework uses an incremental change process that offers several advantages, including the development of

1. A workforce of managers, staff, and physicians who understand the need to change

2. A workforce of managers, staff, and physicians committed to change

3. Staff, management, and physician leadership skills

4. A process for quality improvement

5. Teams willing to take risks to achieve success

6. Appropriate and logical timetables to implement change

7. Key stakeholder involvement and acceptance

The discussion relates one healthcare system's decision to change several of its services. It identifies 10 factors—trust, leadership, shared values, time frame, communication, focus, consultation, commitment, political issues, and learning from mistakes—that are critical to successfully implementing change.

These success factors were based on lessons learned from moving a trauma service from one hospital to another and closing an acute care hospital and reopening it as an ambulatory care-focused health center. These moves were accomplished through an incremental change process, rather than radical restructuring. This process had clear advantages—the hospitals encountered less resistance due to adequate time to adapt to change and more ownership due to participation in both the planning and implementation. The following narrative describes the planning and implementation processes used.

Background

The Sisters of Charity Health Care System (SCHCS) of Cincinnati, Ohio, and the Sisters of St. Francis of Colorado Springs, Colorado, decided to merge their hospitals in 1987 to gain efficiencies. Colorado Springs was the only place where the two orders had competing hospitals. The Penrose system, composed of the 88-bed Penrose Community and 370-bed Penrose Hospital, merged with the 206-bed St. Francis Hospital to form the Penrose–St. Francis Health System, a member of SCHCS. These three hospitals offered the same services in medical-surgical care, emergency department, intensive care, pharmacy, laboratory, radiology, dietary, and environmental services. St. Francis offered trauma, cardiology, obstetrics, and a helicopter service. Two years into the merger obstetrics was moved to Penrose Community, cardiology was moved to Penrose, and behavioral health was moved from Penrose to St. Francis. These moves identified

Penrose as the tertiary center with the exception of trauma. The trauma program was marked as the central activity for St. Francis and developed a positive reputation. One group of surgeons served as the leaders and developers of the trauma service. The program was accredited by the American College of Surgeons as the Level II Trauma Center.

As part of the 1987 merger, governance and management structures were developed and services were realigned to reduce duplication, costs, and to become positioned for capitation. Moving the service and reconfiguring St. Francis Hospital into a health center is the middle step in a long process of incremental change begun in 1987 and continuing today.

System formation

Success Factor 1: To develop and foster trust, maintain open, honest, direct communications at all levels.

The first year of the merger was spent devising and implementing a plan to create a new organization. Trust was identified as a key element in the successful creation of a new system called the Penrose–St. Francis Healthcare System (PSF). Staff and management groups from the three hospitals were encouraged to get together to socialize and share information about personal lives before discussing work-related issues. The necessity of open communication was crucial—its value was emphasized in every meeting and in every document open to discussion. Questions and comments were encouraged.

Success Factor 2: Choose committed leaders who share a common vision to influence and inspire others to achieve the goal.

The next step was to build a system focused on broadening the management control while eliminating duplication. A mix of members from both health system boards were appointed to serve on the new board of the Penrose–St. Francis Healthcare System, including representatives from both orders, physicians, and community leaders. All leaders were committed, shared a common vision, and were visible and supportive.

Success Factor 3: Choose managers who demonstrate shared values, personal responsibility, creativity, and a focus on outcomes.

The chief executive officer (CEO) of the Penrose System became the CEO of the new organization, and the CEO of St. Francis Hospital became the chief operating officer (COO). These leaders created an organizational plan and developed a transition team to design and implement one new organizational structure. The plan sought to minimize duplication, unite medical staffs, and develop one operating license and one Medicare provider number for the three facilities. The result was a streamlined management team and one medical staff.

One management team was to oversee the clinical, operational, and support services for all facilities. The management team (vice presidents and directors) went from 90 to 47. These managers were responsible and accountable for all three hospitals instead of just one campus, developing their abilities to oversee operations in three sites separated by three to six miles. Other staff were offered "assistant" positions or remaining available staff positions, while management positions were eliminated.

Service mix changes

In the early 1990s, clinical services were consolidated to increase economies and efficiencies. Obstetrics was moved from St. Francis to Penrose Community Hospital, allowing for 250 deliveries in one place, decreased management positions, and improved quality of services. Behavioral health programs were moved from Penrose to St. Francis to accommodate space requirements. The cardiac catheterization lab was closed at St. Francis due to low utilization and all cardiology services were consolidated at Penrose.

These actions were not random. A plan for the "footprints" of each facility had been developed that emphasized tertiary services at Penrose: cardiology, cardiovascular surgery, neurosurgery, cancer, respiratory, dialysis, critical care, and general medical-surgical care; women's and children's services at Penrose Community: obstetrics, pediatrics, outpatient diagnostic and treatment; and longer-term care services at St. Francis: behavioral health programs for adults and adolescents, geriatric psychiatry, trauma, rehabilitation, and skilled nursing. All three facilities kept their emergency departments and ancillary services. At the time, the public and some members of the medical staff perceived these changes as radical and controversial—some of whom felt strong loyalties to services delivered at a particular location (especially maternity) and staff whose lives were disrupted.

Success Factor 4: Share the concept and involve stakeholders. Set a time frame and do it.

Listening to each interest group's concerns was key. The focus was on key stakeholders (i.e. physicians, staff, patients, and volunteers). Some of these stakeholders had their own agenda and became hostile. Strong, clear statements of purpose, rationale, expectations, and impact had to be repeated frequently. Time was of the essence so most of these changes were done within a 12-month window. Each change had a team to facilitate the transitions. Target dates for completion of each step of service changes were established.

The success of the first service mix changes stimulated another round of clinical and financial investigation by senior management. All three facilities provided emergency departments and ancillary services, with a trauma center located at St. Francis. A competing hospital, located only a few blocks away, also offered trauma services. Penrose–St. Francis questioned if it should sustain or close its trauma business. If it were to stay in the business, the question was where should it be located? Both St. Francis and Penrose had excess capacity in intensive care and surgery, and financially it did not make sense to keep both open. St. Francis did not have magnetic resonance imaging (MRI) for the neurosurgical trauma patients, while Penrose did. Open-heart surgery and dialysis were not done at St. Francis. Neurosurgery was done at both places but predominately at Penrose.

Quality, service, and costs were all being negatively affected with the dispersion and duplication of services. For example, if a trauma patient needed open-heart surgery or dialysis, the machines and staff would need to be transported from Penrose to St. Francis or the patient had to be moved from the trauma center to Penrose, which was not a designated facility. Ancillary services, high-tech equipment, and trained staff had to be maintained at both places in order to operate the trauma service at St. Francis and other tertiary services at Penrose. Efficiencies and economies of scale could not be maintained with this duplication.

While the trauma service was profitable, due primarily to its predominance of blunt injuries (e.g., those injuries produced by car accidents) rather than penetrating trauma (e.g., those produced by gunshots), overhead costs to maintain necessary support services negated its profit margin. Additionally, public sentiment, as expressed through community groups, indicated it was duplicative and wasteful to have two trauma centers operating within four blocks of one another.

Moving a trauma center

In December 1992, PSF senior managers began to explore the feasibility of moving trauma to Penrose Hospital. This involved four major phases, which included

1. Exploring the implications for each facility of the move

2. Testing the feasibility of the move from St. Francis to Penrose

3. Planning the implementation

4. Moving

Two scenario statements were considered: "What if the trauma service was moved from St. Francis to Penrose Hospital?" and "What if St. Francis was converted from a hospital to a health center focusing on outpatient and prevention services?"

A brainstorming group composed of senior managers and physician leaders was used to explore the potential advantages or pitfalls associated with each scenario. Following the brainstorming, a ranking system was used to weigh the negative and positive implications as well as the likelihood of each scenario's occurrence. The exercise began with the assumption that an action had occurred and then identified the effects the action had on the constituents and hospital. The result was a road map that assessed the positive and negative of each assumption (see Figure 1).

Senior managers were the first group to examine each hypothesis. Although some rather frightening prospects emerged (e.g., losing key physicians to the city hospital), the exploration continued with the belief that obstacles could be overcome. Six teams were formed to further explore the two hypotheses. The internal teams were composed of staff, physicians, and management. A seventh team was formed, made up of leaders from business, government, health and social service agencies, and religious sponsors of the Catholic system.

The six teams were each given a month to deliberate and summarize their findings. The external, community-input team took six months. The internal teams concurred that both scenario statements could be accomplished and were feasible and desirable. However, there were several concerns:

- Staff at both places might lose jobs

FIGURE 1
Brainstorming exercise

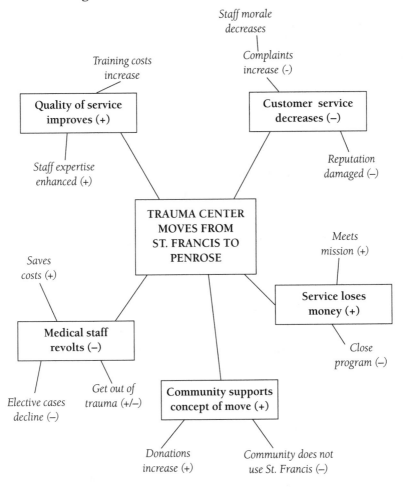

- Physicians might not bring patients to St. Francis (if trauma moved) and might choose to use the city hospital instead

- Penrose might not be able to handle the summer trauma volume

- Following the move, trauma patients might continue to show up at St. Francis

- Both hospitals might lose volume to competitors

- Moving trauma from St. Francis might lead to its complete closure

The community team also recommended pursuing both scenarios but expressed a slightly different view. They identified six major benefits:

- Moving trauma would result in additional space at St. Francis that could be used to meet other community health needs

- The move might be more cost-effective. A wider array of services would be available at the Penrose location. There would be consolidation of staff, less duplication in equipment and potential cost avoidance (for example, not buying a second MRI)

- There could be better access to and distribution of trauma care services with the city hospital serving the southern sector of the community and the Penrose location accessible to northern sectors

- The move may lead to higher-quality trauma care due to the availability of a full spectrum of tertiary care services at Penrose

- The move might lead to more collaboration with the competitor hospital. Moving trauma out of their neighborhood might be seen as more cooperative

- A policy for trauma victims (via ambulance) would be easier to determine because of the distance between the program locations

They also expressed concerns:

- The move could create a negative impact on the neighborhood surrounding Penrose, such as increased traffic, noise, and visitors

- The community would perceive Penrose–St. Francis to have abandoned the St. Francis location. Employees feel that things continue to be "taken away" from St. Francis. Trauma is seen as the focal point for services at St. Francis. This could lead to both an internal and public perception that St. Francis is closing

- The move would be perceived as competitive with the other hospital. It could be construed as an attempt to attract business away from that hospital's trauma service

- Healthcare costs might increase. The move would waste money that had already been spent to renovate St. Francis. Further costs would be incurred to renovate Penrose to accommodate the move to trauma

- If vacancies created at St. Francis were backfilled with more traditional hospital services, a great opportunity for creativity will have been missed

- Patients from the southern part of the city might have to go farther for trauma care

- There could be a negative impact on healthcare available to those in the neighborhood surrounding St. Francis

The internal and external groups exhibited striking differences in the approaches taken and the reasoning behind those decisions. All decisions were reported to the board's planning committee, the Penrose–St. Francis Board, medical executive committee, medical section meetings, the management team, and key employees.

Success Factor 5: Prepare for the unexpected. Plan communication and press releases early.

In the meantime, a leak to the local newspaper resulted in a misleading headline announcing, "St. Francis Closes as Trauma Moves." This necessitated communicating with hospital employees on an accelerated time frame with additional employee and physician meetings, as well as a candid discussion with the reporter and general manager of the local newspaper. A weekly rumor column was included in the weekly internal newsletter for several months following this announcement, and an employee hotline number was established to communicate factual answers to questions. Additional efforts were undertaken to establish communication links with the media so that information could be verified before it appeared in print or on radio or television.

Decision

Senior managers met to review all the input in March 1993. The decision to go ahead with planning the move was made by the CEO and COO. The intent was to accomplish the move as quickly as possible, after the summer trauma season. As work progressed it became apparent to the COO that this time line was not achievable due to construction needs and potential resistance from physicians and staff. Rather than developing an alternate date, it was decided that the move and conversion would occur after the trauma season in 1994. The date would be announced as details developed.

The COO discussed the need with managers and staff to consider St. Francis becoming a health center instead of an acute care hospital. A team made two site visits to other facilities that had successfully converted or changed their facility. As time passed it made sense to call St. Francis a health center.

Implementation

Although feasibility testing and implementation planning are discrete activities, they were accomplished within the same team structures. Nine implementation teams were formed to explore the plan for implementation. The teams represented the functional and physical areas that would be involved with or affected by the move and conversion, including emergency department, intensive care unit, operating room, outpatient services, behavioral health, urgent care, public relations and marketing, construction and moving services, and ancillary services.

Each team included staff, managers, and employees from each of the three facilities represented by the Penrose–St. Francis system. A steering committee was established, led by the COO, and included senior executives for patient care, planning and marketing, and support services as well as directors of critical care, surgery, facilities, and construction. Also included was the administrator for St. Francis and medical directors for emergency room (ER), operating room (OR), intensive care unit (ICU), anesthesiology, and the chief of staff.

Success Factor 6: Realize that derailing and sidebar issues result in delays. Stay focused and get the implementation done as soon as possible.

The role of the steering committee, which met monthly, was to coordinate the work of the implementation groups, solve problems, identify issues, and make final decisions regarding the groups' recommendations. However, problems began to arise within the groups. These included

- Conflicting viewpoints about the purpose of the groups among members. (Some people believed their only role was to find a way to accomplish what had been determined by others, while others viewed the purpose as a thorough analysis of feasibility of the function or service.)

- The feeling that resistance to change could not be overcome. Physician, staff, or management resistance was assumed to be insurmountable

- The assumption of a negative outcome without fully investigating feasibility first. (Time was spent on planning to make the best of a situation already assumed to be bad, rather than tackling the task of thoroughly examining feasibility.)

- Special interest group agendas surfaced. (Surgeons used the move as an opportunity to push for additional operating rooms, an agenda only marginally tied in with the trauma move.)

- Varying interpretations of data arose. (Groups sought information from a variety of sources and received seemingly contradictory answers.)

- Politically correct solutions were desired. (Hospital administrators and physicians wanted solutions that would not offend any key stakeholders. This was unrealistic.)

Success Factor 7: Choose a consultant who is compatible with leaders, has experience and skills, and can relate unpopular realities.

Outside consultants were hired to help the groups synthesize data from an objective point of view. They began by interviewing team leaders and members to determine where perspectives differed. They worked with providers of data to clarify decisions and to standardize the data. For some, the consultants acted as temporary facilitators of the process to refocus their efforts. For example, a debate over operating room capacity ensued. It was discovered that overall utilization of operating rooms was 69 percent at Penrose, which meant that the additional surgical trauma cases could be absorbed without adding capacity. However, on many occasions scheduled surgeries might be delayed or postponed in favor of a trauma case. This "bumping" of cases was identified as a patient care issue, a customer service problem, and an efficiency problem for the physician as well as a morale issue for the staff.

The steering committee also believed that some amount of additional OR capacity should be developed. An analysis of the data showed management that one additional OR should be sufficient, whereas anesthesiologists and surgeons thought four rooms were needed. After much analysis and debate about shifting some surgeries to Penrose Community and St. Francis facilities (a very unpopular suggestion among current users of Penrose facilities) and the costs of remodeling, the COO decided that two new operating rooms would be built. The decision represented a compromise between data that clearly indicated the adequacy of one additional operating room and the surgeons' preference.

Teams evaluated the ER and x-ray space. Three trauma rooms in the ER at Penrose were needed. The placement of these rooms created a need to relocate security services, outpatient registration, patient representatives, and the diabetic clinic. Two new x-ray scanners were needed to accommodate trauma, inpatient, and outpatient needs. It was neccessary that this equipment be located near the ER and radiology. This displaced the outpatient pharmacy. Managers of these areas worked with all those who were going to be displaced and began to search for a home for these services. Work progressed during the summer and October 6, 1994, was established as the new moving day.

The incentive for the management team was to avoid layoffs and provide positions to those whose jobs were eliminated by the move. The directors of critical care and surgery looked at current positions, needed positions, vacancies, and attrition and received permission to hire temporary help for the summer. This made it possible to get through the peak season without adding permanent staff that would then be eliminated following the move. The effort was successful. Additional agency staffing ceased six weeks after the move was complete, and no layoff was necessary.

Success Factor 8: People who are involved and support the concept help create positive outcomes.

Skill sets in trauma, emergency, critical care, and surgery were evaluated with the intent of preparing the staff at St. Francis and Penrose to provide necessary care after the move. The staffs at each place were going to be merged, and the managers wanted to facilitate a smooth transition. Cross-training is a process that takes staff with one skill set and exposes them to other skills through orientation, education, on-the-job training, and a preceptor. Cross-training of staff began early, with St. Francis staff learning to care for open-heart patients and Penrose staff gaining skills in the care of trauma victims. Trauma drills were held at Penrose to simulate various types of trauma situations. Staff from St. Francis served as evaluators and players. This helped prepare the staff for the types of patients seen in a trauma service. The fastest route to the

OR from the trauma center was identified and elapsed time for the trip calculated. Everything had to be synchronized to take advantage of the "golden hour of trauma"—the time during which the probabilities are greatest that the patient can be saved.

At St. Francis, the issues of vacating the ER and moving trauma were vastly different from those at Penrose. Instead of accommodating new volume and activity, the challenge was what to do with excess capacity and how to forge a new identity for a decreased activity in the facility. The behavioral health program, which is housed on two floors of the building, was concerned with not having the resources and support of an acute care hospital as well as the care their patients would receive at Penrose.

Formerly, most psychiatric patients came in through the St. Francis emergency department and were admitted to the behavioral health program as appropriate. Now that the emergency department was closing at St. Francis, with only a 12-hour urgent care service remaining in its place, these same psychiatric patients were likely to show up at Penrose where services were not available. Plans were made to provide psychiatric nurse clinicians at Penrose. Arrangements were made for transport from the Penrose ER to St. Francis behavioral units, education and training for the Penrose ER staff and physicians, and contingency planning for psychiatric patients at St. Francis should one of them have a crisis. In the absence of an ER and 24-hour in-house physician coverage, it was decided that the patient would be stabilized and transported via ambulance to Penrose, if needed.

The medical unit, with a 28-patient bed capacity, closed at St. Francis, and the patients were moved to Penrose or dismissed. The staff accepted vacant positions at Penrose or Penrose Community Hospitals. Many physicians appreciated having one less place to make rounds. Some admissions were lost from physicians who were St. Francis loyalists and not Penrose supporters. The empty unit at St. Francis created questions about what could be done with the space. A local community hospice expressed interest in consolidating its two facilities by leasing space at St. Francis. Dietary, environmental, and maintenance services were provided by Penrose–St. Francis, along with some minor renovations making it possible for the hospice program to lease an entire floor. The program has been successful in its new quarters. It is now seeking to lease 15 more beds and administrative space on another floor at St. Francis.

This move has been well received by the community and by employee and physician groups.

The outpatient reengineering team evaluated the type of patients appropriate for St. Francis. It was decided that low-risk, short-stay (less than 72 hours) patients would be appropriate for this center. Outpatient surgery was to operate Monday through Friday from eight to five with overnight patients kept on the inpatient surgical unit. All outpatient surgery patients are prepared in the former ICU and recover there before going home. It is on the same level as surgery. Current surgeries done at St. Francis Health Center are low-risk orthopedics (e.g., arthroscopies, carpel tunnel, and shoulder); ear, nose, and throat; plastic and minor general surgery. The focus is strictly on outpatient surgery. Two anesthesiologists moved from St. Francis to Penrose to stay with the trauma service.

Success Factor 9: Identify key stakeholders, what influence they have, and who influences them. Address their concerns.

The marketing plan for moving was carefully coordinated. Brochures were sent to St. Francis's former patients of the last three years. Advertisements were placed on radio, TV, and in the newspaper. Notices were sent to all schools, churches, service agencies, fire, police, employers, and libraries. Employees were asked to tell neighbors and friends about the changes. One homeowners' association had concerns over the increased traffic and helicopter noise at Penrose. Public relations, marketing, and the trauma service directors met with these stakeholders and the ambulance company. Information was collected. Decibel readings were conducted of helicopter takeoff and landing. Statistics were gathered and options presented. The ambulance company agreed to a certain route to the hospital emergency department and would shut off the sirens within two blocks of the hospital. Parking and signage issues were addressed and compromises were made even on the color of the covered canopy.

Construction and moving services played a key role in the process. Displacements had to be planned, coordinated, and discussed. Expectations were established that an equal or better space would be offered. Timetables and budget would be met; and once plans were signed, there would be minimal to no change orders. The need for a move coordinator was acknowledged as crucial. This was approved as a temporary position, and an engineer was hired nine months before the move. This person met with staff, managers, and physicians about equipment and move needs and then worked with the construction and contractor team and clinicians to coordinate patient moves. Medical unit admitting at St. Francis stopped 10 days prior to the move, and all patients were dismissed or transferred. ICU patients who could be transferred from the ICU to the appropriate units at Penrose were moved seven days before the move. The week of the move, a few trauma patients arrived at Penrose. Extra ambulances and extra staff were coordinated for move day, and the city hospital agreed to accept any trauma victims during the move. The actual move took less than three hours and was considered anticlimactic due to the work of all the teams and the move coordinator.

Since the move affected ancillary services, the implementation team included radiology, laboratory, dietary, pharmacy, management information systems, environmental services, maintenance, and admitting. This group analyzed the impact on them in terms of services and staffing. Radiology at St. Francis lost trauma volume; however, outpatient radiology was moved to St. Francis so volumes would improve. The lab at St. Francis handled urgent and routine lab work with a courier service to Penrose on the higher-tech tests. Dietary picked up the hospice patients and staff. Pharmacy at Penrose received a new space. All computer changes from St. Francis and cabling at Penrose were coordinated with information systems. All of the ancillary services were able to decrease staff. With some clinical and managerial positions eliminated, the total decrease was 126 full-time equivalents at St. Francis through attrition.

Expectations for the move were met or slightly exceeded. Soon trauma volume was comparable to that of the previous year. Outpatient surgery initially decreased at St. Francis to approximately 12 a day, while Penrose surgery, ER, and general medical surgery were up about 3 percent. This is predominantly due to the trauma surgeons doing their general surgeries at Penrose and the orthopedists doing the big cases (i.e., total joint and hip replacements) at Penrose. Urgent care activity level at St. Francis Health Center has been averaging 35 to 40 patients a day. Behavioral health is status quo, and the hospice is full. It is too soon to evaluate the primary care practice.

The total cost of the trauma move was $5 million, which included two new CT scanners as part of the replacement budget. Two new operating suites and three new trauma rooms were built and equipped. The remodeled ER entrance improved patient flow. Outpatient pharmacy, lab, and admitting are in new spaces, services have been consolidated and quality of care has improved. Staffs have been cross-trained, and no FTEs were laid off.

Interfacility transfers decreased, and two separate physician groups came together as one professional corporation. One physician group at Penrose has accepted trauma responsibility along with the surgeons from St. Francis. This has given a better call schedule with more physicians involved. A new medical director of trauma services was hired in July prior to the move.

The strategic advantages of consolidation have been

1. Ability to partner with the community on appropriate use of resources and work on health initiatives

2. Ability to help another not-for-profit agency (hospice) expand and relocate

3. Implementation of a primary care clinic

4. Integration of cross-trained staff

5. Improved utilization of tertiary services

6. Improved operations

7. Lower cost that allows the institution to better prepare for risk contracting

8. Conversion of an acute care hospital to a health center that better meets community needs

Success Factor 10: Start with a clean sheet of paper. Dream. Design. Take risks and learn from mistakes. Take initiative. Do it.

In all, management, physicians, and staff learned a great deal in this process. However, many things could have been done differently. One designated coordinator should have been accountable and responsible to the COO for the trauma move, instead of nine teams and many other interest groups all demanding time. A clearer mandate with tighter time lines would have helped the move and probably eliminated the need for a consultant. Fewer teams with broader authority for decision making would have made the process smoother. Including community leaders in teams rather than keeping them separate would foster communications. More one-on-one meetings with key physicians may have eliminated some rumors and second-guessing. And managing the press earlier and differently would have avoided the sensational headlines and the resulting need for damage control.

Nonetheless, things were done right. Time and energy vested in managers and staff fostered leadership development. This process also nurtured a strong heritage of participation in planning and decision making. Teams rose to challenges with help from the consultants. Appropriate grieving about the closing of trauma at St. Francis and celebration of opportunities at both facilities was accomplished. Success and positive change resulted from careful planning; a trusting and energized team; and open, honest, and direct communications.

Realigning a service mix can reduce cost and create efficiencies. Eliminating duplication and unnecessary services, however, is not easy to accomplish. Communication at all levels is essential. Incremental change, while not always dramatic or draconian, can achieve results. Change is inevitable and a continuous process that will never be completed. The way to thrive in this new environment is to make "growth" as inevitable as change. Growth does not always mean expanding but includes learning, seeking, experiencing, and using energies to design the system of the future.

▛ 21

Medicaid agencies: Realigning management information systems

Mark K. Shishida
Vice President
Fox Systems, Inc.
Scottsdale, Arizona

THE ALIGNMENT OF MANAGEMENT information systems to support an organization's new business direction is central to the success of business process reengineering. As business processes become more reliant on automation, appropriate systems development is critical. The administration of Medicaid, the federal government's matching of state healthcare programs for the poor, is highly complex and depends on equally sophisticated information systems. As such, it is fertile ground for systems innovation.

Under increased pressure to implement healthcare cost controls, Medicaid agencies are accelerating conversion to a managed care delivery model.[1] This movement represents a reengineering of the delivery of Medicaid benefits because state Medicaid agencies are being forced to find ways to change basic business processes. The reengineering effort involves a massive overhaul of a state agency's infrastructure—its business, policies, structure, business rules, responsiveness to legislative mandates, and manual and automated processes. The administrative and data information systems supporting the agency are often unable to adapt quickly enough to meet the new needs, and the time-honored Medicaid Management Information System (MMIS) model becomes outdated.

This chapter discusses a business application of reengineering in healthcare management information systems. Development of these systems has traditionally been haphazard and disorganized and has resulted in cumbersome, inefficient, and inflexible systems. The approach described in this chapter is more rational and systematic than the traditional systems development methods.

Reengineered Medicaid

The healthcare industry, whose administration has been battered by financial crises, has been seeking solutions and alternatives to overcome them. Encumbered by a myriad of rigid federal and state regulations affecting eligibility, services, financing, and reimbursement, Medicaid, for example, has been slower to adopt alternative delivery methods than the private sector. In recent years, there have been a number of major Medicaid reforms or associated programs, such as primary care gatekeeping and case management, brought about through federal legislation, many of which involved unfunded mandates.[2] As an answer to their financial problems, states are rapidly turning to managed care.

The managed care delivery model is fundamentally different from the existing fee-for-service system (FFS). A full-scale change from FFS to managed care calls for reengineering the Medicaid program. Managed care has changed the basic philosophy of healthcare services delivery and reimbursement from direct payment for services provided to a fixed fee per enrollee per month, placing the provider at-risk for the cost of care. Table 1 illustrates the significant changes Medicaid has had to implement to change from FFS to managed care arrangements.

Each of these changes calls for a complex reexamination of organizational structure, business processes, and information flows within Medicaid and across interfaces between the agency and providers.

In addition to a new orientation to managed care, Medicaid now finds more uncertainty due to factors such as

- Changes in federal funding (block grants)

- Growing uninsured and aging population

- Increasing costs of medical care due to ever-more-expensive technologies

TABLE 1
FFS model versus managed care model

Function	Fee-for-service model	Managed care model
Provider reimburse ment	Providers bill the state for services rendered to Medicaid recipients	Providers receive a fixed, capi tated rate based on enrollment Medicaid recipients; multiple models exist including pre ferred or exclusive provider organization, primary care case management, partial capitation, and full capitation
Program priorities	Focus on controlling services utilized, fraud, and abuse	Focus on accessibility, quality, and continuity of care
State's role	Claims administration and provider reimbursement	Monitor of program access, effectiveness, quality, and out come
Provider's role	Provide direct service and submit claims for reimbursement	Direct service providers who are employed by or contract with managed care organizations that provide reimbursement, administrative, and management infrastructure
Medicaid system focus	Capture, edit, adjudicate, price, and pay submitted provider claims	Maintain data on assignment of eligibles to managed care providers and make prospective capitation payments

As the "payer of last resort" with many recipients having other insurance coverage, Medicaid program policies are complex and intertwined with the overall healthcare industry and changes in other financially pressed programs such as Medicare, Indian Health Services, Veterans Administration, and CHAMPUS.

Program complexity

The reengineering task can be appreciated only by fully understanding the complexities of Medicaid. Although Medicaid is largely a federally funded program with nominal requirements for uniform benefits across the country, it has always been administered by individual states, each with its own unique variations in administrative and operational requirements. For example, each state's Medicaid program must cover inpatient hospital services but can vary with respect to reimbursement methodology, benefit limitations, patient copayment, prior authorization and utilization review requirements, and even claim forms and coding schemes. As a result, each state has developed a system customized to its unique requirements rather than installing off-the-shelf software. These differences between states can only be expected to intensify if federal block grant allocations or some form of capped funding is enacted.

Managed care has forced states to reevaluate existing ways of doing business. Many of the functions performed have become institutionalized from many years of doing things the same way. The first step in business process reengineering is to create the vision of managed care (i.e., Medicaid state agencies must look at the delivery of health services from a managed care perspective and anticipate the change it will have on its business processes). This is not an easy job—managed care models in the Medicaid sector are still relatively new. There is not much Medicaid experience to draw on to help states envision and understand the implications of managed care, either on a broad basis or at the detail level. Furthermore, state agencies are committed to procedures for proposing, finalizing, and implementing new policies, such as those required for managed care. Each Medicaid agency maintains a "state plan" defining its program and all changes must be discussed with all impacted parties during public comment periods: provider associations, welfare clients' rights organizations, and federal, state, and local agencies. Private sector payers are not handicapped by these rules and regulations and have been able to implement change much more quickly and decisively.

For example, there may be legal and ethical concerns that Medicaid program recipients will be disadvantaged by managed care restrictions (i.e., lessened freedom of choice of providers). States must try to overcome provider and community fear and skepticism of managed care, especially in those regions of the country where private sector managed care has not made significant inroads. These concerns must be addressed before Medicaid program changes can be made.

The next step in reengineering is to identify which current and new business processes to integrate, automate, or eliminate. States are looking at what is being done within a process and why processes are performed in a prescribed manner to determine whether the "how" is still appropriate. Rethinking business processes often exposes inefficiencies and redundancies, and this suggests changes in organizational structure, work and information flow, procedures, and management systems.

Automating illogical or outdated ways of doing things because they have always been done that way only results in "faster inefficiency."

Many existing business processes were designed around old systems, technologies, and procedures. For example, older batch processing claims payment systems produced cycles of paper claim receipts, data entry, suspense of processing when errors were detected, return of the claim to the provider for correction, data entry of the correction, and finally, payment. Although technology can reduce processing times with faster and more efficient hardware and software, only business reengineering can revolutionize the way in which providers are reimbursed, such as prospective capitation payments.

Long-established systems and rationale for doing business in a certain way will no longer exist in managed care. Asking "why" leads to redefining and rethinking the business process. Once the process is examined and reconstructed, the MMIS must support these processes. For example, the administration of managed care delivery models is extremely data dependent and time consuming; accurate information will be the key to successful operation of managed care programs. In contrast, current systems often sacrifice data to gain speed in claims processing. The administration of Medicaid has been and will continue to be highly automated, but the MMIS also must be reengineered. New approaches to systems development hold promise for the monumental task of MMIS reengineering.

Medicaid management information systems (MMIS)

In the late 1980s, after more than two decades of patching and mending systems, states began to react to the problem of aging systems. During this period, Arizona developed a custom Medicaid system to support Arizona Health Care Cost Containment System (AHCCCS), a statewide managed care demonstration. This system, called the Prepaid Medical Management Information System (PMMIS), was the first Medicaid system designed expressly to support a managed care program. As with any pioneer effort, the systems development project was expensive and required five years of effort. Other states moving to a managed care model for Medicaid, such as Hawaii, are now also taking up this challenge with the development of new systems.

There have been varying levels of success with recent MMIS developments. Many projects have incurred major schedule and budget overruns. Perhaps more significantly, there have been mixed results in system effectiveness, although it is expected that many problems will be resolved over the first few years of operation. This inability to consistently and successfully develop new Medicaid systems underscores the need for a new approach to be both systematic and effective. While states and their contractors recognize this need, recognition comes at a time when enhanced federal funding may be eliminated in the near future, making it imperative to accomplish more with less.

A number of integrated approaches to reengineering management information systems have proven to be successful in the private sector and can be brought to bear on Medicaid and other federal and state-based programs. The approach is known as information engineering (IE), and encompasses joint applications design (JAD) techniques and automated computer-aided software engineering (CASE) tools. These technologies and methodologies provide Medicaid agencies with a structured framework and techniques for user specification of requirements and software for system design and coding.

The IE approach, and its two main techniques and tools, are summarized in Figure 1.

IE's main features include

- A "top-down" approach, beginning with senior-level management to establish organizational goals and objectives

FIGURE 1
Information engineering

Information engineering
The "methodology" for new systems design and development based on disciplined, structured, and standardized methods and procedures

Joint application design (JAD)
The "technique" for eliciting system requirements using facilitated sessions

Computer-aided software engineering (CASE) tools
Software that supports and enforces the IE methodology

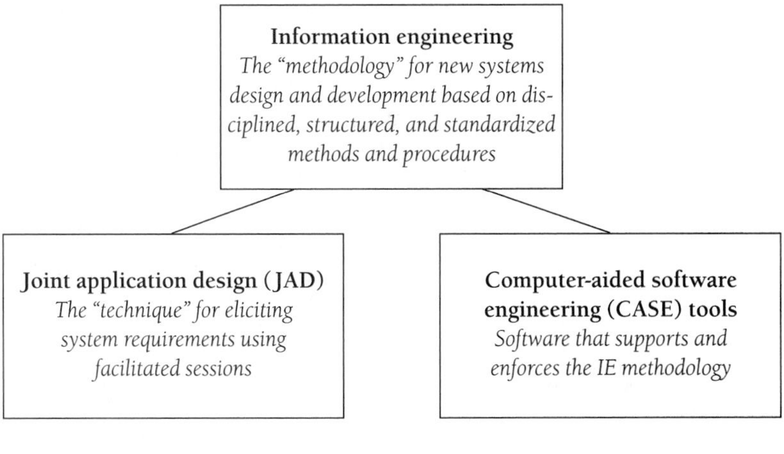

- Involving all levels of the organization in the process, from senior management to actual users

- Facilitated discussions

- Producing models or graphic representations of requirements such as required information and processes

- Using software tools to translate the models into program code

Combining the above steps, this approach produces systems that better meet the strategic, programmatic, and operational needs of the Medicaid program.

Information engineering

Information engineering (IE) approaches systems design and development in a more comprehensive and rigorous manner, replacing traditionally unorganized systems development with rational and systematic techniques and tools. As indicated by inclusion of the word "engineering," an objective of IE is to systematically gather information with appropriate tools and management and control points. The benefits of IE are improved quality, better maintainability, and enhanced user satisfaction.

IE derives system designs from an organization's strategic objectives and develops "blueprints" reflecting them. The traditional model for system development is haphazard at best; that is, it does not consciously link strategic objectives to systems design. In contrast, IE recognizes that the components of system development are interrelated and should be driven from the top down with the results of one phase feeding each subsequent phase of development.

IE can be viewed as a pyramid, incorporating a logical series of activities, beginning at the top with planning, moving to analysis, design, and finally, construction, to translate users' ideas into program data, process models, and ultimately program code. The phases of IE can be analogized to the steps during design and construction of a home. IE starts with strategic analysis and planning based on organizational mission and objectives. In this analogy, a homeowner and the architect work together to define the type of house the owner desires, after deciding (through "reengineering") that indeed, a new house must be built versus remodeling or moving. Once the decision to build is made, the homeowner must answer questions such as what type of structure should be built, time of completion, price, style, size, priorities, and more.

PLANNING

Typical questions asked and answered during the planning phase are

- What is the corporate mission and what are the objectives?

- What is the organization currently doing to support the mission?

- What current functions support the mission and objectives?

- What systems are in place to support the functions?

- How can new technology best be used to enhance the functions?

- What new functions are required to support the new requirements?

The overall objectives of the Medicaid program drive the strategies needed to achieve those objectives. How well the program meets those objectives is determined by strategies used, and identification of the success factors; success is evaluated by using specific performance measures. An example of this process is illustrated below.

Objective:	Control costs, improve access to care, and improve outcomes
Strategy:	Implement statewide voluntary HMO enrollment with default to primary care physician case management
Success factors:	Develop adequate provider network Develop managed care administration procedures Convert to new business model Redesign systems Educate recipients and providers
Performance measures:	95 percent member enrollment 5 percent reduction in overall costs Increase in primary care services Decrease in emergency room and hospital use Increase in consumer satisfaction

Strategic information system planning results in a better understanding of the business, an identification and scoping of needed systems, and the prioritization of those systems.

ANALYSIS

The next level of IE is analysis. It corresponds to the homeowner meeting with the architect to develop the design for the home, which is subsequently defined in blueprints.

During analysis, the specific business requirements for the Medicaid agency are determined. Requirements are described in terms of functions (what is done) and information (what data the functions use). In turn, the requirements are transformed into graphic charts and diagrams, either process or data models.

These models illustrate the information required by the system, how it is organized, and how that data interrelates with other types of information and processes. The following is a an example of a Medicaid business rule that may be portrayed in process and data models.

When a state agency contracts with a new Medicaid prepaid health plan (PHP), the agency may require the following information to be captured and validated:

- Organization address—the street address of the health plan location where services are provided

- Contract master address—the specifics of the contract with the health plan, including the codes identifying type of contract and the optional services provided

- Counties of service—the county codes identifying the county(ies) where the health plan holds a valid service contract

- Correspondence address—the address to which official correspondence is to be forwarded

- Rate codes—the recipient actuarial categories for which the health plan has contracted to provide services in contracted counties

- Zip codes—the zip codes that further qualify contracted counties. This is needed in large urban counties where there are multiple health plans

- Restriction—codes identifying the services that are excluded or restricted from the health plan's contract

Captured data is checked against the valid data values in the health plan's database to ensure accurate entry. The database is continually updated and is used to determine if services are allowable under the health plan's contract.

Once the relationships and requirements are defined and illustrated, both the system engineer and user are able to view the requirements. How the requirements are ultimately implemented are not addressed during this phase of the process.

DESIGN

The next phase in IE is design, where the physical constraints and limitations are considered. The physical design takes into consideration how to best achieve performance, maintainability, and other design constraints imposed by the physical aspects of the system environment. For instance, a database design can appear appropriate from a theoretical standpoint (e.g., normalized with no redundant data,[3] organized efficiently with appropriate access keys, and restricted to data related to the key field). As the system design evolves, however, it may be discovered that the database design will result in a physical database too large and inefficient for the available hardware and other resources. It may be necessary to split the single database into three or four physical databases to make the system operate efficiently.

CONSTRUCTION

In designing a house, the blueprints and specifications have been turned over to the contractor for building. The contractor reviewing the plans may discover the foundation is inadequate for the type of soil it sits upon. To continue, the current house design requires elimination of the home's third story. The counterpart to construction in systems development entails detailed specification of the system's functional capabilities and actual generation of computer program code. This process takes the form of manual coding or, if available, through automatically generated computer code from computer-assisted software engineering (CASE) tool software.

Joint applications design (JAD)

A critical step in reengineering a system is to understand the requirements of the organization and to achieve an organizational consensus regarding how the system should support them. In IE methodology, this step is commonly put into practice through joint applications design (JAD) sessions. JAD is a technique used to structure and facilitate these problem-solving and decision-making discussions. The decisions and agreements reached in JAD sessions are the foundation for subsequent design and development activities.

A JAD SESSION

JAD techniques involve a session leader who facilitates a structured agenda by eliciting opinions, capturing information, and building consensus. The techniques can be used during the planning, analysis, and design phases of IE. In systems-oriented JAD sessions, typical participants include the facilitator, system users, technical personnel who will actually develop the system, and a scribe responsible for documenting results so the facilitator can focus on listening and facilitating. A subject area expert such as a managed care specialist may also be asked to participate. If an organization is using a CASE tool to supplement JAD, a CASE tool technician is also needed. This individual may or may not attend all the sessions but will be involved in taking the results of JAD sessions, entering them into the CASE tool software, and generating the diagrams and models that are then used at the next session for feedback. The optimal number of participants (usually users) is six to eight, exclusive of the facilitator, observers, business area specialists, and scribe.

One of the primary tenets of JAD is that "all participants are equal," so the opinions of managers and their subordinates are both listened to and taken into consideration. Although each organization has its strong, outspoken individuals, the JAD format tends to be democratic and encourages participation from all.

JAD sessions can vary in duration from an hour to an entire day with appropriate breaks to refocus concentration. The number and frequency of meetings varies depending upon the subject. A series of JAD sessions to develop system requirements and design may continue for months or even years in the case of a very large system. A single session may suffice for more limited nonsystem topics where JAD techniques have been adopted for routine corporate problem solving.

JAD VERSUS TRADITIONAL TECHNIQUES

The traditional approach to systems design is unstructured and often performed without user feedback. Analysts meet with users, either singly or in small groups. Users are expected to explain their requirements, often consisting of an unstructured, rambling discussion on how business is currently conducted. The analyst captures the requirements from the user's comments, and later produces a requirements document detailing the problem and describing the perceived system requirements.

Because the traditional approach captures the views of only a few analysts who have interviewed a single user or small group of users, a narrow perspective of the situation is represented. This problem is similar to the parable about blind people describing an elephant after touching it at various locations on the animal's anatomy. In the traditional systems design approach, each user gives a unique definition of "what the elephant looked like" from a personal viewpoint—accounting, purchasing, warehousing of data, and so on. From those separate and disparate views, the business analyst attempts to develop solutions reflecting the true requirements of the entire organization. This approach has often led to inaccuracies and inconsistencies in the requirements document, and, without significant critique of the product, the resulting system can be compromised.

BENEFITS OF JAD

The primary advantage to JAD is that all participants have to agree— consensus must be reached before the session can proceed. Agreement is much more likely to occur in a JAD format if each participant listens to the other users concerning their specific requirements. As pieces of the puzzle are integrated, users often come away from sessions with much more comprehensive views of their organization and its processes. This agreement strengthens each participant's commitment to JAD session results because all participants become stakeholders in the process. The systems resulting from JAD are generally more comprehensive, user oriented, and efficient than those conceived by analysts without the benefits of intense user participation.

JAD also encourages "breakthrough thinking" due to the synergy different perspectives provide. The sessions are an opportunity to invite users to brainstorm, conceptualize new ideas, and look at different ways of doing things. These sessions are an effective forum for users to "get out of the box," look at processes from another unit's viewpoint, obtain an overall view of the system, and participate in redesigning the system. For example, in Arizona, systems designers discovered that the enrollee was the focus of the system and not the provider. Likewise, JAD teams in

Virginia found that program benefit plans were the hub of their new system design. In traditional Medicaid systems, provider claims payment is the focal point.

Computer-assisted software engineering (CASE) tools

The results derived from JAD sessions are entered into software called CASE tool, to produce graphic models and generate program code for the processes, events, and data requirements defined by users.

Models are developed using the software and are then maintained in a centralized repository where they can be continually used, transformed, and modified. These models can be passed from one IE phase to another and will eventually be used to generate actual working program code. In the example of the newly eligible managed care enrollee, the CASE tool would generate code from the model as defined by key "entities" such as data tables and elements, process diagrams, screens, and reports.

BENEFITS OF USING A CASE TOOL

A primary advantage to CASE is its ability to automatically link related objects in the CASE repository such as organizations, functions, or data. This process creates "traceability" that provides a link between organizations and functions and data requirements so that the impact of any future system or operational changes can be easily pinpointed. For example, the CASE tool can answer the question, "Which users are affected if a new data element is added to a data table?" Finding the answer to this question manually would require many hours of labor. Using a CASE tool, however, the task is reduced to a computer search lasting a few seconds.

CASE tools contribute to the success of reengineering MMIS by

- Producing understandable models of system requirements and design

- Ensuring consistency and completeness across all elements of the models

- Enforcing IE methodologies

- Being able to automatically produce system program code

- Providing ease of update when changes to the system are required

- Being easily replicated for use by other state Medicaid agencies, thereby saving time and money

The benefits of using CASE tools increase the value of using IE methodologies and JAD techniques.

Using reengineering methodologies

Although no MMIS development project has yet incorporated or completed all phases of business process reengineering using information engineering, JAD techniques, or CASE tools, several states have implemented different aspects of the process. The following section describes the use of information engineering, JAD sessions, and a CASE tool by a state Medicaid agency. It is a composite representative of groundbreaking advances in systems development undertaken recently in New Mexico, Hawaii, Virginia, and Arizona.

DEVELOPMENT OF NEW MMIS SYSTEM REQUIREMENTS

Several years ago, in anticipation of major Medicaid program changes, a state undertook the development of a management information system capable of supporting managed care and other new business requirements. The original MMIS had been in operation for several years without significant redesign during that period of time. Additionally, with its existing MMIS fiscal agent contract due to expire soon, the state wanted the requirements for a new MMIS to be incorporated into the request for proposal (RFP) for the next fiscal agent contract.

Although the agency staff were not resistant to the announced changes in the Medicaid program or the anticipated systems development effort, they had difficulty understanding (even on a conceptual level) the massive managed care-related changes looming on the horizon. Past negative experience with major and minor systems changes created hesitancy among agency staff to enter into a full-blown effort to reengineer the original MMIS system. The full support of top management obtained in the initial project meeting helped to deal with the staff concerns and build support at all levels of the agency.

Phase one: Planning with senior management

After making the decision to reengineer the MMIS, the state engaged a consultant to assist them with the process of system requirements analysis. The consultant proposed IE methodologies and JAD sessions for developing the systems requirements and a CASE tool for modeling requirements. The consultant first met with the top management to ensure agreement and understanding with the approach. This meeting proved to be of immeasurable benefit to the project's success by interpreting the goals and approach to the rest of the organization.

Next, for several weeks, senior department managers participated in meetings to develop an information strategy plan (ISP) that defined high-level requirements for the new system. The senior management JAD sessions consisted of approximately 10 senior management participants including the Medicaid director, deputy directors, and division directors. In these meetings a trained JAD facilitator met with managers to examine issues in five major areas:

- *Overall system goals.* What is the agency's mission statement? Is the agency's priority to save money or meet federal requirements? What type of managed care program is envisioned? Are the implications of managed care clear?

- *Critical success factors.* What are the specific measurements to determine a successful program (e.g., lower costs, access to care, improved quality of care)? Who will set these priorities? How will these measurements be reported, and to whom will they be reported?

- *Organizational structure.* How is the department currently organized? How can the agency align the system to meet the agency goals? What changes, if any, should be made to support new functions? Which departments within each organization will be responsible for the function? Who is responsible for various functions—the state or fiscal agent or some other organization to whom services could be outsourced in the future? What external organizations are "users" whose requirements need to be taken into consideration when the system is being developed?

- *Business functions.* What is required to support the agency's goals? What sorts of functions does the agency have to perform to meet those objectives? Should the support come from an automated system? Should that automated system be the MMIS or another system within the agency?

- *Information needs.* What data must be captured and maintained to support the business functions? How do those information needs map across the business functions and the organization?

During these sessions, the managers had an opportunity to take an overall look at the strategic program requirements for the agency, determine which should be within the scope of the new MMIS, and decide how system operations should be split between the state and the fiscal agent contractor.

The outcome of this phase was an ISP. It summarized the results of these discussions and documented the visions of the Medicaid agency—its functions, goals, critical success factors, and information requirements. The information from JAD sessions were entered in the CASE software and documented in the form of text, organization charts, high-level process diagrams and data models, and various matrices and tables analyzing relationships and associations between the goals, objectives, organizations, functions, data, and existing systems. This document was distributed to all participants for validation. A diagram illustrating the relationship between and flow of data among various parties involved in managing the medical assistance program was developed and included in the ISP.

Phase two: Business area analysis

The next phase of the project was called "business area analysis" (BAA). Each JAD team comprised a JAD-trained facilitator, a scribe, and a CASE tool technician. The JAD facilitators were very experienced; the primary facilitator had 15 years of experience in JAD facilitation and, in fact, had helped to develop the technique. The facilitators functioned as the traffic cops to keep discussions focused and to be sensitive to interpersonal dynamics and politics within the organization.

The focus of this phase was an analysis of the six major business functions to be supported by the new MMIS. These business functions encompassed claims processing, eligibility, benefit plan maintenance, provider enrollment and maintenance, utilization review and quality assurance, and managed care. A separate JAD was conducted for each business area.

The makeup of each JAD session had to be carefully constructed, balancing the number and types of participants needed for optimal group process and the necessary program expertise. Combined with political ramifications, the task of developing the list of participants was a very sensitive topic and required delicate handling. Based on information obtained from interviews and questionnaires sent to staff and management, both formal and informal leaders and experts in each business area were identified. In this setting, leaders included the acknowledged subject matter experts such as the nurse who was extremely knowledgeable about the prior authorization process and system but was not the department manager. While managers are necessary to discuss program policy and establish business rules, the operations staff responsible for the task were needed to provide information on how things actually worked. This information is needed to eventually build models that are the foundation for program code.

The facilitator played a key role in the JAD sessions. The facilitator began by establishing the session agendas and goals. To begin each session, the facilitator presented the "rules of order" that bound participants to a set of parameters for individual and group behavior. The discussions then commenced. Each topic was introduced by the facilitator who played "traffic cop" with speakers and identified issues that could not be decided upon in the session and required outside discussion. As the last step in the session, agreements were summarized.

Line managers of the functional areas and the staff who did the work in these functional areas were charged with the job of taking the ISP and supplying the detailed data and process requirements. These BAA sessions led by a professional facilitator occurred three days per week for eight weeks. (It was decided to hold the sessions three rather than five days per week so that participants could maintain their regular workloads.) The core group consisted of six to eight individuals and people with expertise in specific areas were brought in as needed to assist the core group in detailing the requirements of the ISP.

While the state was anxious to focus on systems issues, it was soon discovered that there was very little understanding about the ramifications of managed care. In the JAD sessions, a comprehensive exploration of the meaning of managed care was undertaken before any consideration of systems issues could commence. These discussions eliminated a number of issues that would have eventually undermined the successful implementation of the system. For instance, there was

- No common definition of managed care

- Fear and concern about whether it would work

- Disagreement on the need for such a drastic measure

These initial sessions were the foundation to build a managed care mindset. At a minimum, the participants became better educated, and some staff eventually became "champions of the cause," supporting managed care.

For these discussions, a managed care expert was brought in to assist the state through the exploratory examination of this relatively new terrain. The operations staff were anxious to understand program operations details, and management had questions about the handling of program policies.

Each group took the ISP section pertaining to its assigned business area as the starting point for this phase of work. For example, claims processing was one of the six major functional areas identified in the ISP. The ISP identified the processes and data requirements involved in adjudicating claims. During the BAA, the group identified the tasks and detailed data necessary to process claims. Figure 2 illustrates the activities that took place during the ISP and BAA phases of IE to define the claims-processing function.

Occasionally, something discussed in the BAA group demanded an ISP. However, there was generally insufficient time to reconvene the original ISP work group. Rather, the procedure to obtain approval for changes to the ISP was to send a written notification to members of senior management.

To achieve integration of business areas, an integration coordinator (IC) position was created. The IC was responsible for attending all JAD BAA sessions and identifying inconsistencies, redundancies, and data relationships. A simple example, use of naming conventions, illustrates the importance of this position. Often the name for an activity, task, or data element varies from one business area to another. This creates confusion and error. The IC ensured that names for activities, tasks, or data elements were consistent throughout the models created by each business area.

Each evening, the facilitators met to debrief by reviewing the day's events and identifying and resolving problems. The schedule and JAD agendas were reviewed and updated regularly.

The outcome of the BAA sessions were detailed models of data requirements and process. The data models included entity relationship

FIGURE 2
Example of ISP and BAA activities: Claim-processing function and data requirements

DURING THE ISP PHASE	Step one: Identify functions	Example: Claims processing function	Example: Data requirements
	Step two: Identify subprocesses	Pay the claim	Claims data
DURING THE BAA PHASE	Step three: Break down general processes into specific components	Capture claim information Edit the claim for errors Price the billed services Verify provider participation	Patient ID Procedure code Diagnosis codes Provider ID

diagrams (ERDs) that depict the relationships between major categories of information that need to be captured by the system. ERDs were developed for each data entity, corresponding to data tables or databases. The data models also included definitions of all attributes of each data entity such as data format, allowable values and codes, and field size.

The developed process models included process decomposition diagrams, data flow diagrams, and event-driven action diagrams. Process decomposition diagrams define processes and subprocesses and their hierarchy. Data flow diagrams illustrate the logic behind designed business processes and how data are used within each process. Event-driven actions diagrams show how external events (e.g., arrival of a date or submission of a claim) trigger certain processes.

As with the ISP, the various models developed in the BAA sessions were regularly presented to session participants for validation. As the model was updated, new models were then printed and distributed at the beginning of each session and were used as the day's starting point. For the most part, this was pro forma because staff had agreed to them in the sessions. The review usually identified minor corrections.

In both phases one and two, consensus about major issues was reached. This was a major departure from the traditional systems approach where very disparate viewpoints and opinions were never acknowledged or addressed; the sessions involved give and take. Every participant's viewpoint was considered. In the end, there was a high degree of satisfaction with the process and the work products, that is, the ISP and detailed BAA models.

In contrast to the traditional approach where it was not uncommon to hear, "This isn't what I had in mind" at the end of a systems development cycle, this approach resulted in a high degree of understanding of what the system must do and how it would work. At the end of the JAD and IE, users felt more knowledgeable about the system's processes and features. The end product, a new MMIS, will better meet user requirements and expectations.

Phase three: Procurement of the fiscal agent

The agency could have taken an approach different from that described above. BAA CASE tool models could be the basis for documenting the new MMIS system requirements that were to be included in the next MMIS fiscal agent RFP. Prior to this, MMIS fiscal agent RFPs included text descriptions of system requirements. Often there was an incomplete understanding of requirements by respondents to the RFP and key requirements were either incorrectly defined or perhaps accidentally omitted. Since these RFP requirements eventually became the basis for the MMIS fiscal agent contract, subjective statements of MMIS requirements became contractual requirements.

In this scenario, prospective bidders were encouraged to analyze the detailed CASE models developed by the agency to evaluate the scope of work to be performed. The requirements were then incorporated into the RFP to secure the services of a new MMIS fiscal agent. The RFP included the hard-copy CASE data and models representing user requirements and were also available in electronic media "soft copy."

The CASE models provided bidders with comprehensive, objective, and readily understandable systems requirements. The system was developed to the exact specifications of the state at a great cost reduction.

The CASE tool models have been used by the new fiscal agent as the base to design the new system. Using the data models developed during the previous phases of this project, the fiscal agent was able to import them into his own CASE tool. The data models were modified and then transformed into a working relational database by the CASE tool. Preliminary estimates indicate a minimum savings of 25 percent in staff resources and users feel a more complete and accurate database design has been developed. Similar results are expected for development of the program code for system processes. Studies in other industries, such as the military, have found that CASE tool–based system development and maintenance allow organizations to reduce their systems staff effort by half over the life cycle of the information system.

With either approach, the direct line systems development life cycle or the issuance of an RFP followed by systems development, the satisfaction of the state agency user community was much higher than in traditional systems development efforts.

Lessons learned

Based on this case study and projects in other states, the following observations can be made.

JAD is effective—a system design based on requirements defined from JAD sessions tends to be more comprehensive and efficient than one that has been designed without the intense user participation that characterizes JAD. If properly performed, JAD sessions are an extremely useful technique to define requirements and create models. In this case, JAD sessions turned out to be an effective format to discuss managed care concepts and issues and to make decisions on both design and operational issues. The sessions required management from key departments to meet to discuss overlapping functions and conflicting priorities, imagine how the system would work, and design the system. This resulted in an integrated approach to meet the challenge at hand. In the case study, users became very involved, and at the end, there was unflagging management commitment to the process. This reduced implementation problems when the system was operationalized. Another success factor is to ensure ample time for the JAD sessions. In the case study, additional JAD sessions were needed to address the overwhelming concern of agency staff about managed care.

Get users to think logically—users must be retrained to define logical requirements rather than describe system requirements in current terms. Users are accustomed to explaining the hows of their work; it is very difficult to extract their actual requirements in logical and functional terms. Thinking in old terms also tends to limit new system requirements because users believe that current system constraints may not apply to a new system. This is a major problem at the start-up of each analysis JAD session for many users.

Have policies developed prior to JAD—JAD sessions are ineffective when policies are not in hand. JAD participants who do not have the decision-making authority of upper management cannot expect to develop policies. Although the JAD is a good way to identify and highlight those problems, actual policy development should not occur in the JAD sessions. A stand-alone or off-line issue resolution process to which participants can feed requests for decisions in a timely manner must be in place. In the case study, additional JADs were specifically conducted to resolve managed care design issues.

Do not underestimate users—with appropriate training and a skilled facilitator, users quickly catch on to the methodology and are able to read and interpret data and process models. They can understand the implications of such issues as data associations, cardinality, and other model considerations. The facilitator should continue to work with each user until the desired level of JAD proficiency is achieved. Changing the composition of the JAD session can adversely affect group dynamics so such changes should not be made unless they are absolutely necessary.

Use specialized subject area experts—it helps to have on-call subject area experts who can supplement the core JAD user team for specialized subject areas, such as managed care or eligibility determination. These experts can describe what is possible to the group and can be especially useful to help participants envision future requirements. Expertise in other areas such as utilization review or specialized reporting are important in JAD sessions when it is difficult for users to conceive of all the issues related to a future requirement.

Not all facilitators are created equal—the skills needed by a facilitator are considerable. The facilitator must be organized, able to communicate, possess analytic skills, be able to keep discussions focused, and be sensitive to interpersonal dynamics and politics within the organization. When considering contracting for system development services that include JAD facilitation, the qualifications and references of the facilitator(s) are at least as important as other key proposed personnel.

Pilots and proof of concept—when trying new methodologies or techniques for the first time, test them out in a pilot project of limited scope and time. Identify the problems that work against the new design when there is still time to fix them. There is a conservative bent within all organizations and it is necessary to achieve a small success to provide proof of concept before staff are willing to buy into the new process.

Have realistic expectations—IE methodologists and CASE tool experts believe their methods and techniques work. Although the benefits of each technique are undisputed, there is a need to balance optimism with a dose of realism. Many systems developers new to Medicaid, even with other healthcare experience, are unpleasantly surprised by the complexity of Medicaid business rules and systems that must support them. For example, a Medicaid claims-processing system must be able to support multiple pricing methodologies including diagnostic related groups (DRGs); ambulatory care groups; provider or level of care-specific per diem, visit, or encounter, usually subject to maximum allowed; capitation; drug cost plus dispensing; and combinations of all the above.

CASE tool/IE link—by itself, CASE does not guarantee success. CASE is merely a tool and without a sound design, it just implements a poor design. The least effective CASE tool in the hands of good designers is infinitely better than the best CASE tool in the hands of poor designers. Disagreement typically centers around selecting the best CASE tool rather than on more significant issues such as methodologies used and skills of the personnel involved. In other words, the system is only as good as the weakest component—whether it be the design or programming code.

CASE tool use during JAD—do not use the CASE tool during actual JAD sessions to capture models. It is too distracting and requires participants to wait for model update and printing. Use the CASE tools out of the JAD sessions and generate models off-line.

Client/server technology and CASE—if the decision is made to migrate to a nonmainframe client/server platform (i.e., those based on minicomputer, PCs, and workstations), the current state of the art in CASE technology does not provide comprehensive support for the development of client/server applications, graphical user interfaces (GUIs), object-oriented programming (OOP), and the "middleware" connecting and translating between the platforms. It may be necessary to use multiple client/server software development tool sets including combinations of CASE, OOP development tools, GUI prototyping tools, and relational database management systems to support the client/server. Also, do not expect the CASE tool or client/server development tools to generate 100 percent usable code. Medicaid applications are much too complex to accomplish this.

Reverse engineer appropriate legacy systems—reusability is the mantra for object-oriented systems. This concept also applies to legacy systems that are not object oriented. An original system will probably contain reusable components (i.e., modules or programs) that can be updated to reflect new technologies using IE-based reverse or reengineering such as converting from flat file to relational database management system. Because much time and effort is spent defining very complex business rules, retain and reuse them if possible.

Recommendations

In applying the observations and lessons described above, there are several conclusions that can be drawn concerning current approaches to Medicaid system procurement and development. Some of these conclusions are described below.

Incorporate CASE models into procurement—when CASE models are incorporated into system requirements and expressed in a RFP, the subsequently developed models tend to be more concrete and a more objective way of detailing system requirements than any flow diagram or narrative description. The methodologies used, however, support other specifications that may be incorporated into the RFP such as hardware and software requirements and an indication of whether an item is mandatory or desirable. These requirements are difficult to document within standard CASE tool data and process models.

Change in approach to federal models—HCFA and other federal agencies should continue supporting the development of system models based on "best practices" that have been proven to work at the state level or in the private sector. Current practice in the Medicaid system industry is to attempt to transfer and modify code, thereby encouraging perpetuation of current physical structures. However, these models should be CASE tool-based so that states can be flexible with physical design as well as implementation issues. These models could be developed either through reverse engineering of an existing Medicaid system back to a logical model or through developing new logical MMIS data and process models which could then be provided to any state requesting support. Development using industry-leading IE and CASE data formats would increase the reuse of already developed models. States and their fiscal agents could take the logical models, update them to reflect state-specific requirements, convert them to a physical design, and then facilitate new system construction using the models.

Encourage use of off-the-shelf software—current federal regulations require that all MMIS software belong to the state and federal government. This is problematic when there are existing proprietary software solutions that the MMIS developer is reluctant to integrate with the MMIS due to this "public domain" ruling. Various commercial claims unbundling software programs provide functionality that does not exist in most MMIS systems.

Encourage federal flexibility in approval of Medicaid systems—state Medicaid systems must conform to a federally developed system model called the MMIS General System Design (GSD) developed in the early 1970s. The MMIS GSD was designed to support FFS, indemnity-type programs. The federal government provides enhanced federal funding for Medicaid systems that conform to the MMIS model by making MMIS-compliant systems eligible to receive 90 percent federal monies for new systems development and 75 percent for system operation. States have been cautious about straying from the basic MMIS model for fear of losing enhanced federal funds. As a result, states have not been able to easily take advantage of newer, more up-to-date non-Medicaid systems. HCFA should support of non-MMIS models for Medicaid systems and provide enhanced funding for them as long as they support basic program requirements.

Expand definition of the MMIS—a related issue is the need to expand the definition of the MMIS to encompass the enterprisewide system that supports Medicaid program administration so that commercial off-the-shelf software and associated hardware can be integrated with the MMIS. Of particular relevance are local area networks (LANs) and work-stations and software operating on the LAN: Windows or other GUI, word processing, spreadsheet, DBMS, graphics, statistical analysis, geographic information system, or project management.

Reorientation of technical staff—most state technical staff were trained in a mainframe environment and are still unfamiliar with the new enabling technologies, methodologies, and tools. They must be oriented and trained to understand the potential of the new tools and technologies to assuage their fears about these changes. If information system staff are capable of adapting, every effort should be made to retain them so there remains a corporate "IS memory" concerning current and past systems, especially as they relate to knowledge of the original system "business rules." Staff must be made to feel comfortable with the changes so they stay with the organization; it is important that their knowledge of the history of the system remain with the organization.

Just as it takes effort to work with an architect, designer, engineer, contractor, and builder to construct a dream house that suits the homeowner's needs for a lifetime, the process to develop a system that meets the needs of users for a long period of time is complex. When the system is required to be flexible enough to meet ever-changing operational and regulatory requirements, the process becomes even more complicated. The use of business process reengineering, information engineering, JAD, and CASE tools as tools to systematize the process eases the systems designers' challenge.

Many of the recommendations cited above are under review within the Medicaid systems industry by states, HCFA, fiscal agent contractors, consultants, and other interested parties. A white paper discussing these methodologies was presented to HCFA in 1995 by HCFA's private sector Technical Assistance Group. As a result, it is anticipated these concepts will be considered and adopted by the industry to replace the current traditional approach.

NOTES

1. In a fee-for-service program, providers are reimbursed for each service provided, and the recipient has the choice of selecting from participating providers. Utilization is controlled by requiring prior authorization for selective expensive medical services, such as inpatient hospital care and some prescription drugs. Under managed care, costs are controlled by reimbursing a network of providers on a capitated, or per person per month, basis, regardless of the number of services any given individual uses. Managed care emphasizes access to primary care to increase the use of clinical preventive and primary care services with the expectation of reducing the unnecessary use of emergency rooms for ambulatory care and avoiding preventable hospitalizations.
2. Since 1984, federal legislation impacting Medicaid included the Deficit Reduction Action (DEFRA) of 1984, the Consolidated Omnibus Budget Reconciliation Act (COBRA) of 1985, OBRA 1986, OBRA 1987, the Medicare Catastrophic Coverage Act of 1988, the Family Support Act of 1988, OBRA 1989, OBRA

1990, OBRA 1993, Employment Opportunities for Disabled Americans Act of 1986, Immigration Reform and Control Act (IRCA) of 1986, and Anti-Drug Abuse Act of 1986. This list is exclusive of state-level legislative changes affecting Medicaid.

3. A normalized database stores unique data elements joined by "association." For example, a physician is associated with an office location, the patient visits the location to receive service, and the physician bills for the service from this location. The physician's address is stored as a unique data element, linked to the provider and the claim.

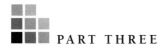

PART THREE

_____

*Quality management
case studies*

22

Academic medical center: Repositioning through TQM

William A. Golomski
President
W. A. Golomski & Associates
Chicago, Illinois

Mark A. Swift
President
M. A. Swift and Associates
Chicago, Illinois

Timothy E. Weddle
Independent Consultant
Chicago, Illinois

FINANCIAL RISK IS SHIFTING to the providers of care because they are perceived as having the most control over the provision of healthcare services. These changes are altering where patients go for care and who provides their care.

Physicians and healthcare institutions recognize that purchasers view healthcare as a commodity. Healthcare institutions that serve the same geographic area stand apart from each other only on cost and access. This structural change means that even the most prestigious healthcare providers, who previously competed on their reputation, must now compete on cost. A look into how one prestigious medical center is responding to the movement to capitation illustrates the depth of the current changes.

Loyola University Medical Center

Loyola University Medical Center includes a 500-bed teaching hospital, an ambulatory care center that receives 250,000 patients a year, a medical school, a nursing school, and several other ambulatory care centers. Like other institutions, Loyola must increasingly contract with insurers and employers to have access to patients. It is anticipated that over time, an increasing proportion of patients will gain access to the medical center through capitated arrangements. Loyola has pursued change by blending together different management approaches and began its transformation by uniting its people and operating units with the initiation of total quality management (TQM) and self-directed work teams.

TOTAL QUALITY MANAGEMENT (TQM)

The TQM approach was initiated by establishing an organizationwide steering committee, whose members included the chief executive officer, chief business officer, and the heads of the hospital, ambulatory system, medical school, nursing school, and physician practice plan. The support areas of information technology, facilities management, and public relations were also represented. The steering committee established the goals of the TQM effort in terms of scope and pace of deployment. An effort was made to work within the existing culture to initiate change while minimizing cultural resistance. The concept was to proceed until cultural barriers impeded progress and then to remove these barriers one by one. The first year was used to develop the TQM mission statement, define and develop the curriculum, train a cadre of facilitators, and take on a few projects. Although there were few tangible benefits, the administration thought that significant progress was being made to support the strategic direction of the institution.

Members of the steering committee had trained themselves and key subordinates in the TQM approach. What was surprising was that cultural resistance to change existed among the committee members in two forms. One form was the reluctance to open up the TQM process to the rest of the organization. Here, the fear of failure was a stronger motive than responding to the needs of the changing marketplace. The second cultural barrier was the reluctance of the leadership group to establish performance measures. One subcommittee had been responsible for establishing these measures. The subcommittee became bogged down and asked to abandon its task. Rather than regrouping and revitalizing the development of benchmarks, the steering committee accepted the subcommittee's "best effort" and abandoned the task of establishing performance measures.

The common theme of the resistance was a reluctance to make public commitments for improvement. It was clear that the TQM effort needed a system of formal targets and support to reach these targets. The approach in going forward was to train the organization how to accomplish improvement goals before establishing commitments. The first year ended with an improvement structure in place, but no goals for improvement.

At the beginning of the second year, the leadership group authorized the initiation of steering committees one level down in the organization. Steering committees were formed in ambulatory care, hospital, finance, medical school, nursing school, information technology, public relations, and physical plant, with each participating in steering committee training. Each committee defined the scope and pace of deployment within their area. TQM projects were selected to address specific issues, and the teams were trained and began work on projects. Additional facilitators were trained to support all of the teams.

The separate committees were asked to develop a list of improvements for their area and were invited to establish a system of performance measures. Each of the areas were able to develop a list of improvement projects, yet none established specific time frames or published performance measures. The result of this rollout approach was mixed between operating units. A few of the component areas made dramatic improvements and involved all of their staff, while others met significant cultural resistance to change and made little progress. As a result, many of the top managers lost interest in the TQM process that was too slow and not focused on results.

SELF-DIRECTED TEAMS

At the same time, the ambulatory care operating unit initiated self-directed work teams with a promise of shared leadership and worker autonomy. These self-directed teams focused on management of processes within each of the ambulatory care subunits. The start-up of self-directed teams represented a cultural shift for the middle management employees. Managers were asked to identify less as managers and more with frontline employees. Some employees were not able to make this shift in how the changing culture reinforced its self-identity. The crisis of change introduced by the managed care marketplace did not afford the time to help employees adjust. Employees were given two choices. They either had to change their behaviors immediately in line with the new culture, or they had to leave. The purging of employees who had developed workplace self-identities under the old cultural norms was considered necessary to assimilate a critical mass of progressive-thinking employees.

The implication of self-directed teams was twofold. First, the teams provided a vehicle for worker participation and self-governance. Second, the implementation of self-directed teams provided a mechanism for purging the organization of vestiges from the prior culture. The message was clearly made to the organization that the move to capitation required that top management absolve itself of responsibility for individuals who had been shaped by the prior norms of academic medicine.

The initiation of TQM had revealed significant cultural barriers to responding to the market movement to capitated payment. Many employees had developed their self-identity under a culture that would no longer serve the medical center. The way to proceed was clear. Goals had to be established and achieved. It was felt that repackaging TQM concepts under the mantle of reengineering would best meet these needs.

REENGINEERING

From a mechanical perspective, reengineering and TQM are identical.[1] However, the way that culture is managed is different. Reengineering as practiced at Loyola gave administration the opportunity to steamroll through the organization to achieve rapid cultural change. Organizational redesign used the "blank sheet" approach, much like the old concept of zero-based budgeting. No positions were considered necessary unless they withstood the test of value analysis. In zero-based budgeting, there is a new budget every year with no amount carried over from prior years. At Loyola a similar approach was used for all management positions. All management positions were eliminated. New positions were created to support a new operating philosophy. The former managers needed to reapply for a place in the new organization. This allowed management to instantly meet fiscal targets by reducing the management payroll and to eliminate all vestiges of the old culture. People could now be selected based on their fit with management norms that were targeted to moving the medical center forward in a capitated environment.

The mechanical aspects of reengineering began by developing a system of measures. Strategic targets were established and widely communicated throughout the organization. Performance targets for finance and operations were established based on the perceived needs of customers. The term "customers" was broadly used to include payers, individual patients, and partners in capitation. Teams were formed to determine how to meet or exceed the needs of the customers. The teams were asked to follow a two-step approach that encompassed assessment followed by implementation. Each of the customer-focused measures was linked to key processes. From among these, those that provided the highest leverage for improving the customer measures were identified. Where appropriate, these activities were broken into component subprocesses. Each team was asked to create a vision for its process. Where available, customer focus groups and surveys provided input to more directly describe what customers expected from the process. The vision was compared to the current process. The teams were encouraged to start their redesign of the process with a blank sheet of paper. Initial customer measures were linked to the new process and additional customer measures were added. The organization and staff were designed to fit into the new process. All processes were expected to conform to an overall operating vision for Loyola and to conform to new cultural norms.

Implementation of the new processes was a foregone conclusion based on the total involvement of the organization in the assessment and design. Management's role in the new culture was to coach and counsel the teams as they met their objectives. It was critical that teams be given adequate training and support to accomplish their task. Training and support included the tools of process analysis and design, as well as the tools of financial measurement and analysis. The new processes positioned the medical center to win significant new contracts with managed care payers and to be positioned for entering into partnerships for serving capitated populations.

Origins of the approach

The idea of value analysis has had a significant impact on the development of TQM. In the 1960s it was recognized that quality and cost improvements could be achieved by asking fundamental questions about core organizational processes.[2] Value analysis originated in the purchasing area, which has traditionally been responsible for processing orders and obtaining the best price. With value analysis, the purchasing function takes on the responsibility of questioning the contribution of items to be purchased to the goals of the organization. For example, what is the value to the organization of having a credenza in every manager's office? Does the credenza help provide a better product or service to customers? Help reduce costs? This line of questioning is credited with reducing costs by eliminating the purchase of items previously thought to be necessities. The value analysis approach was not restricted to small items but was also applied to larger capital purchases. Suppliers recognized that they had a competitive advantage if they could show the value their product or service provided the purchaser. They began to convince purchasers that long-term partnerships were to the advantage of both parties.

The approach is the basis for the field of value engineering. The ideas of value analysis crossed over from the purchase of supplies, equipment, and large capital items to office work and administrative activities. Eventually, it was recognized that value analysis can be applied to all work that is performed within an organization. Value analysis begins by asking basic questions:

1. What function does the work serve?

2. Can these functions be met in another way?

3. Can a function be combined with another function to reduce cost or improve quality?

4. Is the function needed at all?

These questions lead to the radical simplification and redesign of jobs. Value analysis is also applied within a process. The first step is to identify the elements of the process, often by preparing flowcharts. Once the process elements are identified, value analysis poses the following questions:

1. Which steps add to customer value?

2. Which steps add to cost?

3. Where do delays or bottlenecks occur?

4. Where are errors or defects occurring?

The process should then be engineered, or reengineered, to meet or exceed requirements.

The Loyola experience highlights how value analysis and value engineering are the foundation of the analytical approaches used in TQM. Loyola asked the value analysis questions from a top-down perspective about what financial targets needed to be achieved. But the Loyola example shows something more. In accomplishing the object of being cost competitive, Loyola needed to recognize the reality of a capitated marketplace. The changing nature of the relationship between the medical center and the marketplace was passed on to the medical center employees. Just like IBM, the demands of the marketplace superseded implied commitments to individual employees. Healthcare organizations can no longer meet implied obligations to employees, only to the discipline of the marketplace. Loyola demanded more work from individual employees because the marketplace demanded increased efficiency from Loyola. The art of successful change leadership requires organizations to blend together analytical techniques that focus on economics using an approach to engage workforce creativity. It requires an integrated approach and a focus on organizational culture. The aggressive use of TQM allowed Loyola to accomplish these goals.

TQM and reengineering overview

DEFINITION OF TQM

The issue of quality has grown rapidly in recent years. Although some hospitals have been in the mainstream of the quality movement, many got pushed to develop formal quality programs. Due to the increased costs of malpractice awards, physicians rapidly became more interested in quality standards. An independent interest by the Joint Commission on Accreditation of Health Care Organizations (JCAHO) in developing refined standards for quality provided further activity to remain accredited under the new standards. Finally, Medicare, Medicaid, and health insurance providers became concerned about the rapid increase of healthcare costs. All these forces led healthcare organizations to a search for new ways to provide better service at less cost.

The initial approaches in hospitals used concepts of industrial quality control and quality assurance in the clinical setting. Standards were set.

The difficulty in setting standards was that there was no one best treatment for many illnesses and injuries. There was a range of likely treatments where professional judgment was used. Quality review councils worked much as engineers do when a product or system fails. They used something similar to fault-tree analysis, which isolates a problem to determine what went wrong. However, the potential of disciplining someone in engineering and production is far less threatening than in healthcare. The goal was corrective action. The approach was mainly after-the-fact detection.

The next concept to emerge was that of continuous quality improvement (CQI), which improves a product or process in the normal course of work and changes to what is new. CQI often appears in conflict with the economic concept of the law of diminishing returns. Organizations using CQI see if a process change solves the problem. They look to see if the expected improved result occurs. If the change does not help, they go back to what was done before and keep searching. If it does solve the problem, they do not stop, but rather look for further improvements in the normal course of work.

The concept of total quality control (TQC) is an approach where the interrelationships between functions and their processes are reviewed and improved. In its earlier versions, the improvements were directed toward the improvement in products and their processes. Japanese businesses expanded the concept to include "quality improvement in everything we do." This included improvement in all staff, service, and support functions. In Japan this is called TQC or companywide quality control (CWQC). Western managers have added more concepts from the social sciences and call it total quality management (TQM). TQM is both a concept and a set of methods used to tap into the creative energy of an organization. It enables people within organizations to identify opportunities for improvement and to implement them. Management is different in some cases because the concepts of satisfying external and internal customers is the focus of what is done. The organization is not just interested in outcomes, but in improving processes so that desired outcomes are more likely to occur. The culture needs to place emphasis on fixing processes rather than fixing blame. Variability should be viewed as something to control. The causes of variability should be separated into common causes (due to management) and special causes (due to other employees). Individuals and teams should be empowered to do that which they are capable of doing by removing any restrictions they may feel. Cross-functional and departmental teams are formed to solve problems and identify opportunities to improve even if there are not complaints. But the experience of quality circles in the 1980s revealed that teams fail if they are not coordinated through annual and strategic quality plans. Finally, the norms of the new culture should be reinforced through the recognition of good effort and the celebration of success.

What are the benefits of TQM? There is a tendency to exaggerate, but the gains are impressive. Ideally, lower costs, less time to do work, increased customer satisfaction, increased market share, and improved employee morale. These have been achieved by many organizations. The question is, how can this be done? By meeting the rational expectations of customers over the likely period of use by the customer. The elements of TQM are

- Leadership in TQM by officers, physicians, nurses, and managers

- Customer focus

- Taking preventive steps before an error can occur is preferred to checking for errors after the fact

- Never-ending improvement of best practices

- Management by data—facts, not opinions

- Control variation

- Team problem solving

- Recognition of team efforts and team celebrations

- Fix processes rather than fix blame

- Strategic and annual quality improvement plans

- Awareness of the different approaches and using the best one for the situation

A popular line in the musical *Oklahoma!* states, "Everything's up to date in Kansas City; We've gone about as far as we can go!" There is also an old American saying, "If it ain't broke, don't fix it!" Both are contrary to TQM concepts. In economics there is the law of diminishing returns. In the face of all this wisdom, TQM is not only reasonable but essential for survival.

TQM is the process by which those in healthcare identify with the goals of the organizational units of which they are a part or with whom they come in contact. As a result, they are always thinking about how to improve work processes. They then become a part of one successful project team after another.

DEFINITION OF REENGINEERING

Healthcare systems are pushed by competitive pressures and possible reductions in reimbursement by governmental payers to reduce their budgets. The need to make expansive and rapid operational changes in response to fiscal pressure is not unique to healthcare. The automobile, airline, and computer industries have each recognized the need to dramatically change financial structure.

One approach for initiating a surge of fiscal change is to extract from the concepts and methods of TQM those ideas that most directly contribute to the bottom line. An approach based on value analysis techniques allows the organization to give top priority to getting their financial situations under control.

There has been much debate about whether reengineering is something new or if it is the relabeling of TQM. This debate is somewhat academic. The wise organization will build its future on the fundamentals of strategically guided process improvement and cultural transformation.

ADAPTATION TO HEALTHCARE

Healthcare organizations are being acted upon by common structural forces. The accrediting agency for hospitals has a quality assurance system with which organizations must be in compliance in order to remain accredited. Healthcare organizations are affected by federal guidelines and health insurance second-guessing. There is a J-shaped distribution of education levels, which means that physicians and clinicians who have extensive education are outnumbered by service workers with less education. This leads to a desire for professional autonomy and little experience in cross-functional teams. There is also a well-developed system of education and credentialing not found in many other organizations. In spite of these common forces, there is not one common TQM program that will fit all healthcare institutions. TQM is most successful when it is adapted to the organization's history and culture. Thus, a TQM application at the Loyola University Medical Center would be different from the University of Chicago Hospital or the Northwestern University Hospital.

The work performed within healthcare organizations has been divided into clinical areas that require training and licensure and nonclinical work. This historic separation of work has resulted in the creation of a dichotomy between clinical versus administrative quality improvement. This discontinuity is smoothed when concepts of anticipating customer needs are embedded into the work of healthcare centers.

There are five reasons for TQM:

1. *Economic.* Reduce wasted effort, wasted materials, and cycle time

2. *Customer satisfaction.* Provide predictable, hassle-free service that anticipates needs

3. *Reducing malpractice exposure.* Identify critical hazards and get things fixed

4. *Regulatory and external agency compliance.* Comply with JCAHO, HEDIS, federal, state, and local regulations

5. *Increased employee satisfaction.* Create affiliation through involvement

The contribution of reengineering has been to give a name for applying the concepts of TQM to smash through pockets of resistance in the organizational culture.

Overview of culture

DEFINITION OF CULTURE

A simple description of culture is "the way we do things around here." It is based on the organization's history and can enrich the workplace or drive people to fear and desperation. Healthcare organizations are fortunate in that there is a general respect for life inherent in the profession. In a formal sense, the values and guiding principles of an organization are expressions of the culture of that organization. Among those values and principles found in some organizations are

- A respect for every individual and their work

- Choosing the best suppliers and treating them as if their organization is a world-class customer

- Fixing the processes, not the blame

- A customer focus

- Educating and training employees to reach their potential

- Recognizing team efforts

- Not tolerating abusive behavior by management, or management stealing ideas from employees

- Frequently giving recognition and other positive feedback to employees and suppliers

When cultural barriers to organizational change are encountered, it is because the distribution of power is not in the appropriate hands.

HOW POWER IS DISTRIBUTED

Having power means that someone can influence the actions of others. There are three kinds of power:

- *Prestige.* When someone has prestige, other people listen to what that person says. People follow that person's advice because he or she is perceived to have special knowledge based on his or her position. For example, physicians are often writing letters to administrators about parking and billing problems. The physicians feel their complaints will influence action because of their perceived status in the eyes of the organization

- *Economic.* When someone has economic power, that person has the ability to control the economics of a specific situation. The person or group that decides employee salaries has the power to influence employee actions. This is especially true if the economic decision is whether or not the employee will have a job

- *Decision.* Another kind of power is decision power, or the ability to make a decision that has organizational weight behind it. An administrator is granted decision power by the board of trustees, within limits. In healthcare organizations, different types of decision power are possessed by different people. Physicians have clinical decision-making power. Administrators have the decision power to decide the kinds of physicians that should be recruited to work at the hospital

In most healthcare organizations, the lines of power are very confusing. For example, a physician without power to add a new test to the laboratory can use his or her prestige to insist that the test be added to provide quality care. This traditional ability to extend one type of power to attain influence that someone does not formally have could be threatened by TQM if physicians are required to back their requests with data. Or suppose a radiology service refuses to switch to a more efficient means of reading films. The radiologists will be expected to switch as part of the organizationwide improvement effort; whereas in a traditional department-focused approach they had the discretion to not switch. These examples illustrate how culture can change how doctors practice medicine.

Another trait of traditional healthcare organizations is to hoard power at the top of the organization and in isolated pockets. The top administrator and the senior administration team might keep all of the decision power, while the board of trustees have the economic power. The medical staff might keep all of the prestige and create a wide gap between their social standing in the hospital and that of other workers. TQM could be seen as threatening to this traditional distribution of power. Empowerment redistributes power to enable people in the organization to get results.

EMPOWERMENT

Empowerment brings forth different emotional responses based on the individual's place in the organization's power structure. Top managers often say, "Empower the people closest to the work. Cut out the middle managers. That will fix things in a hurry!" Is it a surprise that frontline workers are confused or mistrusting of empowerment? Why do they now have to solve all of the problems that management has caused over the years?

The Rochester Division of IBM, located in Rochester, Minnesota, won the prestigious Malcolm Baldrige National Quality Award. IBM Rochester said the single most important insight that led to improvement of its quality system was the idea of empowering customers. Based on this, IBM Rochester empowered its employees and suppliers to meet or exceed the customer expectations.

When empowerment is used, there is the intention to bring about a culture that provides teams with the ability to get results for customers. The level of empowerment that each employee has can be defined in advance. For example

- What can the employee do without getting permission from anyone?

- What can the employee do on his or her own, but must inform someone about later?

- What should the employee check with someone else before doing?

- What are the things the employee should not do?

FUNCTIONS OF CULTURE

The primary function of culture is to guide people in their daily work lives and to accommodate change. Culture allows the members of a hospital to decide whether or not to purchase a new piece of equipment, helps them decide how to go about downsizing the workforce, and guides people in their daily interaction with patients. It is a task of management to bring culture into alignment with the organization's best interests. The cultural problem facing American healthcare is that organizational interests have traditionally been defined as medical science interests. The capitated healthcare marketplace is causing the expansion of best interest to include the public interests of cost reduction.

HOW THE CULTURE INFLUENCES THE INDIVIDUAL

The individual interacts with the organization culture in several ways:

- *Learn.* It is learned by individuals when they come to the new organization. The employees must learn to function in a new work world where many of the ways to do things learned in prior jobs no longer get results

- *Use.* The employee uses what is learned about culture in going about daily tasks

- *Teach.* An employee teaches the culture to fellow employees. For example, when one employee helps a patient by offering directions, others may see this action and also take initiative to help other patients. This is why quality champions are so important in TQM

- *Innovate.* An employee can add to the culture by finding a new way to do things. Just about every TQM project finds a new way to do something. Some people call finding new ways to do things innovation. TQM encourages everyone to be an innovator

Management often has problems introducing cultural innovations to an organization accustomed to a traditional culture. Leadership can help. In healthcare, the burden of cultural leadership falls on the shoulders of the physicians.

CLINICAL FOCUS VERSUS COMPANYWIDE FOCUS

Healthcare organizations oftentimes place physicians above everyone else in status and think that while TQM is great for administration, clinicians know best about clinical quality. Whether TQM starts in the clinical area and is later applied to administrative functions or vice versa, the lesson is clear: TQM needs to be in all parts of the healthcare organization. There needs to be a companywide or organizationwide focus.

The surgical services at Loyola University Medical Center are an example of an organizationwide focus.[3] Two TQM steering committees were created, one team to focus on logistical and efficiency issues, the other on clinical care provided in the operating rooms. Both teams were chaired by Loyola physicians.

The team focused on efficiency issues, instantly recognizing the need to create a same-day surgery center to improve operating room efficiency. A same-day admission center would help get patients into the operating rooms on time. The team, which included physicians, a nurse, and an administrator, continued the TQM process by defining terms. The team identified nine different opinions about what surgery "start time" meant. Possible definitions included when the patient was brought into the operating room, when the patient was anesthetized, or when the initial skin incision was made. When terms were defined, the team conducted a three-month study to collect data on what percent of operations started "on time." Only 50 percent met the criteria.

The team then brainstormed to create a list of factors that contributed to inefficiency. They prioritized the list to determine which problems were most essential to solve. Many of the barriers to efficiency were easily eliminated: telephones were installed in each operating room so that nurses did not have to leave the room to answer physician pages and personnel names are now posted so surgeons and anesthesiologists know with whom they are working. The team did not wait to implement the obvious improvements.

The next step for the team was to collect data to measure if cases were starting on time and if room utilization was high. Turnover time was more efficient, communication was better, and morale was improved. As a result of the team effort, specific improvements were made, and the operating room suite culture was forever changed.

Guidelines for success in a capitated environment

Healthcare organizations are in a frenzy to align with other providers to form networks for capitated contracting. The organization model of interlocking relationships is not new; healthcare delivery has always crossed organizational boundaries. For example, all major American cities have developed trauma systems that route trauma victims to the most appropriate facility. In a trauma network, the paramedics work cooperatively with the hospital to coordinate the care provided in the field. Trauma centers are alerted to the impending arrival of a victim. In the case of a trauma system, the culture of medicine with a focus on the needs of the patient serves as the basis for integrating the delivery system. It will be culture that allows individual providers to form partnerships for providing capitated care to patient populations.

The problems faced in providing medical services across interlocking networks of care become increasingly complex as the points of service expand. This problem has been faced by companies in other industries such as trading corporations and biotechnology firms. How are quality and cost managed within these networks? For example, there is a Swedish firm that designs firefighting clothing. There is another company that specializes in manufacture. A third company has special skills to test protective clothing and to distribute it worldwide. An American company handles distribution within this country. How do these companies work together across different cultures and languages? The process is defined from design to ultimate product use. The companies work cooperatively to define strategy. The process to achieve quality and cost objectives is jointly managed.

MALCOLM BALDRIGE NATIONAL QUALITY AWARD FRAMEWORK

A worldwide standard for creating a culture for intra- and interorganizational cultural integration is the Malcolm Baldrige National Quality Award.[4] There are two major parts to the guidelines, the core concepts and the criteria framework. The core values and concepts are

- Customer-driven quality

- Leadership

- Continuous improvement

- Employee participation and development

- Fast response

- Design quality and prevention

- Long-range outlook

- Management by fact

- Partnership development

- Corporate responsibility and citizenship

The Baldrige criteria framework includes

- Senior executive leadership

- Information and analysis

- Strategic quality planning

- Human resource development and management

- Management of process quality

- Quality and operational results

- Customer focus and satisfaction

It is important that the organization culture becomes associated with these concepts and criteria. Otherwise, the organization can easily confuse TQM reengineering with a set of objectives, projects, or tools. To cite one example, the AT&T Universal Card Service went from start-up to the second largest credit card company and won the Malcolm Baldrige Award in two years. The company had used the Baldrige criteria as the framework to design its organization and its culture. The lesson for healthcare organizations is that new organizational forms can be rapidly brought into existence for capitated contracting. The culture of the new organization can be based on the concepts and norms of TQM.

Integration through strategic planning

The most helpful Baldrige criteria in providing coherence across an interlocking healthcare network is the strategic quality planning criteria.

A major difference between American service companies and Asian companies is the participation in strategic planning by members of the organization.[5] Asian companies with advanced practices in total quality involve virtually the entire organization in strategic planning. With inclusive strategic planning, everyone in the organization can identify how the effort of their team contributes to meeting the demands of the marketplace. In healthcare, it is increasingly important to have all employees think of themselves as business owners. This perspective can drive the entire organization to reorient its processes and culture to the needs of a capitated marketplace. The development of healthcare networks needs to be driven by coordinated strategic planning. The challenge is to develop a strategy that integrates concerns for customer focus, fiscal performance, and continuous improvement. The strategic plan needs to say more than how the financial risk will be shared and how the surplus will be distributed. It needs to drive the development of care processes that present seamless healthcare services to the capitated population. This change requires the integration of medical practice, often with the aid of new information systems.

In summary, healthcare organizations can thoughtfully shape the future by applying TQM best practices. First in importance is integrated strategic planning sensitive to its goals and organizational culture. All change within an organization is subject to resistance until the power to get results is redistributed to meet new strategic realities. TQM has been applicable across multiple industries to achieve organizational transformation. TQM, based on recognizing the customer, including employees as internal customers, is the basis of all organizational processes and culture. TQM-based approaches are helping existing healthcare organizations transform to survive and thrive in a capitated payment environment. TQM can serve as a foundation for designing organizations of the future to thrive in the era of capitation.

NOTES

1. R. E. Cole, "Reengineering the Corporation: A Review Essay," *Quality Management Journal* 1, no. 4 (July 1994): 77–85.
2. W. A. Golomski, "European, American, and Japanese Practices in Strategic Planning," unpublished study of employee participation in strategic planning, involving 100 companies, 1995.
3. "LUMC Focus," *Loyola World* 14, no. 1 (January 26, 1995): 8.
4. L. D. Miles, *Techniques of Value Analysis and Engineering,* 2nd ed. (New York: McGraw-Hill, 1972).
5. National Institute of Standards and Technology, "The Malcolm Baldrige National Quality Award," 1995.

23

Lovelace Health Systems: Restructuring for quality

John J. Byrnes, MD
Vice President, Quality Improvement

Michael Shainline, MBA
Director, Quality Control

John Lucas, MD, MPH
President and Chief Executive Officer
Lovelace Health Systems
Albuquerque, New Mexico

Margaret Gunter, PhD
Vice President and Executive Director
Lovelace Clinic Foundation
Albuquerque, New Mexico

THE DELIVERY OF HEALTHCARE in the United States is undergoing a dramatic revolution. Healthcare organizations are consolidating rapidly through mergers, acquisitions, and takeovers. Healthcare purchasers increasingly demand that delivery systems reduce costs, demonstrate ongoing quality improvements, and prove value. Similarly, patients and their families demand more efficient service as well as demonstrated quality care. This acceleration of marketplace pressure has created the need for flexible, responsive, customer-driven delivery systems.

As healthcare organizations mobilize to meet these demands, they must move beyond incremental quality improvement (QI) and into a more comprehensive redesign of patient care activities and services. The well-managed organization is focusing more intensely on redesigning its core services—services that directly touch the patients and their families. The strategy's intent is to concentrate the organization and its resources on what it does best—deliver high-quality patient care.

To make these critical decisions and to redesign patient care services effectively, organizations need reliable and valid information. They need a system of comprehensive performance measures as well as the resources to support global service improvement and sophisticated disease management systems.

This new focus is a radical departure from the traditional quality assurance (QA) and basic hospital accreditation requirements of just a few years ago. Yet many organizations continue to support traditional quality assurance departments with traditional QA skill sets. What is desperately needed is a blueprint to redesign the quality management department to help healthcare systems deliver outstanding customer service, improved quality of care, and excellent value.

Lovelace Health Systems, a fully integrated managed care organization located in Albuquerque, New Mexico, recently faced the challenge of designing a quality department to fulfill its quality and service improvement initiatives. Industry literature contained few of the needed examples, and there was no comprehensive blueprint available.

This chapter describes the success in designing a quality management department within a vertically integrated managed care organization. A blueprint is outlined to restructure a quality management department that drives and supports the strategic quality initiatives of a highly competitive healthcare organization. The leadership and structure, initiatives, key components, and products needed to achieve significant strategic advantage in the marketplace are also discussed, as well as review of lessons learned and pitfalls to avoid.

The Lovelace quality program, which started in 1989 using principles of total quality management (TQM), has evolved into an effort focused on clinical practice improvement (CPI), service quality improvement, and a health and disease management program tied to outcomes research. The improvements in cost, quality, and service produced can be attributed in large part to CPI methodology. This suggests that CPI is the major strategic business tool for progressive healthcare organizations that are achieving significant competitive advantage in the 1990s. A well-organized and sophisticated quality department to support these initiatives is key to this success.

The model presented here can be applied to any size or structure of healthcare system with appropriate adjustments. The principal drivers for change include the need for

- Efficiency and cost containment

- Improvements in quality of care and service to patients as well as their families

- Organizational advantage in competitive markets

- Attention to the demands of sophisticated buyers and employer groups

- Systemwide performance measures

- Sophisticated early warning systems to detect breaks in delivery of service and clinical quality

- Increased customer focus

Organizational leadership

The first area to address is involvement of senior management in quality initiatives. Senior management must assume leadership for the design and implementation of the quality program throughout the system. As a group, management serves as role models for demonstrating how quality initiatives can be integrated within every facet of the organization's daily activity.[3] The dedication of senior management is imperative if QI is to be adopted by every employee.

CHIEF EXECUTIVE OFFICER (CEO)

The CEO leads the QI effort and serves as the sponsor for all quality programs. The CEO also ensures that quality initiatives form the core of the organization's strategic plan. Within the Lovelace system, the CEO is also the chief quality officer. It is incumbent upon him to be the active spokesperson for all quality activities within the health system. In this capacity, the CEO chairs all quality governance bodies, such as the board of directors, as well as the senior quality committee. In addition, the CEO is involved in daily quality-related activities including opening and closing quality training sessions, teaching quality training courses, hosting quality award and recognition events, meeting with customers and suppliers, and conducting benchmarking visits.[1]

Through the power of leadership, the CEO sets the direction for the organization and identifies the strategic quality initiatives for the year. This approval is crucial for quality activities to receive top priority from management and employees. Without it, most quality initiatives will fail.

CHIEF MEDICAL OFFICER (CMO) AND CHIEF OPERATING OFFICER (COO)

As with the CEO, it is critical for the CMO and COO to fully and unequivocally endorse QI as the major strategic tool for the organization. They must demonstrate the same unfaltering modeling behaviors listed above for the CEO. In addition, they must drive quality initiatives through their "service lines" and demand accountability for QI objectives from their staff.

VICE PRESIDENT/MEDICAL DIRECTOR FOR QUALITY IMPROVEMENT AND DIRECTOR OF QUALITY MANAGEMENT

Lovelace has adopted a "matrix model" of management for its quality department. This model pairs a medical manager, usually a physician, with an administrator. These individuals function as a team to direct the quality department. This approach combines the best skills of the two administrators while simultaneously demonstrating a teamwork model at an operational level.

One of the major advantages of the matrix model is the division of labor. The primary focus of the physician manager is to drive CPI and customer service initiatives through clinical and service areas. The administrative manager focuses on data measurement, daily management, and analysis functions. Lovelace found it impossible for one individual to fulfill all of the quality department leadership roles with the volume of projects performed. Thus, the matrix model is an efficient framework for structuring quality departments.

Organizational structure

Once senior management's quality roles are defined, the next step is to design an efficient and effective organizational structure to implement

QI programs. This structure should be simple and efficient and should integrate accountability and responsibility within key constituencies. There should be one overall management and quality organization. Redundant and parallel systems need to be eliminated, and committee structures streamlined.

Figure 1 illustrates the quality management structure adopted by Lovelace Health Systems in 1995. It fully integrates quality functions into one seamless structure.

The governance level is represented by the board of directors. System-wide implementation is managed by the senior operating team for quality (SOTQ), one of four senior operating teams that report directly to the CEO and board of directors.

The board of directors provides oversight, review, and approval for all QI initiatives, programs, and teams. This includes approval of the annual QI plan and evaluation of the previous year's quality activities.

The SOTQ serves as the system's primary quality council and is responsible for implementation of the annual QI initiatives. It has five primary areas of responsibility: quality planning, quality oversight, communication of all QI initiatives throughout the system, integration of quality into the fabric of the organization, and systemwide account-ability.

Specific functions and responsibilities within each of these areas include

- Quality planning

   Ensures integration with strategic plan

FIGURE 1
Quality management structure

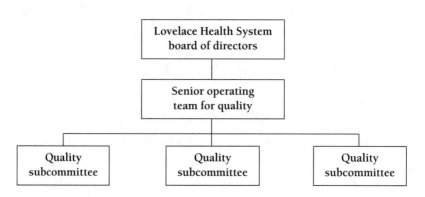

Identifies needed process performance measures

Identifies gaps in quality of care and service through ongoing quality indicator review

Charters all quality programs, initiatives, and teams

Ensures resource availability to successfully execute QI initiatives

- Quality oversight

  Reviews as well as critiques the progress of all quality programs and initiatives

  Prepares as well as critiques the quarterly board report to the board of directors

  Tracks progress on all accreditation initiatives

- Communication

  Holds quarterly quality forums to communicate QI progress to employees

  Celebrates success of the QI program

  Recognizes as well as rewards employee groups for outstanding achievement

- Integration

  Integrates business and quality initiatives in the strategic planning process

- Accountability

  Ensures accountability through a system of rewards and incentives designed and executed within each SOTQ member's area of management and responsibility

The membership of the SOTQ includes all senior physician and administrative executives throughout the system. This ensures that all stakeholders are represented and that accountability throughout the organization is maintained and enforced.

This executive group, as role models for employees, demonstrates the integration of quality activities into daily organizational work.

TABLE 1
Senior operating team for quality membership

- President and chief executive officer
- Senior VP, chief medical officer
- Senior VP, chief financial officer
- Senior VP, chief operating officer
- VP, managed care
- VP, hospital administration and nursing
- Medical director, quality improvement
- Direct, quality management
- Director, care management
- VP, Lovelace Health Plan sales
- Chairman, primary care
- Chairman, medical specialties
- Chairman, surgical specialties
- VP, medical director, Lovelace Health Plan (LHP)
- Associate medical director, LHP and care management
- Associate medical director, LHP and information systems
- Administrator, primary care and regional networks

Quality plan integration

The organizational strategic plan integrates the organization's strategic plan and the traditionally separate QI plan into one. By this simple act, QI initiatives become the core of the business strategy. The quality plan should outline the QI initiatives for the year, targeting both quality of care and quality of service improvements. The initiatives should be focused, easily communicated, readily understandable, and free of buzzwords.

The plan should be conveyed through all organizational levels and be continuously communicated by senior management in all public and private forums. To help ensure success and organizational ownership, it should be developed by all levels of the organization.

The planning process to develop the quality plan begins at least six months before the new fiscal year, allowing adequate time for development, input from all interested employees, and necessary revisions and approvals prior to the start of the new year.

The quality plan should be accompanied by a work plan, a document that operationalizes the quality plan. It highlights in detail the major quality initiatives and their component parts and details time lines, deadlines, accountable individuals, and expected outcomes. In essence, the work plan is a detailed road map that outlines the implementation steps needed to accomplish the quality plan goals.[2] The work plan should also incorporate the steps, process, and theory of change management to ensure greater success.

QUALITY IMPROVEMENT INITIATIVES

It is useful to review Lovelace Health Systems, QI initiatives to demonstrate why the quality management department was restructured. The restructured department's mission is fourfold. It focuses on developing the programs and support necessary to drive competitive advantage through the delivery of QI and outstanding patient care. The department's four imperatives are

- To promote, develop, and support CPI through the Lovelace Episodes of Care Disease Management System

- To create and ignite a cultural shift to provide outstanding customer service to Lovelace patients and their families

- To develop and implement systemwide performance measures

- To provide information management and data analysis expertise

Clinical practice improvement—the Lovelace Episodes of Care™ Program

The Episodes of Care program focuses on improving clinical practice by redesigning the entire continuum of care for a disease process.[4] This includes the entire care process, from prevention and wellness interventions through inpatient and outpatient care. It ends with rehabilitation and patient reeducation. The Episodes of Care continuum includes the following elements:

- Health status and risk assessment

- High-risk case identification

- Prevention

- Primary care services

- Specialty care services

- Outpatient diagnosis and treatment

- Inpatient care

- Rehabilitation and long-term care

- Home health

- Patient reeducation

CPI methodology is extremely powerful. It enables organizations to reengineer care effectively to achieve significant gains in QI and customer service while increasing efficiency to obtain cost reduction.

The Episodes of Care teams established during 1994 by LHS were

- Diabetes

- Low back pain

- Coronary artery bypass surgery

- Pediatric asthma

- Depression

- Birth

- Breast care

- Stroke care

- Knee care

These teams account for approximately 24 percent of total health system costs and patient care service volume.

In 1995, nine more teams were added to redesign care and services around diseases that account for over 50 percent of system costs. These include

- Peptic ulcer disease

- Congestive heart failure

- Hysterectomy

- Attention deficit disorder

- Hypertension

- Adult asthma

- Alzheimer's disease

- Pneumonia

- Epilepsy

The ability to target CPI projects and teams in this manner effectively integrates QI goals with the organization's strategic initiatives. CPI thus becomes a key methodology to achieve strategic advantage in a highly competitive healthcare environment.

The Episodes of Care program requires a tremendous organizational commitment of people, time, and resources. This initiative was the major impetus in the reorganization of the quality management department. The new departmental expertise and resources described below are essential to the success of this program. Based on the experience of Intermountain Healthcare, it is anticipated that the return on investment will be in the 5- to 10-fold range for each team chartered. In other words, for each dollar invested, the institution will save or generate between $5 and $10.

Staff resources dedicated to the Episodes of Care initiative include

- Medical director, QI   .4 FTE

- Director, quality management   .5 FTE

- Senior consultant for CPI   .8 FTE

- Four quality consultants   .7 FTE each

- Four quality analysts   .5 FTE each

- Four Episodes of Care advisors   .2 FTE each

Outstanding customer service

Central to a healthcare organization's success is its ability to provide exceptional customer service to patients and their families, providers, employees, and the purchasers of healthcare services—the healthcare organization's core customer groups.

The healthcare industry has been remiss in assuring that services as well as systems are designed to address the needs of patients, families, and employees. In the hospital setting, services have traditionally been designed to meet the needs of the following groups. The order of listing reflects the priority these customers have typically received:

1. Physicians

2. Nursing staff

3. Support staff

4. Patients

5. Families

6. Buyers

7. Suppliers

As healthcare organizations increasingly realize and embrace the reality of being a service industry, these traditional, and often unconscious, belief systems concerning primary customer groups will change dramatically. The new QI department at LHS has been given the directive to stimulate this shift in customer orientation and to ignite a cultural shift focused on delivering outstanding customer service to all customer groups (with patients and their families the number one priority). Borrowing practices from organizations around the country, such as the Ritz-Carlton Hotels, as well as the customer service literature, the Lovelace patient service initiative has been named "The Ideal Patient Encounter," a term coined by the staff at Johns Hopkins. It is a system-wide program to redesign the patient care process centered on the needs of patients and their families. Because Lovelace is an integrated healthcare system, this goes far beyond the idea of patient-centered care currently popular in hospital settings.

As an example, the surgery department has been challenged to redesign the patient experience around their top three product lines during 1995. This includes the general office visit, the most common office procedure, and the day-of-surgery experience.

This is the most resource-intensive project the organization will undertake in the near future. Lovelace feels it is essential, however, if healthcare organizations are to reverse the current trend of decreasing customer satisfaction.

As healthcare customers become more sophisticated in their demands for outstanding service, organizations must respond effectively and quickly. A well-staffed and knowledgeable quality department is essential.

It can become the key driver in facilitating cooperation with senior management and administration.

As reviewed for the Episodes of Care program, personnel earmarked for the Ideal Patient Encounter include

- Medical director, QI   .4 FTE

- Director, quality management   .5 FTE

- Senior consultant for CPI   .2 FTE each

- Four quality analysts   .3 FTE each

- 20 team facilitators   .2 FTE each

- Department managers and medical directors   4 hours per week

- Clinical and internal department staff   4 hours per week

- Senior management   4 hours per week

Lovelace has also developed an Ideal Employee Encounter to mirror the Ideal Patient Encounter methodology. This program intends to redesign internal support services to better serve the needs of internal customers, employees, and providers.

Performance measures and information management

Nationwide, healthcare organizations are experiencing a void in information that accurately measures how well systems are performing. Because of the lack of a nationally accepted approach and the difficulty in achieving satisfactory results in this area, much has been written on the need for report cards, outcome measures, and performance indicators.

This need for performance measures was an additional driver for department reorganization, especially in the areas of staffing expertise and information systems support. Specifically, staff were recruited with expertise in

- CPI and CQI methodology

- QI study design

- Statistical methodology

- Survey research

- Quality engineering

- Information systems

- Specific clinical service areas

RESOURCES AND STAFFING

Figure 2 represents the quality department structure that was created to help Lovelace Health Systems meet its strategic goals and objectives. Lovelace is an integrated statewide delivery system that includes 10 Albuquerque primary care satellites, a multispecialty group practice with more than 325 physicians, a hospital, the Lovelace Health Plan, and 5 regional group practices. The system cares for a patient population of more than 200,000 and employs in excess of 3,000 individuals.

The Lovelace quality department employs 16 people, including a medical director, an administrator, 6 senior consultants (with major project responsibility), 4 quality consultants, and 4 quality analysts.

The department also recruits volunteers from throughout the organization to serve as facilitators on QI teams. Four facilitators currently serve as CPI advisors and another 20 as service improvement advisors.

FIGURE 2
Structure of the reorganized quality management department

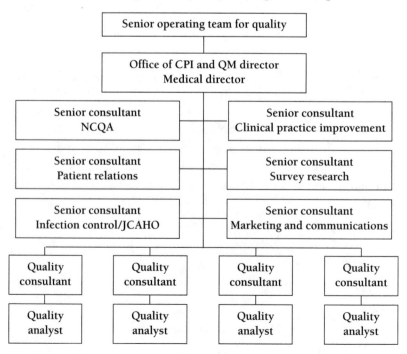

CONSULTANTS AND ANALYSTS

The staffing categories depicted in Figure 3 reflect the varying levels of expertise and experience within the department.

Senior consultants are highly trained professionals with extensive expertise in specific areas of quality management. Their activities are narrowly focused to take advantage of their specific aptitudes and are matched to strategic initiatives or support functions within the organization's QI activities. For example, the senior consultant for NCQA accreditation is responsible for the organization's accreditation activities. She has more than 10 years of accreditation experience and previously served as a quality department director. She directs, motivates, and coaches the managers of health plan departments affected by this accreditation activity.

Quality consultants serve as primary resources for the QI teams that look to these individuals for expertise in QI methodology, QI study design, data measurement, and data analysis. They must be expert in customer service models and function competently as facilitators for QI teams. It is most useful if these individuals come from a variety of backgrounds and experience including nursing, management (MBA level), quality engineering (systems and process expertise), computer sciences, statistics, and biotechnology.

FIGURE 3
Department of clinical practice improvement and quality management
Critical support services and associated departments

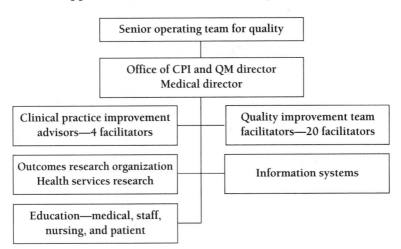

Quality analysts are entry-level staff. They are selected for their potential to become quality consultants. From their first day, they are paired with a quality consultant and are placed in internal training programs and working QI teams. At a minimum, they have basic data management and computer technology skills and are experienced in quality improvement QI methodology. They often have a clinical background.

To assemble a quality department it is essential to obtain individuals from a wide variety of medical and nonmedical backgrounds. The exponential rise in expertise available within the department as a result of this hiring practice has proven invaluable. To develop large gains in service improvement, the necessary expertise and ingenuity will come from a range of disciplines—not just medicine.

To illustrate this point, one of the most valuable additions made to the quality department was hiring a quality engineer with extensive process improvement expertise from a leading electronics manufacturer. This individual's ability to quickly and effectively solve complex process issues within the healthcare setting was invaluable.

There are no training programs currently available to produce individuals with all of the skills and expertise needed to staff the quality department of the future. They must bring complete skill sets or develop them within internal training programs. Lovelace employees possess a hybrid of nontraditional experience and great diversity.

MINIMUM TECHNICAL EXPERTISE

In all quality department staff, there is a need for certain skill sets, expertise, and talents. Individuals hired must demonstrate mastery of the majority of the following core knowledge and skills:

- Quality and process improvement

- Data measurement and management

- Basic statistics

- Advanced computer skills

- Ability to teach and make public presentations

- Mature interpersonal skills

- Good organizational skills

- Creative problem solving

- Systems expertise

- Outcomes research experience

- Change management expertise

- Survey research experience

- Customer service expertise

- Demonstrable record of success in previous leadership positions

- Clinical background (e.g., nursing, medicine, allied health)

- Experience working in healthcare systems

- A natural comfort with innovation and change

Additional experience might include management background (e.g., MBA, MHSA), background in quality engineering, and experience in adult learning theory.

CRITICAL SUPPORT SERVICES AND DEPARTMENTS

In addition to the core quality management department, a number of critical support services and departments are necessary to fulfill the QI mission. As illustrated in Figure 3, these resources play a significant role to drive QI initiatives throughout the organization, give employees the tools to be productive and satisfy QI team members, and demonstrate the positive impact of the QI initiatives.

QI facilitators and advisors

Within the quality system, there are two types of QI advisors. The first group facilitates CPI teams through the Episodes of Care initiative. The second group facilitates service improvement teams across the health-care system. All advisors are highly motivated volunteers who serve as change agents by accelerating QI throughout the system.

CPI advisors lead teams implementing disease management methodology in the Lovelace Episodes of Care program. These advisors are leading physicians and PhDs from clinical or outcomes research areas. They have extensive experience and advanced training in CPI methodology.

Perceived as QI experts, they are in an excellent position to lead, motivate, and encourage the health system's physician leaders and Episodes of Care teams to accomplish dramatic process redesign of clinical care continuums.

QI team advisors are volunteers who lead service improvement teams such as the Ideal Patient Encounter mentioned previously. Coming from all parts of the organization, they include pro-viders, nurses, managers, and administrators with advanced training in QI methodology and serve as advisors and facilitators to QI teams throughout the institution.

It is particularly noteworthy that both groups of individuals are allowed time from their workday to perform these advisory roles for the organization. Since QI is considered part of every employee's responsibility, this is an important organizational statement supporting the high priority given to QI.

EDUCATION

Education is central to QI success and must encompass all members of the organization from the board of directors to front-line employees. Lovelace has created a series of QI training experiences starting with basic orientation to QI and ending with a multiweek class designed to produce QI team facilitators.

Lessons learned

As quality departments have evolved over the last several years, many lessons have been learned. In an effort to help institutions avoid mistakes already made by others, the following list of lessons learned and pitfalls to avoid is offered.

NEEDED EXPERTISE AND RESOURCES

Do not compromise in hiring key personnel. Hire carefully, after clearly identifying the needed skills and expertise for the quality department. Go outside the lines of traditional QA skill sets to hire staff with a wide range of experience, expertise, and training. The recommended areas of expertise listed earlier are particularly useful.

Match staffing levels to the work and do not stretch department resources to the point of ineffectiveness. When designing annual quality initiatives, carefully consider the amount of staffing and resources available and plan accordingly.

When Lovelace initially started its QI program in 1989, many team advisors were selected because of their position in the organization or the title they carried. A more effective approach is to select quality department staff and particularly QI team advisors who have an intense interest in participating in QI. A strong belief in the potential of QI is essential to success.

Leadership issues are one of the most important areas to address in the restructuring of any QI organization. All too often, they are overlooked, and as a result QI departments and initiatives fail. The Baldrige criteria are an excellent guide to the actions needed from senior management and were used in the beginning of this chapter to highlight the daily behaviors needed.

Other senior leadership issues to consider include

- QI should be part of daily organizational life. It is incumbent upon senior leadership to model the behaviors necessary to accomplish this

- Managers must be held accountable for participation and results of QI programs. The structure established to manage the quality process is critical to achieving this very important link. In other words, the quality management structure must be integrated with the daily business management structure and parallel systems must be abolished

- QI leadership must be clearly identified within the ranks of senior management. This is necessary to give the quality directors the organizational clout to be successful

- Quality committees must avoid the trap of becoming "rubber stamp" committees. The quality review process is an extremely important aspect of quality committees as they review team progress, give feedback, help focus teams, ensure resources, and eliminate institutional barriers

- QI must be driven by senior managers. This is a central tenet in both the change management and the quality literature. Lack of commitment at the top will seriously undermine the QI process and the efforts of the quality department

LACK OF TEMPLATES

As is true with many innovations, there are often no comparable models to provide design or implementation guidance to organizations seeking to establish an effective mechanism to support a CPI initiative. Nowhere else is this more true than in the perpetually changing field of quality. Evolving organizations should network widely, benchmark freely, and consult with leaders from around the country who are making similar systems changes.

EDUCATION

There is a distinct relationship between organizational preparedness, training, and the success of QI programs in healthcare organizations. Accordingly, one of the key products produced by the Lovelace quality management department is institutionwide training in QI methodology. This training includes everyone in the organization from the board of directors to frontline employees. A well-trained team accelerates the QI process and achievement of team goals while minimizing team frustration due to lack of insight or direction. Similarly, the ability of the quality department to supply teams with well-trained, effective team facilitators is key.

Although classroom experience is necessary, adult learning theory clearly demonstrates that the learning should not stop there. In fact, classroom training may not be the most effective method to enhance retention. For example, many of the Lovelace QI teams have responded best to "just-in-time" training, where education is provided during team meetings. The training is provided by the team facilitator, highlighting another key talent for these individuals: the ability to teach effectively on the spur of the moment.

CUSTOMER FOCUS

It is important to develop organizational awareness of the importance of customer focus. No matter how often it is mentioned, understanding the true meaning and significance of an organization's primary customers is often a personal process that takes varying amounts of time for each individual. Only through continued repetition will it move to the front of organizational and staff consciousness.

ORGANIZATIONAL COMMUNICATION

Underestimating the need to establish an internal communication program to promote and develop awareness around QI programs is a common mistake.[5] A well-designed communication and marketing plan is central to the quality department's success to move quality initiatives through an organization. To address this need, Lovelace added a communications and marketing expert to the staff of the quality department. This individual designs and orchestrates events, forums, and print media to maintain a continual presence of organizational quality programs in the minds and hearts of all employees and senior leaders.

LACK OF RECOGNITION

To be successful, team members and employees must receive a clear message from the organization and senior management that their efforts are valued and appreciated. Teams must be regularly recognized for their success and accomplishments. There are many ways to do this including public reward and recognition events, institutionwide quality forums, high-profile articles in newsletters, and promotional material.[6] At Lovelace, Episodes of Care teams are now highlighted in regional advertising campaigns. Team members also receive important recognition from presentations to the senior quality committee and the institution's board of directors. The bottom line is to establish and execute a thoughtful system of rewards and recognition for teams.

NOTES

1. Adopted from the National Baldrige Award criteria.
2. NCQA accreditation guidelines, 1995 standards.
3. V. Sahney, "Implementation, Observed Barriers, and Management of Continuous Quality Improvement (CQI)," *National Quality of Care Forum, Bridging the Gap Between Theory and Practice,* 1994.
4. M. J. Gunter et al., "Implementation Strategies in Outcome Management: A Tale of Two Stories," *Quality Source* (November 1994); and M. D. Hornbrook, A. V. Hurtado, and R. E. Johnson, "Health Care Episodes: Definition, Measurement, and Use," *Medical Care Review* 42 (1985): 163–218.
5. Sahney, "Implementation."
6. Sahney, "Implementation."

24

Legacy Health System: Reconfiguring patient flow

Roselyn J. Meier
Senior Program Manager, Patient Flow Management
Legacy Health System
Portland, Oregon

A FTER MERGING FOUR HOSPITALS, a visiting nurse association, a host of community-based urgent care clinics, and a preferred provider insurance brokerage organization, Legacy Health System (LHS) was looking for an innovative way to provide a seamless continuum through multiple administrative steps:

- Patient admitting

- Prior authorization

- Clinical resource management

- Patient records including confidentiality

- Patient discharge and follow-up

- Simplified billing

- Reduction in the number of days an account spent as a receivable

These steps involved handoffs of work-in-progress between departments, caused patient and physician delays, required redundant gathering of information from the patient, and produced bills that were difficult to understand.

A reengineering project, created by LHS, was developed and called

Patient Flow Management (PFM). The initiative produced a case study, methodology, and lessons learned.

In July 1993, a group of 30 LHS senior managers met to determine how reengineering could benefit LHS, key customers, and the community. LHS's vision and strategic pathways defined its key mandates to

- Become an integrated system with convenient, competitively priced, and comprehensive services

- Develop organizational and service capacity through continuous quality improvement (CQI) and learning organization methodology

- Increase market share

- Maintain financial performance at a level necessary to achieve LHS's vision

- Develop relationships with others that would better serve LHS's customers and improve the health status of the community

This context, provided by LHS, helped to focus decision making. The initial senior management session resulted in learning about reengineering, although it was clear that more information was needed for senior managers to have confidence in a decision to reengineer. Using selection criteria listed in Table 1, systemwide reengineering projects were defined and tentative leadership for each project was identified.

Senior managers recommended more detailed consideration and decision making by LHS executive leaders. A postsession evaluation revealed strong support for systemwide focus, coordination of LHS's improvement efforts, and requests for more education on reengineering. Importance of integrating reengineering methodology with its CQI problem-solving process also was stressed. As a relatively new healthcare system, it was important to maintain continuity and reinforce LHS's CQI management philosophy and improvement process.

Two months later, in a meeting of the president's council—which consisted of the CEO, corporate senior vice presidents, and operating unit presidents—organizational readiness, time estimates, and options were considered. PFM was commissioned as LHS's first systemwide reengineering project.

The PFM reengineering project used information from an earlier project, dubbed "Grease PIT," that found that significant cost savings and

TABLE 1
Reengineering criteria for decision making

Implement uniform process throughout system when

1. Customer needs indicate importance of process uniformity and integration across the system

2. Improvement forecast for the project's primary quality indicator is significantly greater by implementing a uniform process throughout the system

3. Strategic pathways or external environmental factors mandate conversion to a uniform process

4. Projected cost to implement a uniform process can be justified by the long-term expected return on investment

5. Projected return on investment for implementing a uniform process is significantly greater than a "high-level only" implementation

6. Information technology and professional support capability is available to implement a uniform process within the project timetable

7. Professional human resources support is sufficient to provide for large-scale job reclassification and description modification, redeployment, and retraining of staff

8. Unequivocal commitment to implementation of uniform process on the part of operating unit presidents is unanimous

improvement could result from increasing the scope of work for staff and reducing inefficiency by consolidating administrative processes.

From the outset, it was clear that a transformational change, not incremental change, would be needed. The current patient flow process was never designed to serve patients efficiently. In fact, the process had never been designed but evolved over the years by adding steps and work as managed care and regulatory reporting requirements demanded more of healthcare systems. The existing process was extremely complex and inextricably interwoven with other parts. It would be more cost-effective to design a new process than try to fix the existing one.

Leadership was to be a critical factor in the project's success. Thus the CEO appointed two of LHS's operating unit presidents to key reengineering roles of champion and team leader. In addition, two internal consultants from LHS's organizational development and quality improvement department were assigned to work on the project full-time, a core team of 12 was identified and recruited, and resource requirements were communicated to team members and their supervisors.

Although external consultants were interviewed, the right "match" for a reengineering coach was never found. PFM was supported with internal consultants trained in reengineering methodology. In October 1993, training of core team members began.

Patient flow management design

The core team's work began with reviewing the results of 34 process improvement teams (PIT), including the Grease PIT, whose charters and conclusions were now within the scope of work defined for PFM. Preparatory work also included developing a comprehensive communication plan and a human resource reengineering plan. Information and human resources leaders were included in the core team and all subsequent design and implementation teams to facilitate parallel development and expert advice in those key areas of infrastructure.

Current departments that handled patient scheduling, admitting, insurance verification and authorization, utilization management, discharge planning, billing and collections, and medical record processing consistently met their quality targets. However, the patient flow process was fragmented, duplicative, and laden with delays and poor communication between functions, levels of care, and operating units. It was necessary to reinvent the process from the customer's perspective.

A high-level idealized design, a design free of the constraints of the current process and of incorporating customers' requirements, was described by 30 individuals working in three teams.

Each design team had representatives from all organizational levels, disciplines, and operating units. The groups met in two-day sessions to describe the features of the work flow from the customer's perspective. Design groups were facilitated by core team members assisted by internal reengineering consultants. Using guided imagery, design group participants set aside what they knew about how work was currently done and alternately assumed the role of a patient, a physician, and a payer. A process free of information gaps, handoffs between different departments, and redundant work was described in detail. Concurrently, patient satisfaction surveys were analyzed to determine recurring customer complaints. The idealized designs from the three groups were integrated by the core team members. Critical areas of needed improvements included

- Develop simple, single-contact scheduling of multiple tests and services for a patient

- Develop methods to interpret complicated health plan benefits

- Gather aggregate outcomes data electronically and prevent inappropriate use of data

- Share clinical, demographic, and insurance information between all providers and payers along with appropriate mechanisms to safeguard confidentiality of patient information

- Manage high-risk individuals not receiving ongoing care through a physician

- Personalize service and education for patients and their family-members

The idealized design was analyzed and adjusted to meet or exceed customer requirements. Key findings included

- Eighty percent of patients were in a managed care program with an automated clinical path guiding all aspects of care during an illness episode. The normal hospital clinical path was extended to include care and patient education provided at all care sites including the physician's office. In addition, payers authorized the entire continuum of care instead of segments of the patient's care. The clinical path began with early identification of a high-risk individual at health plan enrollment and guided patient treatment and maintenance until loss of contact with the system

- One patient contact person supported case management by providing personalized communication, coordination, and education and by electronically generating and interfacing with the patient's medical record to aid the patient and family members in making appropriate decisions

- Scheduling multiple services for a patient or for a physician required only one contact to LHS

- A population-based illness prevention and education model include assessment and early identification of high-risk individuals

- Insurance certification and authorization was accomplished through one payer contact, because payers accepted internal controls defined in clinical paths

- An integrated billing and collection process resulted in simplifying proof of provision of services and billing of payers and patients

- A portable electronic system with shared patient information and an inventory of community resources accessible real time. Patient confidentiality was adequately protected

- Concurrent record completion, electronic transmittal of dictated reports, and physician orders streamlined postdischarge work by physicians

- Workforce competency was increased through hiring and staff education to enable employees to function in jobs with a broader scope of responsibility

- Work was done in the most effective place and point in time for achieving desired results

- A collaborative network between providers, payers, and employers maximized use of an electronic system and standardized methods and tools (e.g., accumulation and analysis of outcome data, educational materials, reports, protocols, and information sharing)

- The collaborative network was flexible enough to meet or exceed changing customer needs and external forces on healthcare

- A single patient information telephone line was established

Following development of the idealized design, the 30 staff members were reconfigured into 4 design teams, and functional experts were added. The detailed design teams included billing and collections, health education and enrollment, access to services, and health information services. Access to services divided into two subteams, transition planning and intake and scheduling. The idealized design was shared with all staff who were expected to be impacted by the changes, and their input was solicited and channeled to the appropriate design team. After two weeks of intensive work, detailed, integrated flowcharts were developed. The core team examined the new flowcharts and determined which concepts were feasible to implement in the first year. Design teams developed plans to define the sequence of work to be accomplished and interdependencies between design components. They also estimated the resources needed and projected a time line for implementation. The design was approved by senior executives for systemwide implementation.

Human resources plan

During the design phase, LHS's human resource council, consisting of the corporate vice president of human resources and the operating unit human resource directors, met to develop a work plan to support the changes resulting from reengineering. Human resource issues included

- Develop a plan to integrate displaced staff into other jobs within the system

- Develop a hiring or selection policy to facilitate transition of staff into new jobs

- Plan and implement an employee skills assessment and a program to help employees decide if assuming a broader scope of work and responsibility would be compatible with their personal objectives

- Prepare managers for change management roles

- Interface with the employee assistance program to support individual counseling needs related to change

- Revise the compensation program to provide team incentives under new process design

- Coordinate communications with employees

- Assure congruity of all human resource policies with planned changes

- Shift organizational perspective to employee development instead of training

- Manage cultural shift of manager and employee decision-making authority to appropriate organizational levels

- Determine job requirements for new positions and write new job descriptions

LHS's human resource directors, who had been involved in both design phases, developed an assessment and transition process (see Figure 1) to involve and prepare staff for the changes.

Other healthcare systems were contacted to determine if they had comparable jobs. Finding none, the human resource staff developed new job descriptions for more than 400 staff whose work would be

FIGURE 1
Patient flow management (PFM)

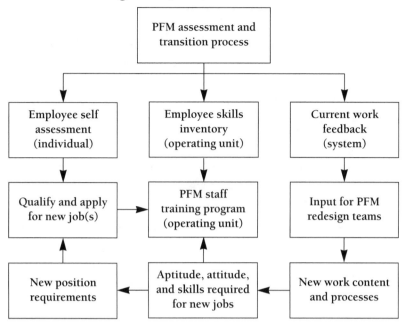

Objectives
1. *Invite input for PFM work redesign*
2. *Collect input for PFM staff training program*
3. *Provide tools to support employee decision making regarding applying for one or more of the new jobs*
4. *Document employee skills and work preferences for employee and human resources*

significantly impacted by the changes. One hundred and two specific job descriptions were reduced to eight. The new job descriptions included

- *Health Services Associate.* Provides general clerical support to administrative and patient care units

- *Health Services Representative.* Performs a wide variety of activities to support patients with service and information needs, patient registration, scheduling of services, and health record maintenance

- *Patient Business Services Representative.* Performs activities related to billing for services rendered, satisfying service and information needs, and patient account collections and reconciliation

- *Medical Transcriptionist.* Transcribes medical reports dictated by physicians, allied health professionals, and staff

- *Health Quality Analyst I.* Performs a wide variety of analytical tasks related to the collection, analysis, and use of data regarding patient information, episodes of care, quality, and long-term studies of treatment effectiveness

- *Health Quality Analyst II.* Performs duties similar Health Quality Analyst I but with greater responsibility

- *Clinical Resource Coordinator.* Provides key services to guide the patient and family members through the continuum of care. Key services include health assessment, coordination of services, interface with payers, utilization management, education, and transition planning

- *Financial Services Counselor.* Assists patients by projecting costs of treatment options, explaining various costs, making payment arrangements, and helping with applications for assistance with their healthcare costs

The new job descriptions reflected a broader scope of responsibility and included many skills that current staff who performed more task-specific jobs did not possess. A multiple-year cross-training program was developed for staff to be fully competent in all components of the new jobs.

Information resources support

LHS's vice president of information resources and selected staff participated in the PFM core team, design teams, and implementation teams. They provided technical expertise, supported expanded use of current information systems, and gathered information on PFM requirements for an integrated clinical information system. In the first year, $500,000 was budgeted to purchase new hardware and software to implement centralized billing and collections, standardize and provide electronic access to new policies and procedures, and streamline communication with physicians regarding test reporting and medical record completion. Concurrently, key information resource staff supported hospital-based, patient care reengineering. Electronic capabilities in radiology, dialysis, imaging, surgery, medication and fluid documentation, and emergency room services also were expanded. All new information resource elements will be integrated into a centralized clinical data repository, making the data available electronically to multiple users at various sites. The clinical data repository integrates patient-specific health data, provides a formatted window to view data in an electronic health record and accommodates both aggregate and patient-specific reporting. Reengineering design was completed in the administrative and clinical areas early in 1995. The design phase was followed by comprehensive planning for the integrated clinical information system that began with demonstrations by software vendors. Organizational readiness testing emphasized educating executives on the potential of the new system and the need to invest substantial time and money. When complete, the clinical information system will accommodate an automated clinical path, documentation of medical interventions against physician orders and the clinical path, charting by exception, and monitoring equipment interfaces. Data will be formatted by patient and by encounter on the computer screen to meet clinician needs. Multiple users will be able to access the information at the same time both on- and off-site.

Other information resource initiatives include electronic forms development, clinical path tracking, on-line lab orders and results to physician offices, remote access to other LHS systems, and an expansion of the information network.

Communication plan

A comprehensive communication and employee involvement plan was developed at the outset of the reengineering project in 1993. The plan assigned frequent communication contacts with key leaders and customer groups to each PFM core team member. Numerous articles were published in LHS's employee newsletter during the design and early implementation phases. A telephone hot line was established to facilitate communication with employees. However, firsthand involvement in the process proved the most effective means of communication. More than 300 staff, 15 physicians, and 20 patients participated in the design phase. With implementation, communication and involvement efforts increased significantly, including all staff affected by the new process. These extensive efforts proved valuable to foster the understanding, ownership, and commitment of a large number of managers and staff whose work would be dramatically altered over time by the massive, five-year PFM project.

Implementation

Each operating unit's senior management team was asked to rate its own readiness to

- Provide continuing staff participation during design and systemwide implementation

- Incur costs associated with staff training through the test period and any necessary design modifications

- Accept timing of change in relationship to other changes in progress

- Provide measurement, control, and documentation of problems encountered while testing the new process

- Accommodate physical relocation of staff related to changed work flow

- Manage human resource issues including intensive communication, fluctuations in staff morale, and probable redeployment of staff

- Adapt to and be flexible in implementing the new process

  In addition, the PFM core team assessed

- PFM staff and core team capability to manage complex changes at the proposed test site, recognizing that an operating unit with a daily patient census of more than 400 patients in 26 inpatient nursing units would require far more resources than one of LHS's smaller hospitals

- If the proposed test site was "typical," not unique or highly specialized within LHS, and would provide significant opportunity for

  Ease of adaptation and transfer of the design to other LHS operating units

  Exercising the limits of the process design not just part of the PFM design

- The operating unit's ability to lead employees through major changes and maintain effective interdepartmental communication and problem solving during complex change

Based on the above criteria, Legacy Meridian Park Hospital (LMPH), a suburban hospital with eight inpatient and outpatient nursing units and an average daily patient census of 60, was selected as the test site. Originally, two test sites had been identified, but expert internal staff time was inadequate to support implementation at multiple sites simultaneously.

With implementation planning under way, the PFM structure was revised by the system CEO who appointed the president of LMPH as the leader for systemwide PFM implementation. The president of Legacy Visiting Nurse Association (LVNA) continued as leader for ongoing design and all operating unit presidents were charged with responsibility for the success of the project. The high level of operational leadership for the project signified the importance of PFM, making it easier to remove obstacles during the implementation phase. An internal consultant was selected to coordinate staff of the PFM project and began reporting to the two PFM leaders. The PFM core team was reorganized. Implementation team leaders from each operating unit joined design team leaders to coordinate simultaneous design and implementation.

The test site's PFM implementation team met weekly to make critical human resource decisions, develop a time line for implementation, identify site-specific issues, and give direction to a series of employee forums. A special "lunch and learn" meeting was held for physician office staff to let them know how the changes would impact them and provide them with materials to help them accelerate patient registration and admission to the hospital. The LMPH PFM implementation team learned to plot its time line for implementation and allow for unexpected delays. In November 1994, the implementation of the new work flow in health information services and intake and scheduling coincided with the grand opening of a new hospital entrance for obstetrical and short-stay patients. By the end of December, health information services was stabilized and staff began to see results from the streamlined flow of work. Intake and scheduling struggled to maintain adequate staff coverage while conducting training in the new process. Staffing was already at a reduced level and a round of flu caused a delay of several planned training sessions. In March 1995, the last segments of implementation in intake and scheduling were completed when new computer hardware allowed the cardiopulmonary unit to admit patients directly into the unit. Transition planning was the most complex component, involving cross-training between preadmitting, utilization management, discharge planning, and LVNA home care consultants. The current process was highly fragmented and patients experienced many handoffs between staff in different departments.

The new design called for a single contact person to handle patient and family education, coordination of services, interface with payers and transfers to other levels of care. Discharge planners assumed the utilization management function. Two staff members, shared by LMPH and LVNA, began cross-training to become equally skilled in handling hospital discharge planning and complex transfers to home health services. Early results included an increase in internal referrals to LHS's home health program. The implementation of the new transition planning process was expected to continue for 12 months due to the extensive skills and knowledge base required.

In February 1995, implementation planning began at Legacy Portland Hospitals (LPH), an operating unit comprising two tertiary facilities, Legacy Emanuel Hospital and Health Center (LEHHC) and Legacy Good Samaritan Hospital and Medical Center (LGSHMC), centrally located in Portland. In May 1995, LPH health information services implemented the new work flow with simultaneous reorganization of the department. Self-managed team development and cross-training of staff is expected to take 12 months.

Initial implementation was expected to continue at LHS through March 1996. Early achievements of the reengineering project include the following:

- Developed quality indicators, established baselines, and designed evaluation instruments to measure physician office and patient satisfaction; employee job satisfaction and turnover rates; salary cost and number of management and staff employed in the impacted functions; the percentage of medical records completed within 30 days of patient discharge; the number of departments issuing separate bills and the number of billing systems; the number of multiskilled, cross-trained staff; the number of high-risk individuals who are identified and referred for physician intervention before receiving hospital services; and the number of clinical paths in place to guide the full continuum of patient care with single authorization from the payers

- Reduced variation in patient flow processes by standardizing the work flow and reducing 350 operating unit-specific procedures to 63 systemwide procedures in admitting, health information services, and transition planning

- Reduced number of job descriptions from 102 to 8

- Cross-functional teams consolidated 24 versions of various forms used to gather patient information to 11 systemwide forms, saving an estimated $35,000 per year in printing costs

- Reduced salary cost per adjusted admission by 6.5 percent

- Consolidated and standardized hospital billing and collection activities to one site. Reduced full-time equivalents (FTEs) by 14.6 and cost by $349,133, by eliminating duplicative functions required to support operating unit-specific billing and reducing billing systems from 23 to 16

- Developed and distributed a comprehensive Community Resource Directory to assist patients, clinicians, and families in accessing community services

- Introduced health information services software products to

   Automate the process of physician notification of incomplete records

   Decrease the interval of time between dictation and receipt of patient records

   Enable physician record completion from the physician's office

   Enable identification and retrieval of current patient medical records across service areas and identify recent admissions to other LHS operating units

- Standardized the medical record abstraction process and retrospective one-pass review to position LHS for computerized patient medical records

- Increased convenience of access for patients by either providing direct admission at service areas or placing new admission areas at entrances closer to service areas when patient volume did not support placing admitting staff on the unit

- Offered redesigned jobs to all employees impacted by work design and retained 90 percent of existing staff

- Reduced the number of calls necessary for a physician's office to schedule multiple services by developing administrative systems to coordinate services, relay patient information to departments who need it, and cross-train staff

- Simplified and automated communication between departments by enhancing and improving use of existing information systems

- Increased patient compliance with pretesting instructions and decreased no-show rate by 30 percent by calling selected categories of patients the night before they were scheduled for diagnostic tests

- Improved physician record completion rate by implementing a form and process to monitor record completion while the patient was hospitalized and the physician was making frequent hospital visits, thereby reducing the work of health information services

- Streamlined the process of assembling and filing medical records of discharged patients resulting in decreased filing backlog and coding delays. Charts are completed concurrent with the patient's hospital stay, are disassembled for filing on the nursing unit, and are filed in the order received from the unit

- Expanded operating hours of health information services from 7:00 A.M. to 11:00 P.M. daily and increased staff coverage on weekends to meet customer requirements with no increase in FTEs

- Developed seamless patient flow between hospital preadmitting, utilization review, discharge planning, and LVNA home health functions through cross-trained staff shared by multiple operating units

- Blended retrospective quality review into the coding function, eliminating a handoff between departments

- Restructured health information service teams to broaden responsibility for managing medical records, eliminated duplication in document pickup and delivery and mail room functions, as well as cross-trained staff

Multiple year project

With the change in design priorities each year, PFM core team members are rotated to include new topical experts and reduce staff whose segments were successfully implemented. At least one-third of the team members are retained to preserve continuity. The fluid nature of the core team works well to maintain enthusiasm, extend the base of expertise, and infuse new ideas. The idealized design will be revisited annually to make sure the changes being implemented are consistent with changes in customer needs.

Design priorities for 1995–96 focus on continuing development within LHS as well as collaboration with payers and private physician practices. These priorities include

- Plan and test a single telephone information line that patients or health plan members can call to obtain information on health plans, bills, community resources, or services scheduled. In addition, access to nurse advice, prerecorded health messages, class registration, and physician referral would be available by calling the telephone information line

- Develop a high-risk assessment process that allows for early identification of individuals who may need prompt intervention by a physician

- Increase the number of individuals who receive and complete Advance Directives, which are patient instructions regarding artificial means of life support. Currently the information is provided at the point of admission to a hospital. It is widely recognized that life-support decisions are better made at a different point in time when the health plan member can receive appropriate family and clinical support and communicate their wishes in a noncrisis setting

- Integrate nonhospital billing functions to include home care, physician, and specialty services

- Develop clinical paths to guide the entire continuum of care for patients during an episode of illness. These clinical paths would include all aspects of care and provider services, have a predictable cost and outcome, and eliminate the need for continuing payer updates and authorization

- Print all appropriate patient materials in foreign languages pertinent to each operating unit's service area

- Initiate collaboration between LHS, physicians, and payers to develop a common clinical information system

- Measure results of implementing PFM through customer satisfaction surveys, employee turnover rate, medical record completion rate, and numbers of standardized procedures and forms, billing systems, and multiskilled staff

Lessons learned

LHS was able to foster commitment in implementing the PFM recommendations by integrating the project into the organization's existing structure. Success was based on the following factors:

- Legacy's CEO advocated for reengineering and PFM

- Senior executives provided consistent leadership for the project

- PFM used the same planning, budgeting, and capital request processes as LHS's ongoing operations

- The project's annual work plan was defined in terms of LHS's vision and strategic pathways

- Reengineering methodology was integrated into LHS's CQI

- Legacy's leadership was committed to becoming a learning organization; PFM provided an excellent arena to try innovative ideas, experience measurable success, and learn from mistakes

Given senior executives' commitment and leadership, investing in external consulting may not be necessary. In the initial stage of the project, LHS interviewed several external consultants to provide technical support to PFM. After several interviews, it was clear that LHS had the internal technical skills offered by external consultants. It also was determined that current LHS staff could learn reengineering methodology and adapt it to the organization's culture effectively. Legacy adopted a "we can do it" approach and redefined the roles of internal consultants from reengineering process experts to technical implementation support. Achieving high levels of customer satisfaction competes with the aspect of diminishing financial resources. Those involved in designing and implementing large-scale change must understand the practical limitations and help everyone, including customers, develop realistic expectations.

During the idealized and detail design phases, staff must become more comfortable with ambiguity. Many times no one knows what the completed design will mean to the organization and its employees. If an organization expects to have all the answers before leaping into reengineering, nothing may happen. A level of trust combined with an in-depth review of implications prior to implementation is needed to move forward into the redesign. Breakthrough thinking and designing an idealized process can be difficult. Staff must be reminded to design from the customer's perspective regardless of the difficulties that will be faced in implementing untested ideas. Potential obstacles should be acknowledged, recorded, and categorized in terms of whether each can be removed or must be accommodated in the design.

Team members as well as organizational leaders need tangible results within a year to maintain enthusiasm and commitment. The pace of the project is a delicate balance between moving fast enough to implement significant change within this time frame and slow enough to develop a well-thought-out design and implementation plan. There is less risk to morale if an implementation date is announced only when readiness can be accurately predicted.

Involving key support functions such as human and information resources in the design process saves time. Providing the infrastructure necessary to support successful implementation of redesigned work and jobs requires complex planning and may require significant expenditures. The work of human and information resources can proceed on a parallel time frame if technical specialists are thoroughly familiar with the design.

Staff who will be impacted by the project may be anxious. Resistance is a normal part of the change process. Leadership should anticipate resistance and communicate with staff who need to understand why and what change is prescribed. Managers and employees need ongoing opportunity to debrief, debug, and communicate with project leadership. The time dedicated to these activities will help uncover process design defects and result in a higher level of commitment from those who are doing the work. When a defect is discovered it is helpful to enlist staff to determine the root cause of the problem, plan the correc-tive action, and monitor the results.

Maintaining ongoing operations while training staff to implement the new work flow requires a temporary increase in the number of staff hours in impacted areas. If staffing margins are tight and new staff needs to be hired, it is less disruptive to hire, orient, and stabilize new staff before beginning implementation training.

A review and documentation of all procedures that will not be changed will assure consistency with the new process. Who will order supplies or make coffee can become critical questions when all staff's attention is focused on the new work flow.

Staff have a high interest in forms. When a form is changed, it is important to involve all users in the design process. New forms are also excellent tools for signaling to staff that change is taking place.

Trainers without operational responsibilities are needed. If the trainers are also managers, they must be relieved from operational responsibilities for at least three months to plan and implement a solid staff training pro-gram (this may vary with the complexity of the process and could take up to a year). A poorly executed training program will result in confusion, low morale, and lack of confidence in the new process. Under these con-ditions, it is easy for employees to return to the old way of doing things. Training does not stop with implementation; the new way of doing work must continually be reinforced to prevent process deterioration.

The degree to which employees initiate improvements in their work and take responsibility for customer-driven decision making is defined by management's ability to redefine its role to support employee learn-ing and risk taking. It is particularly important for the manager to treat mistakes as learning opportunities.

Reengineering is hard work that requires vision and focus on detail. The unwavering support by a CEO who shares the vision and enlists the commitment of key executive leaders is fundamental to project success.

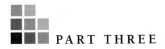

PART THREE

Redesign case studies

25

University of Massachusetts Medical Center: Integrating work redesign and CQI

Steven L. Strongwater, MD
Associate Chief Medical Officer, Clinical Systems

Vincent Pelote, MBA
Senior Quality Advisor, Clinical Systems

Victoria P. Gaw, BSN, MA, RN
Quality Management Consultant, Quality Management Services

Jay Cyr, MSN, RN
Director of Cardiovascular Medical Services

Paulette Seymour, MSN, RN
Director of Cardiovascular Surgical Services
University of Massachusetts Medical Center
Worcester, Massachusetts

DRAMATIC AND RAPID CHANGES in the healthcare system have stimulated reevaluation of the healthcare delivery process. Payers are setting clear expectations for all segments of the healthcare industry to maximize four distinct outcomes—clinical outcomes, patient satisfaction, functional status, and cost/utilization. Segments of the healthcare industry can no longer exist in a vacuum.

By integrating work redesign and continuous quality improvement, the University of Massachusetts Medical Center (UMMC) has adopted a clinical process redesign (CPR) approach that encompasses all aspects of patient care and offers advantages to both the delivery system and the patients it serves. The methodology challenges providers to balance high levels of creativity with scientific, analytical thinking. Over a four- to six-month course, multidisciplinary clinical teams are formed to think futuristically, develop an accurate understanding of their environment, focus on what is important, implement change, and measure results. Teams are driven by an understanding of patients, payers, other providers, and support staff needs to think about alternatives—the best ways to meet those needs.

As shown in Figure 1, CPR is a seven-phase, structured methodology that brings about revolutionary change while helping teams improve quality. It can be used to thoroughly redesign a process or simply to improve one. Phases one through four require innovative, nontraditional, creative thinking that leads to dramatic gains. By repeating phases five, six and seven, teams can deliver CQI.

The art of integrating various approaches may appear to be complex, yet any single approach (e.g., "clean slate" versus "CQI") can result in failure. It was not long ago that many publications were filled with the benefits of total quality management (TQM), only to be followed with their inherent disadvantages. Similar journal articles are today starting

FIGURE 1
Clinical process redesign

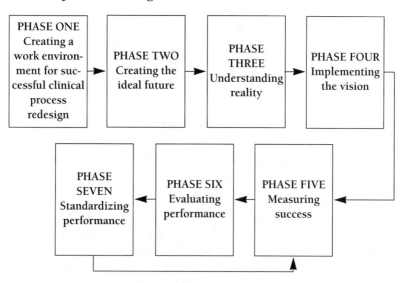

to appear about reengineering. Institutions involved with reengineering or CQI should not stop what they are doing, but should think about an approach that combines the best of both.

Creating a work environment for successful clinical process redesign

There are three components that will produce the best climate for a successful CPR team:

1. Clearly defined goals and a plan aligned to those goals

2. Strong leadership to guide the team

3. Team members who have relevant content knowledge and technical skills as well as the interpersonal competencies to work with a team

CPR begins with upfront development of strong, multidisciplinary support that begins at the highest management and clinical levels and is then communicated, reinforced, and extended to all organizational levels. After upper management support is secured, a consensus regarding key institutional goals and project priorities is developed.

Benchmarking data of key clinical indicators is useful to identify and quantify clinical focus areas. The purpose of benchmarking at the macrolevel is to compare the organization's outcomes with those of relevant peer organizations and to identify potential financial opportunities and quality of care gains. Peer organizations may be chosen from comparable institutions (e.g., similar size, patient mix, geographic area), healthcare leaders (e.g., academic or specialty institutions), or best-in-class performers (e.g., lowest mortality or cost per case, best clinical outcomes or patient satisfaction). Data from similar academic medical centers can be used to identify the high-volume, high-cost patient populations for initial focus. After the potential target areas are identified, the top management group is asked to validate organizational readiness. There must be a clear expectation that the members of the group will continue to be actively involved by

- Monitoring team outcomes as they work through the process

- Serving as advocates for reallocation of resources that may be needed to institutionalize CPR outcomes

- Maintaining personal commitment to serve as CPR champions within their area of influence on an individual level

Project identification, prioritization, and limits are best carried out by a small, knowledgeable, interdisciplinary steering committee that understands the institutional culture.

Healthcare institutions typically have several groups of top managers representing the fiscal, operational, and clinical aspects of the institution. At UMMC, the first CPR projects were initiated without support from the top management. In many cases, the failure to build upon and communicate top management involvement was a barrier to team progress. A second generation of projects was initiated using a new strategy that focused on departmental involvement as part of the CPR process. This strategy contributes to more successful teams.

Physicians are socialized to make independent decisions, create unique management plans for every patient, and maintain independent authority and responsibility. These norms often conflict with the use of standardized patient management protocols, the end product of CPR, and can lead to physician resistance. Even physicians who have previously embraced CQI may have difficulty accepting CPR. Opposition in healthcare is strongest where CPR is viewed as a threat to the institution's educational mission.

Physicians, however, are most apt to change their practice in response to well-validated clinical information from respected peers. Therefore physician-to-physician contact is used to achieve support for both the process and outcomes. The process to select a team leader is used to educate the key physician leaders in the CPR process and institutional goals and objectives and to enlist their support. A meeting with the appropriate departmental or division chairperson and the clinical leader of the institution's CPR program (a physician) serves as the venue for the initial discussion. The purpose of this meeting is to define the expectations of the CPR process, taking into account the institution's goals of insuring quality while controlling cost. All parties should be clearly informed that the CPR process will require a departure from business as usual including

- Introducing organizational best care protocols

- Shifting sites of patient care (e.g., inpatient versus outpatient surgery)

- Changing levels of patient care (e.g., nursing home versus hospital)

- Eliminating redundant testing (e.g., repeat x-rays)

- Developing a more restrictive drug formulary

- Reducing administrative costs and eliminating positions

In academic centers, this often requires balancing intern and resident involvement in protocol implementation with maintaining the educational environment. Once the department-specific CPR goals and potential changes are clearly articulated, the chair's commitment and support is requested. If this support is not forthcoming, the easiest approach is to bypass this CPR project and shift the focus and resources to another CPR project where departmental support is present. This is not necessarily the best alternative. When timely initiation of the project is critical to the institution, a hard-sell approach to persuade the chair can be employed. This includes intensive administrative and peer pressure, building incentives into the project, or as a last resort, some type of negative consequence.

Large departments' chairs tend to delegate the task of choosing and supporting the physician team leader to a senior department member. This can create the risk of last-minute opposition to the team's final proposals from a chair who has not been well informed about or involved in the process.

After securing commitment from the chair, the institution's clinical CPR leader holds a candid discussion about picking the best team leader that covers

- An overview of the CPR methodology and resources available

- The scope of the project and time line for completion

- The role of the leader and time commitment required

- The role of a team coleader

A facilitator assigned to the team sits in on this discussion to act as a process person and give feedback to the project leader after the meeting. In addition to expertise and interest in the area of the project and key leadership competencies (see Figure 2), the designated physician team leader needs to commit a minimum of one to two hours per week for meetings plus an additional two to four hours for preparation, presentation of team progress, departmental meetings to gain consensus on protocols, and report preparation for the duration of the project (usually six to eight months). This time commitment needs to be weighed against the potential candidates' overall commitments. For example, a physician who spends 20 to 30 hours per week in the operating room or seeing patients, as well as conducting research or serving in an administrative capacity, may find it difficult to commit the time that the project requires. On the other hand, a physician who has a flexible enough schedule to commit the needed time might not have the expertise or interest in the project, effective leadership skills, or the personal influence among peers to effectively sell the team's proposals to colleagues. The most successful teams have also had a strong coleader who brings complementary leadership skills as well as a clear understanding of the operational management of the patient population involved. This has typically been a nurse manager.

The physician leader has the specific responsibility to guide the team by providing direction and support. While assistance with the more concrete leadership skills such as assigning tasks and leading productive

FIGURE 2
Team leader competencies

Leadership competency	Description
____ Customer service orientation	Works toward the long-term benefit of patients
____ Directiveness	Uses appropriate positional power Expects high performance
____ Initiative	Takes action Creates opportunities for improvement
____ Team orientation	Encourages and empowers others
____ Relationship building	Develops networks of contracts with useful people
____ Achievement motivation	Strives to improve against standard of excellence
____ Complex thinking	Goes beneath the surface to solve problems at deep levels
____ Interpersonal understanding	Concerned for impact of actions on others

Courtesy of L. M. Spencer, Jr. and S. Spencer, *Competence at Work,*
(New York: John Wiley and Son, 1993).

team meetings will be provided by the facilitator, the leader must possess five key competencies:

1. The ability to envision the future without being bound by current practice

2. Clinical expertise in the area of team focus

3. The ability to provide team direction

4. Setting consistently high standards for the quality of work produced by the team

5. The ability to build team consensus

A candid evaluation of these skills should precede leader selection.

Team development

The newly chosen team leader should meet with the department liaison, project leader, and facilitator for three reasons: it gives the leader an introduction to the institution's expectations from the CPR process including the anticipated benefits from the project, development of outcome indicators, and time lines; it provides the first interaction with the facilitator who will be the key support person for the leader and team; and it provides an important opportunity for a four-way discussion about the support the leader can expect from his or her department, the institution, the facilitator, and a coleader.

After this initial meeting, the team leader and facilitator will begin a series of planning meetings. The first and most important purpose of these meetings is for the leader and facilitator to develop a high level of trust and a complementary working relationship. During this time it is the facilitator's responsibility to bring the leader up to speed on the CPR process and help with the selection of a coleader. An initial literature review is also conducted, a draft macroflowchart of the relevant care process is developed, and clinical areas that should be represented on the team are identified. It can also serve to help the leader develop an initial vision of where the team should be focusing. When a CPR team is created, it can expect to

- Focus on outcomes

- Create enthusiasm for the change process

- Maintain confidence in making changes

- Complete projects in timely fashion

The final steps in leader preparation—review of benchmark data and determining potential gains—are essential but also have serious potential problems. The most widely available benchmarks in healthcare are length of stay, charge or cost per case, and mortality rates. An inherent danger in the early presentation of this data is that it may give the team leader the erroneous message that the team should focus solely on reducing length of stay and cost. The leader may use the data to set a team goal that meets the initial projections, but they might be far less than what could be achieved.

Physicians, particularly academic physicians, are accustomed to the review and evaluation of clinical data. A presentation of detailed data without clear definitions of terms, identification of data sources, description of methodologies, or identification of benchmark institutions will lead to an acute episode of data bashing. Team leaders will balk at being asked to lead their teams to work on projects linked to data they do not trust. Also, when evaluating data, there is generally an assumption that something is wrong and it must be fixed. Whereas if a team looks at the total process, then it has the option of radically changing instead of just improving. Therefore, the best approach is to bypass these concerns by asking teams to consider their vision of best care practices.

Creating a vision

The overriding goal of a CPR team is to create a seamless system throughout a continuum of care that is both evolutionary and revolutionary. The stakeholders and team members need to understand that to accomplish this, the system will develop over time and in various stages. It is crucial that clinicians and team members clearly understand that the driving forces for CPR are patient satisfaction, clinical outcomes, functional status, and efficient resource utilization.

During some stages of CPR, healthcare providers need to take extreme steps to achieve the ideal care. It's important that the leader and the team feel supported through this volatile, risky, and complex phase. This begins by having the team members articulate a clear rationale to achieve a desirable future. They need to use group process techniques to reach a common understanding of the best practices and outcomes as well as external and internal issues. The team then needs to further explore its understanding by conducting a literature search that clarifies best practices, outcomes, issues, and trends. Only then can a best care vision be articulated.

Once the vision is articulated, the team needs to identify the gaps between the ideal future and current reality. The team needs to determine baselines and measure clinical outcomes, patient satisfaction, functional status, and resource utilization. Some global measures for clinical outcomes and resource utilization include mortality rates, cost per case, volume, and readmission rates.

Using a macroflowchart, the team can document the subprocesses of care that support the ideal. This can be done by a using a step table (see Figure 3) to help the team determine value—a reflection of the driving forces (e.g., clinical outcomes, patient satisfaction, functional outcomes, resource utilization). High-value steps may be associated with key process characteristics.

The team should begin the process of choosing outcome indicators once best care has been identified. Having a clear understanding of the purpose and objectives is a prerequisite to determining methods to measure success. Achieving the ideal future or vision can be difficult. Critical factors that will best represent total or incremental successes need to be identified during the planning stage of the project.

Clinical outcomes such as morbidity, mortality, patient satisfaction, functional status, and cost outcomes representing efficient resource utilization are useful categories to draw critical success factors from. Measures may include single or multiple success factors, but eventually

FIGURE 3
Sample value table

VALUE ANALYSIS	CONTRIBUTING FACTORS				Overall value rating
Steps in process	Patient satisfaction	Clinical outcomes	Functional outcomes	Cost and utilization	
1.					
2.					
3.					
4.					

a total outcomes measurement program, addressing both clinical and cost outcomes, is desirable.

Measurement of clinical success traditionally includes morbidity and mortality data. These data alone do not provide direction for improvement and redesign, but they may identify the need for improvement or measure the outcome or effect of changes in clinical practice.

Morbidity data include complications of treatment such as undesired response to medications, infection, unplanned occurrences, or technical and measurement errors by clinicians. These measures may require action such as revising existing protocols or developing new protocols as a part of a larger clinical redesign.

For example, a team focused on a cardiac surgery diagnosis related group (DRG) developed a protocol for extubation of postoperative coronary artery bypass (CABG) patients. The issue was identified by examining data that indicated that a number of patients who extubated themselves did not require reintubation. Each time this happened an occurrence report was generated. The team began to examine the use of diagnostic and laboratory tests for value-added effect on patient care. Arterial blood gases were reported as at 20 per patient per admission for DRG 106 in 1994. Additionally, patient interviews identified the time that they were awake and intubated as the worst part of the intensive care unit (ICU) experience.

The data led to examining the clinical process followed for postoperative weaning in the ICU. The goal was to extubate the patient as soon as he or she was clinically ready. The objectives were to increase patient satisfaction, reduce variance in the process followed to extubate patients, reduce unnecessary lab tests, and reduce clinical resource use.

The critical success factors measured were patient self-report, number of unplanned extubations, rate of adherence to the protocol developed to wean patients, number of arterial blood gases per case, and the number of hours of ventilation time. The latter generated the direct costs of respiratory therapy treating ventilated patients, the use of the ventilator, and the hours of patient care required of nursing, which differs for mechanically ventilated patients versus nonventilated patients.

Patient-driven outcome measures are also important to consider when quality is being determined. Positive results can also reduce costs. Patients who are satisfied with their care and the results of services received will be likely to return to the same providers and comment positively to others about the service. Less-than-adequate responses would provide direction for improvement initiatives.

A Picker Commonwealth patient satisfaction survey is an example of a patient-driven outcome measure that can establish an organization's baseline for patient satisfaction. Changes made in the system can then be monitored for their effect on care as reported by the patients.

Patient satisfaction data can be compared to other organizations nationally or locally. Cost and other clinical indicators could be supplemented with this patient-generated data during contract negotiations with payers.

These measures add consumer-driven data to other organizational success measures and have implications for clinical practice or processes of care delivery. For example, in the CABG systems improvement team, the patient satisfaction survey results indicated that a percentage of patients were in moderate pain more than 50 percent of the actual time they were hospitalized.

Reinfusion of this patient satisfaction data into the CABG CPR team resulted in an interdisciplinary subgroup formed to examine pain management in postoperative CABG patients. This team's goal is to establish a standardized approach to pain management for postoperative CABG patients.

Critical success measures should also include the effect of treatment and services provided on the patient's functioning. For example, is the patient able to return to a productive life postoperatively in terms of self-care and, if appropriate, return to work? In a capitated system it is imperative to measure the effects of healthcare services on the consumer over time. Functional status or health status has many definitions. The service, organization, or team needs to identify an appropriate definition for each patient's situation (e.g., a patient's ability to provide for the necessities of life).

The SF-36 instrument is a survey developed as part of the Medical Outcomes Study and the Rand Corporation. This instrument is an example of a functional status measure for adult patients that has established validity and reliability. It is user-friendly and takes 5 to 10 minutes for the patient to complete. Available standards and norms allow the team to establish their own baseline as well as evaluate themselves against others.

This instrument could be used by clinicians with individual patients or by an organization to measure the effect of treatment on a population of patients over time.

For surgical patients, data is obtained preoperatively, and at 3, 6, and 12 months postoperatively. There are computerized programs now available to collect and collate the data for analysis.

Adequate information is essential to any measurement process. An optimal situation includes an informatics system that automatically integrates clinical, cost, and quality data. This integration is not always available, and it is essential to recognize the time commitment required to make connections to put the data into useable form for clinical and quality decision making. Many organizations may not have these essential linkages in place at the present time. The process of linking the data requires a significant time commitment and can hinder progress at various times. An alternative might be to develop an intermediate database that could handle the linkage.

Many heathcare centers excel at data collection but are not able to translate the data into a meaningful performance evaluation. This may represent a lack of focus when drafting measurement criteria. When the critical success factors are representative of the team's objectives, they are more likely to commit to examining key measures to evaluate performance. An example from a patient satisfaction initiative illustrates this point. The objectives of measuring patient satisfaction are to

- Derive patient-generated reports of the processes of care and their satisfaction with the care

- Establish a baseline for future comparison

- Identify issues that currently exist

The first year's data indicated that patients in general were very satisfied with the care delivered and the caregivers. This initial evaluation produced a baseline that was acceptable to the team. A decision then needed to be made regarding future monitoring on each patient or at regular intervals as a quality control measure.

The team decided to continue with the survey for all patients interested, with a rationale that it gives each patient an opportunity to express his or her opinions and concerns. The results of the survey showed that patients were in moderate to severe pain most of the time they were hospitalized. This data was then reinfused into the quality process. A multidisciplinary team was formed to develop a standard approach to postoperative pain management. The patient satisfaction questionnaire was used to monitor the progress of the pain initiative.

Each organization usually has a regular reporting schedule for quality activities. Regular reporting is important and should not be confused with the intervals to evaluate progress. Time frames will be more realistic if they are based on mutually negotiated time lines. Gantt charts are a helpful tool for planning and evaluating progress.

The results of an analysis should be reinfused into the redesign process at the proper juncture. In the extubation example, the protocol resulted in other changes—a more consistent level of practice, a shorter length of time in the ICU, and reduced utilization of arterial blood gases.

There are instances when evaluation results in reassessment. If revisions are needed, then additional testing and evaluation at a designated time will also be necessary. In a team, available options can be evaluated to determine if revision or redesign is the most likely path to success. Feedback is critical to success; if changes are required, then the team should gather feedback from the those involved and renegotiate the plan.

Clinicians and other departments involved in the care delivery system must have feedback. In the extubation protocol example, the results were reported to the surgeons and nurses at their respective staff meetings as well as the hospital executive committee. Constant communication, involvement, and follow-through are the keys to the competition for each CPR initiative.

Financial success factors should be carefully scrutinized and documented. Not all redesign is focused on cost savings. The expected financial results and rationale should be documented. Clinicians who are working on quality teams may not fully appreciate the cost/charge or reimbursement consequences of the team objectives and participation increases their awareness. Statistical quality packages are available to assist with this effort.

New programs, redesigns, or improved processes of care need to be incorporated into the new organizational norm. If the team is multidisciplinary, then each member should represent and communicate with peers and respective departmental committees to ensure that all organizational and regulating agency criteria is considered and met. Small group discussion, one-on-one conversations, written communication, electronic communication, and teleconferencing are methods to exchange information.

If the change results in a new or revised protocol, then clinicians from the involved disciplines must be oriented. The expectation that the protocol is used can be measured in the clinician's performance review. Ongoing evaluation of the process and a means to communicate concerns should be identified during implementation. A designated individual and method is needed for individuals to comment on the protocol during the implementation phase. The comments should be collated and presented to the team at a predesignated time interval.

The efforts of the group should be acknowledged. The collaboration of the team and the represented departments and services should be documented and when possible rewarded.

The evolution of CPR: A case study (1993–1995)

TEAM DEVELOPMENT

In fall 1992, the University of Massachusetts Medical Center (UMMC) embarked on a cost containment project that focused on a specific category of patients rather than general cost issues. Three key areas were selected for this approach: orthopedics, cardiology, and oncology. All three represented both large-volume and high-cost patient care service lines.

Teams were developed to address the cost containment issues in the focus areas. Each team consisted of three key members: a physician, nurse, and administrator. The team efforts were directed toward four DRGs: DRG 121—complicated myocardial infarction; DRG 112—percutaneous transluminal coronary angioplasty; DRG 127—congestive heart failure; and DRG 141—unstable angina. The case study focuses on the acute myocardial infarction patient.

Team member selection consisted of the physician director of the coronary care unit, a cardiovascular clinical nurse specialist, and the nursing director of cardiovascular medical services. This clinically oriented group proceeded from a clinical perspective to reduce the cost of care for the four cardiac DRGs.

CLINICAL RESOURCE UTILIZATION DATA

Although the task of reducing costs and improving quality seemed clear, the enormity of such a charge was almost paralyzing. In support, the cost accounting department provided a tremendous amount of data directly related to these DRGs. All cost data was organized by the service department and was also presented on a total cost per admission basis. Although this provided important total cost information, its relationship to the patient care process was limited. Reorganizing this data on a daily cost and use basis was the first step toward gaining a better understanding of the resources that were used in caring for the complicated myocardial infarction patient. The team also narrowed the focus, at least initially, to costs generated in clinical pathology (blood work), radiology (x-rays), pulmonary arterial blood gases, and cardiology echo cardiograms (EKGs). This decision was based on the understanding that most of these costs were driven by the physician and nursing practice patterns. Since these were high-volume but relatively low-cost tests, there was little discussion about which test to order and when. Although the total patient charge per admission for these four departments ranged from 10 to 20 percent of the total patient bill, focus on this area provided an opportunity to reduce costs (and patient charges) and, more importantly, to reassess ordering practices and patterns.

RESOURCE UTILIZATION AND THE PATIENT CARE PROCESS

Unfortunately, the cost accounting system was unable to provide a daily usage report. Instead the cardiac care unit (CCU) nurse manager and clinician were forced to collect this information by hand over a four-month period. Although this activity was tedious, the resulting report provided an understanding of cost and resource utilization on a daily basis.

One very important result of this step, which would not have occurred if the cost accounting group had provided a computerized report, was the questioning of the link between the resource utilization and patient information obtained from these resource expenditures (e.g., How do test results impact care? How many positive or negative results are needed to confirm a diagnosis? When do the results become available?). Resource utilization may be effectively evaluated only after a detailed analysis by clinicians who understand costs and the clinical impact of these test results.

From October 1993 through March 1994 this analysis occurred for patients admitted to the CCU under DRG 121. By the completion of this phase of the project, the transition had been made from cost analysis to resource utilization analysis. It became clear that ordering patterns were not based on costs but on past clinical practice. Examining these practice patterns led to a redesign of house officer and nursing staff orientation and continuing education. Instead of telling practitioners not to order a test because it costs too much, clinicians were asked what information was obtained by ordering a certain test. Most importantly, the clinicians were asked if the result of a test added to the quality of patient care or just to the cost of care.

A result of this phase of the project was a clinical pathway for key resources (e.g., clinical pathology's blood work) used in the care process for this patient population (DRG 121). These guidelines are discussed each month during a resource utilization presentation for the house officers and attending physician on the CCU rotation. By using an approach based on clinical effectiveness, most practitioners are more receptive to examining their own practice patterns and accepting changes on clinical outcomes instead of financial spreadsheets.

During this phase of the project, the team leaders also examined resource utilization for the patient admitted with a complicated myocardial infarction. Doing so resulted in a complete redesign of the CCU orientation for house officers and an educational program for the critical care staff nurses caring for these patients.

Nurses and house officers were taught to ask themselves and each other how a test or procedure would affect the patient outcome. If information from a test would not be used to confirm a diagnosis or change the plan of care, it would not be adding value to the patient care process. Although this may seem rudimentary, resource utilization for the myocardial infarction population proves it is not. Instead of ordering by rote, these clinicians are challenged to order only what will have an impact on the patient outcome.

In academic medical centers, the major drivers of care and costs are house officers and, to a lesser degree, critical care nurses. Gaining commitment from these caregivers through regular structured educational sessions is a critical factor for the occurence of clinical process redesign. A structured educational program begins with an overview of past practices. Physicians, specifically house officers, are usually unaware of the total number of blood tests they order, which tests are ordered most frequently, and which are most expensive. Providing detailed information on ordering patterns for patients admitted with complicated myocardial infarctions presents cost information in a tangible and understandable manner. A key aspect of this program is asking physicians what clinical impact or value resulted when these resources were expended. Did they change the care process, confirm an unknown diagnosis, or just add to the cost of patient care?

One question that surfaced frequently during the house officers' and critical care staff nurses' monthly education programs pertained to the total gain from examining resource utilization. Savings generated by reducing the use of lab tests was in fact only a small portion of the cost of care for each patient. However, when the total impact was examined from a hospitalwide perspective, the savings were far more impressive. For example, by setting strict ordering guidelines for a frequently ordered cardiac lab test (e.g., CPK-MB) the hospital realized annualized savings in excess of $ 50,000 for this lab test alone. Although each patient's lab bill may only be moderately reduced, institutional impact is often quite significant.

Additionally, the goal of this project goes beyond the incremental savings from reductions in resource utilization for the complicated myocardial infarction patient. Redesigning the house officer orientation and critical care nurse continuing education leads to a better understanding of the process of care and its direct relationship to patient outcomes.

Success attained in the first phase of this project was important for future efforts and was a direct result of changing the physicians' and nurses' perceptions of their roles in resource utilization, which in turn led to a continued reduction of additional waste and elimination of duplication in other areas.

SYSTEMS IMPROVEMENT AND CPR TEAM

The team began developing a time line outlining the present care process for the complicated myocardial patient population. A macroflowchart developed early on provided a base to begin developing this tool that graphically presented the care process.

At this point the team had used many quality improvement tools such as brainstorming and Pareto charts. Reducing waste and eliminating duplication is a clinical process redesign activity. Initially the teams focused on quality improvements and matured into redesign. Both systems improvement and redesign approaches are needed at different times during a project. Deciding what approach to use depends on several factors including leadership commitment, examining the magnitude of the problem, and the availability of resources.

The systems improvement and CPR team's goals are both to improve the quality of care and to reduce costs. Achieving these goals is possible by applying quality or systems improvement activities as well as redesigning certain aspects of the care process. Understanding that incremental changes (e.g., reducing the number of blood tests) are effective at times while radical change (e.g., redesigning house officer orientation and nursing continuing education) is needed for other aspects of the process was a major turning point for the group.

Instead of being perceived as a cost containment team, it was now envisioned as a CPR team. The transition to basic quality improvement, to systems improvement team, and finally on to CPR was a critical transition. This development enabled the team to begin examining resource utilization beyond just blood work, x-rays, and EKGs. Some of the complex issues that surfaced were

- What other resources influence the process of care?

- When does the care process begin?

- What is the most effective hospitalization period?

With more complex and costly issues at stake a more diverse team with an expanded focus was required.

A second-generation team emerged consisting almost exclusively of clinicians (with only one nonclinical team member) from within the medical center as well as from key referral hospitals. The team comprised the following:

- University of Massachusetts team members

    CCU nurse manager and nurse clinician

    Three clinical nurse specialists from cardiology

    The emergency department medical director and nurse manager

    Quality management advisor

    International cardiologist

Nurse manager, cardiac rehabilitation

Chief of staff

- Referring hospital team members

Four referring hospitals' cardiologists

Emergency and ICU medical director and ICU nurse manager from one referring hospital

NEW TEAM FORMATION

Bringing together this group set the stage to begin redesigning the care process from initial patient contact through outpatient cardiac rehabilitation. After several hours of discussion in the first meeting, four key action items emerged:

1. Communication and patient transfer process

2. Standardized patient care (i.e., patterns or process)

3. Insurance issues, such as required preapproval for care

4. Long term follow-up

COMMUNICATION AND PATIENT TRANSFER PROCESS

Here, the team decided to focus on the communication and patient transfer process since all team members said this was in critical need of redesign. Considering that 80 percent of cardiac admissions are transfers from community hospitals, an efficient transfer system was of paramount importance.

Between the first and second meeting, team leaders examined the present communication system and the shadow system (i.e., a backup system born from the inefficiencies of the main system) that had developed due to numerous inefficiencies. This had evolved over many years with a variety of personal touches aimed at improving access. Incremental changes that had occurred over the years had transformed the original patient transfer and communication system into a cumbersome, nonstandardized obstacle to effective patient care. While most of the users of this system recognized system faults, efforts to improve or redesign were absent. Referring physicians who used the present system most frequently indicated that the number of phones calls required to transfer a patient and to communicate necessary information was a key failure.

During the second meeting, a flowchart of the present process required to transfer a patient was developed (independently of the team) by one of the affiliate hospitals. Although much effort went into the flowchart, team leaders felt that presenting it could lead the team toward more incremental improvements when radical redesign was actually needed. Considering this, the flowchart was not presented. Instead, a blank sheet was provided, giving the team the chance to design or redesign a system without biases or interference from past practice.

According to the referral physicians, an essential component of this redesign was a one-call telephone system. Community physicians transferring critically ill patients wanted to make one call, speak with attending physicians (e.g., emergency medicine, cardiology, and possibly an interventional cardiologist to be brought on-line for a brief conference call), and make a definitive treatment plan, including a decision on the mode of patient transportation (i.e., air versus ground ambulance).

This plan made sense to all involved. However, the system presently used, which had been developed over many years, carried many political trappings. Over the next three months numerous meetings were held between team members, interventional cardiologists, communication specialists, emergency medicine physicians, and hospital administration. After five months of work, the one-call communication and patient transfer system was accepted in principle.

REDESIGNING CARDIAC REHABILITATION

By focusing on the process of care, the team was able to examine the patient care process for DRG 121 (complicated myocardial infarction) from a broader perspective. Instead of just looking at daily resource utilization (e.g., labs, x-rays, and EKGs), issues that pertained to the entire episode of illness, including prehospital and long-term follow-up, surfaced. As the inpatient length of stay decreased, care providers needed to examine the total process of care. Activities requiring hospitalization versus an outpatient procedure were questioned.

One area that became a focal point was cardiac rehabilitation. This service is a necessary and valuable part of cardiac care, but when should the service be provided from a cost and, more importantly, from an outcome perspective?

Clinicians from all cardiac CPR teams were assembled to discuss where cardiac rehabilitation fit into the patient care time continuum. With decreased inpatient hospital lengths of stay, issues that were not relevant in the past began to influence the transition from inpatient to outpatient patient care. For example, most cardiac patients receive antianxiety medication or sedatives as a part of therapy and are often not in a state of mind conducive to learning about the need to make substantial lifestyle changes (e.g., change in diet, increasing exercise, smoking cessation, and stress reduction) during this phase of their recovery. In the past this was not a critical issue, since most patients usually remained in the hospital long enough to allow for their mental faculties to clear (from sedatives and the physiological impact of experiencing a critical illness and the accompanying anxiety and denial).

However, with less inpatient time, many patients are now leaving the hospital before they are fully prepared to absorb important behavior modification information needed to make these lifestyle changes that will reduce cardiac risk factors. This factor, along with high inpatient costs and low inpatient reimbursements, forced the team to reexamine when and where cardiac rehabilitation should begin. Team leaders in each of the four cardiac focus areas have developed clinical guidelines for cardiac rehabilitation, taking into consideration both the cost of this service and the value it adds to the inpatient care process. It became clear to all that a shift from inpatient to outpatient cardiac rehabilitation was mandatory.

A program has been developed that begins with a brief meeting with the patient, while still hospitalized, to discuss the need for outpatient cardiac rehabilitation. What has changed is that this meeting establishes the link between the patient and cardiac rehabilitative services. This meeting, or inpatient cardiac rehabilitation visit, will not serve as a therapeutic session. It serves as a means to identify risk factors the patient may have and expresses the importance of outpatient follow-up to assist in modifying lifestyle. Redesigning cardiac rehabilitation includes the understanding that this is a long-term process, requiring patient commitment toward substantial lifestyle changes, that will not be fulfilled by a few brief inpatient visits during the acute recovery phase.

This dramatic clinical process redesign has resulted in the focus of cardiac rehabilitation switching from inpatient to outpatient (when patients are more able to assimilate the information and participate in plan development), more individualized programs, and a substantial reduction in inpatient cardiac rehabilitation costs from approximately $300 per patient to less than $75 per patient (without an offsetting increase in outpatient costs).

Over the past two years, the cost of caring for the complicated myocardial infarction patient has been significantly reduced as a result of these efforts.

26

Tertiary care center: Using standard treatment protocols to manage costs and quality

John W. Meyer, MPH
Principal

Steven J. Lewis, MPA
Senior Associate
Ronning Management Group
Mammoth Lakes, California

Moira G. Feingold, MPA
Vice President
Oncology Resource Consultants, Inc.
Santa Monica, California

WHAT IS REENGINEERING CLINICAL CARE? It is the fundamental rethinking and radical redesign of business processes to achieve dramatic improvements in critical measures of performance such as quality, service, cost, and speed.[1] While reengineering can improve quality and cost, clinical process redesign is precarious, requiring healthcare to balance the need for radical redesign with the need for patient comfort and safety. Applying the best accepted industry practices as the foundation for clinical reengineering allows healthcare organizations to optimize value (defined as quality divided by cost) without risk to the patient.

The reason for reengineering clinical care is to standardize the complex care process, to create a consistent, reproducible, streamlined, and efficient patient care product. Efficient execution of procedures such as coronary artery bypass graft (CABG) surgery, percutaneous transluminal coronary angioplasty (PTCA), cardiac valve surgery, and total hip replacement surgery require the coordinated delivery of services from a wide variety of hospital departments, medical and nursing staff, and other clinical personnel. Delivery of high-value services means the patient receives clinically appropriate care delivered in the most efficient manner possible. The goal of clinical process reengineering on a product-by-product basis is to improve the value delivered to the customer.

Today, it is essential to reengineer care because the world around healthcare organization has changed, but the processes of care have remained the same and no longer supply products that meet the patients', payers', and providers' needs. Open-heart surgery patients and their family members often feel lost and disoriented as they are passed from coronary care unit (CCU) to step-down to a nursing unit, receiving care from a half-dozen different specialists along the way. Money is wasted and quality is compromised when an overloaded surgeon chronically admits patients a day early because it is the only way the physician can see them prior to the operating room; an old antibiotic regimen is repetitively applied because no one has had time to review the literature and update it; emergency CABG patients arrive unannounced at the operating room from the cardiac catheterization lab; or busy physicians spend time writing orders for patients instead of standardizing their decision making into protocols.

Unfortunately, the clinical and administrative activities of care have grown and evolved to meet the complex operating needs of the departments, providers, and institutions providing them. Thus, caregivers have looked inward and to what works for their professional group, division, or department, instead of organizing input processes around delivery of a medical or surgical product to meet customer and organizational needs.

In the past, clinical services have been delivered via the complex combination of inputs organized to maximize flexibility in the care delivered to each individual patient and to maximize the options available to each physician. Each physician was seen as a scientist-investigator, and it was believed that maximum physician flexibility and individualization of care equaled maximum quality for the patient and the maximum volume of life-improving innovations for the healthcare system. A system that preserved absolute individual physician choice and provided many innovations was built on an assumption of almost unlimited resources to provide care and was predicated on uncertainty regarding the best methods for providing that care. The system also operated on the assumption that maximum flexibility translated into maximum quality. Widespread attempts at innovation that were poorly supported by evidence coupled with processes of care organized around total individuality and flexibility have produced fragmented patient care with wide variability in cost and quality—or inconsistent product value.

Purchasers of healthcare services want to drastically reduce their expenses and reduce the rate of growth in those expenses. Healthcare organizations face a future of fixed or declining operating revenue. The historical uncertainty regarding methods and best practices applied to the average patient has declined with the development of an expansive network of information about the best practices in use for complex clinical care. This radical departure from the past leads to reengineering cardiac care delivery and other specialty healthcare services using a model of adaptive standardization that delivers a product of consistent value to the customers—patients, payers, and purchasers of care.

Reengineering clinical services provides a team-building foundation that supports center-of-excellence development, managed care contracting, cost reduction, and cost control. The redesign effort provides participants with a clear picture of the overall process and individual roles in the process and ownership of both the parts and the whole. Reengineering clinical services is essential to organizations interested in carve-out contracting and therefore essential to program survival.

Falling revenues in conjunction with the prospect of capitation and package-priced carve-out contracting for specialty services has made it important for hospitals to simultaneously manage cost and quality. By using a multidisciplinary group process to develop standard treatment protocols (STPs), hospitals and their medical staffs can address the most important healthcare products provided within major service lines. Using both clinical and financial data, groups of physicians, nurses, department managers, financial analysts, and administrators redesign key patterns of care within their healthcare organization, incorporating the best practices of their own and other institutions. The result is a new, standardized process outlined by a defined set of clinical guidelines that reduce unnecessary variation in care, eliminate redundant interventions, eliminate unnecessary care and resource use, push decision making down to where decisions need to be made and where information is, establish clear lines of communication for all caregivers, and reduce costs and length of stay. The patients, purchasers, medical staff, and hospital all benefit from the improved opportunities for managed care contracting, coordinated care processes, more efficient hospital operating systems, consensus-based quality measures, and reductions in the cost of care.

Improving value

Managing the costs of care while maintaining quality is a challenge physicians and healthcare executives face. Many methods to bring hospital costs under control have been tried with varying degrees of success. Although quality improvement efforts have been formidable, there has been little focus on techniques that simultaneously address quality and cost concerns. The challenge for hospital executives and medical staff leaders is to attack those basically inefficient hospital processes that fragment care, detract from quality, and contribute to unnecessarily high hospital costs.

Healthcare organizations have traditionally approached cost reduction and quality improvement as unrelated issues. Cost reductions have been achieved through layoffs, reductions in inventories and employee benefits, and "cut, slash, and trim" approaches. These methods provide short-term cost savings, but tend to create additional problems in the long run: fewer staff are available to work in an inefficient hospital system.

Quality assurance efforts typically employed what one author has called the "theory of bad apples." Also known as "quality by inspection," this theory holds that by searching out and eliminating "bad" employees, physicians, practices, and hospitals can achieve high-quality care.[2] This is perhaps best typified by the traditional peer review activities of hospital medical staffs, where samples of colleagues' cases are scrutinized for errors and omissions. Instead of searching for and fixing the process failures, most organizations fix something after it breaks, and refix it again and again. Total quality management and continuous quality improvement began the shift to process orientation in healthcare with the idea of incremental change, a concept with which healthcare providers are comfortable. Radical redesign concerns providers with the time and expense of clinical retraining and the patient risks inherent in making clinical process reengineering mistakes.

Managed care is a trend that continues to grow. HMO and PPO contracts encourage many hospitals to compete on the basis of price, rather than cost. Many hospitals had no real notion of what it costs to provide a particular service but agreed to provide care at reduced prices to secure more business. In many instances, this tactic forces hospitals to provide services on a deficit basis, surely a poor long-term strategy. Costs are then shifted or cut indiscriminately to retain institutional viability.

STP clinical process methodology

By using a structured group process, an interdisciplinary group of professionals redesign care for patients with selected diagnoses to create a standard treatment protocol (STP). Care is standardized, quality is improved, and costs are lowered by eliminating valueless or unnecessary tests, procedures, and interventions. The reengineering process that yields STPs identifies and eliminates duplication of effort and problems in interdepartmental coordination. A major goal in the development and implementation of STPs and supporting clinical pathways is the vertical compression of responsibility and authority. The STP allows decisions to be made where the information resides and where a decision is needed rather than forcing it up a chain of command. Once the process is reinvented, process owners and parties responsible for execution are identified and imbued with authority to work from the established guideline or pathway without further management or physician instruction.

STPS' GOALS

STPs' main goal is to increase value by raising quality and lowering costs primarily through defining, streamlining, and standardizing the best process of care for a typical patient in a diagnostic category. Reengineering clinical care entails an interdisciplinary group process focused to develop and implement STPs to increase the value of healthcare provided.[3] Where high-quality healthcare is provided at a low cost, the value to the patient and the purchaser is high. When the quality and cost is average, the value is average as well. When quality is low and cost is high, the value of the care received is a fraction of the value provided by the high-quality, low-cost provider. Figure 1 shows three examples of how value can vary significantly with relatively small changes in cost or quality. STPs are a comprehensive method to raise quality and lowering costs simultaneously.

Secondary goals of STP are to directly involve key physicians to build commitment and partnership with the hospital, to build commitment

FIGURE 1
Value = Quality ÷ Cost

	LOW ──────▶ HIGH			
Quality	0	1	2	3
Cost	0	1	2	3

Hospital A:	Hospital B:	Hospital C:
Quality = 1	Quality = 2	Quality = 3
Cost = 3	Cost = 2	Cost = 1
Value = ⅓	Value = 1	Value = 3

and cohesiveness with nursing and other hospital staff, to identify and correct hospital system inefficiencies that both undermine quality and add cost, and to understand the actual costs of providing care. The emphasis in developing STPs is clearly on process. STPs begin with a clean slate to be filled only with the essential components of care, not with guidelines or protocols gathered from other settings or existing organizational structure. Unlike arbitrary imposition of practice guidelines or standards developed by professional groups or based on statistical norms, STPs reflect the unique characteristics of the institution for which they are developed and the skills and practices of the institution's highest-quality practitioners.

The clinical process reengineering is completed by application of the five phase process outlined below.

Phase one: Data collection and analysis

Either staff or outside consultants collect external and internal data to support targets for identification for clinical process reengineering and average patient characterization. Phase one is also used to support the phase two opportunity analysis and development of the charge/cost model. This data collected includes hospital summary statistics, external clinical guideline and benchmarking information, and information regarding current processes and practices. Target procedures or diagnosis related groups (DRGs) for clinical process reengineering are identified at the end of this phase.

During phase one, three types of data are collected and analyzed, and clinical process reengineering targets are selected based on the information and issues generated.

External data. Clinical process redesign requires balancing the need for radical redesign with the need for patient comfort and safety and is conducted on the foundation of best accepted industry practices. This approach allows optimizing value without risk to the patient. A number of quality improvement tools have been implemented over the past five years. To be accepted, STPs must reflect local practice patterns and concomitantly reflect the useful research that has already been done to define best practices. Applying these tools has yielded industry-validated models, methods, and benchmarks that are useful to committees during the STP development process. These tools are particularly useful when committees work to resolve differences of opinion where the opinion of neutral, expert, and third-party sources may be the best path to resolution. As managed care organizations become more proficient in analyzing quality of care and more sophisticated in hospital scrutiny, they are likely to compare a hospital's clinical paths and STPs to nationally published guidelines. Familiarity with contents of national guidelines and their rationales will be increasingly important.

Available quality improvement tools differ in emphasis, the settings where they were developed, the professions that champion them, and their usefulness in any specific hospital. However, they have three qualities in common. First, they emphasize standardization (i.e., there is "one best way" to provide a service in a given setting, and the best way is also, by definition, the most cost effective). Second, as a prerequisite for adoption, they all require demonstrated effectiveness of a new process, and therefore, protect quality while reducing individualization of clinical care. Third, each method recognizes the shared responsibility for quality within the organization: quality is the responsibility of each person in the organization and in all aspects of the organization's work. The key characteristics of each approach are listed below.

Practice parameters define, from the physician's perspective, an effective means to diagnose, treat, and manage various conditions and diseases. An example can be found in the carotid endarterectomy practice parameter developed by the Joint Council of the Society for Vascular Surgery and the North American Chapter of the International Society for Cardiovascular Surgery.[4] Practice parameters are

- Developed by organized medical and surgical societies

- Designed to have national validity

- Clinically focused and disease or procedure oriented

- Not designed to directly address issues of costs or organizational problems

Outcomes measurements determine the most effective intervention for a condition or disease. Their rationale derives from research indicating that only a small portion of medical care is based on interventions proven to be superior to others.[5] An example is the Medicare Cooperative Cardiovascular Project (CCP), which is evaluating outcomes of cardiovascular procedures among Medicare beneficiaries. Outcomes measurements are

- Costly and time consuming to develop, since they are based on carefully designed health services research

- Designed to have national validity

- Focused on the physicians actions

- Not designed to directly address costs or organizational problems

Clinical indicators are statistically oriented standards or thresholds measuring the occurrence of desirable or undesirable processes or outcomes. For example, the clinical indicators for anesthesia, obstetrics, and oncology established by the Joint Commission on the Accreditation of Healthcare Organizations are[6]

- Imply a threshold of unacceptable occurrences or a proportion of cases that should meet a particular standard

- Focus on physician decisions or actions

- Scrutinize discrete points in the processes of care

- Do not address costs and indirectly address organizational problems

Clinical paths document essential steps in the diagnosis and treatment of a condition or procedure. (See Figure 2 for an example of a surgical clinical path.)

- They document a standard pattern of care to be followed for each patient

- They prompt care to be provided in each time increment (usually days)

- They list care to be provided by category such as x-rays, laboratory tests, surgical procedures, and patient teaching

- They focus on the patient

- They are developed primarily as a nursing tool in some institutions

- They are best developed by an interdisciplinary, collaborative process

Benchmarking identifies the best provider or practitioner of a given procedure, so that high-quality practices can be transferred to other settings. HCFA's Medicare Provider Analysis and Review (MEDPAR) database, state health databases, and hospital system databases such as the Voluntary Hospital Association's Clinical/Financial Information System, are examples of benchmarking.[7] Benchmarking may

- Be done on an individual, one-to-one basis by identifying high-quality institutions and searching out their successful processes

- Involve statistical comparisons of a particular hospital's characteristics of practice with large databases composed of other hospitals' data

Patient-centered care inverts the traditional model of care to place the patient philosophically and physically at the center of clinical functions.[8] This type of care may

- Reorganize the nursing unit to include radiology, laboratory, pharmacy, medical records, and business services functions on the unit

- Require cross-training of staff

- Use protocols and clinical paths

- Decrease nursing documentation demands

- Require a revolutionary rather than an incremental change in the healthcare organization

Indications and patient selection criteria specify which patients are candidates for particular procedures or treatments. As costs, quality, and outcomes are more carefully scrutinized, it is expected that more care

FIGURE 2

Example of a critical path: DRG 112 elective, scheduled PTCA; Length of stay = 1.5 days

	Home, preadmission	Day 1: Day of admit and PTCA; intake/cath
Treatments Consults and discharge planning		Patient to present two hours in advance of scheduled procedure to Heart Pavillion
Tests and procedures	EKG CXR if needed (except within 30 days) on chart, CBC, SMA-7, PT, PTT, platelet count (done less than seven days) Type and screen Notify MD for K+ <3.0, BUN >30, PT >16, PTT >45 (if pt *not* on Heparin), platelet count <100,000	EKG (repeat if available is more than 7 days old or episode of CP)
Treatments		Upon arrival to cath lab holding area: assess VS, CP/SOB, pedal pulses, allergies Consents obtained in holding room or MD office—PTCA/CABG Two hours before procedure, IV with 18ga needle and NS to TKO On-call void, send on stretcher wearing hospital gown Prep—right and left groin Height and weight on chart
Medications		One–two 80mg chewable baby ASA PO immediately preprocedure On-call preop meds per sedation protocol in cath holding or on floor: 10mg Valium PO PRN if patient on floor
Diet	NPO after midnight, check with surgeon if PM case	NPO except meds

Day 1: CV lab

MD assess or confirm this is "Critical Pathway" patient following procedure

Labs checked upon arrival
ACT during procedure
PRN (only after initiation of Heparinization)

Day 1: Sedated, sheath in place, telemetry unit bed

RN reviews patient status, takes appropriate action

Transfer to tele unit immediately on availability of the tele bed less than one hour after procedure complete

12-lead EKG on admission to tele if not done in cath lab holding area postprocedure

Assess IV
Prep and drape per MD order
Upon arrival assess CP/SOB, allergies, pulse
Arterial sheath insertion (venous sheath per MD request)
2–4 L O_2 NC to maintain Sa P_2 >94, DC post procedure
Oximetry
Cardiac monitor

Cardiac monitor
VS every 30 min × two, then every hour × six, then routine
Distal pulses and cath sites every hour and PRN
Follow skin-care protocol
Follow chest-pain protocol
Check groin, pedal pulses with VS
Insert Foley cath if patient has not voided in six hours
Notify MD if BP falls below 90, if pulse rate drops below 50, or no urine output in six hours
Helparinization per standard orders (Heparin infusion: minimum every six hours)
Hand aspirate and flush groin line(s) every hour with standard flush solution

Heparin: 10,000u bolus (range 10,000–15,000u)
ACT: check five min postadministration and one hour after bolus to determine next bolus or drip
Analgesia per cardiologist

NPO

Nubain 5–10mg IV every three–four hours PRN for discomfort, discontinue after patient ambulatory
Inaspine 2.5mg IV every four hours PRN nausea
Enteric coated ASA 325mg, 1 tab now and in AM if not allergic

Diet as tolerated, then push fluids

FIGURE 2 (CONTINUED)

		Day 1: Day of admit and
Treatments	Home, preadmission	PTCA; intake/cath
Activity	No restrictions	Up PRN with assistance
Patient and family teaching	MD office explains procedure	RN confirms preprocedural teaching done and answers patient and family questions. Patient informed of angina symptoms
Patient outcomes		Discuss the procedure. Complies with preprocedure instructions

will be taken to select patients who stand to benefit the most from a procedure. Indications and patient selection criteria can be useful as a starting point to define the average patient for whom the process is designed.

As guidelines, practice parameters, and outcomes measures are published nationally, they have become familiar components of clinical decision making in the community hospital setting.[9] STP process development provides an opportunity to adapt and customize standards from academic centers, using locally developed, consensus-based indications to determine candidates for a wide range of diagnostic and therapeutic procedures. Although the tools discussed above are useful to assist the movement toward a new, more coordinated process of care, adopting an exogenously developed practice guideline does not constitute reengineering. The tools and guidelines mentioned above are merely inputs to the process of reengineering clinical care—a tested foundation to allay patient risk and a means to document best practices and measuring the success of implementation efforts.

Internal data. To redesign care for a specific diagnosis—to create an ideal model of care—participants must first understand how care is currently being provided in the institution. Two types of internal data are collected: summary hospital data and documents that characterize current patterns of care. This information must be scrutinized to

Day 1: CV lab
Restricted

Day 1: Sedated, sheath in place, telemetry unit bed
BR—no bathroom privileges
Turn onto affected side PRN
HOB ≤30° (if flexible sheath, ≤60°)
May use soft restraint PRN

Instruct need for reduced mobility
Encourage patient to notify staff of problems
(e.g., chest pain, bleeding, leg pain)

Describes postprocedure activities, hemodynamically stable, absence or resolution of acute changes and hemorrhage of hematoma, absence of infection, adequate tissue perfusion: skin integrity and level of comfort

understand where redundancies and superfluous activities exist and to document and understand the extent of process variation. Documents maintained in most hospitals that assist to evaluate current patterns of care include patient management guidelines and protocols, preprinted orders, summary of local practice patterns, and practice parameters.

SUMMARY HOSPITAL DATA. To identify targets and develop a picture of the average patient (e.g., average planned admission for a coronary artery bypass procedure), it is necessary to collect all baseline statistics to support target selection, including average length of stay (ALOS), average charge per case, service volume, and Medicare reimbursement rate. Both financial model development and characterization of the average patient are supported by the retrieval and analysis of six months of patient bills for target procedures.

PATIENT MANAGEMENT GUIDELINES AND PROTOCOLS. Many hospital product lines have developed protocols to address their most important or costly diagnoses and treatments. These documents have typically arisen out of a desire to establish quality guidelines for internal use, with perhaps a secondary goal of cost control. Some hospitals have monitored compliance with guidelines as a form of quality review and therefore have some indication of how many patients were actually managed according to the guidelines.

PREPRINTED ORDERS. Many physicians have documented their preferred management practices in preprinted orders that are placed on the medical records of their patients. In any care setting, many versions of orders may exist for the same diagnoses. Some of the variation may be justified on the basis of different training and experience, but much is a matter of personal preference that cannot be justified in terms of quality of care. Comparing preprinted orders has two main purposes: it documents the diagnostic and therapeutic interventions currently provided to patients, and it also may demonstrate that differences existing between the standard orders of physicians are, in fact, easily reconciled.

LOCAL PRACTICE PATTERNS. In spite of professional association attempts to develop national standards of clinical practice, there are still significant differences remaining between practices in different regions of the country and between urban and rural areas. Some of this variation may be attributed to the range of resources available (particularly therapeutic) in a specific region, but a great deal of local area practice pattern variation cannot be explained in terms of resource availability.

The rapidity of the transfer of new medical knowledge from development in research centers to acceptance and use by experts varies significantly.[10] STPs accept the current best medical practice in a community or institution as a starting point, even if it varies from the national standard. The rationale is that healthcare professionals, and physicians in particular, will not adopt and use standard practices that do not reflect their beliefs and experiences or cannot be successfully replicated in their hospitals.

Identifying targets. Selection of target procedures and diagnoses. A process is a collection of activities that takes one or more kinds of input and creates outputs that are of value to the customer.[11] A hospital stay for CABG surgery or the care rendered to a patient for an acute myocardial infarction (AMI) or other episode of illness can be identified as a process. Most hospitals have taken a service-line approach to reengineering, beginning STP development with a small number of procedures or diagnoses and expanding it to other service lines once the first STPs are completed and implemented.

Significant time, effort, and energy are required to begin and complete clinical process reengineering. Physician resistance and concerns about the prospect of engaging in the practice of "cookbook medicine" can be difficult to overcome and the time and passion of staff difficult to marshall. For that reason, great care and attention should be exercised in selecting STP development targets worthy of the investment. Several criteria are used to select target procedures or diagnoses for which STPs will be developed.

VOLUME. Procedures that are done in large numbers in an institution are the logical primary target of STP development. Improvements in the quality and efficiency of the procedure will not only yield larger benefits to patients, payers, and physicians but also will provide greater cost savings, which enhances the financial stability of the institution. This may be particularly relevant to outpatient procedures, which may be relatively low cost, but are done in sufficiently large numbers to yield large overall savings.

HIGH COST. High-cost procedures or admissions, especially those that rely heavily on expensive technology, are also a logical starting point for STP development. Standardizing the use of high-cost equipment and supplies and eliminating their unnecessary use will quickly pay back the hospital for the time and effort involved to develop the STP.

MULTIPLE SPECIALTIES INVOLVED. The more medical specialties that are involved in a particular diagnosis, the higher costs are likely to be. More people also have the potential to increase miscommunication, delays, and errors. Depending on their condition, CABG surgery patients may receive care or services from more than six specialists during their stay, including noninvasive cardiologist, invasive cardiologist, radiologist, thoracic surgeon, pulmonologist, and anesthesiologist. To the extent that standardization can be introduced into the management of complex cases, both cost and quality are better controlled.

MULTIPLE NURSING UNITS. Diagnoses and treatments requiring patients to move to numerous care settings within the institution also lend themselves to STP development. A heart surgery patient who must move from operating room to recovery room, to cardiac care unit, to step-down unit, to the medical floor has a greater chance of being delayed at some stage than a medical patient who occupies the same bed for the entire stay. The motivation to standardize admission and discharge criteria and to streamline communication between units is compelling.

NICHE PROGRAMS. Hospitals that have developed programs targeting specific markets or that have created "centers of excellence" such as heart institutes, sports medicine, or women's health will frequently begin the STP process with diagnoses or procedures contained within those programs. As package-priced, carve-out contracting becomes the norm for specialty services, it will become even more important to demonstrate to payers the quality and cost-effectiveness of a specialty program.

POLITICAL CONSIDERATIONS, CUSTOMER COMPLAINTS, OR PRESSURE. Finally, medical staff or community healthcare politics may dictate a focus on a particular disease or procedure. For example, a local business health coalition may have particular concerns about the high costs involved in caring for pneumonia patients, while the medical staff has another diagnosis for STP development. Such external concerns may influence the procedures and diagnoses selected.

Phase two: Opportunity analysis

Opportunity analysis, which can begin as soon as target procedures have been identified, provides for early identification of major areas where opportunity exists for significant value improvement. Staff or consultants systematically review the current process to identify potential flow problems, cost drivers, system barriers, clinical issues, and interdepartmental communication problems. Opportunity analysis includes consideration of internal data gathered during phase one and staff interviews regarding current processes and practices. Information assembled in this phase supports the committee processes of phase three.

Phase two is dedicated to locating specific operational problems or discrepancies between the benchmark and actual practices and subsequently assigning a real dollar cost to them. This phase seeks to determine which process deficiencies have the greatest need and greatest potential for change as well as where the largest opportunity for redesign efforts lies. It is as important to determine the cost of fixing the problem as understanding the cost of retaining the problem. An analysis can provide focus and depth to the committees' redesign efforts.

The opportunity analysis is a chance to identify barriers to achieve optimal care that may include operational, system, or policy barriers (e.g., AMI patients receive thrombolytic drugs in the intensive care unit (ICU) only at the order of a cardiologist). Initially, internal summary information generated in phase one is reviewed and further analyzed. Then using a generic schematic of patient flow for a specific DRG or procedure, staff or consultants work their way through the care process, systematically interviewing medical, nursing, and technical staff to identify and characterize opportunities for quality improvement and cost reduction.

Staff conducting research would look for flow issues such as the progression of patients through the continuum of care during a hospital stay for CABG surgery. For example, does the average patient progress from the CCU to the step-down unit in a reasonable length of time compared to benchmark values? If the flow is interrupted and patients routinely remain in the CCU for an extended period of time, researchers may examine admitting and discharge criteria to determine if they are too restrictive. Alternatively they would want to examine step-down unit capacity and bed availability to evaluate the possibility of a bottleneck.

In one hospital, treatment for chest pain patients was delayed and CCU expenses inappropriately incurred because of an operating policy of the clinical laboratory. In another example, enzyme studies providing key diagnostic information to confirm or rule out AMI in chest pain patients was being delayed by a half day because the laboratory had established the procedure of running the tests as part of an automated batch process. The reason for the procedure was that it saved $30 per enzyme study, however it resulted in patient-endangering treatment delays or, frequently, an unnecessary $1,200 CCU stay.

Phase three: Committee process

Phase three may begin once targets are identified and the opportunity analysis is complete. Steps in phase three include formation of committees, protocol development, and implementation. Phase three has the effect of combining several jobs into one by unifying responsibility and authority for redesigning the overall clinical process. The committee structure, organization authority, and responsibilities are established and committees assembled. Committees are responsible for engineering the identified care processes and are the bodies that will develop end-product STPs and clinical supporting clinical pathways. Committee representatives provide for a two-way flow of communication during development of protocols and ownership of process. The implementation committee begins formulating its plans at the beginning of the project rather than waiting until after STP development has been completed to allow for rapid implementation (addressed in phase five).

STP development process. The end product of the clinical process reengineering is the STPs, which are developed through a structured group process and carried out in interdisciplinary committee meetings. While each committee structure in a hospital will be unique, a typical structure consists of an oversight committee that supervises and receives input from subcommittees concerned with hospital functions that play a role in the STP being developed. One example of a committee structure used to develop invasive cardiovascular STPs is included as Figure 3. The structure must be customized to each hospital. The subcommittees deal with issues relevant to their functional areas for each of the targeted diagnoses and treatments.

For example, in an STP for modified radical mastectomy for breast cancer, the laboratory committee will consider developing resource efficient operating policies for preadmission and hospital testing, ensuring that the proper tumor assays and pathological studies are carried out and that test results are communicated in a timely fashion. The nursing units committee will address issues of patient and family teaching, range-of-motion exercises, and wound care, in addition to overall issues of how to reduce ALOS and facilitate communication with other departments. The oncology protocol committee reviews, edits, and integrates the output of the other committees into a single STP for modified radical mastectomy, including the target length of stay for the procedure and standard outcome measures.

RECOMMENDED PARTICIPANTS. It is unwieldy and unwise to include in STP development every physician on the medical staff who treats a particular condition. In STP development, the notion of standard guidelines for treating any medical condition runs counter to the beliefs and self-images of many physicians. When the concept of STPs is first raised, it is not unusual to hear some physicians refer to it as cookbook medicine. Rather than convincing these physicians that the process and its outcome are not as threatening to physician autonomy as they fear, most hospitals choose another path. Selecting physicians who have already demonstrated an understanding of managed care contract requirements, a sophistication about the need for hospital practice changes, and a willingness to participate in those changes is the preferred route.

Furthermore, if STPs are to reflect the best practices available in the institution, the best physicians with the most efficient patterns of resource utilization must be invited to participate. These physicians are

FIGURE 3
**STP development committee structure for invasive
cardiovascular services
Example protocol development organization structure**

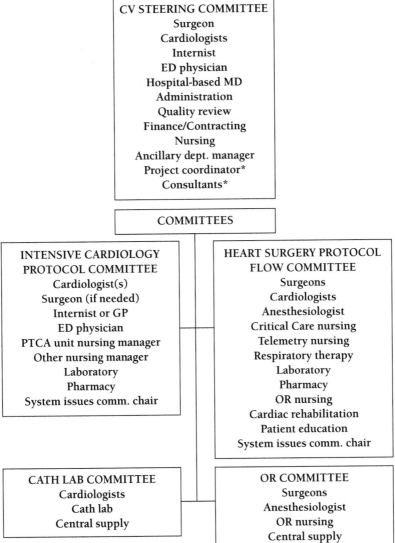

those most likely to understand that increased volume for the hospital
will work to their benefit and that the improvements made as a result of
the STP process will make their work easier and lead to greater patient
satisfaction. Those physicians, initially skeptical, may ask to participate

once STPs have been implemented and their impact on improvement, increased operational efficiency, reduced cost, and increased business—particularly from managed care systems—is determined. They are welcome to participate as long as they agree to use the STPs in managing their patients.

Other important participants include staff nurses; managers of nursing, surgery, laboratory, pharmacy, and radiology; others who play a major role in the process of care; and hospital-based physicians responsible for relevant departments and functions. Departments such as admitting, outpatient testing, and other support functions should be included since the timely processing of paperwork and reports is essential if length-of-stay targets are to be met. Administration should be represented at the oversight committee level, as full and unqualified support of the hospital leadership is essential.

Financial expertise is critical to the overall success of the process, not only in terms of interpreting cost and charge data but understanding billing procedures and reimbursement policies as well. To the extent possible, a finance person with some clinical knowledge is preferable in the STP process. Finally, a project coordinator familiar with the institution and its medical staff, with appropriate interpersonal skills and organizational ability, and the clinical background to coordinate the efforts of a large group of professionals is required.

PROCESS STEPS. The first step in the process is to convene the committees and provide them with an overview of the process and a report of opportunities for improvement developed through extensive preproject interviews with key personnel and review of relevant utilization information. The construction of a clinical path for each targeted procedure or diagnosis is the next key step. The process in each group begins with the question, "What must be done for a patient coming to the hospital for this procedure and when must it be done?" Whether the group starts from scratch with a clean page or starts by reviewing the existing pattern of care in the institution, the initial goal is to design a draft clinical path. System problems are quickly identified and solutions proposed. The charge/cost models, as well as existing preprinted orders, are used to support the process, as unnecessary tests and procedures are identified and removed. Different subcommittees may be responsible for portions of the path, for specific system issues, or for clarifying efficient procedures to streamline the process of care.

The oversight committee is ultimately responsible for ensuring that all issues are resolved and that key issues, including standard outcome measures and target lengths of stay, are addressed. In addition, the oversight committee integrates the work of the subcommittees into a coherent document, which is then refined and revised through additional meetings. A target length of stay is identified based on the aggregate of the diagnostic and therapeutic interventions performed during each day or portion of a day. A revised charge/cost model is prepared specifying only the interventions that remain in the clinical path and noting the cost savings potential associated with each patient managed according to the STP.

The STP document is prepared from the final draft of the clinical path, which reflects the target length of stay as well as the procedures and interventions the patient will receive during each time interval. STPs identify process ownership accountability and location of inputs in the overall process of care. While the clinical path is typically a single-page document, the reengineered STP may be many pages in length, documenting what is to be done for the patient, when it is to be done, and by whom. Editorial comments may be documented, key communications mechanisms highlighted, and new procedures stressed. Additionally, supporting protocols for input processes may be referenced (e.g., "Criteria for Routine Postoperative Extubation in SICU"). Sample pages from two STPs are included as Figures 4 and 5.

The final task of the oversight committee is to develop appropriate quality or outcome indicators for the STP. Part of the required monitoring process is designed to determine if patients are being managed according to the guidelines and which physicians are doing so. At least as important is the knowledge of whether patient outcomes are consistent with clinicians' expectations. Outcomes standards vary with the hospital and the procedures or diagnoses targeted, but at a minimum they should include length of stay, adverse occurrence rates, mortality rate, returns to surgery, and postoperative infection rates.

Time frame for completion. Most hospitals require four to six months to complete the STP development process. Much of the variation in completion time is a function of the extent to which clinical process reengineering and the STP concept are perceived by physicians as helpful to their practices. The actual committee work is typically completed in four to five meetings, held at two-week intervals. Advance data

FIGURE 4
Sample standard treatment protocol
(First two pages of 12-page STP)

General Medical Center

STANDARD TREATMENT PROTOCOL

TOTAL KNEE REPLACEMENT (PRIMARY ONLY)
Length of Stay   = 4.5 Days
AM Admit for Surgery*

Day of Stay   = 0 Day of Pre-Surgical Testing for Total Knee Replacement (target
                = greater than 72 hours before scheduled surgery).

CATEGORY   PROTOCOL

Unit   Pre-Surgical Testing

Dx Tests   1.   Type and screen

                2.   P9 (Creatinine, Albumin, Calcium, Glucose, Sodium,
                     Potassium, SGOT, BUN, Alkaline Phosphatase)

                3.   WHHP (whitecount, hematocrit, hemoglobin, platelets)

                4.   PT

                5.   UA (C & S if white count >5)

                6.   Bleeding time to be ordered only if patient has history of
                     bleeding problems documented by complete bleeding history.
                     History documented on history and physical.

                7.   ECG (if history of heart disease or if otherwise medically
                     indicated). Indications documented on pre-printed orders.
                     ECG to be less than 60 days old.

                8.   Chest x-ray if medically indicated. Indications documented on
                     pre-printed orders. X-ray to be less than 60 days old.

                Note: All labs to be less than 21 days old.

Treatment

Medications   1.   Patient will continue home medications until midnight prior to
                     admit day.

* Refer to Support Protocol entitled, Specialty PPO: Policy Statement on Lodging
          Services for AM Admits and Day Before Surgery Admits

- 1 -

STP - Total Knee Replacement

Activity	1.	No restrictions unless specified by physician.

Diet	1.	Unrestricted unless specified by physician.

Teaching   1. Patient to be instructed regarding the following:

    a. Medications past midnight and/or those to hold on pre-surgery day
    b. Patient to have viewed pre-op video
    c. "Patient News" to be taken home and read
    d. Pre-operative teaching
    e. Physical and occupational therapy
    f. NPO after midnight before surgery (except for prescribed medications). If on medications, they must be swallowed with small sips of water only while NPO
    g. If patient has a walker, instructed to bring walker with them on admit day
    h. IS instruction given
    i. Patient instructed to shower with Betadine/Phisohex PM before or AM of admit day and provided with supplies

Discharge Planning 1. Environmental Assessment Form to be completed as part of pre-surgical testing.

               2. Consult request to social services made as appropriate.

Consults 1. Anesthesia pre-surgical consultation

         2. Orthopedic resident to see patient

         3. Social services PM

         4. Home Health Coordinator PM

         5. Physical Therapy and/or Occupational Therapy to assess patient, overview procedure and rehab course

Other/Misc. 1. Pre-surgical testing staff to complete patient record by 3PM day prior to admission, to include:

    a. Signed consent forms
    b. Diagnosis test results
    c. Indications written for any ECG or CXR
    d. History and physical less than 7 days old
    e. Pre-surgical RN Assessment Form

- 2 -

FIGURE 5
Sample standard treatment protocol
(First two pages of 35-page STP)

General Medical Center

January 1993

DRG 104: VALVE PROCEDURE WITH CATHETERIZATION
Length of Stay = 9 Days

Day of Stay = 0 Day of Pre-Admission for Cardiac Catheterization

---

CATEGORY	PROTOCOL
Unit	Pre-Admission

Dx Tests	Pre-Cardiac Catheterization

1. Profile 7: Creatinine, SGOT, Calcium, Albumin, Glucose, Sodium, Potassium

2. X-ray of chest: PA and right lateral (may come from referral office)

3. 12 lead EKG (may come from referral office)

Treatment

Medications   1. Patients will typically continue on current medications. While patient is NPO, medications must be swallowed with small sips of water only.

Activity   1. No restrictions unless specified by physician.

Diet   1. NPO 6 hours before procedure (except for prescribed medications). NPO after midnight for AM procedures, clear liquid diet in AM if procedure is scheduled for PM.

Teaching   1. Pre-admission staff will provide patient with written materials over-viewing cardiac catheterization procedure and provide a verbal explanation of the procedure.

Other   1. Pre-admit staff to prepare patient admission folder to include the following information:

     a. SPPO patient either "local" or "out of town"
     b. General admission forms

- 1 -

STP - DRG 104

      c.   SPPO authorization form

      d.   History and physical; documentation of need for procedure (result of CV surgeon and cardiologist collaborative review)

      e.   Diagnostic test results from other institutions and physician offices

      f.   Chart sticker identifying "protocol patient"

      g.   Appropriate consent forms

2.   Pre-admission staff will complete social and environmental RN assessment as well as pre-surgical RN assessment

---

Day of Stay = 1 Day of Admission; Day of Cardiac Catheterization; Day of Confirmation of Need for Cardiac Valve Surgery; Day of Pre-Cardiac Valve Surgery Testing

---

CATEGORY	PROTOCOL

Unit   1.   CVL Recovery Room

Dx Tests   Pre-Cardiac Catheterization

    1.   Admitted to CVL Recovery early AM, pre-cardiac cath (all pre-admission documentation collated and available in CVL Recovery at time of patient admission).

Medications   Pre-Cardiac Catheterization

    1.   IV normal saline, 250cc, infuse at 50 ml per hour. Angiocath must be 20 gauge or larger if possible.

    2.   5 mg Valium IV for patients less than or equal to 65 years old, to be given in CVL if no allergy (to be given from CVL stock).

Diet   Pre-Cardiac Catheterization

    1.   NPO 6 hours before procedure (except that prescribed medications must be consumed with small sips of water only). NPO after midnight for AM procedures, clear liquid diet in AM if procedure is scheduled for PM.

Other   1.   CVL Recovery will complete pre-operative check list.

- 2 -

collection, interviews, development of the baseline charge/cost models, selection of participants, and orientation may occupy the first month of the process. Implementation times vary with the hospital's size and complexity, the number of diagnoses or procedures covered by STPs, the number of participating and nonparticipating physicians, and the capability of the institution's data systems.

Phase four: Development of financial models and cost finding
Phase four is primarily addressed through the efforts of the ad hoc committees (such as those on the cardiac catheterization laboratory, operating room, and CCU) that focus their work on the cost analysis and resolution of resource consumption issues that arise during the course of reengineering care to improve value.

Cost and charge information. The STP process uses a tool, sometimes called the charge/cost model, to construct a typical inpatient stay for the diagnosis or procedure under consideration. The charge/cost model serves three major functions. First, because it aggregates data from all discharges within a given diagnostic category over a recent time period (usually six months), it avoids singling out any one physician's resource utilization patterns. Second, it profiles the resource consumption of items chargeable to patients that are typically used. Third, because it lists every intervention, treatment, supply, and procedure received by the typical patient, as well as the direct and indirect costs associated with each, it provides a crude, initial map of current care patterns from which to begin to eliminate redundancies. Figure 6 shows a charge/cost model for an elective or scheduled PTCA.

Most hospitals, even those with cost accounting systems, have difficulty calculating with any accuracy the actual direct and indirect costs associated with a dose of medication, air-splint, catheter, procedure, or service provided to the patient. However, unless the cost of providing a procedure is understood, attempting to contract with payers to perform that procedure is an exercise in guesswork. Therefore, it is critically important to understand the impact of the process on the institution's costs. The charge/cost model begins with the pattern of care before the STP process is initiated to identify potentially redundant or unnecessary steps in the process and presents a second, post-STP pattern of care to be used to calculate actual cost savings. At this point, with complete costs documented, the hospital can selectively reduce prices, passing along the benefits of the STP process to patient and purchaser.

Phase five: Implementation

Phase five is a highly customized process where plans are developed for operating STPs and supporting clinical pathways. Issues addressed include the need for and schedule of formal STP education sessions for clinical and management staff, the content of that training, identification of where the STP and pathways will reside (e.g., medical record, nursing station, ancillary area, business offices, physician offices), and their distribution. Phase five activities include determining how best to make the shift from a highly individualized system of patient management to a standardized process of management by exception where only deviations from the protocol require a unique written order.

Reengineering efforts result in radical change and planning for movement to a new process must begin early. The implementation committee should be established and begin its work on development of STPs. To be effective, STPs must be fully implemented, their results monitored, and the process actively managed over time. Every hospital is unique and all STPs are developed under individual clinical and organizational circumstances. Implementation goals must include the following features: attaining maximum compliance with and reductions in unnecessary variances with STPs, identifying noncompliance and unnecessary variances with STPs, monitoring changes in physician and other caregiver practice patterns and making appropriate adjustments, ensuring that all caregivers completely understand the STPs, and establishing an ongoing mechanism for changing or updating STPs for appropriate clinical, technological, operational, and system reasons.

An extensive orientation must take place to familiarize all caregivers with the new best practices embodied in the STPs and establish a system to document variances from these best practices and monitor defined unnecessary variances. Also, quality outcomes must be measured over time through the design of new or modification of existing data systems and the overall process of care must be fine-tuned.

Perhaps the most significant challenge to implementation is physicians' use of the STPs. For a variety of reasons, not all physicians actively participate in the guideline development process. Successful implementation of STPs demands the widest possible usage, with the goal often

FIGURE 6

Simplified charge/cost model for an elective or scheduled PTCA

Cardiovascular services charge/cost model

Percutaneous transluminal coronary angioplasty (PTCA)—elective or scheduled

N = 125 patients

ALOS per unit: Telemetry unit 2.4 days + Cardiac surgical unit 0.0 days = 2.4 total
   days

Cost center	Item description	Average units	Unit charge
Blood	Blood type and screen	1.0	$26.00
Card	Coronary arteriogram	1.0	$800.00
Card	Coronary dilation (PTCA)	1.0	$3,400.00
EKG	EKG	2.0	$67.00
Lab	CBC without screening differential	1.0	$16.00
Lab	Cholesterol total	1.3	$12.00
Lab	HDL cholesterol	1.2	$9.00
Mon	Monitoring charge/hour	24.0	$35.00
Pharm	Aspirin 5 gr.	4.5	$1.24
Pharm	Halcion 0.125mg	2.1	$4.34
Pharm	Nitro 0.4mg	2.3	$11.00
Rad	Chest x-ray (two views—OR)	1.0	$98.00
R/B	Post-PTCA recovery (hours)	4.1	$129.00
R/B	Semiprivate room (8NW)	2.4	$285.00
Sup	Angioplasty supplies—misc.	1.0	$215.00
Sup	Bag-o-jet	1.0	$2.92
Sup	Catheter judkins (weighted average)	1.4	$132.00
Sup	Catheter pigtail	1.0	$62.00
Sup	CVL arteriogram tray	1.0	$87.00
Sup	Drape—adult angiograph	2.0	$21.00
Sup	EKG electrodes—package	1.2	$9.00
Sup	G.E. covers	3.0	$18.00
Sup	Introducer—sheath long	1.2	$76.00
Sup	Introducer—sheath SH	1.4	$56.00
Surg	OR standby	1.0	$400.00
	Adjustment factor	1.0	$0.00
	Totals		

complicated by political issues and unique circumstances. Often physicians will choose to quietly follow STPs without overtly accepting them,
while others may loudly choose not to follow them at all. This situation
must be managed creatively. While physicians cannot be forced to follow
guidelines they did not create, they ultimately can modify their behavior
as the result of education, peer pressure, and administrative direction

Total charge per vase	Cost/unit		Total vost per case
	Direct	Indirect	
$26.00	$11.00	$5.38	$16.38
$800.00	$360.00	$165.60	$525.60
$3,400.00	$2,100.00	$703.80	$2,803.80
$134.00	$23.00	$20.03	$86.06
$16.00	$4.00	$4.78	$8.78
$15.60	$5.00	$2.65	$9.95
$10.80	$3.56	$1.99	$6.66
$840.00	$21.35	$11.87	$797.28
$5.58	$0.04	$0.21	$1.13
$9.11	$1.56	$0.73	$4.81
$25.30	$3.67	$1.86	$12.72
$98.00	$45.00	$16.56	$61.56
$528.90	$65.50	$21.80	$357.93
$684.00	$194.00	$48.17	$581.21
$215.00	$165.00	$45.15	$210.15
$2.92	$0.67	$0.61	$1.28
$184.80	$43.57	$27.72	$99.95
$62.00	$32.00	$13.02	$45.02
$87.00	$32.54	$18.27	$50.81
$42.00	$12.30	$4.41	$33.42
$10.80	$3.65	$1.89	$6.65
$54.00	$4.48	$3.78	$24.78
$91.20	$26.70	$15.96	$51.19
$78.40	$34.00	$11.76	$64.06
$400.00	$231.77	$110.00	$341.77
$176.89	$65.12	$17.91	$83.03
$7,998.30			$6,285.98

and admonition. In some circumstances, it may be politically important to route all or part of STPs through the organized medical staff for review. The danger of this practice could be dilution of a best practice into a lowest common denominator practice. Ultimate acceptance may rest on the ability of administration to link use of the STPs with participation in managed care contracts or other inducements.

A careful plan must be developed by each hospital to address nonparticipating physicians. The hospital must identify an approach to each physician, individualize the message, and identify messengers to persuade the individual to adopt the STPs. To develop such a plan, administrators and peer physicians will work with resistant physicians differently based on their specialty, personality, practice goals, and the organizational culture. Requiring acceptance and implementation of STPs as a prerequisite for participation in specific managed care contracts, including distinct center of excellence contracts, can be a powerful incentive to participate. All approaches must be highly individualized, and incentives and disincentives need to be creatively structured to achieve the desired results.

Outcomes of the STP process

PRIMARY BENEFITS

Through the STP process, the hospital and its physicians have developed a consensus on how key patient groups should be treated. They also have developed ways to reduce the costs associated with caring for those patients. The hospital and its physicians have increased the quality of care delivered by identifying and institutionalizing best practices in the care of those patients and reducing unnecessary variation in their care. The hospital now has a system to monitor the care actually provided and a means to demonstrate to patients and payers that high-quality, cost-effective care is provided in that institution.

In one institution, length of stay in the five cardiac DRGs was reduced by an average of almost two days. In two of the DRGs (104 and 105, valve surgery), mortality decreased from 10.6 percent to 4.3 percent after STPs were implemented. In the other, lower-risk DRGs, mortality (already very low compared with national averages) either decreased insignificantly or remained the same.[12]

In addition to the cost savings, care processes in this hospital were streamlined. By revising test panels that included tests not used in clinical decision making, the hospital saved time as well as money in the laboratory. Discharge planning was standardized, initiated earlier, and uniformly received by all patients. Surgery preference cards were standardized for many procedures, eliminating redundant inventory and reducing opportunities for error in preparing surgical supplies. Revised preprinted orders were developed that reflected the consensus of the majority of physicians, eliminating the need for individual physicians' standing orders that actually reflected only small differences in practices and preferences. In short, as many aspects of care as could be agreed upon were standardized and set aside, allowing clinical efforts to be focused on the needs of individual patients. Documentation of care by nurses was shifted to a variance reporting system, freeing the nurses from unnecessary paperwork.

FINANCIAL BENEFITS

Financial benefits of the STP process arise from reduced costs and the opportunity to selectively lower prices or develop package pricing or carve-out programs, whereby one hospital reduced both costs and total charges in its invasive cardiovascular services product line by 10 to 26 percent using the STP process described herein.[13] In that institution, laboratory charges were decreased by an average of $800 a patient, operating room charges by $750, pharmacy charges by $550, and radiology charges by $350. Overall, the hospital was able to reduce its annual total costs by approximately $4.3 million on slightly more than 650 surgical procedures and more than 1,100 PCTAs. As a result of these cost reductions, the quality improvements noted in Figures 4 and 5, and the support of physicians, the hospital developed a successful specialty preferred provider organization that now offers reduced package prices for CABG surgery, PTCA, and valve surgery to area employers and insurers.

As a result of the STP process, the hospital has a revised charge/cost model reflecting the new best practice model that can be used as a utilization management tool. On a daily basis, actual resource utilization can be compared to the charge/cost model and, at the very least, comparisons can be made on a retrospective basis following discharge.

SECONDARY BENEFITS

Less easily quantified, but no less important, are increased communication and team-building benefits, as well as the opportunity to solve systems problems that plague every hospital. Communication is increased in two ways. First, the process of committee work breaks down many of the traditional barriers such as those separating physician and nurse or nurse and department manager. Second, the STP document specifies the actual process to be followed in treating the patient, where the treatment takes place, when it should happen, and who is responsible for making it happen. The development process as well as STP adoption eliminate many of the communication difficulties that result in missed appointments, patients being sent to radiology when they are supposed to have blood drawn, or paperwork not being ready when patients present at admitting.

STP team-building benefits are a direct result of the increased communication in committee meetings and part of the new standard process of care. The benefits of bringing together a group of professionals to tackle a common problem are well documented. The positive feelings engendered by a successful team process, evidenced by the solution of common problems, have positive results that extend beyond the immediate STP development process and into daily operations and strategic development efforts.

SYSTEMWIDE BENEFITS

The opportunity to solve hospital system problems is a significant benefit of the STP process. As participants in a product line begin to discuss the barriers to providing efficient care, they will inevitably come upon problems that are not within their power to solve. An example is the widespread problem of late starts in surgery. Typically when STP committees see this problem, they recognize that its solution may involve many individuals who are not part of the STP process. Here, hospital administration commits to finding a solution to the problem or the STP will become just another piece of paper. The active, visible, and visceral involvement and support of senior management is essential to the success of this effort. Identifying all the components of late starts in surgery may not be easy nor will it be a pleasant task to convene the responsible parties. However, if this problem is solved, the administration will have won the loyalty of the physicians who benefit from its solution and will have taken a major step toward securing the success of reengineering efforts in general and the particular STP.

Conclusion

Reengineering clinical services lays the foundation for a close working relationship and partnership between physicians and the healthcare organization. Joint interests are addressed to develop a common understanding of roles and responsibilities to deliver care and control quality and costs to produce a product that meets customer needs and hence organizational goals. By executing STP projects clinicians will learn more about resource consumption and cost, while financial and administrative staff members will increase their understanding of clinical aspects of care. Encouraging and building these relationships can only help a healthcare organization move closer to a common culture and to reach its clinical and business development goals.

Managing costs and quality simultaneously to increase the value of the care delivered is the biggest competitive challenge facing healthcare organizations. Traditional approaches simply have not addressed the issues of cost and quality as directly related. While many professional organizations have actively used various methods to manage cost and quality, they generally lack an integrated approach. Reengineering clinical care can produce significant benefits for the hospital that organizes for change and dedicates itself to increasing the value of clinical care delivered. Using a comprehensive, integrated approach to the cost/ quality interface provides a new and exciting methodology to position healthcare organizations for operational efficiency and competing on the basis of value.

NOTES

1. M. Hammer and J. Champy, *Reengineering the Corporation* (New York: Harper Business, 1993), 32.

2. D. M. Berwick "Continuous Improvement As an Ideal in Healthcare," *New England Journal of Medicine* 320 (Jan. 5, 1989): 53–56.

3. Ronning Management Group, Inc. uses Standard Treatment Protocols℠ (STPs) as part of a Strategic Cost Management℠ process for specialty product lines.

4. Joint Council for the Society for Vascular Surgery, "Practice guidelines for carotid endarterectomy," *Journal of Vascular Surgery* (March 1992).

5. G. Laffel and D. M. Berwick, "Quality in Healthcare," *Journal of the American Medical Association* 268, no. 3 (1992): 407–9.

6. Joint Commission on Accreditation of Healthcare Organizations, *Accreditation Manual for Hospitals* (Oakbrook Terrace, Ill: Joint Commission on Accreditation of Healthcare Organizations, 1992).

7.   E. Gardner, "Putting Guidelines into Practice," *Modern Healthcare* 7 (September 1992): 24–26.

8.   Interview with David Bernd, "Patient-focused Care Pays Hospital-wide Dividends," *Healthcare Strategic Management* (December 1992): 9–12.

9.   B. McCormick, "Can Research Change the Way MDs Practice Medicine?" *Hospitals* (October 5, 1990): 32–38.

10.   E. M. Antman, "A Comparison of Results of Meta-analyses of Randomized Control Trials and Recommendations of Clinical Experts: Treatments for Myocardial Infarction," *Journal of the American Medical Association* 268, no. 2 (1992): 240–48.

11.   M. Hammer and J. Champy, *Reengineering the Corporation* (New York: Harper Collins, 1993), 35.

12.   J. Meyer and M. Feingold, "Using Standard Treatment Protocols to Manage Costs and Quality of Hospital Services," *Hospital Technology Series Special Report* (Chicago: American Hospital Association, 1993) 16.

13.   Ibid., 17.

27

ScrippsHealth System: Redefining appropriate clinical care and financial results

Nancy Lakier
Operations Strategist
Scripps Memorial Hospital
La Jolla, California

SCRIPPSHEALTH HAS ACHIEVED up to 45 percent reductions in length of stay and 18 percent reductions in financial charges by fundamentally redesigning what care is to be delivered and when it is delivered using a process called clinical process reengineering. This process differs from patient-focused care or work reengineering that focuses on who can do the work and whether it is performed on nursing unit or in an ancillary department. A national consulting firm has estimated that between 5 and 15 percent of overall hospital costs can be reduced with clinical process reengineering. These percentages will continue to increase as technology is applied to healthcare delivery.

ScrippsHealth comprises six hospitals, two nursing homes, a home health agency, and various other healthcare support services. The ScrippsHealth physicians are world renowned. The organization is in one of the most competitive markets in the country as there has been a heavy impact of managed care and capitation. There were thirty plus hospitals in San Diego, a city of roughly 3 million people, only five years ago. Now, most of those hospitals have merged into just four healthcare systems.

Improvements in the quality of care delivered and reductions in the cost of delivering that care have been achieved simultaneously at

ScrippsHealth by using clinical process reengineering. Two examples of clinical improvements are reducing ventilator dependent nosocomial pneumonias and enhanced patient involvement in their care. Ventilator-dependent nosocomial pneumonias have been notably reduced to below the national average for the past three years. This was achieved by establishing extubation protocols that reduced the time patients were intubated. In addition to improving care, an estimated savings of $1.2 million for Scripps Memorial La Jolla patients was achieved by reducing the nosocomial pneumonia rate.

Another example that demonstrates greatly enhanced quality of care is seen in the increased satisfaction ScrippsHealth patients express in the patient education tool. This patient education tool is part of the Scripps clinical pathway and case management model called CareTracs. Patients and their families use CareTracs to plan, coordinate, and participate in their care. They know the expected plan for discharge prior to admission and plan accordingly. Frequently staff hear patients reminding family members to coordinate aspects related to their discharge and home health needs. Likewise, the patients know how many times activities are to occur during hospitalization, such as ambulation, and they actively participate in the planning for and completion of these activities. The patient and family participation has led to reducing the length of stay and, therefore, the cost of delivering the care.

Clinical process reengineering creates the environment that allows groups to achieve the kind of breakthrough change that is necessary to fundamentally redesign how care is delivered. It is a process that brings interdisciplinary clinicians together so they may determine the best way to provide care to a given patient population. The clinicians question and challenge existing traditions of delivering care and strive to achieve the most appropriate practice for that patient population. Clinical process reengineering calls for achieving consensus between physicians, nurses, and other clinicians regarding the minimum essential components of care for a similar group of patients.

Reengineering the clinical process is required to eliminate nonvalue-added care, to streamline and simplify systems such as documentation, and to create integrated, interdisciplinary processes. Clinical process reengineering was used to achieve dramatic change at ScrippsHealth, which resulted in the creation of a system to manage and document the predictable patient's progress through an episode of illness. This system is known as CareTracs.

Clinical pathways, case management, and exception-based documentation systems are often thought to serve as models for reengineering the clinical process. However, clinical pathways and case management have been implemented in hospitals without financial savings being achieved. Having these models in place alone does not mean that the most effective and efficient care process has been achieved. To achieve significant financial savings or to redefine how care is to be delivered, it is essential that reengineering principles and processes be used. Clinical process reengineering is critical in adapting to managed care as it is necessary to ensure that the essential components of care are delivered and that they are delivered on time, every time. This allows quality of care to be delivered at the lowest possible price.

Elimination of nonvalue-added work

One goal of reengineering must be to eliminate the nonvalue-added work that does not impact the quality of the patients' clinical outcomes. The organization must determine which activities do not positively impact the clinical outcomes of patients, and which activities should be considered for modification or elimination (e.g., What is important to do for a patient and what is not necessary). "Why" is a critical question that must be asked prior to ordering and delivering care. Some care is currently performed because it is routine; it is how the physician, nurse, or other clinician was trained; it is ingrained in the culture of an organization; or it is tradition within the healthcare profession at large. These routines and traditions must be challenged and changed.

For example, not all the clinical care adds value to patient outcomes. While ancillary testing is usually considered value-added care, does the current volume or frequency of CBCs, chest x-rays, or blood gas panels positively impact the clinical outcome of patient care? It is said that the physician's ordering pen is the most expensive piece of equipment in a hospital. If this is true, then how might a new system be created to ensure that all of the orders given are value-added in that they positively impact the clinical outcome of patient care. A key issue raised regarding the need for ancillary testing or diagnostic procedures revolves around the issue of litigation and defensive medicine. This can no longer be the justification for continuing to perform tests and diagnostic procedures. The key is to determine when it is important to perform a test or procedure and when it is unnecessary and the test or procedure can be eliminated. Defensive medicine can no longer be defended.

Simplification and integration

In reengineering, complex processes need to be streamlined and reduced to simplified processes for providing care and services. The culture of healthcare has valued complex processes more highly than simplified ones in the past. Clinicians have become experts in increasing the complexity of delivering healthcare and have been rewarded accordingly. Often each department has created its own complex systems to perform its specific function, thus yielding inter- and intradepartmental complexity in the delivery of patient care. It is critical to find new ways and new systems to restructure, simplify, and integrate clinical processes across all clinical disciplines and functional departmental lines. Interdisciplinary integration is crucial, and new systems must be founded on this principle.

For example, the documentation process presents a perfect illustration of the need to simplify. Historically, each time new information has been needed, a new form has been created. Independent flow sheets have been designed for each nursing and ancillary area without consistent formats and structures. Current systems require redundant documentation where it is not uncommon to write a given piece of information in multiple places. It is also not uncommon to see various disciplines document the same information, such as vital signs, patient status, and assessment characteristics, on a given patient. Thus, there is repetitive information in the patient record. Too frequently, clinical or critical pathways have not been integrated into the patient documentation system, causing more duplication. Patient documentation systems are typically not read by physicians or used as an important tool by all clinicians, indicating that the tool does not work and needs to be changed.

In summary, new systems in monitoring, documenting, and evaluating care are vital. Interdisciplinary systems that are streamlined to maximize the efficiency of the clinicians using them are needed to reduce the time clinicians spend on the task of documentation. In addition, eliminating useless, repetitive, and nonvalue-added information makes the patient record more useable by the physicians, nurses, and other clinicians.

Standardization of care

Patients clinically benefit the most from standardization of care when there is a predictable surgical course (e.g., total hip, knee, or cardiac valve replacement, cesarean section, or coronary artery bypass surgeries) or when progression through the episode of illness is expected to remain predictable (e.g., vaginal delivery, depression, and stroke patients). Hospitals benefit most from standardization when the most efficient yet effective care delivery process is achieved.

Historically, staff held care conferences to discuss individual patients and determine an interdisciplinary plan of care for specific patients. Clinical process reengineering takes that concept to a broader level and focuses on standardization for groups of patients. The standardization of care is one critical element that has been resisted by physicians, nurses, and clinicians. It has been called "cookbook medicine." Physicians, nurses, and other clinicians were trained to utilize independent critical thinking skills and judgment when delivering patient care. Clinical judgment was left to the individual practitioner to be exercised independently on a patient-by-patient basis. However, it is now essential to standardize care where appropriate. For predictable patient populations, such as patients having coronary bypass surgery or a total hip or knee surgery, it is important to determine best practice and standardize that practice across the patient population as long as patients remain on a predictable course. If a patient develops a complication, then the patient's progress is no longer predictable. Care is then continuously adjusted, based on the patient's needs, through the independent clinical judgment of physicians, nurses, and others. This planning may be minute by minute or over an extended period of time, depending on the patient's stability. This standardization of practice improves clinical outcomes. Best practice approaches are established for the predictable patient, and individual clinician judgment is used to meet the needs of unpredictable patients. Care is, therefore, focused according to patient needs.

Standardization does not mean that the practice should be the same on all units, at all hospitals, or across certain patient groups. There is probably no system that can be implemented exactly the same way in any two hospitals because the patients, physicians, clinicians, and cultures of each organization are different. It has not been possible to implement CareTracs across the ScrippsHealth organization because each Scripps-Health hospital is unique. The focus on clinical process reengineering allows clinicians to work together to fundamentally restructure the episode of illness for a hospital so as to maximize quality and minimize cost for that organization's patient population.

While the system, such as ScrippsHealth's CareTracs, may look different from one hospital to the next, many system components are beginning to be identified as foundational standards. ScrippsHealth CareTracs system is a product of dramatic clinical process reengineering that incorporated many elements critical in achieving breakthrough results. The process of clinical reengineering is critical in achieving quality and cost improvements. The process is what gets results.

CareTracs

What is CareTracs? It is a new method of planning and recording care so as to streamline existing care delivery systems. The template is built on clinical pathway methodology. It is the patient's interdisciplinary plan of care, an interdisciplinary documentation system, and a permanent part of the patient's medical record. It is also a patient education tool that allows the patient and family to have a detailed view of what will occur during an episode of illness and a patient communication tool that fosters communication between the patient, family, and clinical staff.

The ScrippsHealth CareTrac represents a change from a traditional, department-oriented approach of quality management to a systems approach where value can be assessed and cause and effect can be evaluated. The goal has been to create a system for determining, monitoring, and controlling care that allows for optimal clinical outcomes. This is achieved by developing strong partnerships between the medical staff, multidisciplinary clinicians, and hospital administration to maintain or increase the quality of care provided to patients while reducing the cost.

There are four goals to be achieved in a clinical process reengineering effort. It is important not to shy away from any of these goals but to find the right balance among them. These goals include

1. Improve quality

2. Reduce cost

3. Improve service responsiveness

4. Maintain or improve the work environment

There are 11 main concepts built into the CareTracs system. These concepts should serve only as a conceptual model or tool kit to be tailored to meet the needs of an individual organization during clinical process reengineering. The success of the ScrippsHealth model is a result of incorporating the main concepts of the CareTracs system along with the elements that were important to the ScrippsHealth care delivery system.

The 11 foundational concepts, methodologies, and tools built into the CareTracs system are as follows:

1. Outcome orientation; daily and discharge*

2. Patient and family integration*

3. Clinical pathway methodology*

4. Automated case management for the predictable patient populations

5. All-inclusive documentation system; flow sheets, assessments, plan of care, interventions, and evaluations*

6. Integration of ancillary or interdisciplinary systems*

7. Exception charting methodology

8. Standards of practice*

9. Standardized protocols*

10. Labor and supply utilization negotiation*

11. Roy's theoretic model

While the above concepts, methodologies, and tools are not in order of priority, because their importance as tools is dependent on the organization, the critical elements believed to be important in all systems are asterisked.

The first concept is that of an outcome orientation. Historically, care delivery systems have been set up around tasks or activities. It is critical to build care delivery systems for tomorrow around outcomes. Clinicians must constantly focus on how to move a patient toward clinical outcomes. This is important in order to move patients progressively toward a healthier state. Clinical outcomes must be broken up in such a fashion as to be easily understood and incorporated into care delivery. It will not work to have only outcomes such as "the patient will be discharged in four days." The outcome of a four-day discharge should be broken down, and daily outcomes or event outcomes need to be incorporated into the plan of care. This focus will cause staff to think in terms of an outcome orientation instead of a task orientation.

The second concept, patient and family integration, addresses the need to involve the patients and families in a much more dynamic way. Historically, patients did not experience any level of control over their hospitalization or episode of illness. Today, patients want and need a higher level of involvement and control. If it is critical for patients to take responsibility for their health, they must be taught how to be involved and how to take control. A plan must be created and communicated to patients so that they are educated to a level of understanding that allows them to assume responsibility for themselves and participate in improving their health. Patients should have tools at their disposal to maximize their involvement, and those tools should be integrated into their overall plans of care and patient records.

Patients and families of patients should be involved in the development of the care delivery systems. It is appropriate for individuals who have been hospitalized and their families to serve on design teams and evaluation committees. Patients are wise consumers, and their needs and desires should be considered in the reengineering efforts.

The third methodology, clinical pathways, is sometimes called "critical pathways." Many organizations have used this latter term to define their organization's system as synonymous with ScrippsHealth Care-Tracs or with clinical process reengineering. Clinical pathway methodology, as used here, is a template or format on which to create a broader conceptual system such as CareTracs. The CareTracs system uses a template that separates care into daily activities and event activities. An example of the daily clinical pathway template is when all aspects of care to be administered to an open-heart patient are broken down by day. Activities that occur prior to hospitalization, such as preoperative tests and education, are identified. Once the patient is admitted, the activities are divided by day: day of admission, day of surgery, postoperative day one, day two, day three, and day four. The same documentation system, based on the clinical pathway template, is used in the medical and surgical areas as well as in intensive care. Clinical pathways are frequently not the foundation for the documentation system as they are in the Care-Tracs system. Therefore, the key element identified here is the need to integrate clinical pathway methodology with the entire clinical process including the documentation system.

The fourth concept embraces the idea that the CareTrac system is an automated case management system and that the patients on a CareTrac are not in need of individualized case management by case managers. If a patient does not meet the outcomes specified for them, they are evaluated and, if necessary, a case manager is assigned. Frequently, however, patients are able to have minor adjustments to their plan of care, remain on the CareTracs, and not have to be handled by a case manager. Labor savings are then achieved by having some patients who do not need to be followed by a case manager. More importantly, case managers are focusing their attention on patients who are not predictable and need more constant monitoring to most effectively manage their episode of illness.

The fifth area addresses the need for all aspects of documentation to be incorporated into one system inclusive of flow sheets, assessments, the plan of care, interventions, and evaluations. Frequently, it does not work to fully integrate the assessment functions of all disciplines, yet it is helpful to have them be as consistent in format as possible. All disciplines should chart on integrated records rather than having their own form or record, incorporating as much interdisciplinary documentation on the flow sheets as possible. JCAHO has clearly articulated the need for interdisciplinary plans of care and the CareTracs system fully meets this regulatory requirement. Interventions should be integrated so as to capture the benefit of many disciplines working together to meet the needs of patients and to move patients toward achieving their stated outcomes. It also ensures the elimination of duplication among disciplines. The evaluation process improved dramatically at ScrippsHealth when physicians, nurses, and other clinicians began to work together to evaluate patient care. It is crucial to develop interdisciplinary evaluation tools and use them to improve the overall delivery of care for patients.

The sixth component is the need for the redesign work to be interdisciplinary or cross-functional in nature. The critical element is that all disciplines and all areas work together to create care delivery systems that maximize the value that each of the disciplines bring to the point of care for patients. A key question each reengineering team must answer is, "What are the measures to maximize the integration between disciplines and departments or functional areas?" In addition, it is critical to ensure that care delivery processes are smooth and nonduplicative between departments and disciplines. This is best achieved if all involved individuals and areas in any given clinical process are a part of creating the new care delivery systems.

The concept of exception charting is one that frees staff from having to write every observation, activity, and evaluation of patient care in the patient record. For litigious reasons, the norm has been that anything not documented was not done, therefore, everything is written in the chart whether it is important information or not. For example, nurses develop habitual patterns of charting, and batch charts at the end of their shifts result in information being forgotten. This results in pertinent information not being charted while mundane, routine information is. Examples of routine charting are "patient slept well," "vital signs stable," "patient's lungs clear and aerate throughout." Since the patient's medical record does not contain the pertinent information important to pass on about a patient, physicians, nurses, and other clinicians don't find the patient record easy or helpful to use. Exception charting corrects these problems as it allows routine and normal status reports to be standardized. As long as the patients status is within these standards, no documentation is required. Then the information documented is the information pertinent to be communicated between the physician, nurses, and other clinicians to move the patient toward the outcomes necessary for discharge. Streamlining patient information improves the level of care provided by allowing the physicians and clinicians to focus on what is important for the patient.

Standards of practice are necessary elements of any exception charting system. While nursing's standards of practice have historically been kept in binders on the nursing unit, they have not had sufficient depth to be used as the foundation of an exception charting system. In addition, the standards of practice have not been interdisciplinary in nature. Both of these elements are essential. The interdisciplinary standards of practice must have sufficient depth to support the staff's routine charting for the predictable patient's expected outcomes. They must be clear, concise, and readily accessible to the staff. They must also be routinely monitored so as to ensure staff compliance with the appropriate use of the standards. The standards of practice are approved by each appropriate clinical specialty prior to implementation. It is not possible to develop an exception-based documentation system without solid standards of practice. If the standards of practice are not complete, then the exception-based system puts the organization at legal risk.

Standardized protocols are the primary elements that streamline care, communicate the essential components of care for a patient population, allow nurses and other clinicians to exercise their clinical judgment based on clear established physician guidelines, and reduce the workload of the physician. Standardized protocols are developed in collaboration with the medical staff and are approved by the medical staff prior to implementation. These protocols are incorporated into the body of the documentation system so that the information is automatically available when that particular patient is admitted. An example of standardized protocols are extubation protocols. With extubation protocols, a standardized set of criteria is determined to demonstrate best practice for extubating a patient. When the patient meets the established criteria, the patient is extubated without an additional call to the physician to request permission. This practice is what significantly decreases the time patients are on ventilators in intensive care unit and, thus, significantly reduces the incidence of nosocomial pneumonia in patients being intubated.

The tenth concept of labor and supply utilization negotiation refers to the crucial aspect of raising the question of "Why?" regarding supplies and staff support. All disciplines, physicians, nurses, and other clinicians, should challenge each other to identify more efficient ways of achieving patient outcomes. This is the point to discuss whether the supplies used to care for patients may safely be trimmed or exchanged for less expensive options. This is an ideal time to challenge traditions and routines and ask whether there are less expensive ways to accomplish the same outcome. This discussion includes such items as prosthetic devices, catheters, tubing, and staff per case for a particular procedure or treatment. In addition, if significant savings are achieved through decreased documentation, the nurse-patient ratios should be reassessed and new ratios determined to ensure that appropriate levels of care at the right cost are achieved. This is done by using patient classification systems to evaluate the care needs of patients and the staff time needed to meet the patient's needs.

The final component to be addressed is the Roy model of nursing practice—the one selected by ScrippsHealth. It is an adaptation model that all disciplines agreed to use. It is not as important which model is used as long as there is a foundation for clinical practice to be incorporated. This must be well thought out in advance to build on the clinical practice strength that is already in place in the organization, or it should provide the opportunity to strengthen clinical practice by choosing a model on which to build the system. Practice models are perceived to be nursing based. Clinical process reengineering is not a nursing process. Therefore, it is crucial that all disciplines participate in selecting the model to be used.

The process

So how does clinical process reengineering proceed? The first step is to look at what needs to be done for the patient and when the activity should occur. What ancillary services (e.g., lab, radiology, or pharmacy) does a patient need on day one, two, and three? Should the hospitalization for a particular patient diagnosis be two, three, or four days? Should home health visits be made prior to hospitalization or after hospitalization? All clinical components of care that are delivered to the patient and the appropriateness and medical necessity of each component are discussed and a determination is made on each aspect of care that is important for a population of patients.

The reengineering work is achieved by teams of interdisciplinary staff meeting routinely to accomplish the work. Meeting frequency is based on the culture of the organization as well as the urgency to complete the work. Members are selected based on their clinical expertise related to that patient group. Both clinical and support staff are important team members. Additional members are added to the team, who know little or nothing about the clinical process being reengineered, for the purpose of challenging traditional thinking and continually asking the team, especially the clinicians, why they do what they do. This serves to continually challenge the clinicians to achieve the most efficient process of care. Physicians are needed to serve on the teams. However, the teamwork must be organized carefully to involve the physicians where their input is critical but not when other clinicians can make the necessary decisions, so as to use the physicians' time wisely.

The process utilizes continuous quality improvement, total quality management, and reengineering principles. The key is to not stop with small incremental change but to demand breakthrough change. Breakthrough change is what fundamentally alters how care is delivered. Breakthrough change allows value-added care to be delivered while significantly reducing the cost of delivering care.

Once the clinical process or processes have been reengineered, it is crucial to carefully plan for implementation. Implementation planning does not follow the same process as the developmental or design process. Rather, the process is more pragmatic in nature and must ensure that all support systems are in place and aligned. The team needed to plan for the implementation of the designed clinical process will need to include members of the design team as well as new members bringing needed skills, knowledge, and expertise.

The process must incorporate the new system into the organization for sustained change and this should be addressed during implementation planning. If the support systems surrounding clinical process reengineering are not also changed, then the new processes will soon erode and be unable to achieve or sustain the successes intended. One example of this is to consider inventory management systems to support the continued development, duplication, and distribution of new documentation forms. A broader perspective is to consider the need to incorporate the newly reengineered systems into the organization's quality improvement program. The work needed simply to support the new clinical processes designed is also critical and must not be overlooked.

Critical success factors

The developmental process may differ from one organization to another, but there are certain aspects that should be included every time to ensure success. These aspects are fundamental to reengineering.

Clear and specific targets need to be established so that everyone is aware of the clinical and financial goals to be achieved. Targets should be aggressive yet achievable. Targets should be communicated to the team responsible for the work, and the team needs to commit to them and be held accountable for getting the results.

Administration and management must demonstrate support for the clinical reengineering process. A key role for administration is to continually communicate the need for this reengineering process and report on the team's progress. Communication with all staff, especially with physicians, is crucial. It is also critical that administration stay in close contact with the team and take responsibility for removing barriers as they arise.

The interdisciplinary teams should include representation of all key stakeholders. Since the teams should be no more than 12 to 15 individuals if possible, it may be necessary to establish communication systems to ensure all critical individuals or disciplines are represented or, at the minimum, kept in the communication loop. There is typically a champion and a facilitator assigned to each team, and they are responsible for the work of the design team and follow-up after implementation. Expert nurses and other clinicians should be utilized whenever possible.

It is important to define the team's working rules to create team synergy. It is also important to define the level of authority of the team and what the expected result of their work is. For instance, the team needs to know that their recommendations will go to all necessary disciplines for clinical standard and protocol approval prior to implementation.

Frequently, a key question is where to begin. How does an organization decide which patient grouping or diagnostic related grouping (DRG) to begin with when undertaking clinical process reengineering? It is best to focus first on high-volume, high-cost, and problematic DRGs. It is important to avoid complex medical problems until the organization has experience in establishing these processes of care. A standard approach is to start with a specific DRG associated with physicians who are interested in working with administration on clinical process reengineering.

Absolute consensus on clinical protocols or plans of care is not necessary prior to implementation, but it is important to get agreement from key individuals who can move the initiative forward. It is also important to match the initiative to the organization's current market. If the market is not penetrated with managed care, then it is possible that significant process changes are not necessary to drop the cost of care as dramatically as managed care markets have demanded. It is more important to design the clinical process template and methodology to allow the organization to continue to review and adjust clinical processes in alignment with market changes as they occur. Clinical process reengineering is a crucial initiative to undertake to position the organization for managed care. The level of change targeted, ranging from nominal continuous improvement to significant breakthrough change, will depend on the amount of managed care in an organization's market. Ultimately, managed care will likely hit all markets and breakthrough change will be needed.

Data must be provided to and used by the interdisciplinary teams. Important data elements are current practice patterns, the community standard, best demonstrated practice from research literature, and national benchmarking systems. Practice must not be dictated to physicians, nurses, and other clinicians, but, rather, data must be provided so they may make the best decisions for the patients and the organization.

There are two CareTracs developed each time a new patient group or DRG is created. One is clinical, is used by the clinicians, and serves as the patient documentation record. The other is the patient and family CareTrac that is used by patients and their families before, during, and after their hospital stay. The CareTracs system includes documentation tools such as preprinted physician orders, flow sheets, medication and IV administration records, quality indicators, and educational materials.

In the process of reengineering a variety of aspects of the clinical process, clinical pathways, exception charting, and practice models, the significant gains come from integrating all the approaches into one system such as CareTracs. Systems-thinking principles are fundamental to the CareTracs system design. All components of the CareTracs system had to fully integrate with all aspects of the care delivery system.

The design and implementation of new CareTracs is viewed as quality planning and quality improvement. Since quality principles are used to plan and design new systems to improve patient care, this process constitutes quality planning. Significant quality improvements are achieved by the work teams, as well as by the implementation of new CareTracs. These efforts should be incorporated into an organization's quality process. In addition, once a CareTracs system is created, it becomes the template for continued improvement. The practice for a given DRG or patient grouping is then defined and can be reevaluated as often as necessary. If new technology or new procedures are created to improve care, the plan can be easily adjusted. If market conditions change, the plan can be reviewed and adjusted appropriately. Clinical process reengineering is not and should not be a static process.

Results

The results experienced by ScrippsHealth to date have been very positive. There has been a decrease in patient charges of 10 to 18 percent and length of stay reduced by 25 to 45 percent. For total knee surgery patients, DRG 209, the length of stay was reduced by 45 percent at the Scripps Encinitas hospital and by 28 percent at the Scripps La Jolla hospital. Patient charges were reduced by 8 and 15 percent respectively. This example also demonstrates that length of stay and charges are not reduced commensurately. For cardiac valve surgery with and without cardiac catheterization, DRGs 104 and 105, 33 and 37 percent length of stay reductions were achieved along with 6 and 18 percent reductions in patient charges. For cesarean section patients, the length of stay has been reduced by 40 and 19 percent for those patients without and with complications respectively. There are currently 55 CareTracs used in the ScrippsHealth system. New CareTracs are developed on an ongoing basis and continued modification occurs for existing CareTracs to keep current with clinical, market, and technological trends. An example of the advances or continued improvements made through ongoing reengineering is illustrated by Stanford Medical Center's recent an-nouncement that they used a new procedure to perform coronary artery bypass on patients and reduced the length of stay to two days.

Documentation time has been reduced at ScrippsHealth by 40 to 60 percent for medical and surgical patients. Savings have been achieved in all clinical areas, including the surgical areas. The average documentation is 30 minutes per case in ambulatory surgery and 40 minutes per case in inpatient surgery. Most importantly, the patient document is now used by clinicians to communicate pertinent, useful patient information. The percentage of physicians reading nurses', and other clinicians' notes has also dramatically improved.

Patients and families are very satisfied with the CareTracs system. Patients express that the system provides an overview of what to expect prior to hospitalization, a plan of what they are responsible to participate in during hospitalization, and an understanding of exactly what happened during their hospitalization for those who were too critical to follow it as care was rendered. Patients have taken their personal Care-Tracs to the physician's office after discharge and have even been seen to discuss their progress with other patients having the same diagnosis. Patients have expressed that the tool gives them a greater sense of control over their hospitalization and their illness. Families of patients express that the tool gives them an idea of what to expect each day. Knowing this, families have felt confident to collaborate with the nurses and other clinical staff to more actively participate in the patient's care.

Conclusion

Most reengineering efforts have focused on work restructuring that determines who will perform the activities of patient care and where an activity will occur. Clinical process reengineering focuses on what needs to occur and when it should occur to achieve the best clinical and financial outcomes for the patient and for the organization. In all forms of reengineering, "Why?" is the most important question of all. Why is an activity being done? Is it going to positively impact the clinical outcome for a patient? If not, it should be eliminated from the plan of care. The question of why must be asked at each stage of reengineering and asked repeatedly. While the goal is to improve both clinical and financial outcomes, the challenge is to improve the financial status while maintaining or improving quality.

San Diego healthcare operations are still in the middle of transitioning from "what was" to "what needs to be" in the future. The fact that change was and continues to be driven in California by economics creates the need to look at how to approach reengineering from a fiscal perspective as well as a quality perspective. Much emphasis has been placed on reducing costs in order to survive. Reengineering efforts have generated significant cost savings as well as quality improvements. The necessary shift is from providing whatever the patient wants under variable budgets to whatever the patient needs under fixed budgets.

One of the most important redesign strategies at ScrippsHealth was to increase treatment predictability through process and outcome standardization. Where a patient day used to be an asset during the fee-for-service era, a patient day is now a liability under managed care with fixed fees and capitation. It has become a vital necessity to manage every minute of the patient's hospitalization experience to orchestrate all aspects of care. This means increasing the patient's and family's involvement during the hospitalization in order to shift more responsibility to them. This means reducing the time that staff spends documenting care in order to decrease the overall labor cost of delivering care. Salary dollars must be spent on delivering care to patients, not on writing care directions for or duplicating the work of others.

In conclusion, these dramatic quality improvements and cost savings have been a key element of the reengineering at ScrippsHealth. The gains achieved by clinical process reengineering positioned Scripps-Health to compete in a managed care market. The gains achieved by clinical process reengineering also positioned the organization to provide better patient care to the patients it serves, to provide an enhanced practice arena for nurses, physicians, and other clinicians, and to reduce some of the pressures on physicians and nurses by involving them in the creation of systems that more effectively support the practices of medicine and nursing.

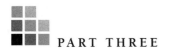

PART THREE

_____

Patient-focused care
case studies

28

Mercy Healthcare, St. Mary Medical Center, Spohn South: Implementing fundamental change in hospital settings

Glenn H. Snyder
Senior Associate
Booz·Allen & Hamilton, Inc.
*San Francisco, California**

J. Philip Lathrop
Vice President
Booz·Allen & Hamilton, Inc.
Chicago, Illinois

IN 1989, SIX INNOVATIVE HEALTH SYSTEMS created a consortium to design, evaluate, and implement a new patient care delivery system and structure aimed at lowering hospital costs and improving service levels.[1] Their efforts resulted in a new approach to care delivery operations called patient-focused care (PFC). PFC reflected the need to change the confusing, alienating, and fragmented patient care system formed to challenge reimbursement mechanisms of earlier decades. These organizations knew they had to change, but were stepping into unknown territory. Using their innovative drive, their strong belief in the principles and philosophy of change, and a fair amount of courage, they began to try a new patient care delivery approach.

Since 1989, PFC has become an industry buzzword. Many waited for proof that PFC concepts did produce outcomes worthy of the energy and investment required to make the change. The original innovators became "national healthcare laboratories" to validate the theoretical cost savings and quality improvements offered by the concepts' developers.

Positive preliminary results from these "experiments" encouraged many others to join the wave of change—anything to offer an advantage in increasingly competitive and overcapacity markets.

A number of hospitals have now taken the PFC concepts from an experiment to a hospitalwide operational philosophy and structure. The following three case studies profile institutions that employed these concepts organizationwide. Each started with a different set of outcome priorities, motivators, and barriers to change, and each has taken a slightly different approach to prioritize the operational and cultural changes. All have experienced positive economic outcomes. These organizations have successfully used PFC to improve care, save money, and increase physician and staff satisfaction.

This chapter is divided into two parts: an organizational case study that highlights three specific healthcare centers and a section on methodology that describes how to implement an organizationwide reengineering effort.

Organizational case study

The three case study organizations are Mercy Healthcare, San Diego, California; St. Mary Medical Center, Long Beach, California; and Spohn South, Corpus Christi, Texas. These three organizations have demonstrated excellence in the healthcare industry by showing their ability to effect change, using PFC restructuring to increase their competitiveness, with outcomes that improved operating costs, quality, and constituent satisfaction. Further, all have used PFC to change their cultures, reaping additional benefits often difficult to quantify.

All three institutions started with a similar set of principles for PFC reengineering, which included

- Deployment or decentralization of selected services to move them as close to the patient's bedside as possible

- Multiskilling or cross-training of staff so that a handful of different staff members can meet the majority of a patient's needs

- Process simplification to eliminate excessive administrative steps, handoffs, complexity, and ultimately work

- Management and organizational restructuring to enable a flatter organization designed around patients' continuum of care

- Empowerment to push accountability, responsibility, and control downward in the organization

- Teamwork to foster a collective focus rather than a functional (departmental) one

These principles were the only elements that were similar among the organizations.

CASE STUDY ORGANIZATIONS

Mercy Healthcare, located in the heart of San Diego, is part of the Catholic Healthcare West system. San Diego, like other cities in California, has seen a rapid evolution of managed and capitated care, forcing numerous mergers and affiliations among the list of contenders: Scripps Hospitals (now affiliated with Mercy to provide managed care services), Sharp Healthcare, University of California San Diego Medical Center, and Kaiser Foundation Hospitals. Mercy decided early on to focus, both internally and externally, on improving the hospital's competitive position. Mercy's desire for competitive differentiation drove it to try the PFC concepts when the original innovators were still assessing the benefits of their early experiments. As such, Mercy started small, as their predecessors had, but quickly embraced a vision to roll out the concepts to all facets of their operation. Today, Mercy is within two operating units away from a housewide rollout of PFC, and has begun to demonstrate the broad applicability of the PFC concepts by employing them in nonclinical areas such as finance.

St. Mary Medical Center, located in Long Beach, is part of the Sisters of Charity of the Incarnate Word Health System. St. Mary realized the status quo could lead to extinction in the competitive Los Angeles metro market. PFC became an effective mechanism to improve their cost and quality position while complementing their reputation as a caring institution with a strong community presence. St. Mary was the first hospital to completely restructure existing patient care delivery systems to PFC delivery, cutting the ribbon for their last phase of rollout in January 1994.

Spohn South fits into a different but increasingly familiar category. Spohn South, a brand-new 102-bed facility located in Corpus Christi, Texas, is part of the three-hospital, 650-bed Spohn Health System, which is considered to be the premier health provider in the Corpus Christi market. To sustain and build the system's leadership position, in light of an increasingly competitive market, the system's leaders felt it was imperative to embrace and implement a unique operational model. After researching the alternatives, they chose the PFC model to reduce operating costs while maintaining or improving service quality. Spohn South opened its doors in February of 1994 as a patient-focused organization after only six months of design and development work. The mother facility, Spohn Shoreline, is currently undertaking the transition to PFC as well.

Due to various factors, each of the three case study organizations chose significantly different routes to implement these concepts. Implementation options can be categorized as either unit-based or functional. Unit-based implementation implies the redesign of jobs, processes, and supporting structures in groups of 40 to 60 beds, changing nearly everything (bedside care, administrative functions, ancillary services, and service functions) for each small group of patients sequentially. Alternatively, functional implementation involves the implementation of new, multiskilled jobs housewide, or changing only a few things (for example, admitting, discharge planning, and coding) for all patients (typically in waves). Functional implementation, for example, would include the rollout of cross-trained service workers, performing housekeeping, food service, and light maintenance; followed by the rollout of cross-trained administrative workers, performing today's unit-based clerical functions, plus admissions, coding, utilization review; followed by cross-trained clinical workers, performing bedside care, therapies and diagnostics, as allowed by legal and personal-capability boundaries. Unit-based implementation allows for greater control of the scope and pace of change, while functional implementation allows for quicker restructuring of central departments (which tends to be the main lever for reducing costs).

DEVELOPMENT

Mercy Healthcare began a unit-based implementation method in late 1991 after six months of design and development. By mid-1995, Mercy implemented changes in all operating units and will have completed its formal restructuring of the remaining central departments. Mercy completed a substantial management restructuring effort in 1994 to reinforce its movement toward shared governance and empowerment. Although California state professional laws and regulations create additional barriers (over federal laws, such as the Clinical Laboratory Improvement

Amendments—CLIA) to cross-training, Mercy pushed hard to decentralize and cross-train (where possible) any commonly employed therapies and diagnostics, such as respiratory and physical therapy, pharmacy services, and basic laboratory and radiology diagnostics.

St. Mary spent more time up front than Mercy on design and development (13 months) preparing for a unit-based implementation. Midprocess, the organization realigned itself along patient-defined "business centers." This realignment was complemented by a complete reorganization of hospital management, placing an executive in charge of each multidisciplinary business center (versus the traditional groupings of housewide functions), thus enabling profit and loss accountability at a level lower than the CEO. St. Mary then started the implementation effort with a three-month prototype of the new approach on one unit. The organization efficiently applied the lessons learned from the single-unit experiment, which proved the concepts, to a fast-paced implementation across the rest of the hospital. The total time from the start of prototype was 11 months. St. Mary held back on deploying and cross-training some of the higher-skill, higher-capital services such as lab and radiology for several reasons: federal regulations such as CLIA, which dictate costly quality control processes that are difficult to manage for multiple lab sites; state licensure requirements, which make cross-training challenging by raising the threshold for educational requirements; and financial requirements, for the duplication of equipment, the investment in smaller and more portable equipment, and the creation of space in already-crowded units to harbor the equipment. Instead, St. Mary focused on decentralizing and cross-training administrative, service, and light clinical functions such as basic respiratory (e.g., oximetry, spirometry, and oxygen setups) and physical therapy procedures (e.g., gait training, hot- and cold-pack application, and range-of-motion exercises).

Spohn decided to adopt PFC for its new facility, Spohn South, to be opened in February of 1994. The organization began the design and development effort only six months before their opening target. Spohn South opened its doors with its new operational design in one swoop, though operational design continued to evolve. Physical therapy capabilities were incrementally deployed in summer 1994 and additional clinical deployment opportunities are currently being evaluated. The key to Spohn's operational evolution was the staff, who, despite being rooted in the "old way" (90 percent of staff came from Spohn Shoreline), embraced the PFC philosophy and actively sought ways to break down compartmentalization. The following pages describe Spohn's PFC savings based on staffing changes relative to a volume-adjusted version of its original (traditional) hospital staffing budget, rather than the actual pre-PFC staffing baseline used for the other two organizations.

A detailed summary of the scope and level of change implemented at the three case study organizations is shown in Table 1.

TABLE 1
Case study center summary

Primary changes	Mercy Healthcare	St. Mary Medical Center	Spohn South
Deployment or decentralization	All services as defined by patient needs	Most clinical services except radiology and lab; all service and administrative	Most clinical services except radiology, lab, advanced physical therapy; most service and administrative (no coding of patient chart)
Multiskilling or cross-training	Administrative, technical and service cross-trained jobs; some clinical cross-training	Administrative, technical and service cross-trained jobs; some clinical cross-training	Clinical, administrative, and service cross-trained jobs; development of case manager role
Process simplification	CQI councils actively review processes	Concerted effort between remaining central departments and deployed functions	No formalized process to root out more ambiguous opportunities
Management and organizational restructuring	Significant management restructuring; no business center structure	Management restructuring along business center lines	Management restructuring along business center lines
Empowerment	Shared governance formally employed	At director levels only; under way with staff empowerment	Shared governance system approved; to be implemented soon
Integrated care team structure	Some self-directed team structures	No formal care team structures	Service and clinical staff work together; no formal assignments

OUTCOMES

Most organizations considering structural change such as PFC ask, "Is it worth all the time and energy?" Many organizations have reaped the benefit of the PFC learning curve associated with the design, development, and operational changes defined by the original innovators. However, the process still requires an often-daunting 10 to 12 months to implement primary changes in high-priority areas, reaching enough critical mass to realize substantive cost reductions and service level improvements. The primary, high-priority changes are generally believed to be those functions conducted most frequently and come in the most direct contact with the patient (i.e., service functions, including housekeeping, light maintenance and nutrition services, admission and discharge functions, and light clinical functions). Thus, the question remains, is the cost for patient-focused restructuring justified?

The research conducted on these three case study organizations indicates that payback will occur within one to six years. Rates of return on investment will average more than 50 percent. Cost per case will decline by an average of 8 percent (including some length-of-stay reductions, which may be attributable to other factors such as managed care, capitation, and the resulting scrutiny of care management practices). Meanwhile, quality and satisfaction will be maintained or improved based on both qualitative surveys of patients, staff, and physicians and quantitative review of clinical indicators such as mortality, morbidity, falls, and nosocomial infections.

Analyses are based on results to date and conservative projections of expected future savings. Table 2 summarizes the investments required for each case organization, which include

- Facility, equipment, and information system capital

- Incremental wages incurred for design, development, and training

- Consulting fees

The range in investments shows the diversity in approach among the case organizations. For instance, Mercy Healthcare chose to incorporate substantial facility changes to enable PFC operational changes, including built-in medical supply cabinets in every room, rooms for unit

TABLE 2
Center statistical summary

Statistic	Mercy	St. Mary	Spohn
Full-time equivalent (FTE) baseline*	1,882	1,730	340
Net present value of investment (at 10 percent)**	$4,400,000	$3,900,000	$1,100,000
Starting admissions	19,500	14,000	3,400
Starting adjusted patient days	126,700	133,800	20,100

*   Baseline may not include all FTEs, such as community service, HMO, or PHO staff.
** Investment includes incremental training, consulting, and capital outlays.
Sources: Client reports and Booz·Allen & Hamilton analysis.

pharmacies and labs, and a new soft-landing tube system. Mercy coordinated these facility improvements and the associated operational changes with their routine refurbishment program, decreasing overall costs on an incremental basis. St. Mary, on the other hand, took a minimalist approach to capital investments, using portable medical supply carts in lieu of built-ins, and deferring the implementation of unit-based lab and radiology. Since the investment understandably varies by size of organization, as well as scope of change, investments ranged from $1 million to $4.5 million.

Despite the large investments, these three organizations realized significant economic benefits.[2] Their net wage and salary reductions (investments have been amortized in the savings) will average more than 5 percent on a volume-adjusted basis. Further, these organizations are realizing substantial reductions in length of stay because of improvements in service responsiveness and decision making. Reduction in hospital stays are due to a quicker turnaround of lab and other diagnostic test results and a higher level of unit-based clinician control over patient care decisions as a result of cross-training. When coupled with wage and salary reductions, these changes are driving overall cost per case down by 8 percent on average.

The size of the savings these three organizations are experiencing is a product of three main factors: the level of change implemented, the size of investment required to effect the change, and the time frame for implementation. Although the level of change varied among the organizations, investment and time frame probably contributed the most to the differential economics of the implementation projects. The progressive reduction in time frame and investment appears to be a result of two things: a willingness to risk housewide implementation (all at once versus within the boundaries of a controlled pilot environment); and a concerted effort to minimize the level of investment through prioritization of the potential changes (i.e., service, administrative, and light clinical first, lab and radiology later).

The move toward housewide, functional implementation has evolved as organizations became confident that PFC was not just an experiment anymore. Further, implementers discovered that they could not complete the bulk of work, job, and organization structure streamlining and corresponding cost reductions until the primary, high-priority changes are completed. (In the pilot implementation methodology, that means the majority of the units must be converted prior to reaching a critical mass point.)

Lower levels of investment also evolved from standardization and prioritization. Many of the early PFC implementers had the luxury of time and cash flow and, therefore, emphasized a "designed and created locally" approach. Since then, PFC implementers have seen an obvious repetition in PFC operational designs, giving comfort to a push toward customization of a standard design rather than a unique redesign effort at each organization. Prioritization has come into play in two regards: a focus on functionality (the ability to operate in a high-quality, consistent fashion) rather than aesthetics, and an emphasis on deployment and cross-training of noncapital-intensive services such as respiratory and physical therapy, versus lab and imaging.

To date, Mercy is the only one of the three case organizations that has completed thorough diagnostics of the differential effects on quality and constituent satisfaction. Its results mirror those of the original innovators, however, and are consistent with the anecdotal information collected at St. Mary and Spohn (Spohn did not have a "before case" for comparing statistics). The Mercy analysis quantified improvements in quality and service responsiveness for each measurement taken.

Further, the majority of staff and physicians agreed that PFC improved their ability to deliver care, the effectiveness of their care, and the patients' perception of care. Mercy also identified significant decreases in length of stay—as much as a full day on average in some care units—measured relative to non-PFC units (to rule out external effects). The reductions in length of stay can be attributed to redesigned documentation and care planning tools, reductions in turnaround times for diagnostic tests, and improved consistency in the on-time delivery of therapies affecting patient recovery. Each of the three organizations captured anecdotal information to further substantiate the improvements attributed to PFC. For example

- A woman in labor tries to phone her husband to tell him she is at the hospital, but the phone does not work. The patient and clinical associate panic. The service associate fixes the phone in 30 seconds and everyone is happy. (Normally, central maintenance would take one to two days to fix such an item.)

- Patients presenting for admission no longer have to wait for a half hour or more in the lobby and answer redundant questions as they are handed off from one staff member to another. Now they are greeted immediately, escorted to their room, admitted in their room, and begin receiving care—all within 15 minutes of arrival

- Administrative associates comment they never used to interact with each other (e.g., financial counseling with admitting) in the old world, so problems were never fixed. Now they meet to discuss them. Everyone tries to fix problems right away

- Clinical associates comment that patient service coordination is now much easier because staff members can either perform all functions themselves or can immediately find others to help

By sensibly decompartmentalizing, cross-training, and trimming process handoffs (e.g., allowing service workers to change light bulbs themselves rather than filling out a work request that routes through numerous people before it even reaches a maintenance worker), these three case organizations have made strides in quality and service, reinforcing these improvements with a continuous improvement mind-set.

COMPLEXITIES OF PFC CHANGE

Despite all the positive results experienced by the implementers of PFC, the process remains challenging and complex. As staff see the impending cost reductions dictated by market and governmental pressures, many resist change. At a minimum, anxiety levels increase until the staff sees how the changes affect them personally. Managers are often asked to help design new organizational structures that no longer include them.

Physicians are asked to adapt to many changes—care is now being delivered to their patients by a few cross-trained generalists rather than a large (and scattered) group of specialists. The specialist ancillary services they once controlled centrally are now fragmented, and they are being asked to standardize their care as part of the implementation of practice parameters. Meanwhile, they are struggling with some loss of independence dictated by market forces, since many are now joining physician-hospital organizations.

PFC also represents a set of philosophies that may not directly impact the bottom line. These cultural changes (e.g., teamwork, empowerment, ownership, and flexibility) are the least tangible changes and, therefore, the most difficult to employ. Change management experts suggest that such a cultural change will not fully engage until five years or more after initiation. Yet Spohn accomplished much of this cultural change overnight, according to staff comments and actions that reflect an integrated, nondepartmental attitude. Ultimately, PFC dictates and is sustained by behavioral modifications, which need to be reinforced with appropriate organizational norms (such as responsible risk taking, empowerment, and teamwork) and incentive structures (such as team-based incentives).

There is a long list of lessons learned, but the most pertinent to this group of second-generation PFC innovators revolve around implementation style and enabling the most desirable outcomes. These include

- Ensure a consistent top-management vision of change by reaching a tangible level of consensus. This can be enabled through the definition of individual roles and accountabilities and tied to incentives

- Lay the foundation for cultural change with communication and leadership by describing the vision and process and acting on the newly encouraged behaviors

- Do not reinvent the wheel; learn what other PFC organizations have designed, operationally and organizationally, and customize as necessary. (Do not assume that if it did not work for others, it will not work for your organization.)

- Start with the high-priority, high-rate-of-return changes (the highest-volume services requiring the least extensive investment in training and capital)

- Make changes in groups of departments (i.e., whole functions: administrative, service, and clinical) rather than one by one

- Implement the high-priority changes throughout the organization as possible to gain the critical mass that enables cost reductions; do not be risk averse

- Establish the tools necessary to measure the success or shortcomings of the change (e.g., information systems capable of recording service delivery on patient units; quality assurance procedures designed for decentralized operations)

SUMMARY

The original innovators gained the interest of the healthcare industry as their implementation of PFC generated positive economic and quality outcomes. But the three case study organizations set new standards for the pace and scope of PFC change. By eliminating work, changing skill mix, and reducing length of stay, they have strategically improved their ability to provide quality, patient-friendly, cost-effective care. The experiment, as defined in the late 1980s and early 1990s, is over. The new challenge will be to expand the horizons for which the PFC concepts are employed to include ambulatory, physician, and home delivery systems to create a more patient-friendly and cost-effective integrated delivery system. Furthermore, organizations will continue to develop ways to sustain the change, including incentive programs designed to reinforce a focus on teamwork and cost-effectiveness; innovative information systems allowing point-of-care access to an electronic patient record and facilitating multidisciplinary, multilocation care settings; and futuristic governance arrangements to foster empowerment, interdisciplinary coordination, and individual accountability. Who will be the next generation of innovators?

Methodology

There is no better way to discover how perfect today's organization is than to propose fundamental change. All of the current problems suddenly disappear, as the organization picks apart every possible difficulty it can imagine about the new world. Implementing change is not easy, but it can be managed.

The process for implementing an organizationwide reengineering effort must be both systematic and holistic in nature, addressing organizational and stakeholder needs. Methodologies for implementing PFC have evolved over the last six years, changing from a pilot-based approach to a functional approach. However, the focus on structural, step-function, organizationwide change has remained consistent versus a total quality management or continuous quality improvement (CQI) methodology that typically focuses on incremental, department-based change. Also, the end-game vision of a PFC operating approach still guides the effort, while the basic methodology of analysis, planning, design, implementation, and assessment has remained consistent. Finally, the recognition that PFC requires a change in individual behavior, group performance, and organizational culture remains the key to successful implementation. This last realization dictates a methodology that fosters trust, respect, communication, and participation by leadership and various constituencies.

A best practice methodology that includes five main steps is recommended. In the following summaries, which define the overall intent of each step, a medical treatment metaphor is used.

1. *Analysis.* The phasing and staging of the "disease" (based on the premise that a diagnosis has already been made, though, like some patients, some organizations have multisystem problems). The most obvious symptoms typically include poor service responsiveness, high delivery cost, and poor continuity of care. Investigation should reveal some of the causal agents, including excessive hierarchy, significant process complexity and fragmentation, functional compartmentalization, and job specialization. Given that a treatment must be applied in a holistic manner, the internal and external condition of the organization must be analyzed as well (e.g., internally, the readiness for change, constituency power and interests, capital resources, and information system infrastructure; externally, the strategic position in the organization's market, as well as local, state, and federal regulations)

2. *Planning.* Similar to a care plan, this step must define a map for transitioning the organization from its current state to some end-goal, which represents an achievable, clearly defined strategic, operational, and cultural state for the organization. To be effective, the plan must define clear and measurable milestones, and it must define individual responsibilities

3. *Design.* In medical practice, the design step equates to defining a surgical or clinical intervention used in the course of treatment. Some physicians or clinicians struggle to pioneer new procedural designs through laboratory or applied research; most choose to learn the designs of other pioneers and apply them to their own practice. The same can be said for organizational design. Many organizations strive to create their own unique designs; others borrow from the experiences of consultants or other reengineering organizations, customizing the results as necessary to reflect their organizations' unique internal and external conditions. The latter (the customizing group) benefits from a shorter design path and a lower level of risk in implementation. However, customization of others' ideas can result in less internal buy-in. The involvement of staff is critical to the successful completion of design

4. *Implementation.* This step includes the equivalent of preadmission testing, preparatory, and surgery (it is not likely that medical treatments alone will be effective). Coordinated, multidisciplinary teams should implement the plan once it has been defined. The preadmission testing analogy equates to the prototyping of organizational changes to surface any unforeseen problems. The preparatory step analogy equates to the development of enablers for the implementation effort—training programs for new skills, facilities retrofitting, information system modifications, equipment purchase and installation, and incentive system redesign. The surgery step analogy represents the changes implemented—the redesign and implementation of facilities, equipment, information systems, service locations, organization structure, job definitions, process flows, behaviors, and culture. Overall, implementation must be coordinated in manageable waves, rather than in a single huge leap

5. *Assessment and continuous improvement.* Essentially postsurgical care and home health. The organization's progress must be measured against the original care plan. Staff and management should be trained to recognize problems and symptoms for future early diagnosis and to use tools and skills to maintain and improve the new state of organizational health

For each of the five steps, it is necessary to focus on both content and process elements. The content (or product) of each step will ultimately define the quality of the overall reengineering effort. The process by which the five steps are applied will affect the ultimate acceptance of the change as well as the quality and speed of the reengineering effort. Process must address leadership, communication, and participation to engage the change agents and the organization as a whole. The following detailed descriptions address both content and process elements of best practice reengineering methodology.

STEP ONE—ANALYSIS

The analysis step will be instrumental in convincing organizational leaders and constituents (e.g., board members, physicians, staff, and patients) that reengineering is appropriate. More specifically, the analyses must help sort and prioritize the change effort. Organizations should begin by challenging and analyzing their strategy (what services are performed), their structure (how services and processes are performed), and their performance (how well services are performed). This three-phase methodology will create the greatest potential for substantive change, resulting in a more significant effect on cost and performance. The following outline refers to the structural elements, the focus of PFC change.

Objectives:

- Determine the current status and the extent of change necessary and identify improvement opportunities

- Educate management and other constituents about the urgency for change

- Assess organizational readiness for change

Content-oriented tasks:

- Conduct internal analyses to define the structural state of the organization, including analyses to determine its

    Structural compartmentalization—spans of control, job specialization, and service fragmentation

    Process complexity

Continuity of care

Service, quality, and cost performance

Demand—segmentation at macro- and microlevels and variability

Cultural cohesion—history of change and participation, and constituent power and resistance profile

- Conduct external analyses to help define guidelines for internal, structural change, including a demand trend, an evolution of service mission and vision summary, and an external constituent needs profile

- Define the opportunity for change in terms of service and quality improvements and cost reduction

- Develop an overall picture of the end-game operating structure, using a thick crayon, not a sharp pencil. The general picture should provide top management with a sense of the overall management structure, functional deployments, and the organizational location of jobs, activities, and accountabilities in the transformed enterprise. This will prove invaluable to make decisions as the process unwinds, especially for human resources issues

Process-oriented tasks:

- At the beginning of the analysis step, appoint a full-time project manager to provide continuity

- Construct a small team to complete and document the analyses, consisting of representatives from finance (to authenticate the numbers), information services (to help generate statistics), and management engineering (to facilitate process flow and other "industrial engineering" processes), and include an organizational dynamics expert (to help measure the cultural and behavioral issues)

- Use the analyses to educate management, staff, physicians, and other constituents on what works well, what does not, and potential opportunities for change

STEP TWO—PLANNING

Planning is a very important component for ensuring the successful implementation of PFC or reengineering changes. This step offers an opportunity to weave in the strengths of the old organization with the vision and spirit of the new one. A plan also serves as a road map from which the organization can measure its progress. Planning should not become a consuming aspect of the change effort, however, preventing change from actually being implemented. Thus, it is useful to keep an action-oriented attitude toward planning.

Objectives:

- Develop constituency acceptance in a set of principles of change (e.g., continuity of care-based restructuring, service deployment, job broadening, process simplification, and empowerment or hierarchy flattening)

- Develop a shared vision of the reengineered organization

- Develop a prioritized plan for change, seeking waves of change that bring the operation to new plateaus of performance where, if necessary, the organization can live comfortably and assess its progress

- Integrate PFC plan with the overall strategic agenda

Content-oriented tasks:

- Draft an implementation framework, which includes phasing of change (milestones), work steps, responsibilities, as well as communications

- Complete a financial pro forma analysis of reengineering effort

- Set new goals for quality, cost, and service performance across the organization

- Define a mechanism and process to measure performance against goals

Process-oriented tasks:

- Organize a change management team

- Begin rigorous communications to all constituents

- Practice new behaviors from the top on down, consistent with the new vision

STEP THREE—DESIGN

PFC is a structured approach to reengineer a healthcare provider to deliver all services in the most efficient, high-quality manner based primarily on the patient's requirements and desired clinical outcomes. PFC should completely redesign the organization from the basic mission, values, strategy, and principles on down. Everything is in play, and no question is too basic.

In practice, much of the design effort should focus on the new multidisciplinary administrative, service, and clinical roles. These roles help define a set of new work practices, jobs, and environments that translate into significant downsizing of central departments (and some corresponding "upsizing" of unit-based staff). An equal amount of design effort will be required to define the organization, policies, and infrastructure to support the new vision, though these aspects of design have less direct effect on cost reduction and service or quality improvement.

Implementation can and should begin in parallel to design. Several aspects of change do not require lengthy redesign efforts, will contribute significantly to reducing organizational anxiety (by making some tough changes early), and can produce significant cost reductions early on. Examples include management restructuring or rightsizing, and nonsalary expense reduction (through implementation of new practices and systems).

Objectives:

- Simplify clinical and nonclinical processes through work and job redesign

- Increase staff efficiency and effectiveness through broadened job designs

- Flatten organization structure through the use of teams and empowerment concepts

- Realign organization along continuity of care through the creation of multidisciplinary business units rather than functional departments

- Reengineer operations and operating strategy along all levels of organization, including corporate departments, business units, central departments, as well as work, job, and process levels

Content-oriented tasks:

- Institutional design—top managers design new management structure, operating policies, systems, and culture

- Operating center design—management teams design the strategy, organization structure, staffing, and service deployment for each new patient care center. (Because of high capital costs and nominal near-term reductions in personnel costs, most hospitals are deferring the decentralization and redeployment of major ancillaries [i.e., lab and x-ray] to later waves of the implementation process. On the other hand, almost all are addressing phlebotomy, EKG, and routine respiratory care deployment in their first wave of change.)

- Work design—multidisciplinary teams develop care delivery models, work flow, work practices, information systems, technologies, and self-directed team principles

- Job design—multidisciplinary teams develop new responsibilities and jobs based on integrating work around three functional roles: service, clinical, and administrative

- Central reorganization—management teams redesign and right-size remaining central or corporate activities to focus on deployed services and supporting the operating centers

- Other (optional but complementary)—nonsalary expenses and practice parameters

Process-oriented tasks:

- Assemble teams and team structure to carry out and facilitate design process

- Define design management and approval process

STEP FOUR—IMPLEMENTATION

The implementation step harnesses the energy exerted in the three prior steps and directs it to its goal. Implementation, like surgery for some patients, is what will save the ailing organization. Functional implementation (versus unit-based implementation) enables a quicker downsizing of central departments (as well as the complementary service and quality improvements realized through process simplification), which can be instrumental in healing the organization.

Realizing that implementation may mean downsizing, employees will grow increasingly fearful and anxious during this step. Change management (everything from basic communication, to involvement, to new incentives) thus becomes instrumental to foster the productive implementation of change. Uncertainty during the transformation is unavoidable, but also highly upsetting for employees. The worst of all worlds, however, involves "unbounded uncertainty" (i.e., "I can't tell for sure what will happen and, further, I don't know when I will know"). This points out the importance of having an overall game plan from the outset, at least to provide a response (e.g., "I don't know what will happen to your department, but we will address it in detail over the next 60 days").

Objectives:

- Complete implementation of the plan's milestones

- Accomplish goals as established in plan

- Involve all constituents

Content-oriented tasks:

- Redesign or modify all of the enablers of change, such as

  Job structure

  Incentive system

  Training program

  Facilities

  Documentation system

  Information systems

  Clinical and nonclinical equipment

Process-oriented tasks:

- Prototype high-risk changes in a small, controllable environment, only long enough to prove the viability of the change and evaluate alternatives as necessary

- Roll out changes as defined in the design stage. Focus on priority changes and on implementing quickly yet safely

- Manage the people aspect of change with carrots, sticks, and plain old communication

STEP FIVE—ASSESSMENT

The assessment step will be critical to evaluate how well the change plan is being implemented and whether the goals of change are being met (these are definitely two separate issues). The assessment step should be viewed as a newly adopted process to improve continually upon the organization's vision of service delivery. Although this may seem similar to CQI, PFC change begins with a much deeper and broader set of changes than is typically associated with CQI. The similarity is more in the use of the words "continuous" and "improvement" in that the organization must be willing to challenge its operating vision as it learns and as its environment changes (e.g., governmental regulations and managed care pressures).

The biggest enemy in change management is the "rubber-band effect," typical during change in any group that values the past. Individual behavior is an important enabler for change and individuals will often lapse back into the behavior patterns that come most naturally to them. The organization must therefore be prepared to administer a reward for new, correct behaviors. But it must first be able to assess whether the change is appropriate or appropriately implemented

Objectives:

- Determine whether the vision or design is appropriate for all aspects of service delivery

- Assess how well the vision or design was implemented

- Look for ways to improve and evolve the vision

Content-oriented tasks:

- Redesign the performance management system to

    Collect information necessary to properly evaluate change and accomplish performance goals under the new vision

    Tie performance into feedback and incentive systems

- Evaluate the effectiveness of change and compare, as applicable, to the analyses completed prechange

Process-oriented tasks:

- Establish a formal team to monitor performance relative to the new set of goals, the environment (e.g., market pressures, labor market changes), and the potential need to change performance goals

- Recognize and value change agents at all organizational levels

METHODOLOGY RULES-OF-THUMB

Effective change requires an intelligent, adventurous, and diligent mindset. Prior to initiating a change program such as PFC, keep in mind the following content focus:

- Create sustainable change—structural change focuses less on individual behavior and more on the system within which the individual works. Change that is less dependent on individual behavior is ultimately more sustainable

- Create step-function change (i.e., strategic and structural changes) rather than incremental change (i.e., performance-based change, such as adjusting departmental staffing to improve utilization). An incremental change approach will not enable simplification of organizational strategy, structure, and processes—a broader and deeper perspective is required

- Change the work required to provide service. Changing jobs and organization structures will not be effective in reducing cost of service delivery unless the work required to deliver patient services and the resulting processes are simplified

Effective change also requires leadership levels that exceed the typical operating-level leadership process. Key process success factors include

- Develop a clear and consistent management vision. Communicate the vision to constituents frequently to solicit buy-in

- Move as quickly as possible toward implementation and be action oriented. This orientation will require individual behavioral changes (healthcare employees are typically risk averse) as well as extremely effective team decision making

- Do not ignore organizational development issues (i.e., the development of a new culture). Cultural and behavioral changes must reinforce the operational vision and normally fit with concepts such as teamwork, empowerment, and responsible risk taking

- Focus the vision and the change effort on the tangible as well as the intangible (spanning the spectrum from facilities to culture)

Other, more specific lessons learned from some of the PFC implementation innovators include

- Make sure to redesign and implement a new performance measurement and productivity system to be able to financially manage the new operations

- Maintain momentum by staying action oriented; once momentum is lost, it is difficult to gain back

- Push past the level of comfort in redesigning jobs and processes. It is easier to pull the structure back toward "the old way" than it is to incrementalize it to a new vision

- Assign dedicated project staff to the effort, and define individual accountabilities for the project staff and operating management. It becomes easy for instrumental people to put this planning effort on the bottom of the stack of important issues to address

- Provide and maintain focus for the project staff and for all constituents (e.g., do not let PFC be one of five simultaneous efforts being implemented)

- Reorganize management upfront to make the new vision more tangible, and increase accountability of the management team to pull the change along. Also, up-front management restructuring releases some of the anxiety of change

NOTES

1. The six systems were Bishop Clarkson Memorial Hospital, Omaha, Nebraska; Crawford Long Hospital of Emory University, Atlanta, Georgia; Lakeland Regional Medical Center, Lakeland, Florida; St. Vincent Hospital and Health Care Center, Indianapolis, Indiana; Sentara Health System, Norfolk, Virginia; and Vanderbilt University Hospital and Clinic, Nashville, Tennessee.

2. Economic outcomes were calculated based on constant wage rates and service offerings. Some data represent centers' projected performance.

* Author Glenn H. Snyder has accepted a position with Deloitte and Touche Consulting Group in San Francisco, California, since the completion of this chapter.

29

Vanderbilt University Hospital and Clinic: Retooling medical care through collaborative organization design

Wendy L. Baker
Business Manager, Primary Care Network
University of Michigan Health System
Ann Arbor, Michigan

Marilyn A. Dubree
Director, Patient Care Services
Vanderbilt University Hospital
Nashville, Tennessee

As early as 1989, leaders at Vanderbilt University Hospital and Clinic (VUH/TVC) considered dramatically altering the way patient care was organized. Consisting of a hospital, children's hospital, clinic, medical school, and nursing school, the medical center is a typically large and complex academic center. At that time managed care was a fraction of the Nashville market, and inpatient admissions were at an all-time high. In spite of relatively stable patient satisfaction scores and reasonable quality marks, staff and patients often complained about the inefficiency of the patient care system.

Hospital and clinic executives joined a small consortium to consider how the concepts of the patient-focused hospital might be tested at VUH/TVC.[1] The decision to apply those concepts in a relocated orthopedic unit was the formal beginning of retooling the academic health center.

In 1989 and 1990 the hospital and clinic received a planning and implementation grant from the Robert Wood Johnson Foundation and the Pew Charitable Trusts to improve patient care and the quality of work life. Originally intended to rethink how nursing care was organized and delivered, the planning groups ultimately involved the range of disciplines and departments responsible for patient care. The grant provided the seed money for the Center for Patient Care Innovation that provided technical and planning expertise to internal teams to improve operations in a cost-neutral fashion.

Between 1990 and 1991 VUH/TVC became increasingly concerned that it was one of the most expensive university hospitals in the country. Anticipating a worst-case financial scenario of a changing reimbursement environment, the hospital and clinic launched a cost reduction and operations improvement initiative in July 1991, which saved more than $30 million. The prime directive to operations improvement teams was to save money. This charge was distinctly different from that given to earlier teams who were directed to improve quality in a cost-neutral or cost-saving fashion.

During the summer of 1993, hospital leadership watched the Tennessee marketplace transform to compete more on cost. The threat of a state-managed care program (i.e., TennCare) to replace Medicaid seemed imminent. With the advent of TennCare, a managed care program for Tennessee Medicaid recipients, the percentage of Vanderbilt's managed care business grew from approximately 6 percent to nearly 30 percent. Although VUH/TVC's cost competitiveness had improved, patient satisfaction scores were declining. The orthopedic project had demonstrated that dramatic reorganization of care around the patient could be done. Operations Improvement had applied the idea of decentralizing management of all patient care services to create RN-led, unit-based teams that used the least expensive, most appropriately trained workers. By focusing largely on discrete inpatient units, both initiatives had not improved the core work processes of the hospital and clinic—admitting, diagnosing, treating, and discharging patients.

With origins in a documentation-by-exception system, which developed in the orthopedic redesign project, the collaborative care system was gradually established between 1990 and 1993. The initiative provided an additional strategy to improve coordination of care and reduce costs by focusing on an episode of illness.

During summer 1993, executive leadership decided on a collaborative approach to improve the core work processes of the hospital and clinic.[2]

The model built on multiple, preexisting improvement initiatives while fundamentally examining and designing a better patient care system.

This chapter describes the individual improvement efforts undertaken by VUH/TVC and the analysis and redesign of fundamental hospital and clinic work processes that constituted the collaborative organization design methodology.

Building blocks of integrated change

ORTHOPEDIC REDESIGN PROJECT

The Orthopedic Redesign Project (ORP) was undertaken to demonstrate that significant work redesign could increase quality, decrease cost, and improve satisfaction among patients, staff, and physicians. The physically and conceptually redesigned unit opened in a new location in July 1990. The redesign was based on the premise that a certain amount of patient care could be done by a variety of workers. Only a small part of the work of each discipline or department is "specialized" (i.e., required by license). Thus, the unit operating philosophy became "never hand off what you can do yourself." By eliminating multiple levels of management and limiting patient transport on and off the unit, improvement resulted. The redesign assumed that the major costs and inefficiencies in delivering patient care reside in the structure of the work or the "how its done."

The steps in the redesign process were

1. Analyze work processes, including

   a. Clinical, administrative, and service jobs and work of patient care from admission through discharge (not including the operating room)

   b. Organizing work into shareable, worthwhile ("value-added"), and deferrable work categories

2. Reconstruct jobs based on the work process analysis and criteria for holistic work

3. Determine the behavioral qualities required to successfully execute the job. These qualities drive the behavioral interviewing questions

4. Develop evaluation parameters, internal and external communication strategies, and plans to manage regulatory and licensure issues (concurrently with steps one, two, and three)

5. Forge agreements with radiology, medical records, and physical therapy to try the model

The planning process produced a unit model with four major characteristics: (1) work shared by staff whose job responsibilities overlapped, ignoring traditional departmental boundaries (e.g., a respiratory therapist helps the patient to the toilet if need be), (2) a unit-based governance and problem-solving system, (3) a critical path, protocol-driven documentation-by-exception system, and (4) decentralized or unit-based ancillary services (e.g. housekeeping, patient transport, radiology, laboratory, admitting, medical records, and nutrition services). Although unit based, the pharmacy, physical therapy, occupational therapy, and social work were still responsible to the central department.

TABLE 1
Shared work by multiskilled staff
July 1990

Roles and responsibilities

Staff type	Clinical work	Ancillary and clerical work
Clinical associates (RNs, LPNs, radiology techs, respiratory techs, med techs)	Bedside care Phlebotomy Respiratory Rx	Radiology exams Lab diagnostics Physical therapy and occupational therapy
Service associates	Supply management Dietary	Patient transport Environmental services
Administrative associates	Unit communication Medical records	Admitting

TABLE 2
Cost/financial analysis
Traditional versus pilot work comparisons
April 1990 versus March 1991

Task	Work time (minutes)		
	Traditional	Pilot	Reduction
Chest x-ray	50	16	68%
Lab: CBC	51	17	67%
Respiratory spirometry	35	9	79%
EKG	34	15	56%
Admitting	115	54	53%
Physical therapy	64	28	56%
Medical records	116	85	27%

The roles and responsibilities of the clinical, service, and administrative associates that constituted the multiskilled staff are described in Table 1.

Lessons learned

The results from this project encouraged executive leadership to further develop the model. Patient and physician satisfaction improved and quality measures stayed constant. The model required implementation on more than one unit to realize substantial labor cost savings. However, comparisons of work time, work steps, and the number of staff participating in various tasks revealed significantly reduced numbers in the pilot unit when compared to a comparable surgical unit (see Table 2).

The pilot also provided experience in managing the transitions between old and new ways of organizing work. A unit board, of the ORP, provided an ongoing forum in which staff could work out issues. Outside the ORP unit, most leadership considered the program an interesting, academic exercise with little application to themselves. The exceptions were radiology and medical records, who opposed the concept on the basis that it would reduce quality.

OPERATIONS IMPROVEMENT

Operations improvement sought to bring the philosophy and lessons learned in the ORP to bear on costly, inefficient care throughout the hospital and clinic.

Cost savings and improvements between July 1991 and September 1993 were realized primarily in administrative, ancillary, laboratory,

Work step			Number of staff participating		
Traditional	*Pilot*	*Reduction*	*Traditional*	*Pilot*	*Reduction*
19	9	53%	6	2	67%
21	11	48%	7	2	70%
16	5	70%	5	2	60%
12	6	50%	3	1	67%
38	25	34%	10	4	60%
14	8	57%	3	2	33%
25	19	21%	7	6	14%

operative services, support services, radiology, and nonlabor areas. Non-labor savings came from changes in supply contracts, pharmacy utilization, and switching from disposable to reusable items. Labor savings were a result of skill mix changes and position elimination coupled with process improvement. Total net value of the savings was $27,841,769. The savings was accomplished through the work of interdisciplinary task forces with broad input from staff and faculty, technical support from external consultants, and internal financial staff.[3] Smaller portions of the total savings were achieved through redesign work in the clinic such as eliminating the clinical-clerical bifurcation, partially decentralizing phlebotomy, and implementing the service associate role. Ancillary and support areas contributed to the savings through introducing efficiencies into pharmacy operations, streamlining management and staffing, shifting patient transport to the patient units, and implementing a reduced-cost linen system.

RESTRUCTURING

The service improvements and cost savings realized between July 1993 and September 1994 were a result of implementing new patient care delivery models on 26 inpatient units and 6 central departments. Although the staffing and service mixes differ according to each patient care area or support service mission, all reflect VUH/TVC's work redesign principles, which included

- Define the best practical clinical care process and outcomes, and manage care to those standards

- Delegate tasks to the least expensive, appropriately trained provider

- Balance workload by redefining jobs to be multifunctional

- Decentralize staff and management of the most highly used ancillary, support, and administrative functions to the patient care units where service and cost benefits can be achieved

- Reduce organizational layers and broaden the span of control to streamline decision making

- Simplify, reduce, and eliminate complexity through process redesign and technology applications

The measures of success that guided restructuring were

- Patient-focused care

- Cost-efficient care

- Holistic jobs

- Fewer work steps

- Fewer delays

- Fewer handoffs

In the new models, the registered nurse delivers care in a team with the care partner (unlicensed clinical worker). Service associates (unlicensed, nonclinical workers) are staff dedicated to the units to provide decentralized housekeeping, dietary, and transport services. Respiratory therapists have been dedicated to high-volume work areas such as surgical intensive care, under joint, central, and unit direction. Phlebotomy has been decentralized to the patient care units. The RN, care partner, service associate, and unit-based ancillary staff (e.g., respiratory therapist) report to the unit manager.

Managing role transitions

While patient unit managers are the local supervisors for the newly unit-based staff (e.g., service associates), they share responsibility with service department managers for key functions, including

- *Clinical support and services.* Providing nonshareable work and services to units without decentralized staff and backup to units with decentralized staff

- *Quality improvement.* Jointly setting performance standards, developing and implementing a quality improvement plan, and upgrading standards as practice and technology evolves

- *Recruitment.* Defining criteria for hiring, providing administrative support for recruitment, and participating in interviews

- *Orientation and training.* Supporting new staff orientation, supporting skill maintenance, upgrading training programs, and arranging student internships

- *Performance evaluation and improvement.* Collaboratively completing performance evaluations, identifying performance problems, and identifying corrective actions and follow-ups

- *Compliance with regulatory standards.* Reviewing regulations, communicating regulations, monitoring compliance, and recommending improvement strategies

Table 3 describes the difference between the old and new management roles. To distinguish the local management role from the historical head nurse role, who supervised only nursing personnel, the nurse manager's title was changed to manager, patient care services. This shift of reporting relationships for former housekeeping, dietary, and transport workers to the unit manager rather than their department head represented a dramatic cultural change. The service department head role (particularly in environmental services) shifted from a traditional line manager, with a large department, to content expert and consultant role. Preliminary cost savings were projected at $3.5 million annually for fiscal year 1995. Preliminary data indicate no change in the quality of patient care or patient satisfaction. Anecdotal evidence, such as reports from staff on the units, indicates that patient care units are cleaner now.

Creating and implementing new roles

New job descriptions were developed for the registered nurse, care partner, service associate, manager-patient care services, and service department head roles. These new jobs were designed around a common set of values including patient/customer focus, organizational systems development, facilitation and collaboration, team learning, and personal learning.[4] Teams created the job descriptions and implementation plans

TABLE 3
Patient care manager role

What is different about the role?

Old	New
Focus on nursing unit	Focus on patient care and all aspects of patient care unit
Supervise RNs, LPNs, MRs, PCAs	Coach and facilitate a broad range of personnel
Work with other department heads to report or solve problem	Work with department heads to develop standards and evaluate performance of services

for the registered nurse, service associate, care partner, and manager roles. An important task of each team was to decide whether work should be shared between or remain unique to each role.

The registered nurse (RN) role transition planning was accomplished within three months. The planning task force was led by the director of patient care services and included staff development and nurse representatives. Focus groups provided broad staff input about the relative composition of the staff nurse job. The Tennessee Registered Nurse and Licensed Practical Nurse practice acts provided a starting point to discuss the roles. "A day in the life scenario" or listing of the average nurse work provided an opportunity to work through the possibilities to delegate work. The group agreed on the role of the RN in the patient-focused team model, which was a leader and coordinator function. After the model was completed a day-long RN role transition workshop was attended by all full-time RNs. These workshops proved to be important forums for staff to hear the vision of leadership and to enable them to voice their frustration.

The service associate role planning built on the role defined in the Orthopedic Project. The planning process for this role and implementation required nine months. The team, led by a senior patient care services administrator, included the dietary, patient transport, and environmental services departments as well as a training design expert and a service associate from orthopedics. The implementation used a "resident match" approach that matched environmental service staff candidates to units hiring service associates. Dietary, patient transport, and environmental services were given unit-level needs and offered an opportunity to meet with unit managers and list their placement preferences. Manager and staff preferences were then matched. Over five months, the implementation staff was gradually moved from its old central department to the new unit. In addition to the three-week central orientation, a coach who was previously a service associate on orthopedics was available to service associates. New service associates formed their own team, but struggled to become a part of the unit team.

The care partner program required nine months of planning. The team first agreed on the core responsibilities and determined what tasks could be added on special units. Complicating the implementation was the need to incorporate an existing unlicensed clinical provider—the patient care assistant. Central to the care team was the idea that a care partner is teamed with an RN and is assigned the same patients as that nurse. The older, patient care assistant role did not partner the unlicensed worker with one registered nurse.

Table 4 outlines the process to transition the managers to their new roles. Patient care manager training included change theory, work redesign, healthcare economics, team building, financial management, professional standards, and negotiation and collaboration skills.

Transition teams

During the transition, unit-based transition teams helped patient care unit members to meet cost-effective, patient-focused care goals while creating a great place to work. The transition teams' premise is that managing change is a fundamental focus of the work of all who support, provide, and manage patient care services. The transition teams provided a structure for staff from different backgrounds, disciplines, and departments to understand one another's jobs. The teams also showed staff how to function as a team. For example, some registered nurses were highly skeptical of unlicensed clinical workers' ability to competently care for patients. The transition teams provided a forum for working through this conflict.

Transition teams were led by the patient care unit managers. Each team started with an initial charter that detailed its purpose, scope, intent, roles, and work time frame. Each unit-based transition team also had a one-day orientation workshop to learn about its role, to practice skills in team communications and handle resistance, and to familiarize itself on specifics about cost, quality, and satisfaction with its particular units (see Exhibit 1).

COLLABORATIVE CARE AND CASE MANAGEMENT

Collaborative care and case management are clinical systems that provide tools and processes to ensure that care provided at VUH/TVC is high quality, cost effective, and satisfying to patients and families. VUH/TVC defines "case management" as the coordination of care during an entire episode of illness by a designated case manager to optimize clinical and financial patient outcomes. Collaborative care is the agreed-upon process to provide care to different groups or types of patients. Collaborative paths (also known as "critical paths" or clinical guidelines) are documents describing agreed-upon approaches to care for a specific

TABLE 4
Manager role transition activities

- Develop assessment tool
- Orient supervisors to tool and assessment completed by managers and their supervisors
- Develop discussions between managers and their supervisors regarding
  Performance expectations
  Current performance strengths
  Development needs
- Address development needs indentified

disease, condition, or procedure. Development of these systems has evolved since its origins in the Orthopedic Project in 1990.

In the past 18 months, collaborative care and case management have contributed significantly to decreases in length of stay and patient charges noted at VUH/TC. Notable components of these programs include

- Developing and implementing more than 300 collaborative pathways

- Change of the clinical nurse specialist to a clinical nurse specialist/ case manger to focus on both clinical and financial outcomes. There are currently 36 case managers at VUH/TVC who focus on systematically selected high-loss, high-volume, high-cost/acuity, or high-preference case types (e.g., trauma cases, because Vanderbilt has a commitment to a level-one trauma program)

- Piloting four staff nurse case management models (i.e., orthopedics unit, burn unit, neonatal intensive care unit, and coronary care unit)

- Developing and implementing Pathways,™ a computerized documentation system to support collaborative care. This system integrates collaborative pathways, nursing flow sheets, charting by exception, and electronic variance data collection, and has resulted in a 40 percent decrease in charting time

- Development of a comprehensive process to define best practices and evaluate opportunities to increase quality, decrease costs, and improve patient focus of care delivery

Internal enablers of change

Effective cultural change requires a clear vision of the desired state, committed leaders, aligned organizational structure, aligned systems, and aligned staff and skills. The structure and programs described below provided that support.

CENTER FOR PATIENT CARE INNOVATION

The Center for Patient Care Innovation was created in November 1990 with joint funding from the Robert Wood Johnson Foundation/ Pew Charitable Trusts and VUH/TVC.[5] The center's charge was to be a catalyst for continuous improvement of patient care and services, integration of hospital and clinic systems, and innovation at all levels.

The center is a physical space with dedicated, expert staff consisting of a director, a shared governance coordinator/organization development specialist, a program design and organization development specialist, an evaluation specialist, director of case management, an administrative assistant, and two technical secretaries. The director of operational improvement and the director of process improvement work closely with the center. Annual budgets between 1990 and 1994 ranged from $325,000 to $420,000.

Center staff consult, coach, and plan with staff and physicians in areas such as project management, group process dynamics, meeting planning, teamwork, and work redesign. Consultation also includes instructional design and development of training and orientation programs. The CPCI supported the planning and implementation of the 26 inpatient and 6 central department patient care models mentioned above, including the role transition process.

FACILITATIVE LEADERSHIP

Facilitative Leadership is a course in collaborative planning and meeting skills.[6] This course was adapted to use healthcare examples and to draw on the experience of participants about current medical center issues. The workshop enables managers and prospective leaders to practice facilitation skills and to receive feedback on strategies from colleagues who come from a variety of areas and disciplines in the organization. Participants are exposed to both the theory and practical applications of collaboration, planning effective meetings, and building consensus.

With more than 200 managers having attended the course, the Collaborative Organization Design effort had a well-developed foundation on which to build.

EVALUATION AND CONTINUOUS IMPROVEMENT

VUH/TVC fielded its first culture survey in September 1991.[7] The organization has based its changes on customer satisfaction, quality, cost, and organizational culture data. Culture data reflects employee perceptions of the values and behaviors that drive and are rewarded by the organization. The organization had excellent patient satisfaction, quality, and cost data for some time, but the data were not regularly compared to each other and were not regularly fed back to users. Further, there was no regular assessment of culture. The system to measure culture was coupled with a cost-tracking system developed during operations improvement. It proved a useful building block for a coordinated approach to examine cost, quality, culture, and satisfaction simultaneously. By drawing on the existing field of cost, quality, culture, and satisfaction data, the team was able to spend more time analyzing work processes.

UNIT BOARD SYSTEM

The unit board system in patient care services consisted of unit boards implemented in fall 1989, with corresponding boards at the administrative level above those units.[8] Unit boards are now developing in respiratory care, rehabilitation services, and distribution services with plans to broaden to other disciplines and departments.

The boards serve as planning and problem-solving forums. They bring administrator, manager, and staff together collaboratively to address clinical and service quality, as well as work-life issues. Boards have been involved in supporting the implementation of patient care delivery models as well as cost-containment efforts. Within and beyond its boards, collaborative decision making across levels and disciplines has been instilled in the Vanderbilt culture. Since its inception, board members and leaders have been trained in effective meeting management, problem solving, and a range of decision-making options, including consensus. These basic group skills allow boards to solve regular operational issues, such as transferring patients between units and advising management on staff morale problems.

Integrating mechanisms

By summer 1993, VUH/TVC completed numerous improvement or cost-reduction initiatives. With the threat of a managed care system for Tennessee Medicaid patients, more managed care, and falling federal revenues for medical education, executive leadership looked for additional ways to improve VUH/TVC competitiveness.

COLLABORATIVE ORGANIZATION DESIGN

Collaborative organization design (COD) offered a way to draw on the achievements and findings of previous improvement efforts while redesigning the organization from a more broad perspective. The approach differed from the narrow, compartmental focus previously used. COD focuses on the work of patient care in the hospital and clinic and beyond. It emphasizes the interdependence of an organization and its environment and the need for a fit among all organizational elements. It pays equal attention to human considerations (e.g., allowing time for staff to discuss and agree on approaches). Phase outcomes are accomplished collaboratively and the appropriate tools are used to diagnose and resolve organizational issues. For example, staff and customer focus groups, as well as work teams, discussing process improvements might be part of the analysis phase. All results are reviewed and agreed upon by representative groups. Customers and their needs are the primary focus for the whole process.

Initial COD activities focused on aligning the leadership team (i.e., executive director of VUH/TVC, patient care services director, and VUH and TVC directors), deciding if collaborative organization design was a desired step, and, if so, how to set the stage for its start-up. The alignment process increased the team cohesion, allowed initial agreement on the organization's draft mission and vision, outlined its purpose, scope, breadth, criteria, time frame, and approach, established team boundaries, and proposed a feedback process on the mission and vision. This process included developing agreement among the executive leadership members about the strengths of the hospital and clinic organization and determining where it was vulnerable. In addition, individual executive leadership team members identified and shared their expectations and clarified the administrative support they needed.

During the early fall, the top management team under executive leadership agreed on the proposed mission, vision, purpose, and process for the change effort, as well as the role of the leadership team. Requirements for design-team member representation and characteristics were agreed on, staff and physicians were nominated, and team membership was established. Table 5 outlines the design team membership.

DESIGN TEAM

The 10-member, multidisciplinary design team, including 3 physicians, worked two and a half days per week between November 1993 and August 1994. Its charge was to look at the entire VUH/TVC system, across traditional boundaries, at the seams between departments, and within each specific center of excellence. The goals were to create an efficient, patient-focused system, to strengthen patient and customer focus, to significantly improve VUH/TVC's competitive position, to enhance staff development, and to decrease organizational bureaucracy.

DESIGN TEAM PROCESS

The design team process consisted of six sequential phases, which often overlapped. These phases included education and planning, definition and analysis, mission and vision, design, implementation planning, and implementation.

During a one-month education-and-planning phase, the team learned the purpose and scope of the change effort, its charter or job,

TABLE 5
Design team representation

Professor and chair, emergency medicine
Associate hospital director, patient care services
Assistant director, financial management
Evening hospital administrator, hospital administration
Practice coordinator, clinic administration, orthopedics
Practice coordinator, clinic administration, urology
Clinical pharmacist, pharmacy
Assistant professor, biomedical infomatics
Assistant professor, medicine
Assistant professor, radiology
Director, center for patient care innovation
Director, operational improvement

its work's boundaries or constraints, and the definition of organizational design including its tasks and tools. The team planned how to accomplish its tasks and how to work and function as a team. It also defined key stakeholders and how and when those key stakeholders would be involved in each of the phases.

During the four months of definition and analysis, the team defined and analyzed VUH/TVC, including assessing opportunities and challenges, determining customer needs and requirements, and examining work processes, inputs, customer feedback mechanisms, and the human aspects of their work, such as how staff are treated by managers. Customers were viewed as patients, their families, physicians, payers, and the schools of medicine and nursing. Core processes were identified as taking patients into the system (access), determining the causes of their problems (diagnostics), intervening to improve their problems (therapeutics), and returning them back to their own homes (exit or follow-up). Strengths of VUH/TVC and causes of the most significant problems of VUH/TVC were identified in the work process analysis (Table 6).

During the mission and vision phase, the team shifted from the past and present to the future. It agreed on why VUH/TVC is in business (its mission) and its future (vision). The mission and vision built on VUH/TVC's current values and on its customer needs and requirements. The mission and vision statement was created specifically to guide the new organization in the design phase. A document was created by the design team, executive leadership, and selected staff at a one-day off-site retreat to provide a concrete reference for the design team's work.

During the design phase, which ended in June 1994, the team developed a new VUH/TVC based on its mission and vision and from the definition and analysis phase findings. Design outlined specific measures that would address root causes including recommendations on work

TABLE 6
Summary of origins of challenges

Accessing VUH/TVC is difficult
Patients and family are not a priority
Data entered incorrectly
Inappropriate or inefficient use of resources
Information difficult to access, no feedback mechanism in place
People only see their own department
Difficult communication

processes, strategy, structure, systems, people, skills, leadership style, and culture. Here the challenge was to get the team to think radically about how the new organization should work. Progress on designing the new organization was made when the team agreed to meet weekly outside the hospital and clinic, away from the normal workplace. Questioning what design approach would solve this problem helped the group focus to develop solutions. A summary of the recommendations is listed in Exhibit 2.

The implementation planning phase focused on how to move the organization from the present to the future. This included identifying the specific steps, responsibilities, resources needed, and target dates to implement the new design and anticipate the stumbling blocks that could be encountered. The VUH/TVC design team, with executive leadership, did preliminary implementation planning in July 1994. As a part of the implementation planning process the design team and executive management, with the assistance of several physician leaders, identified the forces that support and hinder implementation of the recommendations. Executive management decided to defer more detailed implementation planning and implementation until early 1995. In February, implementation team leaders and executive management synthesized individual recommendation time lines into a master time line.

PARALLEL WORK GROUPS FOCUSING ON PHYSICIAN PRACTICE

Meanwhile, a series of task forces was commissioned by the vice chancellor of health affairs to address specific areas of importance to create a successful medical center, including cost containment and capitated care.

These task forces, composed primarily of physicians, focused on managed care, clinical and administrative systems for multispecialty group practice, networking, information systems, education and training, and primary care. The physician leader of the clinical work group for multispecialty group practice was also a member of the design team.

The design team's charge to redesign the hospital and clinic system overlapped with the physician clinical work group's charge to develop a system of clinical management for the multispecialty group practice. Integration was achieved through the physician, as a member of both groups, and through coordinated planning.

Conclusions and replicable concepts

The concepts from several initiatives described here can be replicated. The orthopedic redesign model improved patient and physician satisfaction without interfering with quality. The model also demonstrated potential for large-scale cost savings if implemented on a broad scale. The integrated patient care delivery model concepts culled from that pilot formed the foundation for the models designed on 26 inpatient units and 6 central departments. Early evidence indicates the models improved unit cleanliness, customer focus, teamwork, and reduced cost without hampering quality. Perhaps the most powerful cost savings and coordination improvement results came from the VUH/TVC case management model. Between 1991 and 1995, case management (with operations improvement) significantly reduced gross revenue per discharge.

The following concepts, models, or processes may prove valuable to reduce cost and maintain or improve patient satisfaction and quality.

INTEGRATED PATIENT CARE MODEL

Even at VUH/TVC, operating units applied these broad concepts differently to redesign their unique units. The elements of the model are

- Leveraged (e.g., least expensive, most appropriately trained person) staff

- Decentralized work based on volume and shareability

- Dedicated specialized staff in high-volume areas

- Assistants paired or teamed with clinical staff

- Service associate role to provide transport, supply, environmental, and dietary service

SHAREABLE WORK METHODOLOGY

The integrated patient care models were created, costed out, and adapted using shareable work methodology. This approach requires starting with the work done by each department or discipline that must be done by that group as required by law. For example, according to the Tennessee State Board of Nursing, RNs must create a plan of nursing care for the patient. This responsibility was placed with the RN from the beginning of the work redesign. Other tasks, cognitive and practical, were divided among workers based on what was best for the patient. Focusing on what is best for the patient and assigning work on that basis begins to eliminate duplicate steps.

MANAGER JOB DESCRIPTION AND ROLE TRANSITION PROCESS

The models for new roles for managers of patient care units and service department heads (e.g., respiratory, environmental services, and dietary) and their relationships to one another were a linchpin of the VUH/TVC transition. Deciding the roles for any position is relatively straightforward; however, implementing the position and making ongoing improvements to it is more difficult. Key enablers of the role transition are to develop

- Early agreements on roles and relationships
- Early agreements on the transition process
- Developmental assessment of the skill level
- Collaboration on role development

The transition process for managers and service department heads was useful. Helping managers cultivate the skills and perspectives to develop and coach staff, instead of making the decisions and controlling work flow, required a structured transition process. The steps to support this transition included

1. Developing an assessment tool

2. Orienting supervisors to the tool

3. Arranging discussions between managers and their supervisors regarding performance expectations, current performance, and development needs

TRANSITION TEAMS

Significant change starts with identifying its final goals. The process of the change must reflect future patterns. Transition teams at VUH/TVC fulfilled this requirement, provided the structure for representative staff groups to plan, and worked out the implementation for their own areas.

CASE MANAGEMENT MODEL

Vanderbilt's case management model was composed of several elements:

- Comprehensive analysis of the care delivery process for patients with specific types of disorders or undergoing specific procedures

- Development of pathways or practice agreements to guide high-quality, cost-effective care

- Designation of advanced practice nurse case managers to assist physicians to coordinate care during the entire episode of illness or hospitalization

- Collection, aggregation, and analysis of variance data to drive a continuous quality improvement process focused on refinement of practice guidelines and identification and resolution of system problems

CENTER FOR PATIENT CARE INNOVATION

Expansive redesign efforts require dedicated support. The Center for Patient Care Innovation internal experts in facilitation and complex collaborative change, as well as the external consultants who had used the process before, worked. An effective center requires resources, including space, capital equipment, the time and attention of administrative and clinical leaders, and some dedicated staff that have the following elements:

- Vision and articulation

- Creativity

- Ability to be comfortable with roles and relationships that change

- Ability to move the system

- Personal stamina and confidence

- Effective consulting skills

- Ability to understand complex organizations

- Outstanding facilitation skills

- Ability to understand process improvement

- Ability to be comfortable with multiple levels of the organization such as executive management, staff, and physicians

- Project management skills

- Well-developed written and verbal communication skills

PHYSICIAN INVOLVEMENT APPROACHES

Building authentic physician involvement is a challenge due to the divergent interests of hospitals and physicians. Involving physicians requires identifying the right incentive. Some physicians want to be involved because it is the right thing to do or they believe it is better for their patients. Others are motivated by the potential to author publications arising from the project. Getting physicians on board requires cultivating those with a vision and the ability to articulate it. Sustaining physicians' interest requires leaders who can be viewed as neutral and who work for broader institutional objectives, rather than for their own self-interest.

Incentives can be useful but project leaders must know how to use data to appeal to the intellect, have adequate follow-through, and accommodate physician schedules. Once physicians are on board, effort must be made to avoid losing them, which requires effective meeting skills, group leadership, jargon avoidance, and setting a clear focus and boundaries.

Successful restructuring strategies

Successfully reengineering an enterprise as large and complex as an academic health center requires that all those in the organization learn and change. Recounted below are what the executive leadership at VUH/TVC view as the prime requirements of successful restructuring:

- *Empowerment with accountability.* Empowering people to come up with a better way without clear direction, a clear process, or specific goals invites poor results

- *Including those who do the work in the process.* "No one can effectively plan for anybody else." [9] This is easy to say and hard to do. In spite of trying to represent all levels of the organization, members of many VUH/TVC restructuring teams were department heads and administrators. The team architecture for profound change must honor involving those who do the work, whatever their positions. Effective teams also require members who have vision and will regularly communicate with their constituents. The expectation for communication is often overlooked, even with physicians and executives

- *A clear starting date and finishing date.* This sounds simple but projects drag on without agreed-upon, adhered-to deadlines. Efforts taking longer than six to nine months will lose momentum and their team's enthusiasm

- *Preparation for a significant effort.* The VUH/TVC change mantra has been "go slow to go fast."[10] Many jump to a solution without careful consideration of the problem or planning an effective approach. Time put into a clear charge, boundaries, training, and preagreed-upon goals will guarantee a fruitful initiative

- *Support structures.* In addition to the center for patient care innovation, several other departments provided important restructuring support including dedicated finance and cost-monitoring support, case-type cost analysis, marketing and communications, and human resource consultation

- *Time for groups to take ownership of the vision and the work.* People embrace and own new ideas at a certain speed. Pushing too fast may result in a solution no one will support

- *A neutral person to challenge leaders and teams.* Institutions are political and turf-bound places. Moving forward with new ideas can often happen faster with a neutral staff member who can assist with keeping meetings focused on the goal

Successful restructuring requires individual and organizational self-examination. In addition, regular times to consider progress encourages earnest dialogue between all those involved in the change effort. With the speed of change in healthcare organizations and its incumbent risk, no strategy is risk proof. However, strategies for organizational change and improvement that allow time to develop the staff and group skills build the foundation for sustainable achievement.

NOTES

1. Booz, Allen, Hamilton, Inc., sponsored the invitational meeting to build interest in testing their model for patient-focused care.

2. Collaborative Organization Design is a model created by Gelinas•James, Inc., Oakland, California.

3. APM, Inc., of New York City provided comparative cost data as well as technical support.

4. The job description design draws heavily on the work of Peter Senge, *The Fifth Discipline: the Art and Science of the Learning Organization* (New York: Doubleday/Currency, 1990).

5. Funding for the Center for Patient Care Innovation was partly provided by the grant "Strengthening Hospital Nursing: a Program to Improve Patient Care," a joint initiative of the Robert Wood Johnson Foundation and the Pew Charitable Trusts, a program focused on improving patient care and the quality of work life in hospitals.

6. Facilitative Leadership was developed by Interaction Associates, Inc., of San Francisco, California.

7. The culture survey conducted in September 1991 drew largely on the work of Robert E. Quinn, *Beyond Rational Management: Mastering the Paradoxes and Competing Demands of High Performance* (San Francisco: Jossey-Bass, 1982).

8. The Unit Board system is based on Russell Ackoff's Circular Organization model.

9. Russell Ackoff used this phrase in his lectures to the Robert Wood Johnson/Pew Charitable Trusts, "Strengthening Hospital Nursing: a Program to Improve Patient Care" planning grantees at their September 1989 meeting in Tallahassee, Florida.

10. Interaction Associates, San Francisco, California, Facilitative Leadership course, 1988.

EXHIBIT 1

Purpose of transition team

To develop, plan, and implement with other members of the unit activities that will achieve the desired outcomes for your patient-focused care team during its transition.

- Integration of the new roles on the unit
- Understanding of everyone's role in relationship to all other roles on the unit
- Understanding of the patient care model and how this new configuration relates to the mission of the hospital
- A spirit of patient-focused teamwork on the unit
- A process for identifying emerging issues that seem "ripe" for applied team building skills

Criteria for selection of transition team members

- Select individuals who have knowledge of the model; who have demonstrated skills in collaboration and problem solving
- A representative "slice" of the unit is desirable—however, do not only look at representation of roles—here, it is important to select individuals who are committed to the success of your implementation
- Select a team of 12 members

Individual team member criteria

- Open to learning and applying new ideas and skills
- Willing to speak openly and honestly, challenge ideas, and think independently
- Truly interested in and committed to the success of implementing the patient care model on the unit
- Willing to support consensus decisions
- Willing to listen to others
- Willing to participate actively and fully in transition team orientation workshop
- Willing to support the mission of the hospital and the vision of the unit through words and actions

Selection of transition team members

- Patient care manager in consultation with service specialist and assistant hospital director will select transition team based on criteria and interested volunteers

EXHIBIT 2

Vanderbilt University Hospital and Clinic
Focus of design team recommendations

1. Culture of organization
2. Center for continuous learning and improvement
3. Collaborative care
4. Quality strategies
5. Performance-based compensation and evaluation
6. Computer-based patient record
7. Access and exit process for patients
8. Hotel services
9. Product and supply selection, purchasing, utilization, and evaluation
10. Administrative structure changes

30

St. Charles Medical Center: Streamlining hospital operations

Rick Martin
Senior Vice President, Operations
St. Charles Medical Center
Bend, Oregon

REORGANIZING THE MANAGEMENT structure from more than 50 managers to 16 cluster leaders was probably the most difficult, painful part of reengineering, but essential for patient-focused care at St. Charles Medical Center.

St. Charles Medical Center is a 181-bed not-for-profit regional referral center serving central and eastern Oregon. As the largest acute care facility serving a 25,000-square-mile rural area, St. Charles offers a complete range of services including open-heart surgery, neurosurgery, inpatient rehabilitation, comprehensive cancer care, and the state's only level two trauma center east of the Cascade Mountains.

St. Charles has developed a strong reputation over the years for providing high-quality care in a very caring way. In addition, the hospital has maintained a strong financial base. Reengineering the hospital operations and moving toward a new vision in 1991 was within the context of past and present success. In fact, its longstanding success made it difficult to communicate the need for change. During this time, fee-for-service medicine was coming to an end in the region, and St. Charles was not prepared to deliver care in a managed care environment. The cost of care had become a major issue, in addition to a growing dissatisfaction with the system of delivering care.

Inside, the hospital had become a fragmented and foreign environment, one in which patients felt out of control. Patients in growing numbers were dissatisfied with this type of care and expected to be full partners in control of their care. The challenge was to meet the public's demand for cost control while at the same time meeting the patients' growing quality and service expectations. It was not possible to accomplish both goals by simply tuning up the old hospital. It was time to challenge some of the basic assumptions used in the design of care delivery both within and outside the hospital. Some of these implicit assumptions were based on the following beliefs:

- The care system is the center of care

- Specialization always means better care

- Continuity is something to talk about

- Effort means outcome

- The major way to solve all problems is to either provide more training or hire more staff

Much of what was going on was not by design but rather an outgrowth of gradual change and partial solutions over many years. What was surprising was how loyal staff and management became to procedures and care methods that presented more obstacles to care than solutions. The reengineering effort represented a willingness to set aside old assumptions.

The goals in the St. Charles reengineering effort included

- Restructure care around patient needs

- Develop a stronger external focus

- Improve quality and lower cost

- Integrate a healing healthcare philosophy throughout the organization

It was strongly believed that structuring the organization around the patient instead of around the care system needs would greatly enhance care. With care fragmented among many departments, continuity of care became a major issue. With patients seeing 35 to 40 caregivers during an average inpatient stay, not knowing who is doing what, and unable to develop collaborative relationships, it was not a surprise that patients did not feel empowered. Lack of continuity also created a natural environment for errors in care and high cost. The more handoffs there were among caregivers, the greater the opportunity for a breakdown in communication and a missed observation of a patient's changing condition. Costs increased because more time was spent in communication, scheduling, and coordination among caregivers. Many of the established and well-accepted work practices used every day to provide care were ineffective and actually hampered the caregiver. A typical example of what was found throughout the institution was the same-day admitting process involving the surgical unit. Here a reengineering effort began with customer research, including customer interviews. In an interview with a surgeon, questions were asked about the quality of the staff. The surgeon's response was that quality of staff was excellent when his patients were admitted to the right floor. His response was a surprise to management, since capacity was not a challenge to the hospital. Through data collection and analysis, it was found that admitting surgical patients to the wrong floor was a problem and an example of management focusing on the wrong indicators. While one of the major indicators, midnight census, showed adequate capacity, the process of admitting surgical patients on the morning of their surgery and discharging patients around noon or early afternoon resulted in having many more patients between 6:00 A.M. and 1:00 P.M. than revealed by the midnight census. Because the surgical unit was at full capacity, surgery patients had to be admitted to the medical or orthopedic units and later transferred, often to the wrong unit.

With additional review, the task force found the morning admitting process had little chance of success. During the morning hours, a nurse was expected to admit patients arriving for surgery, find missing paperwork, schedule last-minute tests, provide patient education, and comfort the anxious patient. While preparing patients for surgery, the nurse was also expected to serve breakfast to another group of patients and prepare a third group for discharge. Through an ineffective care design, the nurses at St. Charles were being asked to do the impossible.

The task force's solution was to remove the surgical admit process and replace it with a totally new process that included a presurgery clinic. Now surgery patients are admitted to and by a unit dedicated to preparing the patient for surgery. With the presurgery clinic, documentation completeness went from 30 to 95 percent, lost orders dropped from 13 to 0 percent, delays in the surgery schedule dropped from 20 to 0 percent, and cancellations of surgeries dropped from 2.2 to 0 percent.

Before the new unit, patient waiting times ranged from one to nine hours, then dropped to an average of one and a half hours. Ninety-nine percent of surgical, medical, and orthopedic unit patients are now admitted to the right floor.

Healing healthcare at St. Charles is a philosophy and commitment to address the total needs of the patient—physical, mental, emotional, and spiritual. Creating a warm, caring environment is not just a patient relations issue; rather, such an environment actually plays a role in the body's ability to heal. The healing healthcare philosophy is being implemented through hospital training, life enhancement programs, and facility design.

Examples of healing healthcare training and programs are: life-skills training, life-death transition service, art and music in the hospital, the Mime Clown Ministry, dietary room service, and massage therapy. The programs above are available for patients, their families, and hospital staff.

The architecture and design of patient rooms also play a role in healing, by using warm and familiar patient rooms. Rooms take advantage of the view of the nearby Cascade Range and high desert, and lobbies and admitting areas are designed to welcome and help customers. Family rooms are designed to allow the family to stay with a patient throughout their stay. The patient family apartment in the rehabilitation unit is available for the patient and family to live together for two or three days before discharge to enable patient confidence and practice for newly learned skills. Art was selected for its content, such as the photography collection in the rehabilitation unit that depicts and celebrates life in the region, and the "Yoke of Compassion" sculpture at the hospital entry—a testament to the caring and Christian mission—depicting humanity in the simple yet fundamental act of caring for others. The physical facility can become an active participant in care by encouraging a range of life-affirming activities (e.g., using the facility's fishing pond).

Over the past three years, many changes have been implemented through the reengineering effort. These include the creation of focused units with a stabilized census and multidisciplinary, multiskilled care teams; a new presurgery clinic; and a new medical diagnostics unit. In addition, many services were decentralized to patient care units, such as physical therapy and pharmacy. A variety of modifications to the facility have been implemented to better meet patient and family needs.

At the heart of all these changes is a willingness to focus on what counts and to eliminate what does not. The starting point in reengineering is "what can we do for the patient that will make a difference." By maintaining that focus, the opportunities in improved care and cost reductions become obvious.

One example is with bedside care. When assessing the activities of the care staff, a conclusion was reached that in all the nursing activities, what mattered most was the direct patient care time. Because the overall goal was to improve quality and cut cost, the focus was not only maintaining or increasing the amount of direct care time but improving the quality of that time through using patient education or assessment skills. At the same time, the focus to reduce costs focused on activities that did reduce costs but did not lower the quality of care, such as excessive documentation time or time spent scheduling and coordinating care. When it came to documenting charts, which used 29 percent of the nurse's time, or scheduling and coordinating, which accounted for 19 percent of the nurse's time, every effort was made to find more efficient methods. In the case of documentation, exception-based charting (only charting exceptions to care standards) was implemented, which lowered documentation time to 19 percent. By moving key ancillary staff to be part of the unit's care team, scheduling and coordination time were reduced to 8 percent. The net result was lower costs while improving quality as shown in Figure 1.

While reengineering was intended to review the management structure, it was well into the reengineering effort when it became obvious the current structure would no longer meet the organization's needs. The hospital was moving away from the traditional structure of departments formed around specialties to forming patient care units around patient needs. It also moved from a traditional management model to one driven by leadership focus.

Partially because of its size, St. Charles was never burdened with the multiple layers of management found in many hospitals. However, the organization still suffered from sluggish decisions made by individuals or groups too far removed from the issues that arise at the point of service. This, as with most problems found during reengineering, was not a failure of the individuals involved but rather defective structures, systems, or processes.

FIGURE 1
Time utilization: Orthopedics and neurosurgery

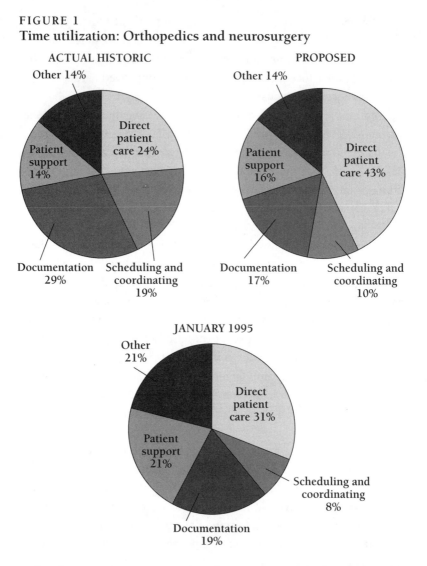

Another serious issue was that the institution was focused totally internally. With fee-for-service and stand-alone institutions shifting to managed care and healthcare networks, it was necessary to direct management resources to managed care contracting and developing a regional healthcare network.

The final outcome was to move from more than 50 departments to 16 clusters and two councils.

Clusters were formed by combining existing departments, such as environmental, material, and facility services into the facility and materiel

FIGURE 2
Prereorganization chart

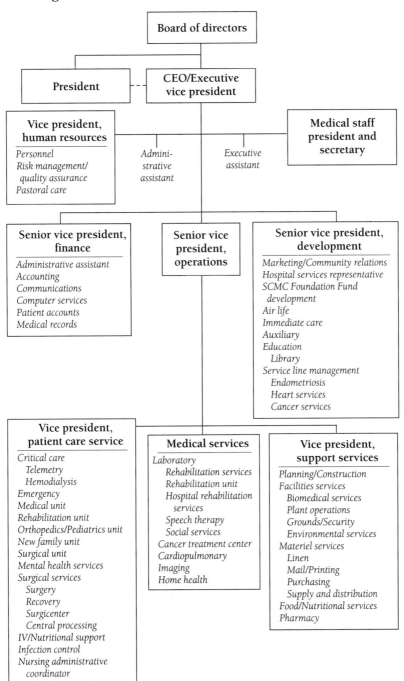

FIGURE 3
1995 organization model

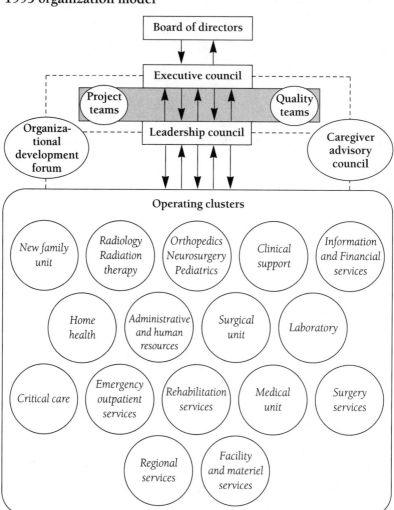

services cluster. Other clusters were formed by eliminating departments and moving their functions into other clusters. In the case of the respiratory therapy care department, respiratory therapy functions were moved to the critical care cluster, while testing and rehabilitation functions moved to the emergency services cluster that operates the medical diagnostics unit.

The primary rationale behind cluster formation was to form them around patients and to maximize the capability of a care unit to provide total patient care. Because of the facility's size, decentralization of all ancillary and support services was not financially feasible. A secondary rationale was to bring like services together.

The current structure, as shown in Figures 3 and 4, is seen as a transition and will likely change in both the number of clusters and makeup of specific clusters. Future modifications will be guided by several factors such as

- Continued changes due to reengineering

- Effectiveness of specific clusters

- Improved understanding of how clusters function

- Changing patient needs

Currently the leadership council, a council made up of the 16 cluster leader/managers, is exploring the possibility of combining three care units (surgical, orthopedics, and medical) into two units—one to focus on chronic care and the other unit caring for acute patients. Rather than using surgery as the main determinant of which unit a patient is admitted to, issues that led to surgery, such as chronic illness, will be used as the admitting criteria. This shift in emphasis will allow the unit to focus on the cause rather than the effect and hopefully prevent the need for future admissions. In the future, the council will also review how functions are organized to serve outpatients. Administration, along with the chair of the leadership council, makes up the executive council.

The primary focus of the leadership council is to oversee the internal operations of the hospital while the executive council focuses on development of a regional health system, managed care contracting, and other external matters, such as provider relationships, development of a community health council, and strengthening relationships with area businesses. The executive council also is responsible for the development of the decision-making parameters by which the leadership council operates. By developing clear parameters within which the leadership council can make decisions, the necessary freedom is created to speed up decision making and become more responsive.

FIGURE 4
Operating clusters

This model shows how the departments (old paradigm) are incorporated into the various clusters (new paradigm). The new family unit, orthopedics/neurosurgical/pediatrics unit, surgical unit, laboratory, and home health have not changed the basic composition of their cluster and are, therefore, not shown here.

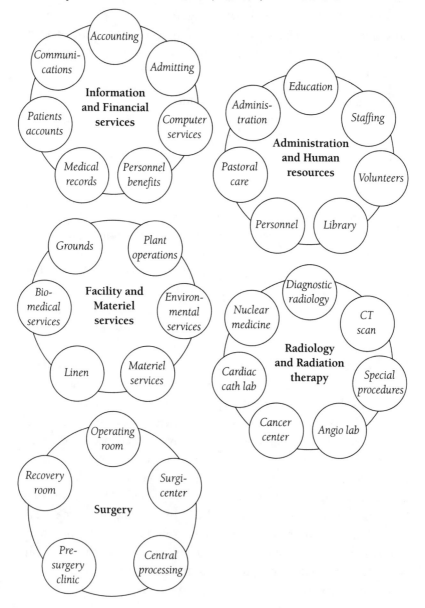

FIGURE 4 (CONTINUED)

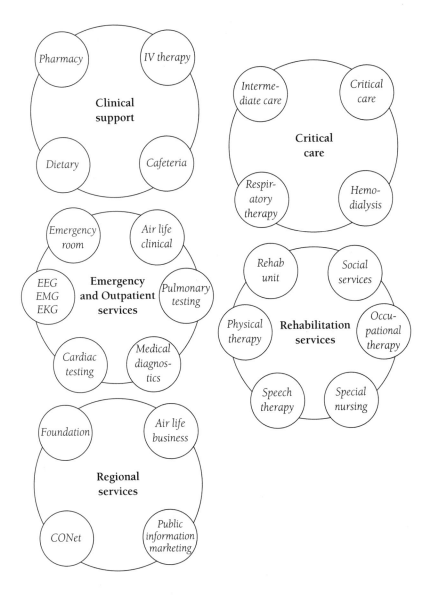

Leader/managers report directly to the leadership council and, as council members, are responsible for their cluster's performance and for the success of overall internal operations of the hospital. Day-to-day decision making remains with the leader/manager, but the vision, emphasis, and decision parameters for internal operations are established and monitored by the council. Monitoring is guided by two matrixes, one on quality and the other on financial indicators. The financial matrix focuses on

Efficiency

- Inpatient hours worked per discharge (case-mix adjusted)

- Outpatient hours worked per outpatient unit

- Hours worked per adjusted discharge (case-mix adjusted)

- Full-time equivalents (FTEs) per adjusted occupied bed, excluding newborns (case-mix adjusted)

Cost

- Total cost per adjusted discharge, excluding newborns (case mix adjusted)

Return

- Return on total assets

- Net margin from operations

The above indicators are monitored monthly to ensure the hospital is reaching annually set targets and that the indicators are improving continually. Many of the indicators are also compared with a national data base and specifically to western states' data. Table 1 shows the quality matrix.

As part of the new structure, nursing administration has been eliminated. Much of the decision-making responsibility and authority has been moved directly to the leader/managers of the units and the leadership council. The vice president of healing health services, who serves as the nurse executive, carries out responsibilities described by JCAHO standards. For specific patient-related issues, leader/managers are expected to work out the issues among themselves or in consultation with the vice president of healing health services. If issues cannot be worked out at the first-line level, the leadership council can take direct action or select a DIG (Do It Group), a group that focuses on a specific objective with a specific time line to develop recommendations.

These changes are also meant to eliminate the territorialism existing between departments. The combination of more than 50 departments organized around specialties and fee-for-service medicine created a competitive environment within the organization. This competition focused on increasing revenues rather than conserving resources and lowering costs, both critical factors in surviving managed care contracting and capitation. An example of this is the case of oximetry (determining the amount of oxygen in the blood) and whether this service should be provided by respiratory therapy or nursing. Rather than focusing on how the procedure could be most effectively provided, it was seen as a revenue source for respiratory therapy. Another example involves admitting and patient care departments. Both groups have important, but often different, needs in admitting patients. Instead of working together to find mutual solutions to create the most effective admitting process, they worked independently—each developing two separate admitting processes. In addition to internal competition between departments, the hospital often appeared to be operated as multiple entities, each under the direction of a vice president.

A project team concept proved very effective during the reengineering process. Task forces comprising individuals from a variety of disciplines with a clear task at hand were found to be powerful tools for change. Each task force was assigned one or more project team member, whose responsibility was to support the task force through data collection such as process flow, cost analysis, and detailed utilization patterns. In addition, the project team assisted the task force in data analysis. Because data collection and analysis skills are necessary throughout the hospital, the project team is also involved in training task force members. Specific tools include process flowcharting, Pareto analysis, cause-and-effect analysis, communicating with graphs and charts, run charting, project tracking, and facilitation. While training the staff how to flowchart a process, it was surprising how little they understood about the processes with which they worked with every day. It was also revealing to see how significant a simple tool such as flowcharting could be when used to understand and gain control over their work routines.

Depending on task force needs, project team members would often work full time for a task force through implementation. Because of past

TABLE 1
Quality matrix

Quality/Satisfaction indicator	Trend chart formula	Source of data
Caregiver satisfaction	1995 rating minus 1994 rating	Employee survey
Caregiver accidents	Lost time; five accident types by cluster	Accident reports
Patient/Family satisfaction: Discharge planning	$\dfrac{\text{1995 month total}}{\text{1994 average per month}}$	Patient satisfaction survey: discharge section
Medication errors	Per cluster $\dfrac{\text{1995 month total}}{\text{1994 average per month}}$	Incident reports
Patient accidents	Per cluster $\dfrac{\text{1995 month total}}{\text{1994 average per month}}$	Incident reports
Hospital acquired infections	Control chart	Infection control report
Unplanned readmits	$\dfrac{\text{Number of readmits}}{\text{Total admits}}$	Admission records
Critical paths (CP) multidisciplinary	$\dfrac{\text{Number of diagnoses per procedures per critical paths}}{\text{Total number of diagnoses per procedures}}$	Preprinted critical paths; DRG printout
Critical paths (CP) with variance analysis	$\dfrac{\text{Number of critical paths with variance analysis}}{\text{Number of critical paths}}$	Count of critical paths
Caregiver time in direct patient care	$\dfrac{\text{Direct patient care time}}{\text{Total caregiver time}}$	Work sample
Documentation time	$\dfrac{\text{Documentation time}}{\text{Total caregiver time}}$	Work sample
Number of caregivers involved per stay	$\dfrac{\text{Average number of caregivers}}{\text{Average LOS}}$	10 or more patient samples
Scheduling/Coordinating time	$\dfrac{\text{Scheduling coordinating time}}{\text{Total caregiver time}}$	Work sample
Service turnaround time: internal customer	$\dfrac{\text{Actual time}}{\text{Desired time}}$	Log/Run chart
Patient waiting time	$\dfrac{\text{Actual time}}{\text{Desired time}}$	Log/Run chart

Responsible cluster	Reporting frequency	1995 target
Administration and human resources	Every 6 months	Increase favorable rating by 50%
Administration and human resources	Monthly	Track and set by 6/30/95
Patient services	Monthly	90%
Patient services	Monthly	Reduce errors by 25%
Patient services	Monthly	Will track during 1995
Healing health services	Significant variances only	Maintain 1994 standard at or below upper control limit ___%
Administration and human resources; case managers	Every 6 months	Track for trends in 1995
Administration and human resources; case managers	Every 3 months	80% of patient population; critical paths; quality per multi-disciplinary
Administration and human resources; Case managers	Every month	100% of critical paths
Patient care clusters and project team	Every 2 months	50% or greater
Patient care clusters and project team	Every 2 months	10%
Patient care clusters and project team	Every 2 months	18 or less in a 4-day LOS
Clusters and project team	Every 2 months	Decrease or maintain time
All Clusters	Every 6 months	Set target through customer interview
All Clusters	Every 6 months	Set target per cluster service

successes and the fact that the improvement effort is now on a continuous basis, the project team has been made a permanent fixture at the hospital. Six improvement projects are currently in the works. Examples of these projects include

- *Materiels management.* The existing system was developed many years ago and has proven to be expensive and ineffective in meeting caregiver needs. Because of the problems experienced with this system an "underground materiels system" (everyone ordering whatever they want from whomever they want without following purchase order procedures) evolved. In addition to improving service, estimated savings are in excess of $608,000 annually (over and above the one-time savings). The majority of savings in this project is found in eliminating the duplicative effort of the underground materiels system, lowering of special delivery charges, automating, increased standardization, reduced inventory and improving purchasing, receiving and accounts payable processes

- *Order communications.* Much time and effort is used to process orders. In addition to wasting time, the manual system was plagued with problems of inaccuracy and lost orders. The task force has developed an automated solution to improve accuracy of orders while saving caregivers' valuable time. Estimated savings are $113,000 annually

- *Clarifying the caregiver role.* The roles of caregiver changed and new categories of caregivers were created during reengineering. Examples include the creation of care associates (nurse aides with expanded responsibilities) and patient support technicians (responsible for room cleaning and supplying the unit). This task force was formed to review, further define, and develop caregiver training, with an estimated $380,000 savings annually. Most savings in this project can be derived from more effective use of skilled and professional staff

The total estimated savings of the six projects is $1.5 million annually.

Over the past two years the hospital has significantly altered its approach to quality improvement. In the past, quality improvement has been an add-on function. Now instead of seeing quality in terms of "what we do" it is seen in terms of "how we do it." In daily operations leader/managers and the leadership council are expected to use quality improvement tools to carry out daily activities. In addition, the board of directors, executive council, and leadership council select the areas of emphasis, assemble multidisciplinary teams to work on selected issues, and monitor progress.

Reengineering has also expanded how the improvement process is viewed. Prior to reengineering, the improvement effort was limited to traditional continuous quality improvement (CQI) approaches. The hospital now uses CQI techniques along with process reengineering and benchmarking. Another change has been in the emphasis in outcomes rather than process. In the past there have been excellent examples of the CQI process but little evidence of an improved outcome.

An organizational development forum and the caregiver advisory council were implemented as major parts to the communication effort, perhaps the greatest reengineering challenge. When the project was first introduced three years ago, it was presented to more than 700 staff members in group meetings. The goal was to reach all 1,100 staff, but 700 was a good effort. The meetings went smoothly and few issues were raised. After the meetings, the task forces were formed and work began. Two months later the task forces began turning in their recommendations to the steering committee and confusion ensued. At the initial meetings a major effort was made to present the reasons for, purpose of, and scope of the reengineering project. However, very little was actually communicated. This was a valuable lesson in that effective communication looks more like a conversation than a presentation.

Three years ago the staff saw a very successful hospital in which few changes were made and what changes were made came very slowly. So the sense of reality of what was being attempted set in very late; from a communications standpoint, the effort had to start over with a greater emphasis on two-way communication. Over time the communications plan included small group discussions, a telephone hot line with all questions and answers posted on a reengineering bulletin board, and a willingness for every level of management, including the CEO, to sit down and discuss the issues.

The change process is similar in many ways to the grieving process. One of the best illustrations depicting this process is shown in Figure 5. Management should be prepared to deal with each stage of transition through two-way, heart-to-heart communication. Discussion at this

FIGURE 5
Transition path

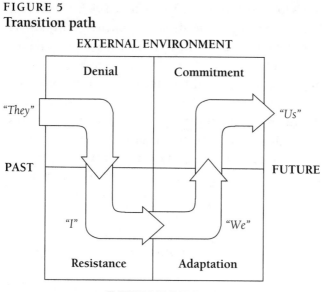

Courtesy of Care Management Consulting, Eugene, Oregon.

basic level was something management was not prepared for nor comfortable with. Part of St. Charles's culture was based in avoiding controversial staff issues. Reengineering and the accompanying changes forced management to address these issues. It was also important to note that individuals and departments move through the transition stages at different paces. The management staff had to work with individuals and departments at various stages of transition. While managers worked with the staff to deal with change, they also had to deal with their own emotions. Much of the work had to be on a one-to-one or on a departmental basis.

Everyone would like to find a consistent, easy-to-manage, effective communication tool, but such a tool has not been found. Because individuals hear messages in different ways and at different times, many communication techniques must be used and the message must be repeated often. In addition to daily communications, special circumstances such as reengineering require an extra effort due to the natural fears that change creates. An effective communication effort is an absolute necessity in reengineering. Without it the effort will slow down and eventually become paralyzed from resistance to change.

The organizational forum is basically a town hall meeting that is open to all—physicians, hospital staff, and board members. The forum meets monthly to discuss the direction of the hospital, changes in healthcare, and other topics of concern. The format is generally 50 percent presentation with 50 percent discussion and questions and answers.

A caregiver advisory council was developed to provide a direct communication link between caregivers and the executive council. The concern by the CEO in eliminating nursing administration was the loss of a valuable communication link directly with the staff.

Some of the most frequently asked questions from other hospitals are "What was the process used to reorganize the management structure?," "What happened to the displaced managers?," "How were changes implemented?," and "What position did the medical staff take?"

Two conditions existed at St. Charles that made the reorganization process smoother. Because the reorganization of management did not occur until the end of the reengineering project, there was more experience with the change process. Secondly, with few alternative management models being widely discussed in print, the magnitude of potential change was unclear and anxiety around such changes remained relatively low. These two factors allowed more time and freedom in the design phase.

As with the rest of the reengineering project, management reorganization was assigned to a task force made up of management, staff, physicians, and a project team member. Unlike previous reengineering task forces, the CEO was a member of the management reorganization group, and as the person solely responsible for organizational design, as designated by the hospital board of directors, would make the final decisions instead of the reengineering steering committee.

The task force began work in March 1993 by researching internal and external sources of information, collecting and analyzing data, and developing possible management models. As with other task forces, the steering committee established goals for the task force to reach. Examples of goals included

- Speed up decision making by flattening the organization and empowering the caregiver for local decision making. Establish specific goals of no more than four levels between the patient and the board of directors

- Reduce management time and cost while more evenly distributing management throughout the facility

- Strengthen working relationships among departments, eliminating internal competition

- Move toward a focus on organizational success versus departmental success

- Organize to better reflect patient-focused care goals

The task force's work was slow initially, partially because of the lack of other available models in use in the industry and partially because of a reluctance to recommend changes that would have such a major impact on a management team that had been together for many years. Progress improved with the addition of a time goal—a specific date for completion of the new organizational design was set. Over the years, time has proven to be a crucial element in change. If rushed, important development work can be left incomplete that may jeopardize implementation, but if a project moves at its own pace, the effort will slow down and often die under its own weight. Many improvement projects never make it out of the planning phase.

In July 1993, the task force turned its work over to the CEO. With additional follow-up discussions with selected managers and vice presidents, the CEO created the draft form of the organization structure that was presented to the department managers and executive council. A two-week period was set aside for additional comments from management staff and a final structure was set within a month. Throughout this period of time the CEO was very direct, interested in a variety of input, but also very decisive. These factors helped minimize the pain involved in such a change.

The final organization structure was announced in September 1993 along with an implementation plan and a detailed displacement plan. Experience proved it was best to address implementation and displacement as separate issues. Rather than implement changes at a pace that would limit the amount of displacement, it was more effective to fully implement changes, addressing the resultant displacement issues separately.

From the start of reengineering, the policy was to do whatever could be done to minimize the negative impact of reengineering on employees and that layoffs would only be used as a last resort. While this policy slowed the benefits of reengineering in that extra cost was incurred by maintaining salaries of displaced staff, it offered a degree of safety and was consistent with the hospital's commitment to staff. How can staff be asked to make a commitment to create a world-class organization without management being willing to provide an equal level of commitment in return?

Displacing managers is a greater challenge than displacing others because there are fewer opportunities to find equivalent positions; turnover is almost nonexistent in management. Attrition has been an effective strategy to deal with displacement in the past but offers little benefit in management reorganization. The most valuable ingredient in management displacement is time. Some examples of the displacement plan are

- Displaced managers with a lower level of compensation will have compensation adjusted over a three-year period with the maximum downward adjustment not to exceed 10 percent. If after three years the existing salary exceeds the target salary, the current salary will be frozen until the target is reached

- Adjustments to compensation for displaced managers accepting positions with lower compensation will be modified based on longevity as follows: managers with service of more than 5 years but less than 10 years will have their current salary frozen for 1 year before adjustments begin. Managers with service of more than 10 years but less than 15 years shall have their current salary frozen for 2 years before adjustments begin. Managers with more than 15 years service shall have their salary frozen with no further adjustments until their target salary is reached

- Managers unable to find employment inside the institution may choose to stay with the hospital for one year at their current salary

Displaced managers ended up in various places. Some found equivalent positions with other organizations, some accepted team leader positions, the manager of healing health care was moved to a vice presidential level, three moved on to the project team, while others accepted staff positions. Every displaced manager found a position either inside St. Charles or with another organization.

When determining the response of the medical staff, it is important not to think of the medical staff as a single group. There may be a wide variety of reactions to the management reorganization. In general, the medical staff viewed the streamlining of management as a positive step, if such a modification would create a more responsive organization. Discussions focused less on the overall structure than on impacts on specific departments. Throughout management reorganization as well as the entire reengineering effort, most physicians were willing to wait and see the outcome of the transformation.

At the same time the hospital was reviewing management reorganization, the medical staff was discussing reorganizing its structure. The medical staff was also interested in finding ways to streamline decision making, better manage the time spent on medical staff business, and reflect the hospital changes.

The new management structure was implemented in January 1994 and over the period since implementation the staff has learned a great deal. Perhaps the most important lesson learned has been that changing the structure is far easier than changing long-held beliefs, patterns of behavior, or culture. Reorganizing the management structure to accelerate decision making or to become more responsive to changing conditions does not translate into managers being more comfortable with rapid change. Even with the setbacks and unexpected issues, St. Charles has made progress.

Once the new management structure is in place and all the displacement issues worked through, the estimate is management time will be reduced by 29,650 hours (22 percent), with a total cost savings of $683,000 annually. These estimates include the addition of three project team members, a vice president of healing health services, a vice president of information services, and a vice president of medical affairs. The estimates also include reductions in some existing executive-level position hours. At the present stage of implementation, actual savings being realized is $374,000 annually. Total management time, all levels, represents 5.7 percent of total payroll hours. In addition, management time dedicated to external issues, such as development of a regional hospital

FIGURE 6
Modifications in management levels

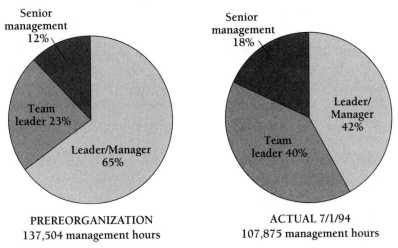

Senior management 12%

Team leader 23%

Leader/Manager 65%

PREREORGANIZATION
137,504 management hours

Senior management 18%

Leader/Manager 42%

Team leader 40%

ACTUAL 7/1/94
107,875 management hours

network and managed care contracting, has increased by 85 percent without having to increase total management cost, as shown in Figure 6.

While benefits have been achieved through a reduction in management cost, it is a mistake to reorganize solely for cost reduction. By reducing management time and cost there is also the risk of reducing the operation effectiveness. Saving a half-million dollars in management costs could create a loss of millions in reduced productivity. Overall goals had to far exceed cost reduction in order to justify such action. The primary goal at St. Charles was to create an organization that could be far more responsive to a changing environment. With respect to the effectiveness of operations, every 1994 budget goal was met or exceeded.

Today 95 percent of all daily operating decisions are being made at the leadership council level or lower. In the near future the intent is to focus on caregiver decision making and empowerment. Many of the daily decisions thought to be the traditional role of management can be more effectively accomplished with caregivers, providing there is agreement on goals, outcomes, and decision parameters. Focus is a key word: simply stating a goal to move more decisions to the point of care will not make it happen. There is a need to structure the decision-making process—to determine what will it look like, what the expected outcomes are, which decisions are made more effectively at the bedside, what parameters the caregivers will utilize in decision making, and which decision-making tools will they need additional training for. There is an inherent risk in setting up a group of caregivers to fail if enough time, effort, and planning are not devoted toward their success.

One final key to success is a unified vision of where the hospital and care system are going—not the vision necessarily on the wall but the vision that is in the hearts and minds of the organization. The ultimate goal is to improve the quality and efficiency of decisions, creating a more efficient, responsive organization.

Management reorganization let St. Charles reallocate resources to critical areas such as information services, healing healthcare, and a variety of improvement projects such as the materiels system reengineering. By reallocating management resources rather than hiring new management staff to meet these needs, there is an additional cost savings.

Prior to implementing the new management structure, a substantial effort was made to develop new teams and clarify roles. However, it is not until actual implementation that the full array of issues becomes apparent. Most of these issues fall into three general areas.

- *Additional role clarification.* There has been a tendency to move decision making to a committee process, which is not the goal. The expectation is that the majority of decisions are to be made by the individual closest to the issue. In addition, there are the normal start-up questions such as, "Who do I go to for what?"

- *Implement leadership model.* While much time and effort has gone into leadership training, the process of moving from theory to reality is continuing. Because old management behaviors are still being maintained, leader/managers are buried in decision making. Sixteen leader/ managers cannot possibly accomplish what more than 50 managers accomplished unless they break from the old management model and move more decisions to the caregivers

- *Redesign of some systems and processes.* Because of management structure modifications, many existing management approaches—such as new employee selection, evaluation, and compensation systems—no longer apply

Despite these issues, St. Charles is beginning to see the light at the end of the tunnel. Individual managers and the councils are gaining ground on clarifying their new roles. Rapid progress on external issues, such as networking and managed care, is being made with noticeable results.

It is far too soon to say the medical center's goals have been reached. Judging from past experience, further modifications will need to be made. The organization is willing to modify any part of the reorganization that fails to reach expectations. What works today may not work tomorrow. In the long run, the organization's increased flexibility and openness for change may be the greatest legacy of reengineering.

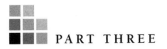

PART THREE

*Customer-focused
case studies*

31

Group Health Cooperative of Puget Sound: Improving customer satisfaction

Judy Morton, PhD
Vice President, Quality Resources
PREMERA (Blue Cross/Blue Shield)
Mountlake Terrace, Washington

A S HEALTHCARE ORGANIZATIONS are challenged to create value for their customers and stakeholders, they are shifting from strategies designed chiefly to attract new business to those intended to create long-term customer loyalty. In the healthcare industry, success depends upon satisfied customers who continue to reenroll and who communicate their satisfaction to others.

Creating and maintaining high levels of customer satisfaction, however, is not a simple feat. While it may appear straightforward, there are few examples of organizations that have wildly satisfied customers— within or outside of healthcare. There is still much to learn about providing care and service that predictably satisfies and even delights customers.

This chapter is based on work done at Group Health Cooperative (GHC) of Puget Sound, a large, mixed-model managed care organization in Seattle, Washington. It describes a six-phase strategy to improve customer satisfaction across an entire managed care system. The strategy continues to be tested and refined at GHC. The ideas described in this chapter are intended to stimulate further dialogue among those interested in accelerating their ability to systematically improve customer satisfaction in a large healthcare organization.

The Plan-Do-Study-Act cycle provided a method to build and refine the strategy over time.[1] The strategy was initially developed based on secondary research and discussions with leaders in various service organizations across the country. It was then implemented over a several-year period. As each phase was implemented, key participants were asked to reflect on what worked well and to identify ideas for refinement. The strategy described in this chapter provides a snapshot of the state of development through the first quarter of 1995.

Customer-driven management

An important observation that helped set the context for this work was the recognition that GHC wanted to do a better job of satisfying customers. GHC leaders recognized the need for an improved approach to this area of strategic importance.

To begin, a group of consumer, physician, and management leaders was asked to develop recommendations for continuously improving customer satisfaction over the next decade. This team began by reading about strategies for providing excellent service and identifying a number of organizations that had earned a reputation for excellent service quality. They set out to learn how these organizations achieved this goal. The ensuing work required the group, and subsequently managers and teams across the organization, to examine basic organizational beliefs and to explicitly state assumptions about the organization's reason for being, the definition of quality, and responsibilities of those in the organization for improving satisfaction. Beliefs that came out of this process are summarized below.

> Our mission is to enhance the well-being of our patients and other customers. Customer satisfaction is a key measure of our progress toward this mission, and, as such, is a key measure of organizational success and performance. In this area, quality is whatever customers think it is.

Most definitions of quality include the concept of customers and the idea of meeting or exceeding their expectations. Karl Albrecht, a service management writer and consultant, suggests that the basic product in service organizations is the "moment of truth," defined as any time when the customer comes in contact with an organization and forms an impression of quality.[2]

Frontline staff manage the thousands of moments of truth that occur every day within a managed care organization. The ability of each frontline staff person to meet or exceed each customer's unique expectations is key. For customers, the frontline staff person is the organization. Customer perceptions of their interactions with staff drives their satisfaction with the organization.

This fact substantially affects the role of management. It means that the manager's main job is to support frontline staff who manage these moments of truth. The way that managers demonstrate that support is by building systems and processes to help staff consistently and reliably manage their daily interactions (or moments of truth) with customers. Key processes and systems that support staff in their efforts to manage these interactions include

- Knowledge of the organization's mission, vision, and commitment to its customers

- Measurement systems

- Improvement methods and tools

- Management practices and policies that ensure that improved customer satisfaction is continuously pursued and achieved

By building such systems and by treating their staff as important customers, leaders create an environment that allows and encourages staff to effectively manage the quality of care and service they provide. The process of developing and describing this managerial philosophy and working with various consumer, physician, and operational leaders across the organization to refine it was essential in laying the foundation for the development and implementation of the strategy described below.

Strategic approach to improving customer satisfaction

Figure 1 illustrates how the six-phase strategy contributes to the systematic improvement of customer satisfaction. The key outputs of this approach are delighted customers. The measure of success is customer satisfaction. The figure shows key inputs including what is happening in the marketplace; the organization's mission, values, and people; and resources committed to this area of organizational performance.

FIGURE 1
Improving customer satisfaction

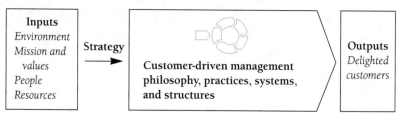

The foundation of this strategy is a customer-driven management philosophy, supported by management practices, systems, and structures aligned to meet the goal of delighting customers.

Strategy for improvement: Six phases and competencies

An overview of the six-phase strategy to systematically improve customer satisfaction is illustrated in Figure 2. Together the phases make up a systematic business planning and implementation process requiring organizational attention and resources to be directed to a few high priority areas that, when addressed, can help the organization achieve its

FIGURE 2
Road map
Improving customer satisfaction

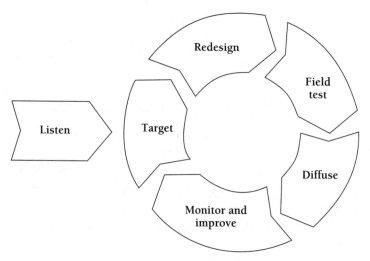

vision. Adapted from principles of policy management, policy deployment, or *Hoshin Kanri,* this approach focuses an entire organization on the vital few challenges and serves to align divisions and departments around the achievement of a set of shared high-priority goals.[3]

Each phase represents an organizational competency that is necessary for improvement. The progress of each phase depends on successful implementation of previous stages, the existence of specific managerial practices and systems, and the execution of specific roles and responsibilities.

The key product(s) of each phase are listed below.

Phase	Key products
1. Listen	• Standardized, ongoing listening system for each key customer group
2. Target	• Agreed-upon list of high-leverage breakthrough improvement goals
	• Plan for addressing each strategic improvement opportunity
3. Redesign	• Customer requirements
	• Supplier goals
	• Supplier requirements
	• Ideal process
	• Philosophy
	• New mental models
	• Support systems
4. Field test	• Summary of best practices
	• Tested tools, methods, and training materials
	• Diffusion plan
5. Diffuse	• Evidence that breakthrough improvement has occurred at all appropriate sites

6. Monitor and improve
- Outcome and process measurement system
- Evidence of continuous improvement at all appropriate sites across the system

This model is most useful for improving cross-functional processes or systems that contribute to strategic goal achievement. They require

- Breakthrough, as opposed to incremental, levels of change
- Standardized outcomes or processes across different parts of the organization
- Fast, real-time change

This model is not intended to replace continuous quality improvement efforts in local work units but to augment local efforts to identify, improve, and control daily operations.

For each phase, the following topics will be discussed: challenges encountered, key steps, supporting managerial practices, and key roles and responsibilities.

PHASE ONE: LISTEN

Success is measured by customer opinions.

Challenges encountered

Developing an ongoing customer-listening system requires an organization to identify the specific customer groups to whom it will systematically listen. It also requires the organization to identify

- Metrics to use for different customer groups and for subpopulations within each group
- How customer-derived data will be used
- How the information from customers can be provided to those who can best use it for improvement purposes

The development and implementation of a system to measure customer satisfaction represented the first tangible opportunity for many at GHC to assess how or if quality concepts and tools would impact their daily work. The agreed-upon need to develop a measurement system generated a combination of interest, fear, excitement, and concern. Many wanted to be involved in the development of measurement systems that could potentially help them in their work.

Key steps

A system to measure customer satisfaction in outpatient facilities was selected as the first main element of the organization's systematic listening system. It was selected because the majority of moments of truth occur in outpatient facilities.

The following steps helped build a systematic way to listen to outpatient visitors.

1. *Discuss key foundational questions with future users of the data.* Issues requiring discussion and systemwide agreement included

   - Topic areas to be measured

   - How the data would be reported

   - How the data would be used

   Gaining agreement required initial discussions with future data users, circulating summaries of initial thinking, discussions of each issue, and a restatement of key agreements. Extensive discussions were held with leaders of all outpatient facilities about the content of the instrument and how the data would be reported to the leaders and teams in each outpatient facility. Due to the strong interest and concern about how such a measurement system would work, six months were invested in developing agreements and plans with the eventual users of the data. The extended discussions with various stakeholders resulted in agreements about the instrument, data reporting methods, and a statement describing how information would be used once it was produced. These preagreements set the stage for excitement about the subsequent appearance and use of the data and helped to minimize concerns about invalid data.

2. *Identify and continuously improve methods for meeting the requirements of the users of the data.* The main users of the outpatient satisfaction data are leaders and teams at three different levels: facility, regional, and systemwide. These users want reliable and valid data, facility-specific, if not unit-specific, information, easy-to-understand information, and timely information

3. *Work hard at meeting or exceeding the requirements of the users of the data.* The requirement of timeliness proved to be the most challenging. To meet this requirement, report production was automated, interview cycle times were reduced, and the time required for internal printing and distribution was decreased

4. *Invest time working with leaders and teams.* Time is needed to help them understand the data, identify how the information could be more usefully presented to them, and identify improvement opportunities or monitor progress over time. In general, managers and teams who regularly discuss and use the data with their entire team tend to improve more than those who do not share and use the information as aggressively

The use of the data and the discussion generated by the data changes over time. GHC conducts an outpatient satisfaction survey twice a year. For the first few times the survey data were discussed, there were many questions about the methodology used and data validity. There was also a great deal of interest in differences among sites. As staff became more comfortable with the methods used and the way the data were being used, they began to demonstrate more curiosity about what customers really mean by dimensions such as "coordination" or "thoroughness of treatment." They also began to wonder what processes or behaviors contribute most to satisfaction with key dimensions. By the fifth administration of the survey, some improvement efforts were designed and implemented, and there was great interest in learning whether improvements had resulted in increased satisfaction levels.

Early on, staff in different clinics agreed to share their data with each other so internal benchmarking opportunities could be identified and pursued. However, it was not until the third year of surveying that such efforts began to occur with much frequency. Data are currently being used to evaluate the extent to which significant improvements have been sustained.

Supporting management practices

The regular review and discussion of data—as part of regular management meetings—is the main management practice supporting the listening phase. In many high-performing organizations, senior executives look at their key service/quality indicators and set action plans for the next steps in the continuous improvement journey.[4] The regular review of customer-derived information is part of a massive shift in performance measurement. Many high-performance organizations are moving from treating financial figures as the foundation for performance measurement to using them as only one element of a broader, more prospective set of measures of organizational performance.

Key roles and responsibilities
During the listening phase, senior line and quality leaders are jointly responsible for

- Developing agreements about the importance and role of customer satisfaction measurement and its relationship to improvement

- Identifying resources required to support the measurement and educational effort, including staff with background and expertise in measurement, analysis, and education; funds to support the required level of data collection; equipment to analyze and present the data; and time for line leaders to learn about what the data say and do not say

At the systemwide level, service quality assessment staff are responsible for

- Working with potential users of the data to identify key requirements

- Using proven scientific methods to gather and analyze the data

- Presenting the data in user-friendly ways

- Helping line leaders to understand the data well enough to help staff in their teams to interpret and use the data

PHASE TWO: TARGET
It is not enough to just do your best work or work hard; you must know what to work on.[5]

The targeting phase makes this approach strategic. The focused use of customer-derived information helps direct improvement resources to areas that will optimize system performance in the eyes of key customer groups.

Challenges encountered

There are two major challenges when developing an agreed-upon list of systemwide breakthrough improvement goals. The first involves developing agreed-upon methods to identify the "vital few" strategic priorities in the eyes of the organization's customers and translating those priorities into appropriate goals. The second challenge is managerial and involves gaining organizational alignment around the vital few. Agreement about the organization's improvement priorities helps ensure that each targeted area is appropriately resourced.

Key steps

1. *For each key customer group, identify the importance levels of specific factors and describe each level of performance.* For example, for enrollee customers at GHC, specific dimensions are identified that most strongly correlate with a variable labeled "customer loyalty." This variable includes respondents' levels of agreement with the following four statements in an annual enrollee survey:

   - "I intend to reenroll at the next opportunity"

   - "Joining GHC was a good decision"

   - "I am very satisfied with the medical care I receive"

   - "I would recommend GHC to my family and friends as a place to receive medical care"

   Performance in key items within each dimension can be charted on an importance-performance matrix to graphically illustrate the relationship between the importance of different factors to enrollees and organizational performance in each area. The matrix, adapted from Albrecht and Bradford and illustrated in Figure 3, assists users in beginning to identify the major gaps between what customers value and what they perceive to be delivered.[6]

2. *Where possible, gather comparable performance data from other organizations.* As employers, national organizations (such as NCQA and The HMO Group) and purchaser/plan coalitions gather comparable satisfaction information across different healthcare plans, it will become easier and less expensive for individual plans to gather comparable information from other organizations

FIGURE 3
Sample importance/performance matrix

IMPORTANCE	*Higher importance and lower performance* **Essential improvement opportunities**	*Higher importance and higher performance* **Strategic/differentiation opportunities**
	Lower importance and lower performance **Relative indifference**	*Lower importance and higher satisfaction* **Irrelevant superiority**

PERFORMANCE

FIGURE 4
Targeting the "vital few"

MORE IMPORTANT AREAS	Below others	On par with others	Higher than others
LESS IMPORTANT AREAS	Below others	On par with others	Higher than others

Figure 4 shows one way to present data that highlights areas where major gaps exist between the plan's performance and the performance of other organizations.

3. *Identify gaps between actual and desired performance for each customer group.* Areas important to key customers and those where performance is low or average in relation to other factors or other organizations represent improvement opportunities. Likewise, areas that are important to customers or those where performance is high in relation to other important factors or in relation to other organizations represent potential areas of strategic opportunity and differentiation. For example, access to routine care may be identified as an essential high-priority improvement opportunity for the enrollee customer group—if it is strongly correlated with customer loyalty and if satisfaction levels for

this factor are significantly below those of comparable plans or lower than other areas of importance to enrollees. A prioritized list of major improvement opportunities for each key customer can be derived by using this approach

4. *Explore customers' perceptions in high-priority areas.* Focusing the improvement agenda requires a deep understanding of how customers evaluate quality in each area of interest. Focus-group research represents one way to efficiently gather such qualitative information. [7] For example, if a plan had targeted access to routine care, access to specialty care, and coordination of services as possible high-priority areas, more information could be gained by inviting randomly selected groups of customers to share their views about how they evaluate quality in each of these areas. A trained focus group facilitator could probe for information about how customers judge quality in each of these areas. Information from such discussions can be analyzed from two perspectives: to discern issues that relate to all three topics, and to identify themes unique to individual priority areas

5. *Target high leverage processes for systemwide improvement.* The idea of leverage is key to identifying the vital few systemwide improvement opportunities. Leverage points are places where a little change has a great impact.[8] Identifying organizational leverage points requires a thorough knowledge of the voice of key customers, the organization's vision, and the interrelationships among different elements of the entire system of care and service[9]

Identifying the extent to which major improvement opportunities for different customer groups overlap can help the organization identify areas of strategic importance. This concept is illustrated in Figure 5. Areas that two or more customer groups see as very important help the organization identify its core processes.

By using such an approach, organizational strategists can identify the top three to five priorities for each of their key customer groups and identify which priorities coincide. At GHC, for example, complaint handling was identified as a top priority for two of the three key customer groups.

6. *Set "stretch goals" in key strategic areas.* Setting satisfaction goals requiring a performance level substantially beyond current levels challenges

FIGURE 5
Targeting the "vital few"

Areas that address the high-priority needs of more than one key customer group point toward a customer view of core processes.

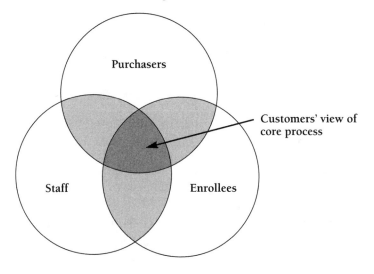

the organization to achieve an unprecedented level of performance. Targets should be aggressive. Satisfaction information from other organizations can help identify what is currently possible. However, it is important to recognize that other high-performing organizations are also improving; thus setting and achieving a goal only as high as today's highest performer may not allow the organization to differentiate itself from other choices the customer may have in the future. For example, if a plan decides to improve significantly its enrollees' level of satisfaction with ease of seeing providers of choice, comparative satisfaction ratings from other plans could be used to identify a targeted level of performance. In examining this data, it might see that the percentage of enrollees rating this dimension as excellent ranged from 11 to 28 percent. If the plan was performing at the 15 percent level and wanted to significantly differentiate its performance, it might set a stretch goal of having 30 or 35 percent of its enrollees rate the ease of seeing the provider of choice as excellent

7. *For every selected goal area, develop an improvement plan.* The improvement plan includes a summary of essential background information

and an overview of the proposed approach to goal achievement. Specifically, it includes

- The rationale for selecting the area as a strategic improvement opportunity

- A description of the gap between current and desired performance

- Measurable stretch goals

- A proposed approach and time line for addressing the strategic improvement opportunity

- An estimate of resources required for all phases of improvement

- Expectations for implementation in all appropriate sites (if field tests yield significant gains)

An example: Targeting a high-leverage improvement opportunity. Through an analysis of the results of annual enrollee surveys, access to specialty care was identified as one of the factors most strongly associated with loyalty to GHC. Moreover, this factor was rated less positively by the organization's customers than other loyalty areas. Comparable health plan data also showed customer satisfaction in this aspect of care was below some other health plans. Additionally, this general area was identified as a high-priority area by enrollees, purchasers, and staff. For these reasons, this area was one of the few targeted for systemwide improvement.

To identify the main processes underlying satisfaction with access to specialty care, focus groups were conducted with enrollees who had rated access to specialty care either very positively or negatively. Focus-group participants were asked to give examples of what they saw as evidence of excellent access and poor access to specialty care. Their responses indicated that four interactions provided enrollees with evidence of superior or poor access to specialty care: scheduling an appointment with a primary care provider, getting a referral from the primary care provider, scheduling the appointment with the specialist, and waiting for the appointment to occur.

Initial improvement work focused on the referral process, a process that begins when the primary care provider and patient agree a specialty appointment is necessary and ends when the patient has a confirmed appointment. This decision was based on two considerations. First, survey and internal data indicated the referral process was taking an unacceptably long time. Second, a major systemwide improvement effort was already under way to improve primary care appointment access.

Supporting management practices and processes

A well-designed and executed strategic planning effort can facilitate dialogue needed to help organizational leaders understand key issues from the perspective of different customer groups and select the vital few priorities for emphasis. Financial and staff resources are needed to design, test, and implement improvements across the system.

Key roles and responsibilities

The targeting phase requires leaders from different parts of the organization to collaborate. Those with data from each customer group, in conjunction with leaders from the planning area and the line, need to discuss and agree about the key breakthrough improvement goals for the organization. Once senior leaders have agreed upon targeted strategic directions, medical and operational leaders need to identify cross-functional or departmental processes to be marked for breakthrough improvement. Designated leaders then become accountable to ensure progress toward the agreed-upon goals.

PHASE THREE: REDESIGN

"Most service failures are not failures; they have been designed into the system."[10]

Achieving and sustaining unprecedented change in a specific area begins with either a redesign or a new design. The specialty referral process will be used to illustrate how the steps outlined in this chapter apply to a specific systemwide targeted improvement opportunity.

Research and initial development is conducted during the design phase. The intent is to develop a new process that will substantially improve organizational performance from the customer's perspective.

Challenges encountered

Major challenges encountered in the redesign phase include

- Defining clear roles and responsibilities for individuals participating in the systemwide design team and the sponsoring leadership team

- Describing the products to be delivered by the redesign team

- Developing supplier support systems

- Lengthy cycle time from the beginning to the end of this phase

- Transitioning to the next phase of the improvement strategy

Key steps

The steps outlined below describe key actions that need to occur during this phase.

1. *Develop a charter.* The team charter provides detailed information about the first phase of improvement, including information about

   - Products of the design team

   - Expectations of the key players in the design process

   - Proposed membership for the systemwide design team (including the estimated time commitment required for each contributor to the design process)

   - Resource estimate (in addition to people's time) required to support work in this phase

   Progress can be significantly delayed if involved individuals do not begin with a shared understanding of these mutual expectations.

2. *Discuss the improvement plan and the proposed charter statement thoroughly with the sponsoring leadership group.* Such a discussion allows the sponsoring leadership team and senior quality staff to develop a shared understanding of the full extent of the strategic challenge, the resources and time required to address the challenge, and the level of support (in terms of personal time, staff time, money, and leadership) each person will be expected to contribute. The discussion also provides an opportunity to further refine and clarify the improvement plan and the design team's charter

   A senior manager (or managers) should be identified to lead and champion each major change effort. Ideally, the process owner for each targeted change effort will be a person with line responsibility for this activity, who is willing to invest a substantial amount of time in the long-term improvement effort. This level of senior leadership accomplishes three important objectives. It signals the importance of the targeted effort to the entire organization, it increases the likelihood the effort receives the needed level of support and resources, and it provides senior leaders with an opportunity to further refine their improvement and implementation skills.

3. *Ensure that appropriate resources are allocated to adequately support improvement work in targeted areas.* In the majority of cases, the most important resource needed is the committed time of key players. During the design phase, these players include at least one leader (or process owner), a highly-skilled and trained facilitator, and five to seven team members from across the organization, who are familiar with different aspects of the process and who agree to participate in developing and testing the new design

The design phase time can be shortened and momentum can be optimized if teams meet frequently, over a short period of time. Typical time commitments include four hours per week for three months for team members and six hours per week for team leaders and the process coordinator. Skilled analytical staff can accelerate the work by coordinating and facilitating focus groups, analyzing data for team use, and documenting the team's work. Depending on the project, the time commitment for an analyst can take up to 20 hours per week for the duration of the design phase.

4. *Select, enroll, and orient members of the systemwide design team.* Members of the systemwide design team should come from different parts of the organization where the improved process will eventually be implemented. Ideally, the team includes a customer, suppliers who work in different parts of the process, at least one person who is known for thinking "outside of the box," and a person from each site where the improved process will be tested

Design team members are expected to attend regular design meetings, contribute their views, complete assigned homework between their meetings, and communicate with colleagues about progress and emerging challenges. Although time commitments will vary with the scope, approximately four hours per week for a three- to four-month period is usually sufficient.

An approach that enrolls team members and ensures they will have the time to contribute will increase ability of the team to complete its design work within the targeted time frame. Members of the sponsoring leadership team play key roles in paving the way for full participation of design team members; they can identify potential team members and help potential design team members (and those to whom they report) understand the importance of the design effort and expectations for participation. Since participation in a systemwide design effort requires team members to take time away from their ongoing responsibilities, senior leaders can help them plan for how existing work will be reprioritized or done while the individual is participating in design team work.

The team charged to redesign the specialty referral process at GHC was co-led by three senior leaders: a regional vice president with broad operational responsibilities and two regional chiefs of staff (a primary care physician and a specialist). They identified the following staff to work with them in the redesign process: specialty and primary care managers from regions where the process would eventually be tested, a primary care physician, a manager of the internal audit function (a person known for thinking outside the box), and a senior-level quality analyst. Before membership was finalized, the coleaders spoke directly with the individuals they were hoping could participate and those individuals to whom the potential members report, explaining the importance of the effort and the need for full participation for a three- to four-month period. Where appropriate, they also assisted in reprioritizing the existing responsibilities so team members would be free to participate. In some cases, they arranged for the ongoing work of design team members to be managed by someone else for the period the design team was scheduled to meet.

5. *Develop key products.* Figure 6 shows where the design phase fits into the overall improvement strategy and summarizes the products to be completed by the end of this phase

The following key products are needed to transition to the next phase.

- Customer requirements are key attributes desired by customers. Members of the redesign team went through a structured process to identify the key customer requirements for the specialty referral process. They reviewed literature and relevant studies and viewed

FIGURE 6
Products: Redesign phase

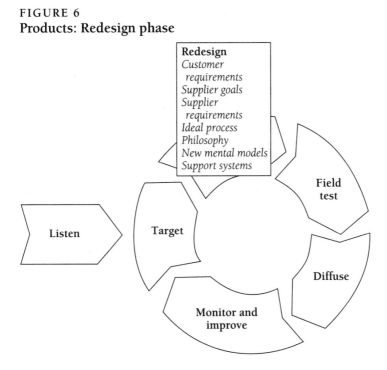

focus groups. This review helped them to understand that once an enrollee agreed with the primary care physician that a referral is needed, the enrollee wants to know where the specialty appointment will be and with whom; he or she also wants to know all of this information within a reasonable time

- Supplier goals are specific targets that must be consistently met by those who ensure that customer requirements are reliably met or exceeded. Based on an analysis of survey and focus-group data, the design team identified one key supplier goal for the specialty referral process: 100 percent of the time, the specialty appointment will be confirmed by the end of the business day following the referral

- Supplier requirements include a list of processes, systems, or materials needed to enable those working in the process to reliably meet supplier goals. For the specialty referral process, supplier requirements included training in carrying out the new process and a fast way to communicate referral information between primary care and specialty sites

- A flowchart of the ideal process illustrates the sequence of steps needed to ensure that supplier goals are consistently met or exceeded. Initially, two process flows were developed to describe the ideal specialty referral process: one was a "today tech" option and the other was a "dream tech" option. Several meetings with both primary providers and consulting specialists were held to critique and refine the process flow. The suppliers in the process provided essential input to the final design of the ideal process. A high-level flowchart of the improved process is shown in Figure 7

- A philosophy statement describes why individuals in the organization care about this outcome and the basic beliefs driving the improved design

- Old and new mental models[11] describe the explicit assumptions underlying the current process and those underlying the newly designed process

- Supplier support systems include a list of those materials, tools, or systems needed to adequately test the improved process. Since training materials, information systems, or other key support systems are often required, this part of the process may require a substantial time investment if major development work is needed. Since the redesigned specialty referral process required rapid communication between the primary care and specialty site, an improved e-mail system was devised to ensure that the supplier goal could be reliably met

6. *Regularly communicate progress, challenges, and emerging lessons.* Early communication with future implementers lays a foundation for success in subsequent phases. It also provides members of the systemwide team with an opportunity to hear and incorporate good ideas from outside the design team.

Several tools and methods have proven helpful at GHC. One is a quarterly internal newsletter called *Quality Update.* This organizationwide publication for managers and leaders provides the following information about each targeted systemwide improvement area: progress, emerging lessons and challenges, next steps, and the names and phone numbers of key contact people. Many design teams have also found it useful to circulate brief meeting minutes (summarizing draft products and plans) to

FIGURE 7
High-level flowchart
Appointment scheduling process for consultant (specialty) care

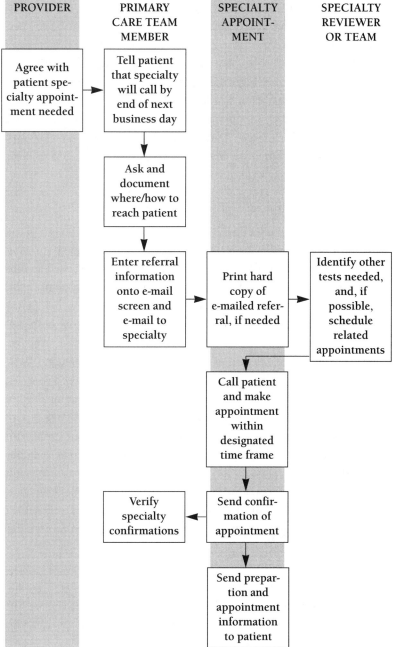

| PROVIDER | PRIMARY CARE TEAM MEMBER | SPECIALTY APPOINT-MENT | SPECIALTY REVIEWER OR TEAM |

those who will be involved in subsequent testing or implementation. Many design teams report that this practice increases the likelihood that future implementers will share ideas or issues that need to be considered before design products are finalized.

The specialty referral redesign team paid special attention to communication issues. They formed a subgroup of the team to develop a communication plan. The plan identified key groups that needed to receive information, messages that each group should receive, and target dates by which information would be exchanged. Materials were then prepared to be used by senior leaders and members of the subgroup to communicate with all targeted audiences. The plan was staged to raise early awareness and increase involvement from sites targeted to begin testing or diffusing the redesigned process.

Supporting management practices

Two management practices contribute to success in the redesign phase. The first requires senior leaders to include the chartering, sponsoring, and support of redesign teams as part of their ongoing work. The integration of these functions into ongoing leadership work ensures that design efforts get the attention, support, and resources needed. Senior leadership of design teams also communicates the importance of the targeted effort to the entire organization.

The second management practice involves the promotion and facilitation of continuous communication and learning about progress and emerging lessons. Leaders can facilitate this type of organizational learning in several ways. One strategy involves incorporating progress reports and discussion of design work into regular agendas. When sponsoring leadership teams hear back from design teams about progress and challenges, they can ask team members to reflect on what they are learning and how design work could be streamlined. Such management practices accelerate the ability of individuals and the organization to improve the content of the design work in a specific area and the design process that will be used in the future.

Key roles and responsibilities

Individuals with different sets of skills and roles bring unique contributions to each phase of improvement. Two different leadership roles are important in this and subsequent phases: the process owner and the process coordinator.

The systemwide process owner is accountable for achieving specified results for each phase of work. This person is usually a member of the sponsoring leadership team or has line responsibility for the process targeted for improvement. During the design phase, the process owner ensures that the design team has the required resources, chairs design team meetings, updates the sponsoring leadership team about progress and emerging challenges or lessons, and removes barriers that threaten success.

The process coordinator brings expertise in quality measurement, quality management, and organizational change to the improvement effort. During the redesign phase, the process coordinator works closely with the process owner to ensure that appropriate measurement, analytical, and improvement methods are used in the design process. The process coordinator facilitates key segments of the design meetings, while the process owner leads the meetings. The process coordinator for major systemwide design efforts needs in-depth knowledge of quality concepts and tools, and a high level of skill in helping cross-functional teams apply these concepts and tools. Additionally, during the design phase, the process coordinator ensures that the work of the team is documented and analytical work is completed between meetings.

Since the successful execution of the specialty referral process required the joint ownership of several different parts of the organization, three senior leaders were identified to co-lead this redesign process. During the redesign phase they were jointly accountable for ensuring the design team produced the specified products within a three- to four-month time frame. They worked in partnership with a senior quality improvement consultant to plan the agendas for the design team meetings. A quality improvement consultant and a senior quality analyst served as system-wide process coordinators for this phase. The quality improvement consultant ensured that appropriate methods and tools were used to achieve the targeted goals, and the senior quality analyst documented the work of the team, provided high-level analytical support, and ensured the overall process was effectively managed. While the three leaders rotated responsibility for chairing the meetings, the quality improvement consultant facilitated major segments of the agenda. As the design process unfolded, the process coordinator spent less time facilitating different aspects of team meetings, while the process owners assumed greater responsibility.

PHASE FOUR: FIELD TEST

"Testing is absolutely key."[12]

The research and development work that began in the design phase continues during the field-testing phase. The work completed during this phase makes it possible to learn how the conceptual design can be implemented by those who work in the process. Several successive tests occur during this phase to allow a number of products to be developed. Figure 8 shows where the field test phase fits into the overall strategy and summarizes the key products of this phase.

Emerging challenges

Several major challenges are encountered while field-testing the conceptual design and completing the three key products, including a description of best practices, a diffusion plan, and tested training materials. First, many staff who are suppliers in the targeted process fear that improvements in external customer satisfaction may occur at their expense or may create other unintended consequences. For example, some providers feared that making specialty appointments within a targeted time period could preclude needed triage or scheduling that should occur before a specialty appointment is finalized. Thorough field tests help address and assess the concerns of those who will eventually implement improvements.

Second, providing sufficient time and resources to adequately test an improved process can be difficult in an environment that concurrently requires lower costs and fast improvements in key outcomes. Before an adequate field test can occur, the staff testing the new process need to be oriented and trained. Often, new or different information systems or patient education materials need to be developed. Sometimes new or different roles or even jobs need to be developed. In the case of the specialty referral process, schedulers at the specialty centers needed to incorporate more frequent referral reviews into their daily routines. It can be difficult to accurately predict the amount of energy, resources, and time that is required to adequately support and test the redesigned process.

Lastly, field-testing of new or improved processes can suffer when

FIGURE 8
Products: Field test phase

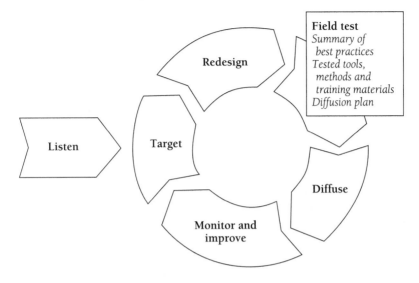

changes in pilot site leadership occur during the field test. Such changes can significantly interrupt or delay progress.

Key steps

1. *Select several sites in which to field-test the improved process.* Testing in several different types of sites accomplishes three things. First, it provides the organization a way of anticipating the range of possible barriers that can arise during implementation. Second, it can help identify the extent to which different process variations can achieve the same outcome. Third, it can help identify if unique implementation strategies should be considered in sites that vary by model (e.g., staff or network), size, or types of population served. At GHC, selecting the test sites for the redesigned specialty referral process required thinking through a range of options. In the end, the specialty referral process was tested in one of the three geographic regions served by the organization. Three different primary care sites and all specialty sections in the region served as test sites

Because the first time a new process is implemented may take more time, energy, and persistence than later efforts, it can help to identify sites where leadership is stable and there is evidence of strong interest in the targeted area of organizational performance. Staff in potential field test sites may have already tried some innovations in this area or may have contributed ideas to the design process. This positive energy and prior improvement work proves to be a huge asset in doing critical research and development work on behalf of the organization.

2. *Identify a process owner for each test site.* Local field test process owners lead the implementation efforts in their site and ensure that staff receive the implementation assistance they need. During the early part of implementation, these individuals often invest many hours planning the rollout and then coaching staff as they try the redesigned process. They also spend significant time with staff learning about what works and does not work, as well as strategizing about how to remove barriers to full implementation. Lessons identified are very important to share with the systemwide coordination team so emerging knowledge can be further exchanged across the system

3. *Create a systemwide coordination team to systematically support and learn from field test experiences.* Although most of the work in this phase occurs in the designated field test sites, key work is also carried out by a systemwide coordination team. This team, composed of several members of the initial design team and individuals from each field test site, periodically meets to review progress, identify and share emerging challenges and lessons, develop strategies for collaboratively addressing barriers, and help the sponsoring leadership team understand about progress and needs for additional or different types of support. If staff join the systemwide coordination team who did not participate in the earlier design work, it is important to invest some time helping them gain an understanding of previous work and the thinking behind it

The systemwide coordination team for the specialty referral process learned about the operational difficulties of gathering data to assess how well the process was working. Together they developed a more efficient way to gather and report the data to individuals working in the process.

4. *Before any field test starts, assess the staff's level of confidence.* The staff must have confidence in their ability to meet customer requirements and their perception of the level of support they receive to meet those requirements. Not only does this practice provide a baseline from which initial progress can be assessed, it also identifies areas that require attention before and during field testing. When staff in future implementation sites see evidence that staff who implemented the redesigned process in field test sites report improved confidence levels and satisfaction in their ability to meet customer requirements, their willingness to test improvements developed elsewhere can be increased

5. *Further refine the supports needed to test the redesigned process.* Educational materials, tools, and information systems are often needed to enable the improved design to be tested. Adequately testing and refining these foundational supports increases the likelihood the field test sites can achieve significantly improved levels of performance. Investment in developing such support helps to address the fear that staff requirements will not be considered

During the field-testing phase of the specialty referral improvement effort, several tools were developed for and by field test teams. For example, a standardized referral form was designed and refined. With support from the information systems part of the organization, an existing e-mail system was customized and installed in test sites. Appropriate individuals were trained to use the new forms and systems. This effort required a large amount of unanticipated resources. Questions such as, "Who will pay for printers?," "Who will do the training?," and "Who will pay for release time for staff to receive training?" needed to be answered.

6. *Implement and stabilize the improved process.* Several adjustments and refinements are required before an improved process begins to work as originally planned. Measuring the achievement of key supplier goals helps to identify the extent to which the new process works as designed and has achieved a level of stability over time

7. *Continue to test ways to improve the redesigned process.* During this period, different sites try new ways to meet supplier goals. As mentioned earlier, constant reflection and dialogue within and between

field test sites can significantly accelerate the improvement of the redesigned process or the methods used to implement the process

8. *Once it appears the process is working as designed and is stable in all field test sites, conduct a thorough evaluation.* The evaluation should assess both customer and staff satisfaction with the process and the extent to which the targeted outcomes are being achieved in each test site and across the system. The evaluation also allows supplier goals to be rechecked and modified if necessary. The results help the systemwide coordination team to refine the generic design and identify implementation strategies and tools associated with strong performance. Such an evaluation also helps field test sites identify areas requiring additional attention. For example, the evaluation of the specialty referral process showed variation within both primary care and specialty sites. Such information allowed process owners in individual sites to identify gaps between their performance level, the goal, and what was possible. The variation in performance represented an opportunity to learn more about what implementation practices were associated with higher levels of performance

9. *Summarize the best practices that emerged from the field tests, and develop a diffusion plan that incorporates lessons learned.* Through field test evaluations, it is possible to learn which practices are associated with improved outcomes and if the number or content of supplier goals required to meet customer requirements can be reduced or refined. Such lessons can significantly simplify subsequent implementation efforts

Therefore, a diffusion plan can be built that addresses the following questions:

- What is the process to be implemented?

- Where is variation permitted and not permitted?

- What has been learned so far about how to best implement this process?

- Which sites across the organization should implement this process?

- Who will be accountable for implementing this process in each site?

- How will process owners and their teams know when the process has successfully been implemented and is working as designed?

- What are the targeted dates for implementing and achieving specified outcomes?

10. *Assemble tools, methods, and training materials that have helped test sites achieve targeted outcomes.* Sites being asked to implement improved processes can significantly minimize their initial development work if they are provided with tools, methods, and training materials that have already been tested and refined. These generic materials can be adapted to address local needs and issues

Supporting management practices

Field test sites carry out important research and development work for the organization. Compared to the initial design work, which can be intellectually exciting and visible to many in the organization, this work involves careful planning, attention to detail, and concern for a myriad of change issues at local sites. During this phase, visible interest and support of the sponsoring leadership group is key.

Those working in the test site need to know there is continued interest in this work. This interest can be demonstrated both formally and informally. Members of the sponsoring leadership team or the systemwide coordination team can visit test sites to learn about progress and emerging challenges. In addition, representatives from field test sites can be invited to leadership meetings to share progress and concerns. Providing additional or different resources, if needed, represents another important type of support during this phase.

Key roles and responsibilities

In addition to chairing the systemwide coordination team, the systemwide process owner is responsible for ensuring that the field test sites receive the resources they need to adequately test the process. In the case of the specialty referral process, the owners ensured that all affected staff in field test sites had an opportunity to learn about why the process was targeted for improvement, the targeted performance levels, and the time frame for testing. The systemwide process owners also ensured that affected staff received training in how to implement and evaluate the effectiveness of the new process. When it became apparent that additional resources were needed from information systems to further refine the e-mail system, they arranged for an information specialist to be assigned to the team.

The systemwide process coordinator continues to facilitate segments of the meetings of the coordination team. This person also shares with all field test sites the refined materials, tools, and methods that begin to emerge from individual sites or from the collaboration of several sites. One strategy that proved helpful at GHC was to develop a tool kit for field test process owners and teams. The kit is regularly updated as new assessment instruments, training materials, or methods are developed.

The tool kit developed for the improved specialty referral process included a range of information and tools, including

- Background materials (i.e., information about why the process was selected for improvement, targeted levels of performance, a description of how the specialty referral process was redesigned, and expected time lines and products of the redesign team)

- Implementation tools designed to help local staff

   Create district and local teams

   Ensure equipment readiness

   Prepare the clinic for change

   Monitor performance to stabilize and continuously improve the process

- List of the names and phone numbers of people who can serve as resources

PHASE FIVE: DIFFUSE

"We're different."

Diffusion involves transferring a targeted outcome or process to all appropriate locations. As demonstrated in Figure 9, this phase is completed when there is evidence that breakthrough levels of improvement have occurred at all appropriate sites. In the case of the specialty referral process, breakthrough performance was deemed to have occurred when

FIGURE 9
Key product: Diffusion

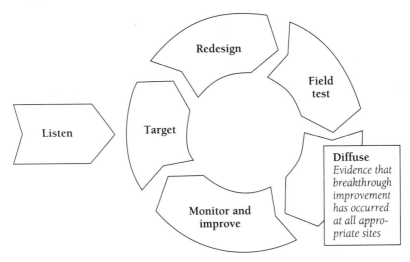

all sites were achieving from 70 to 80 percent of the targeted goal. The remainder of the targeted goal was to be achieved in the monitoring and continuous improvement phase.

It is during diffusion that the work done in the earlier phases begins to show results. With concurrent replication occurring in all appropriate sites and performance levels rising simultaneously in many sites, systemwide performance begins to accelerate quickly.

Emerging challenges

Many challenges in the diffusion phase relate to a set of unstated assumptions or beliefs that appear when staff at various sites are asked to implement a process or reach a targeted outcome that has been developed or achieved elsewhere. These beliefs include the perception that "We're different." Differences in populations served, delivery models, and resource configurations are often seen as limiting the applicability of practices from other locations. A second belief is the perception that implementing a process tested at other sites is not as important or as creative as developing a new improvement at one's own site.

Another challenge involves integrating the use of process measures into daily work. Regularly gathering and using process data to identify the need for adjustment represents a new set of behaviors for many local teams. Establishing these new behavior patterns is no small feat.

Implementing a new process in several different locations within an aggressive time frame can be difficult. Such an effort often competes with other local initiatives, and other systemwide improvement efforts.

Key steps

1. *Review and commit to diffusion plans with the sponsoring leadership group.* Once the systemwide coordination team has developed a proposed diffusion plan, the sponsoring leadership group needs to thoroughly discuss the plan. This discussion provides the opportunity to further develop and commit to agreements about

- Specific systemwide goals (including measures of success)

- Where variation is and is not permitted

- Expected time lines for initial implementation and the achievement of specific outcomes

- How this change effort is coordinated with other high-priority systemwide efforts

Explicitly clarifying where variation is and is not permitted is especially helpful. This decision depends on the targeted process or outcomes. For example, to improve primary care appointment availability, it was decided that all primary care sites were expected to meet systemwide satisfaction outcomes and specific supplier goals. The process to achieve those goals, however, could vary. In this case, process variation was allowed because inputs and processes were very different in each primary care site, and the process was managed independently by each primary care site. On the other hand, the goals for the specialty referral process involved achieving both a systemwide satisfaction level and implementing the same process in all sites. Since the specialty referral process requires coordination between different sites, the implementation of a standard process was necessary.

Simultaneously implementing an improved process in all targeted sites, rather than one site at a time, significantly speeds the diffusion process. Concurrent diffusion can also create a kind of synergy and teamwork among sites working to achieve goals at the same time.

2. *Clarify accountabilities for key parts of the diffusion.* The roles of sponsor, process owner, and coordinator are key. The roles and responsibilities section will highlight areas particularly important during diffusion

3. *Orient local process owners and coordinators.* It is especially important to ensure that those who are responsible for implementing strategies to improve specific outcomes in their areas understand

   - Why this change is important to the organization's success

   - How the system and individual sites will measure success

   - The expected time lines

   - What flexibility each site has (e.g., where standardization is required and where it is not)

   - What has been learned from the field test experiences

   - Plans for assessing progress and challenges

   - Resources are available to help carry out this effort

Kick-off sessions, attended by members of the sponsoring leadership group and local process owners and coordinators, are an efficient and fun way to ensure that expectations are clearly set. At such sessions, those who will be implementing improvements can ask questions, identify concerns, and share ideas. The kick-off session can start the development of a community committed to extending the ability of the whole system to improve in the targeted area. Achieving such a goal means recognizing that there is a great deal to learn about how to achieve targeted outcomes and that each site can help the system learn how to do this work more effectively.

Evaluations of these kick-off sessions indicate that several features are important to participants. Local leaders appreciate knowing that the person to whom they report supports this goal and understands the amount of time and energy such an effort requires. They also are interested in gaining an understanding of what worked and did not work in implementing the improved process in the field test sites. Hearing both leaders and frontline staff from field test sites tell stories about their experiences adds reality and humor to the session.

During this session, it is helpful to share copies of the tool kit developed in the previous phase. It should include copies of tested materials that can be used or adapted to speed the implementation process. Materials that local process owners and coordinators have found especially valuable include

- Copies of overheads they can use with staff to describe the nature of the challenge and the approach to change

- Tested pre- and post-staff satisfaction instruments

- Training materials

- Process measurement tools

- List of the names and phone numbers of people who can serve as resources

4. *Implement and stabilize the improved process at all targeted local sites, and ensure that staff at each site have the opportunity to make the process theirs.* Part of the orientation needs to highlight the need for continuously learning how to do this work better. As local sites adapt a generic process and implement it in their area, they will identify innovations that can benefit the entire system

5. *Systematically share progress, as well as emerging challenges and lessons, with those involved across the system.* This step must be successfully implemented if outcomes are to be achieved within targeted time frames. There are many structured ways to facilitate and encourage this kind of cross-team learning and dialogue. The following ideas have been implemented or are being considered at GHC.

  - Staff at each site are encouraged and expected to review progress and to identify emerging challenges and new ways of approaching the targeted goal. They are also expected to share their progress and observations with the systemwide coordination team. Several coordination teams have developed standardized formats that allow local process owners to easily summarize progress, identify ideas that are being tested or are working, and recognize barriers being encountered

- The systemwide process coordinator summarizes this information and shares it with the systemwide coordination team, the local process owners, and the sponsors. The systemwide coordination team reviews these summaries, identifies ideas worth sharing, and develops ways to tackle systemwide barriers. This summary is included in tool kit updates

- Use voice-mail and e-mail technology to request real-time consultations or share emerging lessons, questions, and challenges among sites

Once these kinds of support systems are in place, staff from local sites often increase the frequency with which they exchange ideas with each other about successes ideas and challenges.

Supporting management practices

When local sites need additional assistance to achieve the targeted goal, members of the sponsoring group must provide that assistance. While that assistance may involve providing money or identifying additional consulting help, it also may mean spending time in a local site or working with a local process owner to help staff further understand the importance of improvement in a targeted area.

Management processes that facilitate the exchange of information about progress and challenges in the vital few areas of focus support successful diffusion. Vehicles that are used to supplement ongoing face-to-face communication at GHC include regular letters from the CEO to all employees, regular reports from the medical director to all medical and affiliate staff, a quarterly video highlighting major developments and change efforts, a biweekly internal newsletter, and the quarterly *Quality Update. Quality Update* includes progress and emerging lessons about all major quality initiatives at GHC. When frequent messages about each key improvement area are sent through multiple vehicles over time, it builds and sustains continued focus in key areas.

Recognition of diffusers, improvement efforts, and progress is key. Formal and informal recognition not only sustains continued effort, it builds momentum and confidence. It is important to recognize the ability to quickly replicate best practices is a key organizational competency for the future.

Key roles and responsibilities

Because the improved process eventually needs to become part of ongoing operations, implementation needs to move from a project structure to the existing line structure. The systemwide process owner's chief responsibility during diffusion is to ensure that specified goals are met within targeted time frames. To accomplish this goal, the systemwide process owner ensures that local process owners understand the outcomes for which they are accountable, that progress is reviewed, and that necessary support is provided to local sites when needed.

The systemwide process coordinator ensures that those with line implementation roles receive the information and consultation assistance they need to carry out their work. Additionally, the systemwide process coordinator works with local process owners or coordinators to describe progress in each area and identify emerging challenges or concerns. From this input, the process coordinator surfaces ideas that are speeding progress and pinpoints those areas that require the attention of the sponsoring systemwide leadership team.

As was the case during field testing, local process owners and coordinators are key to diffusion. They lead the implementation efforts in their area and ensure that staff receive the help they need to implement the improved process. They also help the systemwide training and coordination team to identify

- Major barriers or concerns that require systemwide attention

- New learning, ideas, or approaches

- Systemwide strategies that could either minimize barriers or increase supports to goal achievement

PHASE SIX: MONITOR AND CONTINUOUSLY IMPROVE

"Maintaining the gains from improvement eventually boils down to a focus on methods—what will we do differently to maintain the gains, to prevent the recurrence of a problem, and to achieve new, consistently higher levels of performance."[13]

FIGURE 10
Key products: Monitoring and improvement

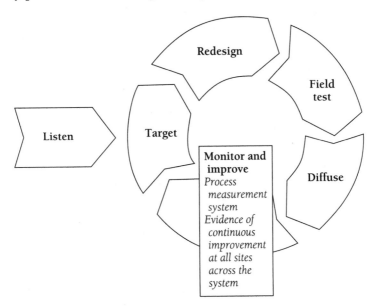

Once the targeted outcomes or processes have been implemented and stabilized at all appropriate sites, it is important to ensure that the significant gains are not only maintained over time but are continuously improved. Figure 10 illustrates where this phase fits into the entire cycle and the products of this phase.

Continuously improving satisfaction levels in the targeted area in all appropriate sites provide evidence that the work in this phase has been successful.

Key challenges

Given the excitement of design, the achievements of testing and diffusion, and the continuing call of new and seemingly more urgent new challenges, sustaining the requisite energy to maintain gains and to further improve them can be difficult. Without focused attention to the less visible phase of monitoring and continuous improvement, the substantial investments made in achieving breakthrough improvements can be lost.

Several challenges appear while monitoring and continuously improving the newly designed or redesigned processes. The first involves the development of methods to continuously monitor outcome and process performance. If key outcome measuores are not already included in the ongoing service quality assessment system, they need to be added. For example, for the specialty referral process improvement effort, a question designed to assess visitors' satisfaction with the specialty referral process was added to the ongoing survey of outpatient visitors. Additionally, the process measures developed and implemented during diffusion need to be integrated into the ongoing practice of teams managing the process. This has proven especially difficult when these measures require staff to collect data.

As was the case in earlier phases, continuously exchanging information among the sites about progress, challenges, and emerging lessons continues to represent a challenge. A designated individual or team is required to ensure that this function is carried out on an ongoing basis.

Key steps

1. *Identify local process owners to be responsible for continuously improving the process in their designated area.* Working with their teams, local process owners ensure that data about outcomes and the process are regularly collected, interpreted, shared, and used to identify if or when further interventions are required. This responsibility needs to be written into this person's job responsibility statement. During this phase, individuals or teams may need help understanding and using the data. As they carry out this effort, they may discover improved measures, as well as easier ways to gather, display, and act on the data

2. *Identify a systemwide process owner or team to monitor and continuously improve the performance of the process over time.* This individual or team plays a similar role to the local process owner but on a systemwide level. This person monitors outcomes over time and works with local process owners to exchange information about emerging challenges and lessons. The process owner or team also identifies what can be done to improve process capability; this may require increasing supplier goals or further modifying the process. For example, the specialty referral team is currently looking at challenging primary care to send referrals within one hour after the referral agreement. Success in this phase is measured by the continuous improvement of customer satisfaction over time

Supporting management practices and systems

Much of the success of continuous improvement depends on the extent to which staff and managers at local levels can use statistical process control methods. The availability of user-friendly training in the use of these methods is key. Staff often need help in translating these methods to their daily work. This phase provides teachable moments for staff working on maintaining and further improving the performance of the targeted process. For example, when individuals are accountable for ensuring a targeted level of performance with the specialty referral process, training in the use of statistical process control is often seen as more relevant than a general class that covers the same content.

Another kind of management support involves investing resources to develop automated process measurement systems where appropriate. Useful process measures and reports can often be generated through the organization's existing information systems. Automated process measures can speed the gathering and reporting of process measurement data at local as well as systemwide levels. For example, an automated appointment-making system used by all schedulers can be programmed to generate information automatically for local staff about how well different aspects of the appointment-making process are working.

Without ongoing management review and discussion of process performance, improvements will be difficult to continue and sustain. As was the case in previous phases, when data reviews show progress, it is critical to recognize and celebrate success.

Key roles and responsibilities

Systemwide and local process owners are pivotal in this phase. They are accountable for working with appropriate teams to regularly review progress, exchange emerging challenges and refinements, and identify methods to continuously improve performance over time. For the specialty referral process at GHC, systemwide process ownership is invested in a team.

Results

Although this strategy is early in its application, GHC is beginning to see improved satisfaction ratings in targeted areas. Significant improvements in overall satisfaction with the outpatient visit have occurred.

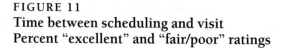

FIGURE 11
Time between scheduling and visit
Percent "excellent" and "fair/poor" ratings

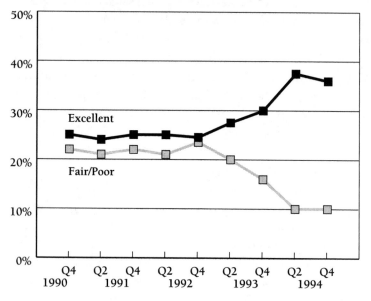

Statistically significant increases in the percentage of excellent ratings and decreases in the percentage of "fair/poor" ratings in the following targeted areas have contributed to this overall improvement.

- Getting through on the phone to make an appointment

- Time between scheduling and visit

- Ease of appointment making

- Ease of seeing provider wanted

- Specialty referral process

- Lab test notification

For example, Figure 11 shows changes in the percentage of "excellent" and "fair/poor" ratings of the time between when an appointment was requested and a visit occurred.

Not surprisingly, improvements show up sooner and more dramatically in encounter-specific surveys than they do in surveys of all enrollees, some of whom have not had recent interactions with the system.

Reflections and observations

There is much to learn about healthcare customers and their expectations. There is also much to learn about how healthcare professionals can work together to meet and exceed those expectations. Reflections and observations about the overall strategy are offered below.

- The speed of implementing systemwide change can be dramatically improved. Actions that are accelerating this work at GHC include reducing the total time needed to complete each phase, reducing substantially the time it takes to execute the handoffs between one phase and the next, clearly specifying the role of process owners and coordinators during each phase, and concurrently implementing best practices

- Carrying out this improvement strategy profoundly affects management assumptions and practice. It requires leaders and teams to

  Challenge basic assumptions about how managed care should work

  Learn more about how to implement and diffuse quickly

  Develop systematic ways to help staff across the organization learn how to learn

- Progress is seldom linear; there is often a lag time between when improvements are implemented and when customers notice improvements

- Even though this work requires persistence, attention to detail and substantial personal effort, it provides staff with an opportunity to work toward goals that have great personal meaning

NOTES

1. W. E. Deming, *The New Economics for Industry, Education, Government* (Cambridge, Mass.: Massachusetts Institute of Technology, Center for Advanced Engineering Study, 1993).

2. K. Albrecht, *At America's Service* (Homewood, Ill.: Dow-Jones Irwin, 1988).

3. W. H. Brunetti, *Achieving Total Quality* (New York: Quality Resources, 1993).

4. J. Clemmer, *Firing on All Cylinders* (Homewood, Ill.: Business One Irwin, 1992).

5. W. E. Deming, *Out of the Crisis* (Cambridge, Mass.: Massachusetts Institute of Technology, Center for Advanced Engineering Study, 1986).

6. K. Albrecht and L. Bradford, *The Service Advantage* (Homewood, Ill.: Dow-Jones Irwin, 1990).

7. K. Riley and J. Rohrl, *Locally Managed Assessment Methods: Surveys and Focus Groups* (Seattle: Group Health Cooperative of Puget Sound, 1994); R. A. Krueger, *Focus Groups: A Practical Guide for Applied Research* (Newbury Park, Calif.: Sage, 1994); and O. W. Stuart and P. N. Shandasani, *Focus Groups: Theory and Practice* (Newbury Park, Calif.: Sage, 1990).

8. B. L. Joiner, *Fourth Generation Management* (New York: McGraw Hill, 1994).

9. P. B. Bataldan and P. K. Stoltz, "A Framework for Continual Improvement of Health Care," *The Joint Commission Journal* 19, no. 10 (October 1993); and G. Capozzalo, "Quality Improvement Principles Power New Strategic and Financial Planning," *Quality Leadership* (September 1993).

10. L. Schlesinger, "The Service Driven Company," *Harvard Business Review* (September–October 1991) 73.

11. P. C. Senge et al., *The Fifth Discipline Fieldbook* (New York: Doubleday Dell Publishing Group, 1994).

12. D. Berwick, Presentation at Total Quality Management Conference, HMO Group, Boston, Mass., July 1994.

13. Joiner, *Fourth Generation Management,* 202.

32

Health maintenance organization: Reengineering member services

Ann Gillespie Pietrick, JD
Vice President and General Counsel
The Scheur Management Group, Inc.
Newton, Massachusetts

A T THEIR INCEPTION, HMOs were a radical departure from the traditional mode of providing healthcare services; they focused on what the purchasers needed in terms of service and all clinical needs rather than solely addressing acute clinical needs. The growth of HMOs is a response to consumer needs, even before consumers had articulated those needs. The earliest HMOs were founded in the recognition that the healthcare system was deficient in reaching out to those who needed services. As the center of the healthcare system evolved from the family doctor to the specialist, patients were left without a guide to assist in accessing healthcare services. Thus, HMOs developed as an alternative to the specialist-dominated healthcare system by packaging patient convenience with clinical expertise at reasonable and predictable costs.

In the last decade, HMOs have been reshaped in response to purchasers' needs. This time, however, the focus has been primarily on the large group healthcare purchaser—the employers, Medicare, or Medicaid. Instead of focusing on the convenience of individual consumers, HMOs have shifted to the group purchasers' needs to provide healthcare benefits: administrative ease, multiple benefit designs to appeal to a broad spectrum of beneficiaries, and reduction (or at least stabilization) of health benefit costs as a percentage of their total budgets.

A by-product of the shift from consumer to purchaser, as well as of the rapid expansion of many HMOs from single-service areas to regional or national companies, is that many HMOs today are bureaucratic, complex organizations that have lost their entrepreneurial spirit. These HMOs have gone from being the simpler alternative for obtaining and paying for healthcare services, to becoming a maze of barriers. Instead of being an aid to the consumer in navigating the healthcare system, the HMO is being viewed as another hurdle to overcome.

Thus, many HMOs have been experiencing stagnant membership (i.e., the number of disenrollments equal the number of new enrollments) or net membership losses. In competitive markets, where the variation in price among competitors is slight and network composition is comparable, HMOs perceived as being quality organizations are those experiencing enrollment growth. This consumer perception of quality is largely based on service components rather than clinical expertise. Member satisfaction is primarily measured in terms of ease in getting appointments, waiting times in provider facilities, proximity of providers to the home or workplace, office hours, and physicians and staff demeanor. Since most members use clinical services infrequently, their contact with the HMO is sporadic. However, if they find it difficult to use the services when they finally need them, they are less likely to be satisfied with the HMO regardless of cost or clinical excellence.

The following case study involves an HMO in a competitive market experiencing stagnated or loss of membership. Its price is competitive and it is considered the market leader in terms of consumer awareness and size (i.e., high brand-name identification). Member satisfaction surveys and employer group information revealed the HMO's member service was inferior to its competitors although it delivered high-quality clinical care. The HMO had implemented numerous "fixes" over the last several years to improve member services, and senior management was frustrated to find that none seemed to have improved overall performance. It became clear that the HMO needed to embark on a complete member service function reengineering.

The case study describes the functional analysis the HMO undertook to determine what was wrong, the recommendations made to achieve genuine change and improvement, and the process to implement those recommended changes.

Functional analysis

The functional analysis reviewed each area in the organization where significant member contact occurs. Member service processes include all of the activities related to the resolution of a member need or problem, beginning with the identification of a need or problem. All actions, statements, policies, and documents related to finding a resolution to the member need or problem are part of the process. An example of how the functional analysis of member services processes crosses organizational lines is illustrated in the HMO's response to eligibility inquiries. Rather than reviewing only its member services department's response to eligibility inquiries, all activities relating to eligibility—from new group enrollment to eligibility verifications—were evaluated. These activities occur in a number of departments, including marketing, finance, management information systems, member services, government programs, and clinical facilities. When member services activities involved providing clinical care (e.g., appointments, referral authorizations, or resolving complaints regarding physicians or other clinical staff), the functional analysis was extended to all service tasks and functions related to the point of clinical service.

The HMO then decided to focus on "member" rather than "customer" service. The word "customer" had two problems. First, it carried a double meaning: everyone (except physicians) viewed customers as including both enrollees and physicians, making it difficult to focus on what needed to be improved in servicing members. Second, "customer service" was viewed negatively by physicians as business school jargon appropriate to the retail industry but not to healthcare. The provision of member service was analyzed from the perspective of member satisfaction and the attitude of the HMO's personnel. The significance of the member contact was measured not just by frequency but also by the importance of the contact to the member's perception of the HMO. It included telephone, in-person, and written communication with the member or the group purchaser on behalf of the member. "Member contact" also included all nonclinical contacts wherever they occurred—in the HMO offices, in HMO physician offices, and in HMO hospital facilities.

The functional analysis methodology included three components: document review, interviews of clinical and administrative staff, and project team observation of the operations and interrelationships that exist within areas involved with member service activities.

Document review included the following: completed member service audits, member service departmental performance standards and reports, customer survey and satisfaction reports (member and purchaser), sample member communications materials, organizational charts, material relating to member service improvement efforts in the field offices, provider agreements, employment policies and incentive programs, member grievance policies and procedures, and employee and provider orientation and training materials.

The interviews of clinical and administrative staff took place at HMO corporate offices and at provider facilities. Two standard interview questionnaires were used, allowing interview responses to be compared more accurately based on the extent of the individual's involvement in member service. One was designed for member service department personnel and the other for all other personnel. The categories of personnel interviewed included: member services (i.e., corporate and field staff deployed to major provider facilities), enrollment and billing, marketing and sales, group service, government programs (e.g., Medicare, Medicaid), legal, communications and media relations, market planning, human resources, utilization management and quality assurance, urgent care units, claims, physicians and their office administrators, and hospital admitting personnel. Interviews were also conducted among the HMO's MIS personnel, due to the central role it plays to support member contact technically and by providing information needed to resolve member issues. Interviews were conducted with a cross-section of management and line staff to provide a well-rounded perspective of issues and opinions.

Areas targeted for observation were selected based on information obtained in interviews and from the document reviews. Observation by project team members was performed to provide an objective counterpoint to information and perceptions gleaned from interviews. Observation was carried out in the following areas: clinical appointment centers in larger (as measured by HMO enrollment) physician offices, member service department phone banks and walk-in areas (corporate and field offices), reception areas in provider facilities, and in the enrollment and eligibility department.

The interviews, on-site observations, and review of customer satisfaction surveys provided important data regarding member's service expectations. Through these tools, both subjective (i.e., the HMO employee's view of member expectations) and objective (i.e., the member's expressed expectations) data were obtained. The expectations data became the basis to determine the organization's service goals and establish revised service processes.

MEMBER CONTACT POINTS

The first step of the functional analysis is to identify the member contact points within the HMO system. Large organizations frequently lose sight of the fact that from the customer's perspective, the quality of the organization's service is measured at a customer contact point. This is particularly true in healthcare organizations, where service and quality issues usually are muddled together. Most of the HMO's personnel viewed the member services department as the only area where member service contacts are made. Thus, all types and locations of significant member contact must be identified before attempting to analyze the function.

In-person member contacts occured primarily at clinical sites and the member services department, while mail and phone contacts occurred in many different areas, depending on the nature of the contact. Figure 1 illustrates the various points at which members contacted the HMO system.

Members were forced to contact a variety of different points within the HMO system about a single issue. Figure 2 depicts the multiple contact points available for a single issue. Member contacts for problem resolution were overly complex, as illustrated by Figure 3.

Problems in member services

The interviews, observation, and document reviews indicated significant member services problems as described below.

Complex organizational structure. The organizational structure of the HMO was very complex, often making it difficult for members to obtain information and services. The complexity of the organizational structure, relative to resolving member problems, is illustrated by Figure 3. There are multiple departments with member service units or functions (e.g., member services, claims, enrollment, and eligibility). Such

FIGURE 1
Member contact points

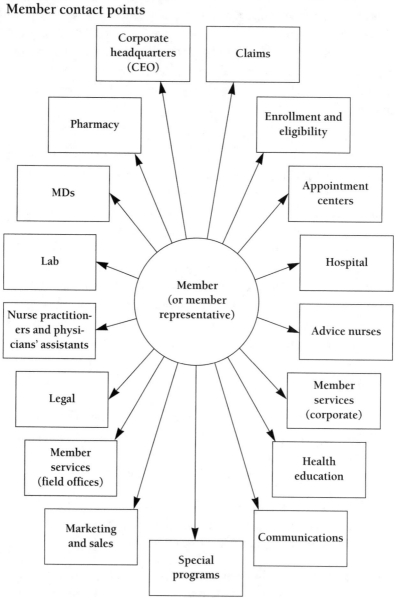

FIGURE 2
Member contact points by type

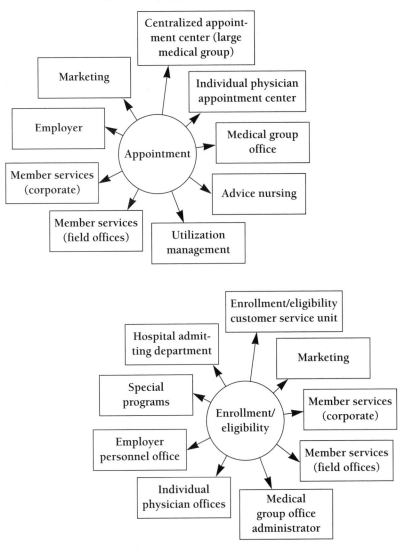

FIGURE 2 (CONTINUED)

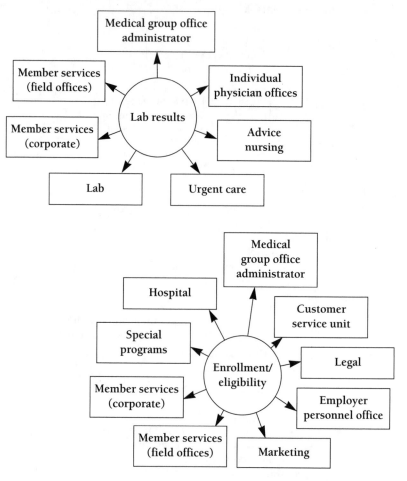

FIGURE 3
Current routing of member inquiries

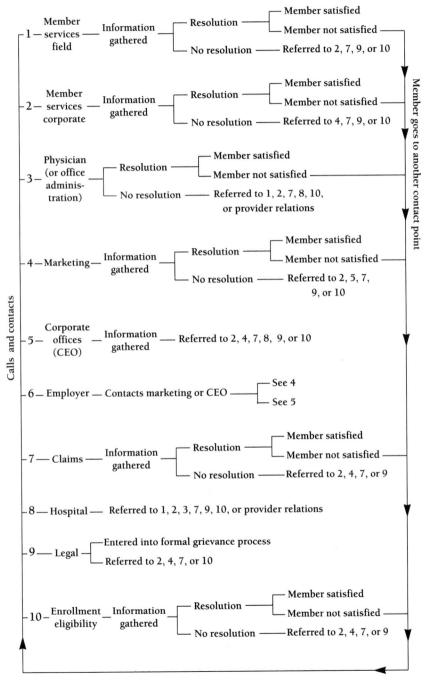

overlapping responsibilities and labels caused confusion for members and employees. Alternatively, the overlaps in responsibility frequently gave rise to one of two phenomena: de facto abdication of responsibility (an individual's hesitancy to exercise authority to resolve member issues because of the confusing dynamics) or a fierce preservation of turf. This complex structure resulted in both members and employees resorting to working the system rather than having the system work for them.

Strained relations between the HMO and its providers. The project team found the HMO and its large provider units to be distrustful of each other. This often resulted in direct conflicts over appointment scheduling, the appropriateness of member service standards, and the process for resolving member complaints and injuries. The strain was most notable in the appointment-making process and accessing clinical services. The provider unit's goal was to accommodate the physicians' work schedule preferences and to tightly control member requests and access. The HMO's goal was to accommodate members by making access to appropriate appointments and services more convenient for members.

Although this dynamic is present in many HMOs, the conflict between the providers and the HMO was more severe in this HMO and very visible to the member. These conflicts and resulting frustrations were directly and indirectly communicated to members. For example, it was communicated when appointment clerks told members they were doing their best to assist the member, but that the physician did not work and the office was not open in the evening, on weekends, or during lunch hours. It was also communicated by staff who were frequently observed commiserating with members that such appointment schedules made it difficult for members to get appointments without missing work. The effort to be sympathetic to the member is laudable and usually appropriate, but it often results in communicating to the member that there is conflict within the HMO system. This visibility of the conflict leaves the impression that something is not working, particularly when HMOs are supposed to be one cohesive organization rather than an administrative and a separate provider network. The perception of the HMO and its providers as a unified organization is based, in part, on the HMO's own marketing and member communication. Thus, when the conflicts and tension become apparent to the member, the HMO did not live up to its self-promoted image.

Lack of corporate support and understanding. Due to the concentration of large segments of the HMO's enrollment in a few larger provider units, the HMO had displayed foresight by placing field member services representatives in these large offices. However, field representatives uniformly stated that they operated with little or no support from or contact with the corporate headquarters. The primary interaction between field representatives and the corporate office was through the reporting of monthly telephone call answering statistics. Field representatives questioned the usefulness of such reports to assess how services are delivered to members and whether the reports have any impact on member retention. The representatives received little if any feedback as to how the data were used or if it actually impacted operations or corporate decisions.

Inadequate technological support. The existing telecommunications and information systems were found to be inadequate and a barrier to serving member needs efficiently. The HMO relied on a patchwork of outdated, separate systems that precluded the use of common databases and frustrated access to information. The result was that the members were forced to take responsibility for what should be an internal communication, such as updating the many membership databases, obtaining member identification cards, or having to call several departments to resolve an issue rather than having an HMO representative access the necessary information or at least transfer the member to the appropriate department.

Limited commitment to member service. Although there is a verbal commitment to member service in many of the HMO communications (both internal and external), the commitment is not carried through in employee orientations, training programs, or performance or salary reviews. Rather, the HMO developed into a bureaucratic culture, where staff who are committed to member service must bypass the system to achieve their goals. There was no universal understanding of what member service is—the most common statement was that member service means to "make the member happy." The observation sessions revealed that while services were provided with courtesy, most members were treated impersonally. Both in corporate and clinical areas, members were not greeted or asked for their name until after they were asked for their HMO identification number. Many of the field member service offices maintain hours of operation that were significantly shorter than those of the adjacent medical center. The message this activity conveyed was that service is not important to the HMO.

Although there was discussion at all levels of management and staff about the need to be more service oriented, these words appeared hollow without the accompanying implementation and integration of service standards within each operation, job, and task. For example, to have an organizational slogan of "put the member first" has little meaning to line personnel. However, an organizational commitment to member service is demonstrated when responding to member needs and inquiries is made a part of every job description or when compliance with service standards (e.g., telephone answering within 30 seconds or required follow-up calls to members to determine if a problem has been resolved) is a basis of employee reviews. Many of the fixes that management had tried to implement were dismissed by personnel as cosmetic changes.

Multiple, overlapping initiatives. To stem the membership losses and jump-start growth, the HMO was engaged in several corporatewide initiatives to improve planning and performance at the time the functional analysis was performed. Most of these initiatives involve some facet of member service or the systems supporting member service (e.g., MIS, corporate communications, and infrastructures). Significant resources, primarily at the management level, were diverted to these multiple and often overlapping initiatives. The interviews revealed the initiatives were confusing to the HMO's staff and were viewed as diverting staff time and corporate dollars from daily HMO operations for an unclear purpose.

Member service was not acknowledged as a process. Member service was not recognized as a responsibility inherent to all positions within the organization. Instead, when the term "member service" was used, staff commonly thought of the department of the same name rather than each individual's role to serve members. One consequence is that the core functions that provide value to members—determining eligibility, enrolling members, and providing primary care—are conducted more from a focus on which department is responsible rather than a focus on what the member or purchaser needs. Thus, member and employer group surveys indicated the HMO performed poorly in these service areas. As an example, the scheduling of urgent care appointments may be more important from a clinical perspective, but members appeared to be more concerned with their ability to access the system for an initial, physical assessment. Perceived problems with initial access into the system were further demonstrated by the fact that there was a higher rate of attrition among members enrolled in the HMO for fewer than five years. The management of initial member contacts, from enrollment to primary and preventive care appointment scheduling, needs to be conducted with a member-focused service perspective because of the immediate impression these basic functions have on the member.

Management style raising barriers to change. The document reviews, interviews, and observation sessions revealed an overall management style of control rather than support. The complex organizational structure inhibited staff from raising problems and suggestions for change beyond their department coworkers. Additionally, often burdensome oversight mechanisms were imposed (e.g., reports on telephone-answering statistics) without providing adequate resources to perform the function being overseen (e.g., adequate staff and equipment to answer telephones in a timely and unrushed manner). The management culture was characterized by control and conflict avoidance. Repeatedly, "solutions" to issues were offered by the HMO management that treated only the symptom rather than its underlying cause.

Resulting service problems

The organizational, personal, and management issues described above translated into the following service problems for members and staff:

Eligibility

- Delays in receiving identification cards (i.e., initial, corrected, or replacement cards)

- Repeated need for members or providers to confirm or assure eligibility and enrollment (e.g., when making an appointment, arriving for an appointment, processing a claim)

- Member embarrassed upon arriving at a provider office or facility and having eligibility questioned

- Surgical and diagnostic procedures are sometimes delayed until eligibility can be determined

- Outdated membership databases

Access

- The time between scheduling an appointment and the appointment itself is too long

- Not enough appointment availability (e.g., restricted, inconvenient hours versus evenings, early morning, lunchtime, weekends)

- Difficulty in getting same-day appointments

- Wait time in offices for appointment too long (e.g., it was not uncommon for physicians to be 30 to 45 minutes late for an appointment; long pharmacy waits were also common)

Patient relationships

- Patients were not always treated with courtesy

- Apparent lack of or inadequate respect for patients

- Little recognition of the person before the identification number (e.g., eye contact, greeted by name)

- Time spent with physician perceived to be lacking in quantity and quality (e.g., rushed, terse responses to questions)

- Inadequate communication and follow-through or follow-up

Claims

- Difficulty reaching a person with definitive information about the status of a claim in process or when processing may be completed

- Repeated requests by the HMO to the member for the same information (e.g., referral authorization number)

- Lost documentation requiring resubmission (e.g., emergency room reports)

- Delays in processing time (e.g., more than 30 days)

- High initial denial rate with high rate of reversal upon appeal (e.g., 80 percent)

- Poor phone access to claims customer service unit (e.g., busy signals, long time on hold)

Communication and problem resolution

- Lack of clarity about where to go and who to contact to get issues resolved (e.g., multiple phone numbers and locations)

- No communicated standards for service responses and resolution (e.g., observation sessions revealed that members were often told that they would be called back but were not given any time frame)

- Confusion about where to go to get appointments and services

- Inappropriate billing by HMO for copays that were paid at provider's office

- Communication that was often one way (e.g., canned responses to member questions), indirect, and too complicated

Recommendations

At the completion of the functional analysis, it became clear that the problems in member service were pervasive and crossed all HMO organizational lines. The problems were not limited to the HMO's member services department but were present in the health plan administration as well as larger provider units. They could not be fixed by "cutting and pasting," as evidenced by the repeated attempts without positive results. The functional analysis confirmed for the project team and some of the HMO's key leaders that the entire process of servicing the member must be reformulated and upgraded. The following is a summary of the major recommendations made to senior management by the project team.

REACH CONSENSUS ABOUT THE PRODUCT

Before defining what member service should be, the HMO must first answer the question, "What does the member believe is being purchased?" The answer reveals two key ideas behind member service: what the HMO member (or group purchaser) perceives to be the package of services that was sold and what the HMO communicated, intentionally or unintentionally, about what it is selling. Member service is, in large part, a question of meeting expectations.

The interviews, document reviews, and marketplace analysis indicated that members believed they were purchasing the following when they enrolled:

- *Access and availability.* Members expect to have ready access to appointments with their chosen primary care physician, rather than whomever may be on call

- *Physician-patient relationship.* Members expect to be able to build or maintain a relationship with the primary care physician and the clinical team working with that physician. This means an expectation for an ongoing interaction in which, over time, the caregivers will know the patient, if not from memory then at least from having reviewed the patient's medical record prior to each contact

- *Help in staying healthy.* The member expects to receive preventive care (e.g., physical examinations) and education (e.g., asthma care for children, smoking cessation) soon after joining the HMO

- *Simplicity.* The individual joining the HMO believes the representations made by the HMO that there will be "no hassles," a statement generally made relative to claims submission. The member expects the "no hassles" pledge to also mean that information (e.g., how to make appointments, get referrals) needed to use the HMO system easily and efficiently will be made readily available

- *Financial security.* The member expects the HMO to protect him or her against catastrophic healthcare costs and high annual rate hikes

- *Experience.* Members expect the HMO to be experienced in delivering healthcare services in addition to insurance-type administrative services, such as claims payment on a timely basis. Given the HMO's age and size in the market, its members' expectations in this area are high

- *Value.* The members expect to receive value, generally perceived as a combination of affordable price, scope of benefits, and quality of service for their premium. This expectation is generally heightened for HMO members due to the restrictions in choice of providers they are accepting when joining the HMO

- *Service warranty.* Most HMO members do not expect perfection at all times, yet, expect to have any problems they encounter resolved promptly, correctly, and courteously

- *More than fee-for-service.* Members generally expect more from an HMO system than they expect from a fee-for-service system. This is in part due to the promises HMOs make, such as preventive care for health maintenance, quality oversight, lower cost, and comprehensive benefits. However, it is also perceived as an offsetting benefit to giving up control over provider selection

Clearly, some members' expectations are unrealistic in HMOs. However, many of their expectations are derived primarily from statements and promises made in marketing activities to members and literature distributed to potential members. When the expectations are based on statements made by the HMO, failure to meet those expectations is blamed on the health plan.

The goal of member service, therefore, is to ensure that the members' reasonable expectations regarding the package of services being purchased are consistently met. Unfortunately, the findings showed that the role of member services in the HMO was viewed as changing the members' expectations to conform to what the organization was currently able to deliver, rather than meeting the members' expectations. The real service goal was being lost. Rather than addressing members' concerns by reassessing the relevant process to prevent the concern from arising again, the member is either informed that the concern is not appropriate and therefore will not be fixed, or shown a solution that merely teaches the member how to get around the problem. With either approach, members are left with a perception their HMO cannot meet their expectations. This leads to members becoming dissatisfied with the purchase they made when enrolling in the HMO.

Granted, no HMO can always meet a member's expectations, particularly with regard to medical services (e.g., the member cannot be given a referral to a specialist on demand). By its very nature, part of the package of services an HMO sells to purchasers is the management of healthcare services; ensuring that necessary services are available and that unnecessary utilization is reduced. This inevitably results in the HMO sometimes telling the members that their expectation for a particular medical service is unrealistic. However, because there is often a need to say "no" to members regarding requested medical services and providers, it is even more important that the HMO meets member expectations when it comes to nonclinical services. In other words, the failure to always meet one expectation must be offset with the ability to consistently meet others. Otherwise, the member becomes dissatisfied with the entire HMO system and may disenroll when presented with alternatives. The member does not always have to be given an appointment with a physician when the member requests one but should always be able to navigate the appointment-making process swiftly and with ease and courtesy.

The reformulation of the member service process begins with an accepted definition of "member service." The definition must be realistic and must take into account that the HMO member is not a happy vacationer but rather is generally apprehensive and very concerned. Also, the acceptance of the definition by physicians is essential to convince them to join in the delivery of member service as well as clinical care. The definition, therefore, cannot be made up of hyperbole and management jargon. Furthermore, the definition must be concrete so that those within the organization understand the standard they are expected to meet. Statements such as "the member is always right" are fine sentiments but do not express an achievable goal. Nor do they help the organization understand what steps need to be taken.

The project team recommended the following definition of member service: "We will reliably deliver the purchased package of benefits and services at all times." This means

- We are collectively and individually responsible for guaranteeing the delivery of promised benefits and services

- We ensure that the optimal infrastructure is in place to support that delivery

- We resolve deviations from service standards promptly

- We continually improve performance against established standards that are flexible and adaptable to changing member needs

This definition offers a realistic goal—reliable delivery of the benefits and services purchased. Second, it describes how the goal is to be achieved—through collective and individual responsibility for delivery, establishing an adequate infrastructure (e.g., information systems that can support the activities necessary to reach the goal), and prompt resolution of any deviations from service standards. Third, the definition provides benchmarks against which successes and failures in meeting the goal may be measured—prompt resolution of problems and continual improvement in performance measured against established standards.

The definition is not one that an advertising executive will rave about but is intended to serve as the guidepost to reengineer a core operation.

ELIMINATE THE DIVISION BETWEEN THE HMO MANAGEMENT AND THE LARGE PROVIDER UNITS

The member expects the HMO to be one unified organization. When the divisions become apparent at the operational level, the member sees it as an organizational failure.

Also, the distrust serves as an impediment to resolve member issues quickly or make improvements in member services. In some cases, the divisions are so intimidating that ideas for improving services are automatically rejected because they are perceived as having been generated by "the other side." At a minimum, the divisions between HMO management and the larger provider units must be eliminated to design and implement new member service activities because the functions cross organizational lines. The member is caught in a game of "monkey in the middle" where the HMO and the physicians toss blame and accusations at each other around the member. Figure 4 illustrates the relationship with the member when the HMO and providers work together to service

FIGURE 4
Communication postreengineering

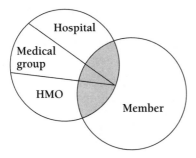

the member. There will always be a certain degree of separateness, which is often beneficial for checks and balances, but management and physicians must work as a unit when interacting with the member.

For the purposes of member services reengineering, eliminating divisions within the health plan requires the following:

- Teamwork needs to be fostered and demonstrated in resolving member service issues (e.g., eligibility verification) and problems (e.g., appointments and obtaining referrals) at upper levels between the HMO and the providers

- Communication between the HMO and the providers needs to be open at all levels to enable rapid identification and resolution of service issues

- Operations need to be considered and redesigned in total rather than piecemeal, without regard to existing functional and organizational lines. Each member contact must be examined—from initiation to resolution—as one process rather than as a series of departmental contacts. From the member's perspective, contact regarding an issue is one process until the issue is resolved. The HMO and its providers must recognize this perception and meet it, so that the member experiences the health plan as a well-run organization

THE ORGANIZATION'S LEADERS MUST DEMONSTRATE
A RENEWED COMMITMENT TO MEMBER SERVICES

The commitment to member service must be actively demonstrated on a regular and frequent basis. Both employees and members of the HMO are skeptical of jargon—they have heard it all before. Therefore, the organization's leadership, from the CEO to provider leaders to middle management, must demonstrate commitment in a number of ways.

Leaders must demonstrate to administrative staff and providers what member service means to the leaders and to the organization by actions, not just words. For example, the CEO can make a regular practice of talking directly with the health plan's employer group contacts or periodically visiting member service locations to obtain feedback from line personnel. This tangibly demonstrates service is important.

This type of approach is challenging, but the potential payoff is tremendous. The leader becomes more aware of member issues, the staff and providers become more motivated to be actively involved in member contact and service, and the member and group purchaser feel good about and important to the HMO, thus increasing their loyalty to the organization.

Employee training that emphasizes member service, as a part of the orientation and as an ongoing program, is a necessary core activity that the HMO's senior management should support. Staff should be trained and made aware of the current perceptions of members and learn how they can play a role in changing any existing negative perceptions. Employee and provider orientation programs should, wherever possible, include explanations and demonstrations of how service issues that arise can be resolved.

Rewards for outstanding member service should be considered. Meaningful rewards are an important element to recognize the importance of a member-focused staff to a member service-focused organization. Motivational posters or certificates by themselves are not meaningful, whereas receiving a write-up in the employee newsletter or a bonus for excellence in member service is meaningful.

INTERCONNECTING INFORMATION SYSTEMS MUST BE DEVELOPED AND IMPLEMENTED

Internal and external studies over the last five to seven years show amazing consistency in the reasons for member complaints, dissatisfaction, and disenrollment. The majority involve eligibility verification, timely issuance of identification cards, family coverage issues, access to providers, and impersonal service. The studies show that 35 to 50 percent of all customer contacts related to eligibility, enrollment, and benefit use.

A major component of providing member service is an information system that allows complex internal operations to function invisibly to the member. The HMO needs to determine an organizationwide systems strategy to set standards for file structure, data access, data retrieval, updates, and reporting requirements to ensure that system initiatives align with and support the rapid response to member service issues. For example, the system should allow any area contacted by the member (e.g., large provider units, claims, or enrollment) to answer questions regarding enrollment status and simple benefit coverage issues such as copayments. The member should not be shuffled between departments because the databases are so separate and incomplete that basic questions cannot be answered.

The quality of services provided to members is closely linked to the quality of the enrollment process, benefit package, eligibility systems, databases, and the telecommunications system. Improving these systems should be the first priority of the HMO. The systems must have complete data on a single, relational database (not multiple databases) and be available for decentralized access and limited updating (e.g., address changes). Such a database should contain all pertinent information about a member's eligibility status, eligibility history, and record updates pertaining to his or her individual or group eligibility, product and covered services, and payment history. The file then serves as the source for any requirements to distribute data throughout the HMO. Whether such information is distributed via periodic routine download or real-time direct or client-server connection can be determined based on each administrative area's requirement for timely information. Consistency in terms of member responsiveness is greatly enhanced through the single information source.

ADDITIONAL RECOMMENDATIONS

Related recommendations regarding specific functions included the following:

1. *Develop and implement an ongoing new member outreach program.* Statistics show that HMO members are most vulnerable to disenrollment within the first five years of membership. Thus, an outreach program was recommended to take place over the member's first year of enrollment. The program should actively acknowledge, contact, and begin to educate members about the HMO's philosophy, member service commitment, and exact scope of benefits purchased. Key features of this 12-month outreach program include

   - Periodic wellness education (e.g., newsletter, seminars)

   - New member health status screening and communication of age-, sex-, ethnicity-, and disease-specific health information (e.g., at least three calls or letters to each member within the first three months of enrollment to set up a screening appointment)

   - Periodic phone calls to solicit feedback and determine HMO customer satisfaction

2. *Institute member self-servicing capabilities.* Key member services functions can be decentralized and relocated to high-traffic areas where members routinely congregate (e.g., reception areas in the large provider offices) so that members can access assistance to handle the highest-frequency service needs (e.g., obtain information on facility locations and hours, make address changes)

3. *Develop methods for constructive use of wait times for service contacts.* Given the amount of time members can wait in certain provider offices, the HMO can adopt the approach of successful theme parks and make waiting times as enjoyable and beneficial as possible. Well-made health education videos, as well as using the time to routinely survey members' service needs and satisfaction at the point of service, are two examples to make the wait times more productive

4. *Conduct telephone and mail surveys of member satisfaction after key contacts with the HMO.* Examples of triggering contacts include after emergency room visits, urgent care visits, office visits where no return visit is scheduled, when an appointment is missed, after a nurse postpartum visit, or after laboratory or diagnostic tests

5. *Charge an organizationwide group with analyzing member service information to make rapid decisions about service improvements.* To make member service a seamless process, emphasis needs to be placed on continuous information assimilation and analysis. Service standards and benchmarks must be communicated throughout the HMO, including providers. Performance to meet standards and service trends across the organization should be tracked and analyzed to identify service breakdowns and changing member needs and perceptions. The information obtained should be analyzed to predict service issues and identify new, improved approaches to delivering member service. Most importantly, the results of the analysis should be regularly communicated throughout the organization to provide feedback to administrative personnel and providers

6. *Make representatives or roving ambassadors available at high-contact points.* This would provide a personal contact for members to immediately resolve minor problems and answer questions. Examples of high-contact areas include the lobby of the HMO's primary hospital, large provider office reception areas, and in or near HMO-owned or -operated pharmacies

7. *Establish service quality managers.* These managers are responsible for resolving issues within a specified and published time frame. This should be easily available to members by telephone and in high-traffic areas such as large provider offices

8. *Develop a telephone hot line or call center available for resolving service issues.* Care must be taken to ensure that the member is in contact with a human being as often as possible. Hot lines or call centers should not be seen as a replacement for personal contact. The use of member service personnel at large provider facilities is an investment that demonstrates to members and providers the HMO's commitment to service

9. *Maintain uniform standards for access to medically necessary and appropriate healthcare.* Examples of such standards and their use in member service include

   - Maintain and monitor compliance with uniform appointment standards (e.g., emergency care the same day, urgent care within 72 hours, routine physicals within three to four weeks of request, follow-up appointments within two weeks

   - Communicate appointment wait-time standards (and successes in complying with those standards) to members in a way they understand (e.g., publishing standards in member newsletters and new member kits)

   - Appointment hours should be available at convenient times for members. Members should be continuously surveyed regarding appointment time of day needs (e.g., 5:00 P.M. to 8:00 P.M., weekends) and large provider unit schedules should be adjusted to meet member preferences

   - Consider providing service guarantees such as a $5.00 voucher (to be used against copayments) for patients who experience a wait of 20 minutes beyond the time their visit is scheduled. These vouchers can be given to members by any of the medical or administrative team

Implementation

The implementation steps necessary to reengineer the member services function will be different for each HMO. However, there are common principles to guide all HMO reengineering efforts.

NAME AN INTERDISCIPLINARY TEAM TO INITIATE AND OVERSEE THE REENGINEERING PROCESS

The participation of representatives from all functional areas in the HMO is necessary. Because HMOs are a service business, everything they do is to serve members and group purchasers. There is no area in an HMO that does not have some member contact, directly or indirectly. Thus, without the participation of all areas, the reengineering effort will be incomplete and will fail.

CEO, COO, and provider representatives' participation is key. Reengineering is a major change and can be threatening to employees and providers. Employees and providers need to know that the effort is supported by every level in the organization before they look beyond existing departmental lines.

DEFINE THE PROBLEMS AND GOALS

Reengineering is not reorganizing existing departments but determining basic goals and then designing the work processes to best achieve those goals. By definition, reengineering will ignore existing departmental lines to create the new work processes. For example, if one goal is to deliver an HMO identification card to every new member within one week of the effective date of coverage, than all functions that affect the delivery of ID cards must be examined. In a typical HMO, the following areas would be included:

- Sales (staff submitting the new group or reenrolled group forms)

- Billing (staff preparing the billing forms based on enrollment lists)

- MIS or printing (staff processing the cards)

- Member services (staff preparing new member kits)

- Mailroom (staff preparing the mailings)

By defining the end goals at the beginning, the process steps for reengineering can be identified.

REORGANIZE AND ACCEPT THE FULL SCOPE OF MEMBER SERVICE

Everyone within the HMO, including providers, must understand that member services is more than one department. Early in the reengineering process an educational program should be launched to include all personnel and provider units. The program should include statistics showing the importance of member service (e.g., disenrollment rates, member survey responses) and should identify member contact points and service goals. The CEO should be involved in the educational effort in some manner—in person, by letter to all employees, by videotape.

TRACK IMPLEMENTATION PROGRESS AND EFFECT

Once a reengineered process has been implemented, its effect on achieving the service goal should be measured. Using the goal of delivering member ID cards within one week of the effective date as an example, the mailing date of ID cards should be tracked from the beginning of the implementation activity. Progress in reducing the lag time from enrollment to mailing cards should be seen. Also, new members should be surveyed beginning one week after mailing the ID cards to determine if the cards were received and are accurate.

MAINTAIN CONSTANT COMMUNICATION

The case study clearly revealed that failure to communicate throughout the process is the most damaging obstacle to the reengineering effort. When employees know that major changes are being developed but they are not kept informed of the nature and status of those changes, rumors begin circulating. At that point, confidence in reengineering is lost and the entire effort begins to unravel. Biweekly (or monthly if the process is lengthy) update memos should be sent to all employees and providers.

Conclusion

Member interaction is a dynamic process. Service standards and benchmarks evolve along with individual and group members' needs and build upon the HMO's organizational improvements and innovations.

Regardless of the point at which the HMO begins its member service reengineering program, it must emphasize and recognize the following:

- A mindfulness of the members' needs and circumstances at the time of contact

- The member is a fellow human being, an equal partner in his or her care, and requires honest care and service

- The HMO's need for immediate feedback on member satisfaction

- All members of the healthcare team (i.e., physicians, nurses, and other clinical and administrative personnel) are engaged in every member encounter

33

Blue Cross and Blue Shield of Massachusetts: Integrating financing and healthcare delivery

Matt Kelliher

Executive Director, Health Care Division
Blue Cross and Blue Shield of Massachusetts
Farmington, Massachusetts

IN 1992, FOLLOWING A CHANGE in corporate leadership, Blue Cross and Blue Shield of Massachusetts (BCBSMA) set in motion a series of strategic initiatives to transform the company from its traditional role as a third-party processor of medical claims to a company increasingly engaged in the delivery of healthcare.

Among the first steps taken by the new management team were a reorganization of the company's market lines, adoption of a new team-oriented approach to business, and development of a new strategic vision for the company—a vision that would commit the organization to delivering high-quality, cost-effective, customer-focused healthcare.

To underscore this new corporate vision, the company took two important steps. It launched HMO Blue, Massachusetts's first statewide managed care network, and forged a strategic partnership with Bay State Health Care, then the state's second-largest HMO. These initiatives not only accelerated the process of transforming the company into a multi-product organization but also positioned BCBSMA as New England's managed care leader.

Perhaps more important (and certainly more intensive in terms of the level of involvement throughout the company) have been more recent efforts to create a management system and improved operating processes to strengthen and sustain BCBSMA's leadership position.

Reengineering core business processes

The organization's initial reengineering efforts focused on improvements in the areas of quality, service, and cost, with particular emphasis at the outset on cost. BCBSMA began by looking at operating areas that were more heavily staffed than others, where operational redundancies existed, and where incremental improvements could be realized to improve the company's costs.

The expectation was that by adopting best practices from a business and operating point of view and rolling them out across the whole company, immediate cost benefits could be achieved.

Indeed, improvements were realized as a result of these early reengineering efforts. In the enrollment process, for example, improvements were achieved by reducing overstaffing and decentralizing steps that could be accomplished more efficiently and more accurately at locations closer to the customer. These improvements led to an overall cost reduction of nearly 10 percent. While the cost factor was improved, the fundamental data flow in the enrollment process remained overly complex, time-consuming, and, thus, potentially problematic in activating members' health coverage in timely fashion.

Later, it was discovered that these early efforts were just tinkering at the margins. The efforts to redesign processes and pare down costs were undertaken somewhat hastily. Management had not fully anticipated the extent to which changes at one level of operation might impact administrative behavior or other staff; that is, they did not take fully into account that what seemed to be simple redesign in one area might cause disruptions elsewhere. So, while costs were lowered in one area as a result of process redesign, they increased in other areas. Over a nine-month period, the initial cost savings began to level off, and the organization was still not realizing all the improvements needed to deliver superior quality service. It was becoming incrementally better, but not fundamentally so.

A different approach was indicated. Management knew what needed to be done: costs had to be reduced and service quality and efficiency had to be improved. But it was not until the organization actually went through the formal exercise of analyzing its major operating processes that it truly realized where to concentrate.

From the analysis, four critical processes rose to the top: claims, product development, business acquisition, business enrollment, and provider network development. These operating processes accounted for about 80 to 85 percent of BCBSMA's costs, including staff resources, thus fitting the textbook definition of core business processes. The focus then became obvious.

CLAIMS PAYMENT

Claims operation cost was hardly a surprise. Claims payment is typically the largest cost factor, mainly because it is the most labor-intensive operation. Of the company's approximately 6,000 staff, more than one-third were dedicated to claims processing. Analysis indicated that the overall claims process cut across 51 functional units in the BCBSMA organization, some of which were in different geographic locations in the company's statewide network.

To support this decentralized claims-processing function and administer a product portfolio that included managed care and indemnity-oriented products, the company needed nine different computer systems before the reengineering effort began. Not only were there obvious cost redundancies, but with different systems in place, time was wasted simply coaxing information from the system. For example, to respond to customer inquiries about managed care claims, customer service representatives had to log in and log out of three different systems to access information on members' eligibility, referral history, and claims status. Meaningful information to manage overall business operations could not easily be generated.

To address these problems, the company undertook a massive systems consolidation effort in 1992. An outsourcing partnership was formed with Electronic Data Systems (EDS), which began to put all claims processing systems onto a single data processing platform. This systems consolidation effort, which took about 12 months to complete, resulted in a reduction of nearly 35 percent in the company's information services costs, while also facilitating the creation of better information needed to manage the business.

The consolidated claims processing system also enabled the company to create an uplink to the information superhighway, which was an essential element of the company's overall business development strategy. The unified system now enables the company to share basic information with its providers through a linked network of electronic point-of-service terminals, giving medical practitioners a valuable tool with which to speed up the claims process.

By year-end 1994, BCBSMA had installed more than 5,000 of these point-of-service terminals in physician offices. This interactive system now allows providers to swipe a patient's identification card through a box connected to their office's personal computer to receive immediate confirmation of eligibility status, receive immediate claims approval or denial information, or administer referrals to other providers. The company is continuing to refine this system so that providers may also access information on patients' overall file status and medical history. The goal is to improve provider cash flows by processing claims and paying them more quickly and to equip providers with up-to-date patient information to help them deliver better quality care.

PRODUCT DEVELOPMENT

Another discovery made during the initial analysis of the BCBSMA product portfolio was that the company was offering nearly 6,000 different benefit configurations. The breadth of this huge portfolio had risen out of the company's efforts to accommodate the special needs of its group customers. Nearly 80 percent of the company's members were enrolled in only about 250 of these benefit configurations.

Clearly there were problems with this approach from a product management point of view. Not only did it present an administrative nightmare for the 50 to 75 people in the company's product management group, it also created substantial problems in the downstream enrollment and claims operations. With so many different benefit configurations, it was difficult to assure the accuracy of information on member identification cards during the enrollment process, and inaccurate identification information could cause associated problems as a claim moved through the payment process.

With such a broad product portfolio from which to choose, it was not easy for the company's sales staff to know the most appropriate benefit configurations to suggest to group customers. Recognizing that the product platform needed to be streamlined, the company adopted a manufacturing model that suggested the creation of six or seven basic product "chassis," with options that could be added as needed to accommodate member preferences. This approach would strike a balance between being able to administer the portfolio effectively while also continuing to offer a broad range of choice.

The effort to streamline and simplify the portfolio began with an analysis of the company's overall market, with emphasis on market share and profitability factors. The market analysis indicated there were several discrete consumer segments the company should be targeting. Among these were physician loyalists, value shoppers, families, young adults, and the HMO market, whose members make up the fastest-growing segment (see Table 1).

Through these customer surveys within market segments, the company gained a fuller understanding of what drives customer satisfaction and then dedicated itself to adopting a new customer-focused service orientation. Among the most important drivers of customer satisfaction identified were the overall ease of doing business with a health plan, the speed and quality of claims processing, and the sincerity of customer service efforts.

The process of streamlining the product portfolio began by bringing together teams of staff members to share in the product management matrix. These cross-functional teams were represented by product management, finance, actuarial, underwriting, sales, and information systems. Using data gleaned from the customer survey analysis, these teams were charged with developing product enhancements or new offerings to meet market demand and could be administered by the company in an effective and efficient manner.

The product redesign process, however, was not without challenges. In addition to the administrative and operational effort of bringing new offerings on-line, it was also understood that great care must be given to assisting customers through the transition to a new form of coverage. It was important to assure them that these new product offerings would continue to meet their needs, while making them easier and less expensive for BCBSMA to administer.

To manage product changes effectively, the organization focused on developing communications materials and work site support and training programs to make it easier for members to understand and accept new product offerings. For example, user-friendly product certificates were developed to help members understand the coverage offered under new benefit configurations.

TABLE 1
Market analysis

Overview of consumer segment	Size and BCBSMA penetration	Demographics and health status	Cost-versus-coverage
Sophisticated physician-loyalists	Largest market Best penetration	Wealthiest Least in excellent health	Least cost-conscious
HMO naturals	Small Fastest-growing market	Highest percent in excellent health	Will pay more than average for "extra benefits"
Mainstream families	Moderate size Moderate share	Oldest mean age High utilizers	Focus on coverage without "extra benefits"
Bargain hunters	Medium size Strong presence	Most likely to have no utilization	Want it all; low cost and "extra benefits"
Cost-sensitive young starters	Small and decreasing Low penetration	Youngest and least wealthy	Cost-conscious More benefits

BUSINESS ACQUISITION AND ENROLLMENT

In an elementary form, the process of enrollment was understood as simply getting out an identification card to new members. Deeper analysis revealed, however, that mailing an identification card was really the final step in the larger process of business acquisition and renewal. First, a sales effort was conducted, followed by actuarial analysis, underwriting, and contract administration. Only then, once the actual sale was completed and a member enrolled, was an identification card produced. From a member's point of view, receiving the identification card was what mattered most.

Business acquisition operation spiked activity during open enrollment periods in January and July, but the enrollment function is not always able to stay ahead of these peaks. Too often, new members did not receive identification cards until well after the effective date of their new coverage, and sometimes the information on their cards was inaccurate. These deficiencies caused disruptions in the claims processing operation.

Reengineering efforts focused on solving the problems of: compressing the time cycle in issuing cards and assuring greater accuracy of information. This process redesign effort was addressed on a number of levels.

Multiple cross-functional staff teams were formed to look at critical points in this paper-intensive process, from the initial sign-up by a member to the final mailing of an identification card. Eight to 10 different operating units within BCBSMA were involved in this enrollment process, and 25 to 34 different pieces of paper were generated to open one account. The improvement teams were not only charged with identifying problems and delays but were also authorized to resolve difficulties immediately, at the functional level, often without the time-consuming process of receiving managerial approval.

On a temporary basis, until a workable, automated solution to paperwork backlogs could be achieved, teams of implementation specialists helped the sales force get enrollment information into the system. These specialists actually walked paperwork through the system, taking administrative pressure off the sales force and letting them concentrate on the selling process. In addition, a reporting system was introduced to identify where backlogs were occurring, measure turnaround times, and determine causes for delayed processing, which were most often associated with incomplete, inaccurate, or late-arriving paperwork. A continuous improvement approach was adopted within these units to ferret out problems and put permanent remedies in place.

Redesign of this process is an ongoing effort. The amount of paperwork to open an account has been reduced by more than 50 percent, but the process is still too paper intensive. Further refinements to the automation process are necessary to reduce this drag on efficiency. The goals are to achieve complete accuracy for member identification cards and to get them to new members about one week before their effective enrollment date.

Producing new member identification cards that accurately record members' names, types of coverage, and account numbers has shown dramatic improvement, with overall accuracy levels approaching 100 percent. Similar improvements have resulted in issuing cards within the one-week-prior time frame. Turnaround times in processing new enrollments have also improved. Where once it had taken more than 50 days to process enrollments, by mid-1994 the task was completed in about 20 days, with continuing progress toward an ultimate goal of 5 days.

PROVIDER NETWORK MANAGEMENT

In a third-party payment system, the accuracy of provider information is equally as important. If any information is inaccurate or incomplete, the claim cannot be reimbursed. This not only affects the patient but also interrupts the provider's cash flow, which is a key determinant of provider satisfaction.

In analyzing its provider network development operation, BCBSMA found it was not simply the inaccuracy of information on providers that sometimes delayed the payment of claims, but more fundamentally, the whole process of acquiring providers as part of the network and entering them into system files in a timely fashion.

This is a complex process because it involves verifying provider credentials as well as establishing contractual agreements. One of the principal delays in this process was the requirement that providers enroll separately for each of the products offered by BCBSMA. While most of the information provided was identical, separate forms were required for each type of patient coverage.

For instance, there were occasions in which some provider applications actually traveled a circuitous route of about 250 miles, through three locations (for different points of processing), sometimes taking as long as four to five months for completion. Processing facilities have since been merged, and the work content has been reduced significantly. Now, the process is completed within two weeks.

The solution was to redesign the provider enrollment process to enable the sharing of basic provider information on applications for all products. The provider credentialing process also was streamlined and, in keeping with the company's quality assurance standards, a recredentialing effort is under way to update provider information biannually.

Two other provider management refinements were developed as a result of reengineering efforts. A new contract was developed for the company's relationships with specialty care providers. As part of its fee capitation agreements with specialists, the company now receives contractual assurances that these providers will cooperate in BCBSMA's utilization and quality management programs and that their annual compensation may be adjusted according to their performance in meeting goals in these areas.

The company has implemented a new performance management program for its staff physicians, tying individual compensation to established goals and achieving specified levels of competency in five critical areas of performance. These include patient focus, which measures patients' satisfaction with the care provided by the practitioner; care management, which evaluates how well a physician plans a course of treatment, particularly when it involves consultations with other physicians or specialists; practice management, which judges how efficiently the provider uses the organization's resources; clinical excellence, which critiques physicians' performances in maintaining and enhancing their depth of knowledge in their clinical discipline; and collaboration and teamwork, which assesses how well physicians work with others to provide care and meet organizational needs.

Evaluations of these criteria are made using surveys and other measurement data. Performance is scored against established benchmarks, with compensation linked to overall scoring and performance rating.

CREATING AN ENVIRONMENT FOR CHANGE

The primary obstacle to reengineering these four core processes was cultural. Change can be threatening, and as BCBSMA began to look at its business differently and institute new ways of managing it, organizational reluctance became apparent almost immediately.

Feedback from staff members demonstrated a concern that efforts to transform the company were driven primarily by outside consultants with cookie-cutter solutions. More than simply a response to the implied threat of change, this was the feeling that the people closest to the company's operating procedures should take active part in facilitating changes that would affect them.

Basic tenets of the total quality management (TQM) approach to reengineering suggest that staff must be an integral part of the process of change and that fundamental change cannot be dictated from the outside or in a top-down fashion. Rather, it must emanate from within. This approach was adopted by the BCBSMA organization early on and has been an important ingredient of the company's successes thus far.

An important part of this effort was to ensure ongoing communication within the organization. Much time and effort were spent working with staff members, through face-to-face meetings in small group environments, to assure their understanding and acceptance of the company's business vision and process objectives. By being up-front with staff about the reasons and need for change and making them an integral part of the goal-setting process, management broke down much initial defensiveness. Management successfully engaged the entire organization to facilitate sweeping changes to the company's core business processes through the following actions: seeking direct staff participation and supporting their training in team-based, problem-solving techniques; empowering them to resolve problems; and tying their successes to compensation incentives.

The next step was to translate these process improvements to the delivery system and to redesign clinical care delivery.

Improving the delivery of healthcare

BCBSMA operates nine staff-model health centers throughout the state, serving the healthcare needs of more than 100,000 managed care members. The health centers were structured primarily to provide service to members of the company's HMO Blue, Bay State Health Care, and Blue Choice managed care plans. To strengthen its competitive position, the company recognized it had to redefine and broaden the health centers' mission to include a wider cross-section of the healthcare market. This would enable the centers' multispecialty group practices to deliver care to members in other managed care health plans, as well as to those with other types of insurance coverage.

In 1992, as BCBSMA was assimilating its regional HMO insurance products into a single, statewide managed care network, the health centers functioned as a disparate group of clinical facilities, geographically dispersed, with few cohesive bonds beyond their regional HMO ties. As clinical facilities, the centers were key to the company's strategic goal to become more involved in the delivery process. But first, a direction and road map were needed. A management system had to be developed to focus clinical staff energy to achieve significant improvements in performance.

The first organizational step was to form a Health Centers Division to unify and coordinate this effort. Looking toward the year 2000, management established goals and a broad vision for the health centers that were closely aligned with those for the entire organization. Specific annual goals were established, with special emphasis on cost, quality, employee involvement, and profitability. Next, a management system was developed to focus and coordinate efforts at all levels of the organization, across all nine health centers.

TABLE 2
Looking toward 2000
Our vision of the future

From the members' perspective:
The health centers will be the best place in the region to receive and coordinate care

From the employer/purchasers' perspective:
The centers will be considered effective partners in lowering the overall cost of healthcare by continuously improving the quality of care and promoting health lifestyles

From the perspective of other providers:
The centers will routinely collaborate to improve integration of the care process across our organizations

From the staff's perspective:
The centers will be recognized as the best place to work in our business

TABLE 3
1994 Health center division goals

1. Achieve customer satisfaction that is a least 15 percent higher that the local community
2. Demonstrate our ability to prevent illness and reduce avoidable hospital admissions
3. Increase the percentage of employees who would recommend the health center to family and friends as the place to receive care
4. Maintain sustainable profitability of 4 percent for the region

ALIGNING GOALS OF THE DELIVERY SYSTEM

The initial step for the Health Centers Division was to create a leadership process, a framework to translate corporate goals through the organization to the level of clinical care. A new management organization was developed and structured into four levels: a statewide leadership forum, regional quality councils, health center leadership groups that would operate across all functions at the individual centers, and departmental lead teams that would operate at the clinical level (e.g., internal medicine, surgery, pediatrics, OB/GYN), coordinating goal-oriented initiatives as well as daily operational issues at the patient level.

Through these management structures, broad corporate goals were converted into specific objectives on a statewide, regional, center-specific, and departmental basis. Those agendas were then translated into resource planning, budgeting, implementation processes, and individual action plans at the operating levels. Quarterly, the statewide leadership forum meets to review performance to plan. This review process is repeated at each level of the organization down to the individual departments.

FIGURE 1
Overview of the management system

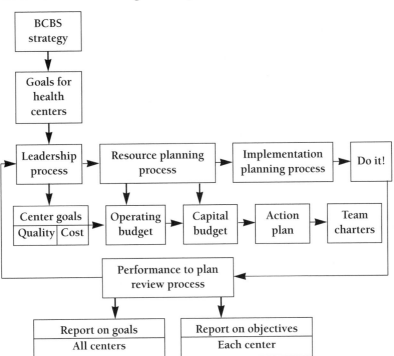

In addition, functional leadership teams were established to coordinate broad improvement initiatives across the Health Centers Division, operating in such areas as clinical systems, training, measurement, performance management, and business growth and promotion. Each of these functional leadership teams has a specific charter that directs it to accomplish improvements that benefit the entire delivery system and that assist individual operating units to accomplish their own particular goals and objectives.

The growth and promotion team, for example, is represented by a cross-section of technical, operational, and clinical fields, including marketing and market research professionals, advertising and public affairs specialists, and physicians and nurses. This team's charter focuses on developing competitive strategies to help the Health Centers Division build membership growth, add new fee-for-service business, and retain existing business relationships (see Table 4).

TABLE 4
Sample charter

Growth and promotion lead team charter

Project: Health center growth and promotion plan

Problem: The health centers need to know more about their competitive break-points and how to take advantage of them. Breakpoints are those product features that are so valued by potential customers that they cause them to choose the product over that of a competitor.

Beyond the question of breakpoints, the health centers need growth strategies based on thorough analysis of local competition and identification of benchmarks against which to measure competitiveness. The health centers also perceive a need to educate areas with the company as to the existing and potential "value added" that the health centers offer.

Effective growth strategies are vital to the future success of those centers with insufficient capacity as well as those with excess capacity.

Opportunity: Identify and capitalize on competitive breakpoints which can significantly increase membership growth and retention and fee-for-service business at the health centers. Increase awareness with the company of the value-added elements in the health centers.

Expected output of team:

1. Design a growth and promotion planning process that focuses on competitive breakpoints. They should be at the levels of the account and the member—both sales and retention—and the fee-for-service patient. The process will incorporate three organizational levels: statewide, regional, and center-specific. The design should address the following:
   a. Key players in the process
   b. Resource needs and opportunities
   c. Potential barriers and means of minimizing them
   d. Potential interdependencies and impacts of planning process
   e. Time frame for completion of initial plans
2. With the advice and consent of statewide, regional, and local health center decision makers, set the planning process in motion
3. Guide the planning process to keep it on track and on schedule
4. Evaluate the initial growth and promotion plans that result from this process

Measure of success: Each health center implements "quick hits" within 30 days and an initial breakpoint strategy during 1993; health center growth occurs as a result of these efforts. Team makes recommendations on planning process to health center decision makers by 4/30/93.

Barriers: Cooperation of company's core business units in the midst of their ongoing reorganization. Identifying funding source for outside professional support for research and planning. Gaining commitment for funds to implement plans absent capital funding plan/process.

Expectations and support: Initially, team meets biweekly for two hours over the course of six to eight weeks; members complete additional work off-line for two hours per week as needed. Upon completion of planning design, team meets as needed to guide implementation, evaluate, and revise.

Senior Health Center management will assist as needed with gaining participation and support of other divisions within the company.

BUILDING ORGANIZATIONAL CAPABILITIES

Performance reports provide valuable information to measure progress in meeting goals and to identify barriers to progress. Understanding the barriers that exist is particularly important, because all barriers are related in one way or another to the organization's capabilities or limitations. By understanding its limitations, an organization can build new capabilities or enhance existing ones to effect improvements and achieve performance goals.

Barriers to progress have three basic characteristics.

- *Structure.* Do the appropriate forums exist to enable staff to interact effectively to achieve superior performance?

- *Skills and knowledge.* Does staff have the level of training needed to achieve their goals?

- *Motivation.* Does staff accept the need to change, and do they demonstrate the initiative to improve performance?

To build capabilities, the health centers began by identifying and removing barriers that existed. This meant building the previously mentioned cross-functional teams and focusing their efforts on achieving specific objectives. As illustrated in Table 4, these groups were given written charters that specified tasks at hand, opportunities to be gained, management's expectations, constraints team members would face, and the measures by which success would be gauged.

The ongoing process of building skills and knowledge is accomplished through extensive training and development programs. These programs offer staff a variety of classroom opportunities to improve skills in such areas as leadership, customer service, medical interviewing, process management, improvement methods and tools, and team effectiveness.

Motivation can be addressed in three ways: by involving staff in the goal-setting process for their own area, soliciting input and valuing their suggestions; by providing staff with compensation incentives linked to achieving their goals; and finally, through a process of performance review based on achieving certain core competencies.

No prescriptive model exists in healthcare to instruct the development of this management system. The approach taken by BCBSMA was designed by looking at the best practices of many world-class business organizations, from auto manufacturers to financial services companies, and by applying what were deemed the best management techniques for achieving BCBSMA's corporate goals.

DESIGNING IMPROVEMENT SYSTEMS

The primary goal of the health centers division and the entire BCBSMA organization is to improve continuously upon the quality of the company's healthcare products and services.

The health centers' newly developed management system engages individual participation in a variety of ways. First, through training efforts, staff are encouraged to approach improvement projects by using step-by-step methodologies that specify objectives, identify and measure core processes, develop new approaches, and design, test, and implement solutions.

Process management has been the approach taken to achieve improvements in clinical operations that cut across different functions and department lines (see Figure 2). Under this management model, cross-functional teams from operating areas across the organization are chartered to develop and implement improvement projects.

Organizational research has shown a strong correlation between the level of employee involvement in an organization and the quality of its products and services. The research demonstrates that overall product quality increases in direct proportion to the number of employees actively involved in improvement initiatives.

Within individual departments, the health centers use two approaches in improvements to involve individual employees, rather than teams. These approaches invite administrative as well as clinical staff to participate and measure results without interrupting daily operations in their departments.

The first is a model known as CEDAC (cause-and-effect diagram with the addition of cards). As the acronym implies, the heart of this model is a large cause-and-effect diagram, prominently displayed within a work area for all to see. On one side of the diagram is a brief statement of a problem that needs solving; opposite that is a statement that identifies the goal of the improvement effort, together with a graphic display that measures the impact that problem-solving suggestions are having on the area's operations. The two statements are linked in the diagram by

FIGURE 2
Process management approach

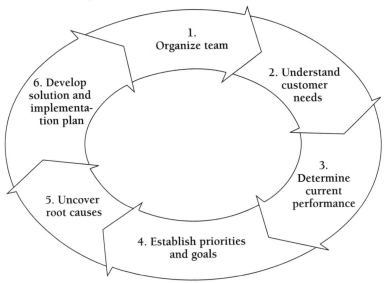

a straight line along which staff members affix their problem-solving suggestions (see Figure 3).

Using yellow cards to identify what they believe may be the cause of a problem and green cards to indicate a possible solution, staff members are immediately engaged in an interactive process-improvement exercise. If a green card contains what appears to be a plausible solution to the problem, it is marked to show the solution is being tested. If the test demonstrates positive, measurable results, the card is marked again to indicate the idea has been successful and will become a standardized operating procedure.

At the company's Agawam Health Center in western Massachusetts, for example, a CEDAC project was undertaken to improve the accuracy and completeness of information contained in patient encounter forms. These forms, initially filled out by a receptionist, contain such basic information as the date, patient's name and medical record number, critical details of the patient's symptoms, the provider's diagnosis and recommended treatment, and a notation as to whether a copayment is required for the visit.

Among the numerous suggestions received to ensure more accurate encounter form information were three suggestions that have now

FIGURE 3
CEDAC diagram

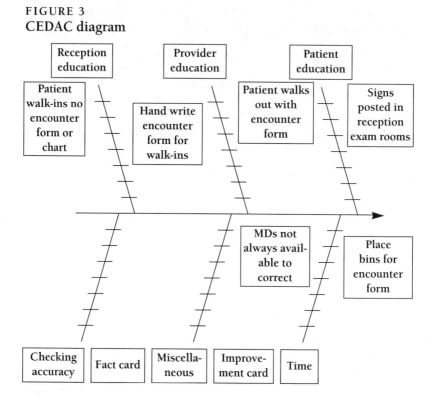

become standardized: a training session for administrative and medical staff who use the form, emphasizing the importance of filling it out thoroughly and accurately; placement of signs reminding patients to turn in their forms before leaving the health center; and a quality control system where individual staff members routinely check forms for accuracy and completeness and make corrections on the spot as needed. As a result of this improvement process, the accuracy rate on encounter forms has increased from about 95 percent to more than 99 percent, reducing duplication of efforts in updating information after the initial patient visit.

The second approach taken by the health centers to encourage individual participation is an employee idea system that encourages all staff to share ideas for improving the quality of their daily work. The ideas need not be directed at or aligned with any of the centers' specific goals but can be focused on anything staff and providers believe may be improved.

For instance, a nurse at one BCBSMA health center suggested the practice of sending a letter and postpaid return envelope to patients treated outside the company's service area, reminding them to provide information about their treatment so that the health center would have a record of it. The nurse's recommendation is now standard practice. With this information recorded in its claims system, the company avoids having an outside provider's bill denied for payment.

This idea system encourages individual initiative by giving staff members the authority to test their problem-solving proposals before submitting a formal suggestion. Staff are invited to identify potential problems, measure their impact, develop and refine solutions, and quantify their effect.

The health centers division also has created an administrative process to communicate the hows and whys of newly developed processes and practices, and transfer that knowledge throughout the health centers network so that best practices may be replicated and standardized.

MEASURING PERFORMANCE: DASHBOARD INDICATORS

Most organizations create management reports, but few use them to manage daily operations. This is often because information contained in these reports is not presented in real time nor accurately collected at the outset. It may not always be current enough to make immediate, on-the-spot improvements, and it may not be as valuable as a speedometer, turn indicators, or fuel gauge are to the operation of an automobile. But, it should be.

BCBSMA's health centers division has used this automotive analogy to create a performance measurement system that relies on dashboard indicators to provide real-time feedback on individual operations. This dashboard model has four categories of indicators: health status of members, efficiency of the practice, process quality, and customer satisfaction. These measures facilitate the monitoring of progress on an immediate basis and enable the organization, when necessary, to take remedial steps toward improvement.

The current set of dashboard indicators includes

1. Health status of members

   - Mammography screening (see Figure 4)

   - Hypertension screening

- Immunization rates

- Cesarean section rates

2. Efficiency of practice

- Primary care visit utilization

- Outside referral rates

- Admission rates (see Figure 5)

- Absenteeism

- Staffing rates (see Figure 6)

- Home care utilization

3. Process quality

- Quality in daily work

- Telephone call handling

- Appointment access

- Unused appointments

FIGURE 4
Mammography screening

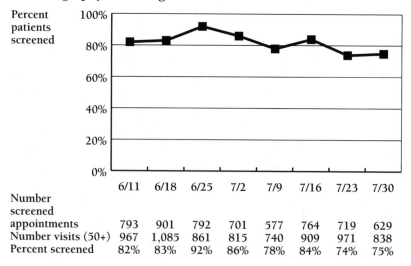

	6/11	6/18	6/25	7/2	7/9	7/16	7/23	7/30
Number screened appointments	793	901	792	701	577	764	719	629
Number visits (50+)	967	1,085	861	815	740	909	971	838
Percent screened	82%	83%	92%	86%	78%	84%	74%	75%

FIGURE 5
Admission rates

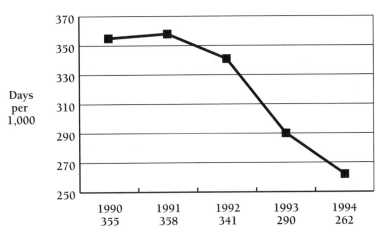

FIGURE 6
Staffing rates

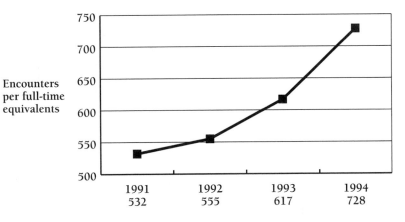

- Pharmacy wait times (see Figure 7)

- 24-hour discharge rates

4. Customer satisfaction

- Complaints and customer-service guarantees invoked

- Visit satisfaction

- Member satisfaction (see Figure 8)

An example of the health status indicator is contained in the company's practice of mammography screening. All women over 50 years

FIGURE 7
Pharmacy wait times

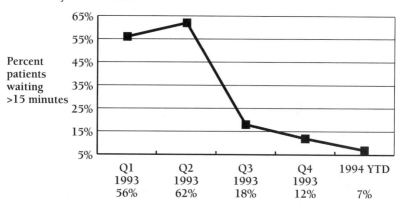

FIGURE 8
Member satisfaction

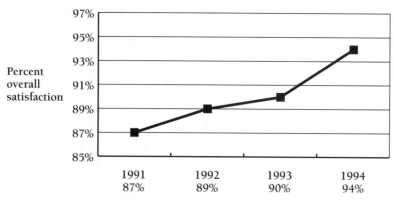

old seen by health center medical staff are checked to determine if they have had a recent mammogram: if not, they have one scheduled. In either case, the data are recorded in the dashboard measurement system. Reports are generated on a daily, weekly, and monthly basis and circulated within the team structure of the Health Centers Division. This information forms the basis of comparative analyses that helps determine, from a clinical management point of view, the overall health status of BCBSMA members, how the company's individual health centers are performing in the application of an important care protocol, and what action may be needed to improve the delivery of care.

As another example in customer satisfaction, the dashboard indicator model is used to measure responses to on-site surveys regarding the quality of patient visits. In addition, the company performs quarterly telemarketing surveys of its members to determine their overall level of satisfaction with the delivery of care. Feedback from these customer satisfaction surveys can help validate successes, as well as prescribe remedial action when necessary.

PIONEERING THE SERVICE GUARANTEE

By mid-1994, with a redesigned management system in place, BCBSMA decided it was time to test its quality improvement efforts in terms of ultimate customer satisfaction. Breaking new ground, BCBSMA extended a service guarantee.

The guarantee promises that if a customer is not completely satisfied with the level of service received, BCBSMA will not only strive to remedy the problem as quickly as possible, it will also pay the patient's contribution to the next month's health insurance premium.

An obvious objective of this service guarantee was to increase member loyalty and retention. Perhaps less obvious, the guarantee also served as another dashboard indicator of customer satisfaction. It identifies potential problem areas and facilitates quick responses to customer feedback, while also providing a tool to manage the company's business and stimulate its quality improvement efforts. The financial impact might be viewed simply as purchasing valuable consumer research.

The results of the service guarantee program have been encouraging. In a retrospective sample of patients who had invoked the guarantee, the majority of patient concerns were satisfactorily addressed. Most members indicated their intention to remain in their health plan and were

TABLE 5
Service guarantee

Our health center committment to you

Your health is one of your most treasured possessions, and we are pleased that you have chosen us to help manage it. We are proud of what we do and we are committed to providing you with excellent care and service.

So, when you visit us at Medical West Associates, Braintree Medical Associates, Framingham Medical Associates, Peabody Medical Associates, or Valley Medical Associates in Methuen, we will

- See you when you feel you need to be seen
- Avoid inconvenient delays in serving you
- Treat you in a competent, compassionate, and friendly way
- Listen to you and understand your needs
- Care for you as a person and as our patient
- Provide you with information to help you maintain or improve your health and lifestyle

Our health center service guarantee

If, as a patient in our health center, you are not completely satisfied that these services meet our commitment, please tell us immediately. We will strive to resolve the problem and promptly forward to you next month's health insurance premium.*

*The amount we forward to you will be equal to the value or approximate value of the monthly individual employee contribution.

pleased at the company's level of responsiveness. Less than 1 percent of all patients who used the health centers' services have invoked the guarantee, which compares favorably with other service-oriented companies whose guarantees are invoked at an average rate of around 2.5 percent. By comparison, these results were well worth the year-long effort to bring the guarantee to market.

LESSONS LEARNED

A number of valuable lessons were learned from the development of the guarantee program, as well as from all of the preceding efforts to build and refine a quality-focused system to deliver healthcare within the BCBSMA organization.

First, the benefits of retaining a loyal, satisfied customer base far outweighed risks of seeking new ways to run an operation.

Second, to be truly successful, improvement efforts must involve the creative energies of an entire organization.

Third, there needs to be a universally embraced commitment to change within an organization for a new management system to work.

Next, in order to achieve long-term, sustainable gains, a health plan must invest significant financial and human resources to increase its organizational capacity (e.g., administrative systems, operating processes, and individual skills training).

Finally, there needs to be a general tenet of breakthrough marketing strategy: the true beneficiaries of new business ideas in any industry are those who do it first and stick with it over the long term.

It is not enough, however, to focus an organization's energies on continuous, incremental improvements. Organizations must always look ahead and develop new competitive strategies to enable them to anticipate and respond to the changing needs and marketplace demands. Indeed, with its service guarantee initiative, BCBSMA has achieved a breakthrough strategy to secure and build market share.

Through its corporatewide reengineering efforts, the company has created a management structure and a system of measurements to enable the organization to compete more effectively on the basis of delivering quality healthcare. It has set in place operational methodologies and developed a cultural ethic among its staff aimed at assuring continuous improvement in delivery of care. And in the process, the company also has lowered its costs.

BCBSMA has come a long way in transforming from a traditional insurance carrier to an integrated deliverer of healthcare services. The company has approached this transformation in a systematic fashion. It has refined its core operating processes to bring greater efficiencies to its continuing role as a third-party processor of medical claims. And it has streamlined its portfolio of healthcare products, while broadening its ability to serve a wider cross-section of the health benefits market. It has made a strong commitment to balancing the critical issues of cost containment and quality care through a series of initiatives aimed at more fully integrating the financing and delivery components of its business operations.

The company's shift toward a more customer-focused, quality-driven approach to healthcare hinges on a keen awareness of two indisputable points: that competition in the field will inevitably become more intense over time and that organizations expecting to thrive in this challenging environment must constantly improve the quality of care they provide.

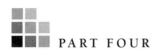

MANAGEMENT TOOLS

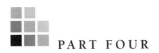

PART FOUR

Communication

34

Communicating change through employee involvement

Margaret Jordan
Vice President of Healthcare and Employee Services
Southern California Edison
Rosemead, California*

L IKE MANY LONG-ESTABLISHED COMPANIES, Southern California Edison encouraged its employees to think of
their employer and fellow workers as family. "Uncle Ed," as the company
was affectionately known by many on the payroll, could be counted on
for lifelong employment and benefits that would take care of workers
and their families for the rest of their lives.

Healthcare was high on the list of what Edison employees expected as
part of the covenant that existed between them and their employer. For
more than 90 years, the company made accommodations to provide
healthcare that was practically free and allowed an almost limitless selection of providers. It was expected that this tradition would continue.

Healthcare could not be any more intrinsic to an organization than it
is at Edison. Historically and through policy, healthcare is a cornerstone
of Edison's corporate culture.

By 1989, Edison had one of the best-known self-administered corporate healthcare systems in the United States. But, like many employers
who have opted for self-administered healthcare, Edison underestimated
the true cost of administering its own program. Self-administration was
also limiting Edison's ability to stay in sync with the tremendous structural changes evolving in healthcare delivery and financing systems.

By the start of the 1990s, under the CEO's leadership, a new vice president of the healthcare department was brought in to assess the company's

healthcare system and drive any necessary changes. It did not take long to determine that the company's entire healthcare system needed to be redefined with a fresh perspective to honor the commitment of Edison to its employees but not be limited by tradition. Planning and implementing such a major restructuring over three years would be complex, particularly dealing with the "people side" of the change equation.

Analyzing and managing the operational changes would be difficult enough, but these tasks paled in comparison to explaining the changes to Edison's 17,100 active employees, 6,800 retirees, and their family members and garnering their approval of the new system. What was to change at Edison was not just a workplace benefit, it was renegotiating long-held beliefs about what employees considered to be an integral part of their unwritten contract with the company. The conversion was sure to bring into question the company's values and principles—the reputation for trust, loyalty, integrity, and honesty it had cultivated for more than 90 years.

The proposed healthcare changes would also mean a reduction in Edison's own healthcare staff from a high of 240 to about 50 and a totally different management structure for those who remained. Other Edison employees and retirees might be distressed about rethinking the way they choose and use health benefits, but the change would be genuinely traumatic for individuals in the healthcare department who were destined either to lose their jobs or to stay employed in a workplace environment different from when they started with the company.

The healthcare change leader had many goals for restructuring Edison's program: decreasing costs, providing choice and quality services, and continuing to influence regional and national healthcare reform. But equally as important was handling this major corporate transformation in a way that was sensitive to the needs and feelings of the individuals affected by the change. For this transition to occur smoothly and to achieve the desired results, Edison staff needed to contribute their energy, time, thinking, patience, hard work, and commitment. Transition management determined that adhering to four principles would allow Edison to accomplish its ambitious agenda in the least painful way possible. The guiding principles were

- Communication with all stakeholders (executives, senior managers, the unions, current employees, retirees, and family members) must be open, direct, candid, and factual

- Involve employees in the transition process whenever possible

- Encourage employees to look at their situations realistically and to take charge of their own future by making career decisions based on objective criteria, not emotional responses to unemployment or misperceptions about the job market

- Treat each individual with dignity and respect

Adhering to these principles allowed the change leader to execute a rapid corporate transition while not losing sight of the affects these changes had on individual lives.

Edison's healthcare history

In 1902, Edison agreed to provide first aid and medical care for workers at remote heavy-construction sites where no other medical services were available. When staff in the main office complained that they were not receiving the same benefits as their field colleagues, the company extended healthcare benefits to all union and nonbargaining employees. A clinic and pharmacy were opened at Edison headquarters and other clinics were opened later at various other sites.

Edison employees saw company physicians for free and had prescriptions filled free at the Edison pharmacy. Edison physicians were general practitioners, not board-certified specialists. If an employee needed to see a specialist, a referral was made to a company-designated physician in private practice. Physicians were added to this referral network in a number of informal ways.

Edison employees began contributing to the cost of their care in the 1950s. For 50 cents a month (10 percent of the premium), they would receive medical services coverage within the Edison service territory. During the 1960s, with the offering of Medicare, Edison became the intermediary and provided Medicare-eligible retirees healthcare services. Edison then billed Medicare for reimbursement and accepted whatever payment Medicare made as payment in full.

In the mid-1970s, 12 specialists were hired as independent contractors to visit the headquarters clinic for a half day per week. Employees received 100 percent free medical coverage if they limited their healthcare providers to the Edison general practitioners, the visiting specialists, a physician who had obtained company-designated physician status, or any provider to whom these physicians referred. Edison offered an 80 percent benefit for service outside the network and the company began to offer HMOs as an alternative.

Although not billed as such, Edison was, in effect, trying to operate a managed care system. The gatekeeping was not obvious to employees and retirees and, in fact, many participants were successful at working the system so that they could see their own physician outside of the network. All that was required for them to receive 100 percent reimbursement was a referral from an Edison provider, most of whom readily gave referrals upon request. Other than loss of revenue for Edison services, there was no financial impact on the referring provider.

Edison eventually extended healthcare benefits to employee families and dependents but did not want to burden Edison physicians with treating nonemployees. Thus employees and their families were given a choice of indemnity plans or HMOs. Dental coverage was added in 1973, an employee assistance program started in 1977, mental health was covered through the indemnity plans, and vision care was included in 1987. Edison employees were happy with their healthcare benefits.

By the middle of the 1980s, healthcare was big business at Edison. The company managed eight clinics, a pharmacy, x-ray and laboratory services, a claims unit, and a utilization review function. The cost of healthcare provided through the indemnity plan was increasing at an average of 20 to 25 percent each year.

In 1989, Edison made a major attempt to contain costs with the elimination of the indemnity plan and the much-heralded introduction of HealthFlex, a self-administered, self-insured preferred provider plan for active employees and their families. In addition, it introduced Prime-Care for retirees and their dependents. Both plans were administered using the existing resources, plus a newly established PPO network of 7,500 physicians and 85 hospitals, and 7 HMOs. Employees and retirees who selected the PPO could opt to see an Edison physician in one of the company clinics or an outside physician in the massive PPO network and could make use of the Edison pharmacy. The program also added preventive care benefits, a wellness program, and cardiovascular health risk assessments. Edison's company-run health facilities were the first corporate systems in the country to be approved by the Joint Commission on Accreditation of Healthcare Organizations.

This complex corporate healthcare program seemed to be the next logical step in the evolution of healthcare at Edison. If the programs worked well, management even speculated that the healthcare department could turn into an Edison profit center by selling its services to other employers in southern California. From management's point of view, this program was accomplishing its goals of providing Edison's employees, retirees, and their families with one of the best healthcare benefits programs in the United States at a lower price to the company— although costs were still at an overall growth rate of 13 percent.

But the new program was not welcomed or endorsed by all at Edison. Many employees believed that HealthFlex reduced and restricted the corporation's traditional healthcare benefits in a number of ways. For example, monthly contributions were implemented and the premiums increased for dependent coverage, particularly for the HMO options. Precertification for some services such as hospitalization and specific outpatient surgeries were introduced. Employees had more paperwork requirements and greater cost sharing in the HealthFlex plan.

The unions that represent almost half of the Edison workforce protested the HealthFlex Plan, and its collective bargaining reached an impasse. The programs were implemented by the company despite this opposition, and for the next two years, unions pursued every legal remedy to get this healthcare decision overturned. It did not take long for such hard feelings about healthcare to permeate and taint the broader relationship between the unions and management. Healthcare soon became such a divisive issue that it led to problems in all aspects of union-management relations. The number of filed grievances increased and the unions challenged and actively opposed Edison's proposed merger with San Diego Gas and Electric before the public utilities commission (which was not approved).

A joint healthcare committee (JHCC) was formed in 1991 made up of management and union representatives from the International Brotherhood of Electrical Workers (IBEW) Local 47 and Utility Workers of America (UWA) Local 246. This committee's mission was to work out a mutually acceptable healthcare approach. After studying many different healthcare options, the committee recommended

- Introducing a point of service (POS) plan by January 1994

- Reducing employees' share of overall costs with continued cost containment

- Improving plan benefits, with benefits competitive with HMOs

Although the committee agreed the administration of the revised program should be handled by outside professionals, the direction was to develop an Edison-designed program. It was in this context that Edison's CEO decided the company needed to evaluate its healthcare approach. In 1992, new leadership was recruited for the healthcare department to reassess and redefine healthcare at Edison and to drive the resulting changes through these turbulent corporate waters. Hovering overhead was the 1994 implementation deadline set by the JHCC.

The first agenda item had to be a postponement of the 1994 implementation date to allow time for redesigning the company's healthcare approach. A one-year reprieve was granted. The change leader focused on data gathering, reflection, and analysis. After several months of intense work, many decisions were made regarding healthcare at Edison. Edison was in the electricity business, not the healthcare business. It was time to take full advantage of outside experts and the many qualified healthcare delivery programs already available. The self-administered HealthFlex plan for active Edison employees would be replaced by a choice of six options: two POS plans and four HMOs. Two POS plans was a first for an employer.

The method used previously to calculate employees' contributions to healthcare benefits would be changed. Previously, employees paid a fixed dollar amount that had not been altered for three years. Employees would now pay a percentage, starting at 9 percent for 1995 and escalating 1 percent per year up to 11 percent in 1997.

Healthcare benefit levels for Edison's retirees and their families would not be changed, but the way they were delivered would be. Once the PPO network for Edison's active employees was dissolved, the company needed to find a substitute way for the retirees to get healthcare services comparable to what they had come to expect.

Edison also decided it would turn over four clinics and the pharmacy to an outside medical group to operate as a healthcare resource for Edison and for patients from outside the company. Edison healthcare staff at these facilities would be interviewed and, hopefully, hired by the new management. Edison would continue to operate the remaining clinic at the site of the San Onofre nuclear plant, but it would be limited to occupational medicine related to requirements of Nuclear Regulatory Commission, OSHA, and the utility industry.

In addition, Edison decided that the healthcare department would be downsized to a quarter of its previous size, from 240 to about 50. The purpose, function, and structure of this department had to change from an insuring entity and delivery system to an organization that would negotiate and manage relationships with external providers. Individuals would no longer be needed to develop Edison's network of physicians, maintain relationships with doctors, pay claims, make precertifications, and review controls.

It was also decided that the healthcare department and employee services department would be merged into a single new unit to bring together a continuum of services to maintaining a healthy, productive, and competitive workforce.

Specifically, the domain of this new department would include the administration of health and disability benefits and services; occupational medicine and safety services; and related policy, planning, research, and evaluation activities.

These radical changes were decided upon during 1993 and the first part of 1994. The remainder of 1994 was devoted to detailed planning and comprehensive communication programs designed to get buy-in from all the stakeholder groups. In 1995, the old organization would be dissolved and the new organization built.

The reconstruction planned for Edison's healthcare had the potential to be traumatic and painful, but leadership strongly believed that a well-thought-out strategy could manage the transition in a way that would minimize the pain and unpleasantness of change. The change strategy would emphasize the personal aspect of the change equation and focus on employee involvement, skill building, and especially communication. The latter is most frequently criticized by employees as being faulty during significant organizational restructuring. For the new healthcare system to be implemented smoothly, Edison needed all of the stakeholders to understand the need for these radical changes, to accept the company's decisions, and to cooperatively assist with developing the new system.

Communicating the new reality

Healthcare is one of the most intimate services an employer provides to employees. Any time health benefits are discussed—regardless of whether the group represents senior executives or workers from the line—it is difficult to keep the topic at a policy level. Conversation almost immediately deteriorates into personal preferences, concerns, and anecdotes (e.g., "Will I have to give up my doctor? Will my children still be covered? What about a preexisting condition? How far will I have to travel? Will I get the best quality care?").

In an entitlement environment where lifetime employment was once the norm, the attitudes and emotions involved in the proposed changes to healthcare benefits could not have been more intense. An underlying theme at Edison had always been a paternalistic sentiment that "Edison takes care of its people and Edison knows how to do it best." In fact, the persuasive argument for the self-administered HealthFlex plan had been that Edison could do it better than anyone else. Now the company had to reverse its longstanding tradition and convince employees, retirees, and their families about the benefits of this new way of approaching healthcare benefits.

Early in the planning phase, key phrases about the healthcare changes were developed so that each and every communication piece would reflect the core messages.

- Healthcare benefits are changing as part of the company's overall strategy for staying competitive in a fast-changing, deregulating business environment

- Edison must change its atmosphere of entitlement to more realistic expectations

- Healthcare is changing throughout the nation by competitive forces and the prospect of reform

The next question was to identify who needed to be on the receiving end of these core messages and what Edison's communication goals were for each of these stakeholder groups. This matrix, shown in Table 1, provided the framework for developing communication strategy and tools.

UNIONS

The anger and resentment felt by the unions since the company introduced the HealthFlex plan in 1989 made communication with the unions the top priority in redesigning healthcare at Edison. There had been no agreement on healthcare benefits with the unions since 1988, and it had become a bitter subject between management and unions. The first step was winning the one-year reprieve on the January 1994

TABLE 1
Communication goals

Stakeholder group	Communication goals
Executive leadership	• How can we deepen the understanding of health-care issues among the top level of management, and prepare them to concur with the radical change recommendations that would be coming?
Unions	• How can we show a good faith negotiating effort and still achieve the changes we need?
Active employees	• How can we obtain their support for the changes we determine must be made? • How can we preserve the continuity of care Edison employees have come to expect and count upon?
Retired employees	• How can we convince these faithful employees that Edison is remaining true to its commitment while changing the way in which healthcare is delivered? • How can we help them take full advantage of the excellent healthcare system Edison will be making available?
Healthcare department staff	• How can we involve these employees in the transition? • How can we help them make a successful move to the next step of their career—whether that is inside or outside of Edison?

deadline in order to implement a new program. Using those extra 12 months to forge a new, positive working relationship with the unions was the next step.

The same philosophy that was to guide Edison in dealing with its employees was applied to the unions: communicate directly and honestly, build trust, educate them about the need for change, and involve them in the transition. If rapport was to be established, the unions and the new leadership had to get to know one another and narrow the knowledge gap each had about the company and healthcare in the 1990s and beyond. The unions were acknowledged to represent many of the recipients of Edison's healthcare benefits and to have a legitimate concern and point of view. In turn, the unions were requested to spend time evaluating and understanding the benefits of selecting an external plan versus designing an Edison plan. They also kept an open mind about revising their role in restructuring healthcare. Edison management was frank in admitting many differences of opinion about what the company should do, but that there would be an honest effort to work for compromise acceptable to both sides.

The program to educate the unions and staff about healthcare took many forms. Union representatives and department leaders visited a number of the possible health plans for presentations, and speakers were brought into the company to put Edison's changes into the context of the broad healthcare issues being discussed all across the country, such as quality management. For the first time, union leaders were invited to jointly visit congressional offices in Washington, DC, to deepen their comprehension about how healthcare was evolving on the national scale. This was not negotiation, but rather education and preparation; and it served to further build the foundation of trust before Edison and the unions ever sat down at the bargaining table. By the time real negotiation was to begin, a long list of tangential points was narrowed to those issues everyone knew needed to be hammered out. Every suggestion made by the unions was taken seriously and given prompt and thoughtful consideration.

In the end, the new healthcare benefit program at Edison received 92 percent ratification by the unions' membership.

ACTIVE EMPLOYEES

Employees can tolerate major change if they know it is going to come, if they have as much information about the change as possible, and if there is a context for the change. Like it or not, employees can at least then understand why there needs to be a change. In other words, employees should be treated respectfully, as adults, and given as much power as possible over their own destiny. This was the philosophy adopted by the change leader in dealing with Edison employees.

A 1990 study of the corporate culture at Edison analyzed internal correspondence from the healthcare department to employees in 1989 and found it was often arrogant, condescending, and seemed to assume that employees were dull and childlike. Under the new leadership, the department's communication style was deliberately shifted to a respectful, collaborative approach. This change was necessary for Edison to convince employees the healthcare changes would be beneficial to all.

During the time a new healthcare approach was being formulated, employees from the healthcare department were recruited to study key issues and propose alternatives for change. For example, one group charged with analyzing the future of Edison's eight clinics recommended the immediate closure of three clinics because they were no longer used enough to warrant the expense. A second group of employees convened to work with a consultant to define what the mission should be for the remaining five clinics and the pharmacy. As a result of the group's work, the decision was made to seek an outside medical group capable of and interested in assuming ownership and operation of the Edison pharmacy and clinics at Big Creek, Long Beach, Rosemead, and San Bernardino. The belief was that these sites could be converted into profitable, private business ventures. The remaining clinic at San Onofre, the nuclear plant, would be run by Edison but confined to providing occupational medicine.

For many employees, Edison's clinics and pharmacy were sacrosanct. A remote site clinic was, after all, how the company first provided healthcare to its workers 90 years ago. The clinics were a symbol of Edison's healthcare commitment to its people. To have made any drastic decision about the fate of the facilities without the involvement of employees would have evoked a bitter response.

Employees also were invited to participate on teams involved in other phases of research and planning, such as studying the true costs of providing healthcare services in their traditional form as well as developing proposals for phasing out some soon-to-be-unnecessary functions such as claims and delivery units. Oddly, no one at Edison could say how much was actually spent to provide these services to each employee. A new in-house unit was established to collect and analyze financial data related to healthcare, a task previously delegated to an external firm.

As soon as employee groups were formed to explore healthcare changes and people were reassigned to cross-functional work teams, rumors began. The change leader's communication policy during the transition was straightforward and strict: managers were to quell rumors as they surfaced by disclosing complete and factual information. If rumors touched on situations that must remain confidential, then managers were directed to fully explain the need for confidentiality at this time and promise to relay information as soon as it could be made public. Quarterly all-hands meetings were held with the vice president of healthcare to convey information, answer questions, and, most importantly, to allow everyone to hear the same thing at the same time. This was a communication device seldom used at Edison and never before in the healthcare department. Employees were impressed with the vice president's forthrightness.

Complicating the communication effort with employees was the fact that the Edison family was more than just a warm, fuzzy feeling in many cases. In the company's early years, family members expected their offspring to follow in their footsteps, and the company actively recruited new employees from among family and friends of current workers. Growth and an increasingly tough regulatory environment changed this somewhat, but there is still a high percentage of employees related to fellow workers and retirees. These personal relationships increased employees' concerns for how the changes would affect them and other family members and friends. Healthcare was speculated about not only at work but also at home, at family gatherings, and at social events with friends. There was more opportunity for misinformation to circulate more quickly and more broadly than at an organization where contact between employees was more conventionally defined by the boundaries of the workplace.

The long tenure of many company managers and the circuitous route many took to reach management status were both a blessing and a curse. It was a longstanding custom for Edison to promote management candidates from within, so a great number of the company's leaders actually started in entry-level positions, working their way up the organizational chart to management positions. Long history provides credibility to reassure employees of the company's intent in making these massive changes, but it can also snarl change activities with personal feelings of loyalty and concern for the effects the changes will have on long-time colleagues.

A special effort also was put forth to keep executives informed and involved. The executive team had long been aware that something was wrong in the way Edison was approaching healthcare, but they did not know what. Executives needed to be educated about the rapidly changing healthcare market and ways to measure quality healthcare. They needed to understand the components of healthcare benefit design and hear the advantages and disadvantages of each plan option. They needed familiarity with both broad concepts and enough detail to be able to answer questions and support the planned healthcare changeover at Edison with candid, factual information.

Senior executives were briefed in periodic special sessions by the healthcare department vice president. The CEO received monthly, in-person updates on the status of the conversion program. These extensive presentations helped to demystify healthcare for the executive level while building trust and support for change. The resulting depth of comprehension among the executive branch and its endorsement of the changes added an extra level of credibility to communication efforts with employees and retirees.

Direct communication of the proposed healthcare changes to active employees was assigned to a newly designed group of managed care specialists. Workers from the healthcare department applied and interviewed for these new positions. Those selected were trained on how to communicate changes to the many employee strata of Edison and how to deal with a wide range of employee concerns—everything from simple questions about the facts of the changes to confusion and disgruntled anger. In less than six weeks, more than 400 meetings were held for active employees to describe the proposed changes to healthcare benefits and assist individuals to make the changes. Meetings were held at many work locations at many different hours, including weekends.

Each of the new healthcare plans had a toll-free telephone number for questions from employees. In addition, Edison put together a telephone help line specific to the healthcare changeover as a supplement to the company's regular healthcare information center.

It was a challenge to obtain so much buy-in from the employees in the healthcare department that they could communicate the benefits of the new health plans to active employees and retirees even though they knew they were likely to lose their jobs. But it was also effective for a healthcare department staff member to stand before a group of angry, hostile fellow workers and say with sincerity, "My job is going to go away as a result of this change, and I still think it is a good idea for you and the company. This is the right thing for Edison to be doing at this time."

RETIREES

The 6,800 retirees and their dependents were about to have an abrupt change made to the healthcare services to which they had grown accustomed. Those who had retired before 1991 had specifically been guaranteed through the PrimeCare program "full healthcare benefits for themselves and their dependents at no cost to them for their entire lives." These PrimeCare benefits were delivered through the same PPO network used for active employees in the HealthFlex program. Edison took care of every detail for retirees and their dependents. If there was a question or problem, a retiree could call up the Edison staff and get all the help they needed to fill out the forms. Edison paid the bills.

Again, Edison found that the company-as-family concept was a double-edged sword. Retirees think of their former workplace as part of their extended family. Edison retiree clubs are organized all over the state. Retirees who have moved out of the area often schedule vacations to come to southern California in order to have their annual physical at the Edison healthcare department and visit old friends. This is not the typical employer-employee relationship, and the close, personal identification with the company complicated the process of making changes in the way retirees' healthcare benefits were administered. There were many communication hurdles to leap with this group of stakeholders.

First and foremost was the emotional reaction of many retirees when they first heard of the proposed changes, especially those who had accepted early retirement offers specifically in order to qualify for Prime-Care benefits. "In my mind retirement under these circumstances [early retirement] constituted a deal whereby we gave up our right to future earnings in exchange for a vested right in PrimeCare," wrote one retiree to Edison's CEO. "I do not see how anyone at Edison can interpret our retirements and feel morally or legally justified in seeking to impose one of the new options on us without our consent."

Most retirees had never had to choose a plan before because Edison's 7,500-member PPO network practically guaranteed they could go to any doctor they wanted and Edison would pay 100 percent. The retirees and their families did not know how to go about investigating the differences between the plans selected to administer their future PrimeCare benefits and choosing which would be right for them.

Despite the possible pain and confusion it might cause, the way healthcare would be administered for Edison's retirees and their families had to be changed. The internally administered PPO network was being dissolved and something had to be selected to take its place. An internal company committee studied the options and recommended an approach that would be the least disruptive and the most legally defensible.

Under the new healthcare program, the retirees could choose from among two POSs and six HMOs. Offering eight different plan options was a deliberate attempt to cast a far-reaching net in hopes of snaring as many of the retirees' current primary care physicians as possible. Even so, this meant that as many as 40 percent would have to find a new physician because the one they had been using was not included in any of the networks now available. Every reasonable effort was made to minimize the number of retirees who would have to switch healthcare providers because Edison knew that those retirees whose physicians were no longer on the list would be enormously upset.

The retirees' initial reaction to the announcement of the new program was not positive; they perceived it as a change in their healthcare benefits, not in the way their healthcare benefits were being delivered and administered. A retiree action group was formed to protest the changes, and Edison did, indeed, modify the program in response. Edison retirees and their families were still to receive 100 percent coverage, and there was never any attempt to take that away from them. But for some retirees, the only thing that would be satisfactory would be an exact replica of the existing PrimeCare program. Any change would be an unacceptable change; there was threat of a class-action suit that never materialized.

Many of the retirees had only worked for Edison and had no understanding of the generosity of their healthcare program compared to what was available from other employers. In casual conversations with retirees from other companies, they heard stories of how retired workers had lost benefits. They were highly suspicious and afraid that this was going to happen to them.

As the formal communications program kicked in, retirees began to understand what was really being proposed and their apprehensions were assuaged. The same core group of healthcare-department-trained presenters that explained the new program to active employees was expanded to communicate directly with retirees. Approximately 85 meetings were scheduled and more than 6,000 retirees and their dependents attended them. Information meetings were followed by 10 enrollment assistance clinics to walk retirees through the selection/enrollment process. Retirees also had access to each plan's toll-free telephone number and to Edison's healthcare hot line. An average of 500 to 600 calls was received each day at this information center during the two-week period that followed the introduction of program changes for retirees.

In retrospect, the retirees needed a much more custom-tailored communication plan than was originally launched at Edison. Although there was always the commitment to treat retirees with respect and sensitivity, the company underestimated the level of resistance retirees can have to change. The median age of the retiree population was 71 and, in general, they did not absorb new information easily. This group required much more repetition of key information than was necessary to educate active employees and needed consistent reassurance of the intentions and integrity of Edison to bridge the emotional riptide that accompanied any discussion or thought of change.

The media, which so often headlines flagrant abuses by other companies in the treatment of their retirees, fanned the fears and anxieties of Edison alumni. Once the new program was well under way, and retirees could see how it worked, they were calmed and, for the most part, pleased with Edison's quality of healthcare. It was, however, a difficult few months during the transition that could have been smoother with a more carefully crafted communications program to address retirees' fears directly, quell their apprehensions, and repeat key messages in easy-to-understand language.

HEALTHCARE DEPARTMENT

Of all of the stakeholders affected by the transformation in healthcare being planned by Edison, the employees of the healthcare department were the ones whose lives changed most drastically. The change leader asked many of these people to design an organization they might not be part of and, in some cases, to actually plan the phase-out of their own jobs. Even the vice president knew she was working herself out the door.

As with active employees, the communication strategy concentrated on making individuals in the healthcare department understand the external conditions that made this major corporate change inevitable. Placing emphasis on the big-picture business game plan behind the decisions and the importance of these decisions to Edison's competitive future reinforced the "it is nothing personal" message. People who would lose their jobs as a result of the restructuring needed to hear this message many times while they dealt with the trauma of change.

Another goal was to involve healthcare department employees as much as possible in the planning and implementation of the change process since their structured involvement would deepen their understanding of the reasons for change. This effort was helped by companywide emphasis on encouraging team performance and inspiring a spirit of entrepreneurship. Workers at all levels and in all departments were already being told to look for ways to cut through bureaucracy and find more productive ways of doing work.

Managers often fear that employees will slough off once they know their tenure is limited or even try to sabotage a corporate restructuring. Edison discovered the opposite can be true if the employees who will be affected are given honest, direct communication. The change leader's message to the healthcare department was: "For the time you are working here, you have work to do. You are getting paid to do it. You are expected to perform at the highest level during that period of time, and in return you will gain skills that are transferable and useful in the next phase of your career." Staff did.

Managers within the healthcare department were provided with guidelines to help them communicate with employees during the transition. The company also provided training and coaching on how to stay focused on the task at hand and not take personally employees' anger or emotional reactions to change. The guidelines were as follows:

1. Don't take employees' feelings personally

2. Don't be defensive

3. Don't inject your personal feelings or "cop out" by criticizing the company or saying "I don't want to do this but . . ."

4. Don't discuss motivations of "why"

5. Don't argue about anything

6. Don't say "I know how you feel," because each person feels differently

7. Don't get on the topic of your needs, feelings, or problems

8. Don't guess, speculate, give your own opinion, or attempt to give advice

The restructuring of the healthcare department from the ground up gave employees a unique opportunity to become aware of all the interconnecting jigsaw pieces that go into the creation of an organization. They had a new realization of how their individual jobs connected with the role of the department and the overall success of the enterprise. They were able to see beyond their daily "to do" lists and consider the real value their function held for the organization.

In addition to this insight, healthcare department employees gained or improved specific skills during the transition, such as public speaking, effective communication techniques, conflict resolution, and cross-functional team building. Furthermore, employees fully participating in the transition received a condensed education on the evolution and current state of healthcare in America.

The following letter was sent to healthcare department employees in July 1994, a few weeks before they were needed to help explain the new healthcare program to the other active employees, retirees, and their families. This correspondence was one of many points of communication between management and affected workers that treated all concerned with integrity. The memo worked well in answering questions and clarifying the situation without setting off an explosion of fear, anger, and lessened productivity.

> As part of our efforts to keep you informed of the progress of our department's reorganization, you met with your manager today to discuss the following points.
>
> As the healthcare department transitions to an externally administered healthcare plan, several changes are required to meet our business needs. The attached chart illustrates the planned new organizational structure. We plan to move toward this new structure over the next several months.
>
> As you can see from the attached chart, we plan to eliminate some units. Several units continue to be under study. Still other units will continue to exist in the new organization. We pledge to inform you of decisions that affect you as soon as they are made.
>
> We anticipate that certain positions will no longer be needed in the new organization. If your job is one we currently believe will be eliminated in the new organization, your manager has shared with you the earliest date such job elimination may occur. This is a projected date, however, at this time we do not expect that it will be any sooner than then . . . Today's communications are merely an early warning of expected changes that may affect you. We are providing you with this information to allow you some time to plan for your future . . .

This appeal to employees' integrity and professionalism was supplemented with the sensitive, caring acknowledgment that these individuals were likely to experience the typical emotional roller coaster (i.e., denial, fear, anticipation, grief, excitement) of pending job loss. The most effective triage came from a team of employees who volunteered to develop and provide support and training opportunities. Workshops covered stress management and constructive conflict management skills and many employee meetings included small group exercises to bring out different perceptions and reactions of employees to changes in the healthcare department.

Most of the healthcare department staff who were about to lose their jobs had been hired under an assumption that they would be working for Edison until they retired. Many of the employees who were about to be unemployed had never written a resumé, had an interview, or looked for a job. They were hired at Edison right out of school, usually as a referral from a friend or relative who already worked at the company. Many lacked the skills to seek employment in a competitive job market.

Severance from a company once considered a lifetime employer must be managed as a major loss. Individuals are likely to pass through the same emotional stages as in the loss of a loved one: denial, anger, grief, and, finally, acceptance.

It was important for Edison both to acknowledge employees' emotions and to provide them with practical information useful to plan the next phase of their careers. The goal was to help employees feel they were in control and to empower them to determine their own futures. They may not have had control over their jobs, but they could prepare themselves to live with that eventuality and to do something to control their futures.

Consultants at career development workshops for employees of the healthcare department used a variety of tools such as the chart of career paradigm changes (shown in Table 2) to emphasize that the reorganization under way at Edison was typical of significant changes occurring at companies throughout the United States. It was important for employees to understand that individuals universally have a new responsibility for taking control of and managing their careers.

An extensive campaign was sponsored to help affected employees recognize and deal with their tumultuous feelings, study career options, and make successful transitions. Career development workshops were created by employees serving on the career team and led by employees with the assistance of outside consultants who were able to reassure them that their reactions to diminished job security were normal and to alert them about what feelings to expect in the coming days. Job search clinics, outlined by a group of employees and delivered by career management consultants, covered a broad range of topics: career development plans, skills assessment, job networking, job research, resumé writing, and interviewing skills.

On the practical side, employees were issued "take charge" cards that allowed them to take an hour of company time for every hour of personal time they spent in workshops to be more competitive on their present job and in the job market. The underlying theme of every workshop was to encourage employees to evaluate their situations realistically and to make choices about their futures based on objective data, not emotional responses or misperceptions.

As the following example shows, career development workshops focused on providing practical skills to help affected workers with their job search campaigns. Some had never worked anywhere but Edison; others had been with Edison for many years. Across the board, job-search skills were rusty or nonexistent. Table 3 describes a few of the dozen different workshops offered.

Incentive cash bonus programs to ensure commitment until the changeover was complete were limited to a very few individuals. Only those with highly marketable skills whose contribution to the healthcare department would be extraordinarily difficult to replace were offered incentives—a group of about six individuals. Some employees chose to leave before the transformation was in place, but the majority of the healthcare department stayed and participated in an exciting enterprise

TABLE 2
Trends 2000: Career paradigm changes

Old paradigms	New paradigms
Job security	Employability security
Longitudinal career paths	Alternate career paths
Job and person fit	Person and organization fit
Organizational loyalty	Job and task loyalty
Career success	Work and family balance
Academic degree	Continuous learning
Full-time employment	Alternative employment
Retirement	Career sabbaticals
Single job/career	Multiple jobs or careers
Career stability	Career instability

rebirth. Because of the depth of career assistance available to them, virtually every employee in the healthcare department moved to the next phase of their career with poise and grace. These next steps went down a variety of different career paths: continuing roles in the newly defined healthcare and employee services department, early retirement, returning to school for additional education, starting their own businesses, positions in other departments of Edison, or jobs with other

TABLE 3
Career development workshops

Self assessment

Participants complete a self-assessment of interests and skills that will be explained and interpreted. In addition participants will complete inventories of values, attitudes, work habits, and performance in order to understand their strengths and weaknesses.

Resumé preparation

Participants will learn the most recent trends in resumé preparation. Most importantly, participants will learn how to highlight their marketable skills and accomplishments in order to create a strong, attractive, stimulating, competitive resumé.

Networking and informational interviewing

Participants will learn how to use networking as a valuable job-research tool. By the end of the workshop, participants will have created the beginning of a networking list and will know how to conduct informational interviewing.

Resumé writing

In today's competitive job market, individuals must have resumés that grab attention. This workshop will build on the information presented in the resumé preparation workshop and will teach the art of resumé writing—how to focus on measurable accomplishments and achievements that will attract the recruiter's interest and win the interview.

Becoming a STAR

While your resumé might get you the interview, it will not get you the job. How well you interview can make the difference between getting the job and being "runner-up." This workshop will focus on the art of using the STAR system of answering interview questions so you will feel confident in communicating important information in any situation without feeling intimidated.

Exploring your work style

This workshop builds on the information you gained about yourself in the self-assessment workshop. Earlier you completed a very brief and simple values questionnaire. This time you will complete a much more detailed and comprehensive values inventory. The results specifically concern how your values and personality are reflected in your work style and what to look for as you develop your career so you optimize your work style.

Using the career center

This workshop will be offered in small groups in the new career center. The purpose of the workshop is to introduce you to all of the services and resources available to you to pursue your career development in a professional, safe, supportive environment. You will also learn more specifically how to use the job research materials in the center.

organizations. As a result of the intensive career development work, several individuals made significant shifts in the direction of their careers, changing fields or industries.

One group of healthcare department employees that experienced a slightly different kind of transition was the healthcare professionals at the four clinics and pharmacy that were taken over by an outside medical group. The Edison staff members who worked at these facilities were interviewed and all were offered positions. Those who accepted the jobs were still employed, but faced a rough transition nonetheless. They continued to work in the same place as they did when they were "Edison people," but now they were "Friendly Hills people" with a new employer and new ways of doing things. They also were treating non-Edison people in what used to be exclusively Edison surroundings. There is no blueprint for this kind of transition and the first few months were confusing and stressful.

Summary

More than half of the major corporations in America considered significant organizational changes in the late 1980s and early 1990s in order to keep up with a radically shifting business environment. Edison was no exception. As senior management charted a new course of action for the company in the twenty-first century, the company's efforts to redefine and reorganize its entire premise of healthcare benefits dovetailed with three critical business imperatives.

First of all, Edison's corporate strategy for staying competitive in the fast-changing utility industry returned to "sticking to our knitting." Edison's core competency is in providing electrical power. Recent regulatory developments appear to be hastening the day when Edison and other electric utilities will find themselves in openly competitive markets, after many years of operating with exclusive franchises and careful regulatory scrutiny. The traditional utility business of supplying electricity to a customer's meter is not a new enterprise, but there are burgeoning regional needs for energy efficiency, electric transportation, environmental improvement, and connections to the information superhighway. The company also has opportunities in the global marketplace where there is a huge unmet demand for electric power, particularly in developing countries. The changes in Edison's healthcare system allowed the company to once again focus these resources on its core competency, rather than on providing a service to employees that could be outsourced or provided through a partnership alliance.

Secondly, meeting the challenge of the future also meant that Edison had to contain costs wherever and whenever possible. For Edison to be a strong competitor in this new marketplace, it needed to improve productivity, streamline the organization, and aggressively control costs. Healthcare had become Edison's fourth largest cost center behind the company's core business and added no appreciable value to its four million customers. Reengineering its approach to healthcare contributed to a better financial position to meet the company's business goals and future vision.

Lastly, healthcare reform was targeted by government as a prime goal for the decade. As the advantages and disadvantages of different healthcare systems were debated in and out of government, it was clear that the wave of healthcare reform was going to wash over large corporations like Edison. While the exact implications for the company and its healthcare department could not be determined, there was no doubt that the changes would be significant and probably costly. Edison had historically taken a leadership role in healthcare and wanted to continue to be on the forefront. The achievements of the three-year restructuring give Edison a competitive edge to meet the business challenges of the future and stayed true to the corporate philosophy that "a healthy company is equal to healthy employees, and healthy employees will keep our company strong."

Edison drew national attention and recognition as an innovator in the creation of a corporate healthcare system and as one of the major corporations calling for national healthcare reform. But like many other employers, Edison needed greater cost controls and increased accountability for quality.

The changes made in healthcare at Edison felt uncomfortable to employees and retirees when they were introduced, but the disquieting transition period quickly became part of the lore of the company. The healthcare transformation at Edison managed to accomplish what seemed to be an almost unrealistic goal: increased benefits and choice for employees while decreasing employees' out-of-pocket healthcare expense and the cost to the company.

---

* Author Margaret Jordan has accepted a position with Dallas Medical Resources in Dallas, Texas, since the completion of this chapter.

35

Gaining physician support for cultural and professional change

Diana Weaver, DNS, RN, FAAN
Senior Vice President for Patient Services

Richard J. Nierenberg, MD
Associate Director, Emergency Services
Yale–New Haven Hospital
New Haven, Connecticut

THE DECADE OF THE 1990s in healthcare may well become known as the "collaboration by necessity" era. In fact, the forces at work strongly suggest that collaboration and integration of purpose are essential for survival. The development of high-performing teams who ensure that all members contribute equally and fully to the best of their ability is paramount. The principle that cooperation or collaboration among individual caregivers is important to the care function is not disputed. However, using an institutional value philosophy that promotes equal voice and accountability may violate the hierarchical tradition that the physician holds the deciding vote in any care decision. Institutions that seek to change the clinical decision-making culture should be prepared for strong and often negative physician reaction.

The purpose of this chapter is to describe the challenges Yale–New Haven Hospital encountered when multidisciplinary thinking was incorporated into the operational care philosophy and was perceived by a powerful medical staff as disruptive to traditional caregiver relationships.

An organizationwide redesign process, known as patient-focused operational redesign, was undertaken in 1993. A planning goal to redesign care was developed to capitalize on the strengths of all hospital employees. The belief was held that effective redesign must reflect the underlying values and culture of the whole institution and that these shared values would be instrumental to meet the institution's goals. The leaders of the redesign process were committed to using the input of all disciplines to arrive at an underlying framework for change. In particular, the intent was to avoid allowing one discipline to articulate goals and practices that would be practiced by other disciplines, since that approach would only promote the segregation of management structure and not facilitate an organizationwide alignment. For such a restructuring to have enthusiastic participation and support at all levels, it was imperative that physicians and hospital staff be involved in the redesign process. The redesign committee made a number of assumptions regarding the new environment that was to be created. The first was that power is not finite; empowering one discipline on the team does not diminish the power of another discipline on the same team. Second, shared values and visions are operationalized similarly by all team members, regardless of their role socialization. And, finally, past behaviors are easily shed in favor of a new improved approach to care. In retrospect, these assumptions, although altruistic, were naive.

To facilitate multidisciplinary thinking and ensure broad participation, a care management team was created. The charge to the group was to develop a conceptual framework to redesign the care environment at Yale–New Haven Hospital. Integral to that process was the need to look at current practice—comparing and contrasting it to care that was deemed to be optimal from the perspective of patients, physicians, payers, and providers. The care management team then developed a set of guiding principles that were to facilitate consistent delivery of high-quality, cost-effective care. Inherent in the work of the team was the review and revision of a number of roles on the team, including those of physician, nurse, and ancillary staff who interacted with the patients on a day-to-day basis. New roles were also created, using the redesign concepts of cross-training, decentralization, and systems thinking. The final outcome of the care management team's efforts was a draft document titled, "Guiding Principles and Implications for Patient Focused Care."

Key redesign principles

Pivotal to the concept of team development was the belief that individuals from different disciplines would work in harmony and synergy to improve patient care delivery. Each professional was viewed as a team member, with the team striving to achieve optimal care while focusing on the coordination and integration of all direct and indirect care activities. Patients were the focal point of service, and their interests primary. The team was accountable for and committed to solving patient care problems while embracing the ideal that leadership was a shared function, dependent on the expertise needed within a specific patient or clinical situation.

The document stated that the primary nurse is identified by the patient as one principal director of care throughout the patient's hospital stay. The primary nurse collaborates with the physician in decision making, setting goals and priorities, monitoring outcomes of care decisions, and ensuring that clinical effectiveness is combined with efficiency and optimal resource use.

The care management document also stated the actions of the team would be facilitated and monitored by specially trained and experienced care coordinators who would have the authority to cross traditional discipline lines to ensure care was of high-quality coordination and delivered in a timely, cost-effective manner.

Notably absent in the guiding principles was the traditional concept of one discipline, physicians, unilaterally giving orders that are carried out by a second and subordinate discipline, nursing. The team was deliberate in identifying areas of responsibility for each discipline, while maintaining the primacy of the team concept. For instance, while the physician was to be responsible for formulating the medical plan of care, identifying medical and other problems, and formulating the diagnostic and workup plans, it was also stated that the physician would function as a member of the team and medical decisions would not take place in isolation, but would be shared with the entire team.

After giving careful consideration to the interests of various caretakers, the team produced the final draft of the document, one that the team agreed was complete, comprehensive, and fair.

Reactions of the medical staff

One of the most interesting, and perhaps the most powerful, lessons learned from this experience came out of the unexpectedly strong, sudden, and almost singular negative reaction from the hospital's medical staff shortly after a draft of the care management document was circulated under the auspices of the chief of staff.

When the care management team met, six physicians were invited to the meetings. Few came to more than one meeting, and some never came to any. However, after the draft was widely circulated, a group of physicians organized to voice objections and rewrite the entire document. Participants included a dozen of the university's and community's most powerful physicians, virtually all of whom showed up at the early morning meetings scheduled specifically to hear their objections to the document. The physicians presented a proposed redraft of the original document, and the group went line by line through both the drafts to address objections and arrive at a compromise document. It should be noted that the hospital's attorney had participated in crafting the language in the original document to avoid an implied legal contract. However, one physician did share the document with his attorney, who inserted additional legal language. It is instructive to examine some of the language changes, which, while subtle, had important implications for the perception of multidisciplinary thinking in patient care.

In reviewing the definition of optimum care, the very first section that had been presented in the original document, members of the medical staff wanted to change the wording of two lines. The first proposed change was from "care which holds all caregivers accountable" to, "care which establishes accountability." The second proposed rewording was from "care which redefines the role of the nurse and physician" to, "care which uses the skills and knowledge of those disciplines."

These proposed changes suggested that some members of the medical staff objected to redefining the nurse's role to assume more accountability for patient care. This impression was supported by several further proposed changes in the document's cornerstones of care management. They were: a change from "the process will be under the supervision of a care coordinator" to "will use the skills of a care coordinator, who, instead of being responsible, now will assist in the application of case management principles" and instead of stating that "critical pathways are used as guidelines," it was insisted that "critical pathways should be developed with physician leadership."

The substance of the objections of the medical staff seemed clear in specific proposals for rewrites in passages regarding the role of the nurse. Many insisted that the initial statement, "the primary nurse is identified by the patient as one principal director of care," be changed to read, "the primary nurse assumes responsibility for the delivery of much of the care to patients." The initial document had stated that "the nurse uses professional judgment and discretion to be responsible and accountable in planning care, setting goals and priorities, selecting among appropriate interventions, making decisions, and solving problems." The proposed rewrite had a very different tone. It now reads, "the nurse will act in collaboration with physicians to monitor outcomes of care decisions and to solve problems at the bedside."

In reviewing this proposed redraft by members of the medical staff and in initial meetings with representatives of the physician staff, the major point of contention was the perception that the original document endorsed amplifying the nurse's authority at the expense of the physician. The phrasing was viewed as a challenge to the autonomy traditionally held as central to the physician's role.

The realization that the initial document had engendered such a reaction created a conundrum for those on the original care management project who wished to promulgate a multidisciplinary culture and to endorse the responsibility, autonomy, and collaborative nature of all disciplines. It was difficult to promote these values in the face of what appeared to be relative unity of purpose. The redesign leaders were caught, strategically, in a difficult bind since a fundamental principle of the redesign philosophy was now in jeopardy.

Bowing completely to the demands of this powerful constituency would have a negative impact on the entire process of redesign. Many members of the hospital staff had worked very hard for a long time to develop a guiding philosophy that reflected the interests and values of these diverse segments. If that work was discarded, then faith in the importance of their participation would be lost and the majority of hospital staff would question the sincerity of the redesign effort. This dynamic was not in the best interests of the institution, the patients, or, in the long run, any of the individual disciplines.

On the other hand, certain cultural and structural realities needed to be acknowledged. Practicing physicians are seen as credible primary advocates of patient interests and quality of care. In addition, physicians continue to wield considerable power, both through role authority and through the continued ability to control the dispositions of patients. Therefore, it was essential to address the concerns of those who initially perceive a diminution in their authority through multidisciplinary restructuring. The redesign team recognized that when a culture change runs into the determined opposition of the consensus of medical staff, it is stopped as if by a brick wall. This was a lesson in realpolitik, one based on practical and material factors, rather than theoretical or ethical objectives. To be effective, serious change in the clinical roles of caretakers must be acceptable to significant clinical stakeholders and, most certainly, to the physician staff.

At this point, a subset of members of the original team sought to determine how to promote a multidisciplinary culture while trying to recognize the voiced concerns of the physician staff. Any progress in such negotiations had to be based on the legitimate interests of all clinical stakeholders coupled with sincere and consistent efforts. Quelling these concerns, while still preserving the intent of the initial document, was key to the negotiations.

Protecting the bond of the physician-patient relationship is a legitimate interest for physicians and healthcare institutions. Progress will not occur if physicians view multidisciplinary participation as eroding the essential nature of that bond. Physicians and the public value the physician-patient relationship. The current national dialogue regarding optimum healthcare delivery systems shows that Americans desperately want their own physicians. Both patient and physician view it as essential to the relationship that one particular physician manage a case. This central feature of having one person primarily responsible for a patient is a source of tremendous comfort to both the patient and the physician.

It is a legitimate interest for the physician to insist that a choice of treatments be honored, subject to certain checks and balances on medical appropriateness. However, those legitimate interests do not imply that physicians have unquestionable and completely unfettered control over all diagnostic and therapeutic resources. Any attempt to increase the collaborative nature of the clinical relationships among all health professionals must be presented to enhance the accountability of all. This principle, applied appropriately, will not prevent nursing or involved disciplines from taking an active and collaborative role in patient care management. Rather, it will maximize the responsibility and accountability of other disciplines without displacing the physician. This will require both sensitivity and insight into the professional psyche of both disciplines. Nonetheless, physicians must begin to come to terms with the fact that no one discipline can or does possess the clinical expertise to address all care and treatment decisions. Providing the best and the most efficient care demands input and knowledge of the entire clinical team. Within the bounds of any professional role, authority to act in the patient's best interest must be granted by the entire team.

Through careful consideration of the physician community, a document was negotiated that created a framework for the input and participation of all professionals involved while preserving specific patient care interests of physicians. In fact, those nonphysician healthcare professionals who had worked hard and were committed to the original document had no cause to believe their work was overturned. Additionally, physicians who perceived the original document to be an attempt to erode their legitimate and appropriate position as primary arbitrators of their patients' medical care accepted that their concerns were heard and addressed. The unexpected opposition encountered after presenting the original document and the efforts expended to moderate that opposition are fundamental cultural elements that must be recognized and managed in the change process.

Conclusion

Some of the most important lessons learned from this initiative include the following:

1. Developing multidisciplinary thinking in patient care and promoting a multidisciplinary culture that will continue to grow in importance in any care redesign initiative

2. Shared institutional and professional values must drive redesign

3. Core values must be fully explained to and discussed with all members of the team, if redesign is to succeed

4. Developing effective teams in care delivery may threaten physicians who are increasingly fearful about encroachment upon their perceived authority and autonomy

5. Effective management of these reactions requires several steps. First, significant members of the physician staff must be integral to the planning process; although difficult to effect, flexibility is of paramount importance. Hospital management must impress on physician staff that it is in their interest to be part of the process early on; otherwise, they are virtually certain to be resistant and react in a counterproductive manner, thus undermining the common good of the institution

6. The legitimate interests of all stakeholder groups must be carefully assessed and viewed realistically from each stakeholder's perspective. In the case of physicians, relationships cannot be seen as antithetical to such traditional and entrenched principles as the physician-patient relationship and the capacity to practice medicine without undue or unnecessary interference

7. Promoting a team-oriented, multidisciplinary approach to patient care may erode the autonomy of all stakeholders to some extent. However, using the concept of the patient's needs as primary offers leverage for negotiating through the territorial concerns of all disciplines

The process of restructuring care along patient-oriented lines mandates the formation of broad-based, multidisciplinary hospital teams. Accomplishing this new alignment is not an easy task. However, when certain caveats are recognized as important and necessary, the effort can yield a heightened awareness of the interdependent nature of effective, efficient patient care. Such awareness is a basic building block to any improvement process. In the case of Yale–New Haven Hospital, the frustrating and time-consuming steps that were necessary to get physician buy-in could have been short circuited somewhat; however, they could not have been skipped.

In fact, during this time the volatile healthcare market was replete with changes that were assailing physicians and heightening their sense of loss of autonomy. The team, particularly the administrative members, should have been more tuned in to these significant developments. For example, in the meetings to redraft the document, physicians who appeared to be very role secure were citing statements from the press about the escalating healthcare opportunities for midlevel providers. Indeed, HMOs and other healthcare organizations were, in increasing numbers, using nurse practitioners to provide clinical care for patients who were formerly seen by physicians. In addition, teaching hospitals were introducing acute care nurse practitioners to provide additional clinical resources for patient care management. In some cases, this change was the result of unfilled residency slots, and in other cases, the role was a true replacement for physician coverage. At the national level, polls were suggesting that physicians were losing public confidence as a profession. Given these factors, the physicians' reactions to the proposal of team and collaborative decision making should not have come as a surprise.

Hindsight planning would suggest that more care should have been taken to ensure that key physicians across the institution were engaged in dialogue about the need for increased teamwork in healthcare treatment and delivery. Powerful physicians who held leadership roles in the organization could have been used through a train-the-trainer approach. This approach would have allowed the team leaders to work, one on one, with key physicians who could be expected to carry the message of the new care philosophy and its benefits to their professional colleagues. In fact, that message could have been scripted by the team, and a feedback loop that directly linked the team with physicians could have been established, providing a safe place for physicians to be able to talk out loud about their fears and concerns. When a representative group was ultimately assembled, only one nonphysician was permitted to attend. On multiple occasions, physicians voiced the need to be able to discuss their insecurities when only understanding and supportive colleagues were present. In hindsight, Yale–New Haven Hospital learned the importance of supporting a physician group facing enormous cultural and professional changes, and the resulting impact on patient care. Reflection on both the dynamics and the process of this work offers lessons for the future.

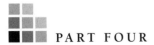

PART FOUR

Teamwork and training

36

Designing and implementing teamwork programs

Adrian Tibbetts, MBA
Director of Service Innovation
AvMed–Sante Fe HealthCare
Gainesville, Florida

MANAGED HEALTHCARE IS A DYNAMIC, competitive, service-oriented industry. Organizations must be responsive to the changing environment and innovative with service personnel and operations. The current management trend is to accomplish more goals and objectives with fewer people. As competition increases, the challenge to retain qualified service representatives also increases.

An October 1994 survey of 150 executives from the nation's 1,000 largest companies found that people leave organizations for five reasons:

- Limited opportunities for advancement

- Lack of recognition

- Unhappiness with management

- Inadequate benefits and salaries

- Bored with their job[1]

Teamwork programs can provide a structure to address the issues to keep service representatives from leaving the organization and to improve customer service. Team programs are small groups of motivated people that manage the delivery of service to external or internal customers. The teams may share various management and leadership functions.

Traditional theory states that planning and control are management activities. Planning and controlling work processes such as scheduling of work shifts and breaks, monitoring and adjusting staff levels to reduce telephone abandonment rates, and cross-training can be handled by the service representatives. Representatives can monitor the costs involved in correcting mistakes in quality, such as identification cards printed with an incorrectly spelled customer name or assignment to an incorrect primary care physician.

The teams may assume responsibility for the quality of their service by enacting new ideas to improve the service or the working conditions. For example, service representatives may be cross-trained between telephone-answering and claims-paying functions. Cross-training allows claims representatives to assist with answering telephone calls on the busier days, and on slower days of the week the telephone representatives can assist with processing claims.

This chapter will outline how the design and implementation of teamwork programs can be beneficial to healthcare organizations. The benefits of a team program include improved communication, commitment and motivation among employees, and retention of trained personnel. Preparation is necessary to anticipate the benefits and potential pitfalls through planning and design. There are five critical planning and design concerns to be addressed:

- Corporate philosophy and managerial commitment to the teamwork concept

- Team composition

- Meeting schedule

- Group dynamics

- Training

Corporate philosophy and managerial commitment

A key element in the transition from the traditional hierarchical work structure is managerial commitment to the teamwork concept. Managerial actions, both verbal and nonverbal, must communicate support of the program. For example, a manager may learn how to use the teamwork concepts but really believe that the only management methods that work are the traditional, hierarchy-based approaches. The manager may talk teamwork approach, but employees see the daily actions carried out by the management authority practice. Management philosophies that do not emanate from a genuine belief in the teamwork concept come across as insincere, artificial, and phony.

There should be a requirement that managerial performance be measured by support and promotion of the teamwork program. Measurable ways to assess performance include

- Demonstrate costs or processing times have decreased, such as the processing time from application being entered or the production of a membership packet and identification card

- Demonstrate service times have decreased, such as reduction in customer hold time and abandoned call rate

- Evaluate service representative annual performance reviews based on the team's performance instead of on the individual representatives

- Survey the customer service representatives on managerial performance and commitment to process and tie management's bonus to scores

- Monitor the types and number of training sessions and sources used to develop employees' skills and abilities.

- Conduct customer surveys with newly enrolled members. The enrollment objective should be flawless entry of new customers' information

- Monitor consistent and timely communication flow of the organization's mission and objectives. Communication should be conducted verbally and in writing and in language the employees understand. The communication should focus on the program's benefits to the organization and the employees and address their concerns. Communication will need to occur on a regular, scheduled basis

- Track the number and types of new ideas and corrective action suggestions put forth, as well as the number implemented. Even if the idea is unsuccessful, innovation and implementation shows risk taking and support to let customer service representatives develop skills and learn from mistakes

- Track the money spent to generate new suggestions for improvement and to implement team programs

Organizations should commit to a minimum of 24 to 36 months to realize consistent and continuous benefits from a teamwork program. It is a learning process for employees and management and it requires time. The learning process encompasses the need to evaluate the organization's mission, determine how it can be translated into the service process, develop short- and long-term objectives, and plan for training sessions. The organization and management should view the concept as a cultural shift, rather than a short-term program.

The successful transfer of power and responsibilities from management to the teams will only occur in an environment of trust. Trust fosters the loyalty and commitment from the team that are necessary to achieve team and organization goals. The employees must perceive managers as fair, honest, and supportive of the transition. They need to have confidence that managers will stand by the team because of their belief in the teamwork program. In the best case, management will have an established track record of commitment and support for the employees to build upon. However, it may take management a period of six months to a year to prepare a foundation of trust. This ingredient is essential prior to program implementation.

It may be difficult for management to accurately assess whether a trusting environment exists. Managers inherently believe their title automatically implies trust and respect from the employees. However, employees may be suspicious of new programs, especially if management has had several failed management projects. Employees also may view management with the latest program with skepticism—"Top management is often like a group of seagulls. They come in, raise a lot of noise, mess up the place, and then leave."[2] Poor commitment and implementation of past programs may have left employees with the sentiment illustrated in the seagull analogy.

An accurate, objective assessment of the environment for trust may be obtained through the use of an anonymous, confidential survey soliciting employee perception of the organizational environment. The survey should seek to obtain answers to the following questions:

- Does management have an established, positive track record for meeting commitments and keeping promises?

- Does management believe that frontline employees should make the majority of decisions that affect how they conduct their work?

- Does management understand that developing the teams is a lengthy, time-consuming, and labor- and financially intensive process? Are management and the organization willing and able to make the investment?

- Does management listen to what other people have to say about the working conditions, product service delivery, and customer feedback? Does management try to appreciate and understand the individual viewpoints and demonstrate respect for the person and ideas?[3]

Exhibit 1 shows a sample of a feasibility survey.

Productivity may decline as the team works through the dynamics of group interaction, requires training to learn new skills, and reevaluates the existing work processes. One of the greatest challenges will be to resist reverting to past habits and performance standards. Managers and teams may try the program for a month or quarter, then want to abandon the concept when the novelty or pressure from top management subsides. However, as team members learn and bond, the productivity should return to the original level and eventually improve beyond the original performance level. For example, empowering the customer service representative with the authority and responsibility to be the contact point for customer concerns may slow the resolution time. The representatives may have to work directly with other departments, such as provider relations, to receive information for issue resolution. Unlike the past, the customer service representative is not transferring the decision responsibility to another department or management for resolution. Initially it may take the representative longer to determine the right thing to do and assess the implications. Over time, the customer service representatives will gain knowledge and improve response time based on their learning experiences. Management will need to be supportive throughout the transition process to build and maintain trust and commitment. The team must have the confidence that management will provide support through the transition.

Team composition

The reorganization process begins with reorganizing personnel from individual workers into groups. The distinction between groups and teams is made at this point. Teams are groups in which participants have bonded and are working as collective, cooperative, cohesive forces. Careful planning and well-thought-out groups are important because the members will be working together for an extensive period of time. The objective is to make the group experience interactive, especially if past group experiences were not successful in achieving objectives.

The groups may be structured by product, department, or function. The groups may be organized by type of healthcare product delivered: health maintenance organization, point of service, indemnity, Medicaid, or Medicare. The groups also may be organized by company department, such as marketing, accounts receivable, customer service, and provider relations. Cross-functional groups incorporate several products or departments into one group.

Successful group arrangements take into account the organization's geographic locations and interdependence between departments. There must be synergy between the groups and the organization structure for the teamwork program to succeed. Organizations that are geographically dispersed may have difficulty meeting in one physical location or on a regular basis if extensive travel is required. Conference calling may allow people to talk; however, some of the essential nonverbal communication cues may be missed using this method. A video conference is an effective alternative because it allows verbal and nonverbal communication.

Organizations or departments that have low interdependence (i.e., not needing to work together to accomplish the department's goals) may have minimal incentive for group meetings or cooperation. For example, the accounts receivable or member application processing departments may not have to interface with the customer service representatives to conduct operations. It is the customer services department that is dependent on the efforts of the accounts receivable department to send timely, correct statements and of the member application processing department to accurately enter the application information. Departments that are not interdependent should find the mutually beneficial connections and develop internal customer responsiveness. Integration of these departments' efforts will influence the team's and organization's success or failure.

Determining the group size is a critical consideration in the planning stage. The group size can be too large or too small. Effectiveness tends to diminish when more than 12 people participate. Ideally the group will consist of four to eight members; an uneven number of members eliminates deadlock in decision making and voting.

Meeting schedules

For a group to train, function, and bond as an effective team, a consistent and frequent meeting schedule is required. A minimum meeting time should be at least once every two weeks. A group that convenes less often is essentially a new group each time. Infrequent or irregular meetings will result in repetitious review of previously discussed activities that are carried over from meeting to meeting with minimal resolution. Detailed minutes recording and an agenda are essential to reduce the time spent reviewing previously discussed issues. A group meeting is more effective when it meets twice per week, for one to two hours per session. The substitution of other department or temporary workers to assume the customer service responsibilities is essential to the consistent and frequent scheduling of meetings and training sessions conducted during business hours.

Group dynamics

Once the group's membership has been structured, the individuals must learn to work together and develop cohesiveness. The first introductory meeting should lay a foundation by discussing the corporate philosophy and commitment to the teamwork concept, outline the benefits for the participants, and develop communication channels. Participants will be looking for sincerity from management and peers. The participants will be searching for confirmation that this team experience will be personally rewarding and have value for the organization. It will be difficult to implement a program without a solid foundation built on trust and a sincere belief in the concept.

During the introductory meetings, the group should discuss the expectations of management and the individual participants. The discussion topics should include

- What experience do the participants want to gain from the group interaction?

- What leadership styles might exist in the group? Will the group designate a leader on a permanent or rotational basis, or not have any official leader?

- What responsibilities do team members have within and outside their group? What tasks will the teams be responsible for?

- What is the team's primary purpose? How is the team's purpose integrated with the organization's mission? Do team members know their expected roles, feel a sense of ownership, and perceive that they can make a difference?

- How will accomplishments be measured? At what intervals will measurement occur?

- What criteria will be used to assess when the team has met the primary purpose and completed the objectives? At what intervals will the evaluation for possible disbanding occur?

- How will positive and constructive feedback be communicated among team members?

After several meetings, a written covenant should emerge. This is an important step to unify individuals into a team. The covenant will specify the team members' mutually agreed-upon standards of conduct. The guidelines may require periodic updating. In the beginning the guidelines should be limited to fundamental points and should be consistent with the organizational team philosophy, such as

- Team members will support each other 100 percent. A receptive environment will be established to discuss ideas and dialogue between members. Contrasting viewpoints will be reviewed in a positive and constructive manner. The signature for each member on the covenant signifies commitment to other team participants and the team concept

- Decision-making agreement will be reached by a prespecified percentage of the group's participants. Although the members agreed to support each other, consensus does not have to be at 100 percent to implement a decision or idea. Consensus at 100 percent may often be an impossible standard, and the team would be stalled in dissension and deadlock. The agreement percentage may be set a point above 51 percent. The 75 percent agreement level works well in groups of four people because it is easy to determine that three of the four members reached consensus. A 60 or 80 percent agreement level works well in groups consisting of five members for the same reason. Once the agreement percentage is reached by the membership, the dissenting members must support any team's decision 100 percent, as specified in the first guideline

- Team members are expected to participate consistently and offer suggestions. Members are expected to be prepared to discuss the issues that affect the group. Consistently sitting quietly at the meeting and being nonresponsive to the discussion is not acceptable team behavior. Positive and constructive input is required from each member

- Members who do not participate constructively or who demonstrate demoralizing behavior can be voted off the team. Samples of unacceptable behavior include members who talk while another member is speaking, monopolization of the conversation, negative nonbusiness remarks about another team member, and a "we've tried that before and it didn't work" or "I told you so" attitude. Some individuals may not wish to participate in the team concept or may not try to bond with the other group members. An individual voted off a team can be assigned to tasks that are less than popular or less prestigious than those on which the team works. For example, teams will be creating and implementing ideas to change working conditions, such as flexible work hours. A former team member may wish to participate in the flexible work hours. However, as the former team member was unwilling to participate in the team process, the individual is ineligible to participate in the trial phase of the flexible hours. The former team member may be reassigned to routine functions such as filing or data entry. The nonteam individual may feel left out and reevaluate wanting to participate with the team or request permanent reassignment to a department with a more traditional type of work structure

- There will be no "parking lot" or after-meeting agendas by team members. A parking lot agenda occurs when one or several members pursue a topic in a negative manner outside the group forum.[4] The member may have been stating agreement during the meeting but vocalizes dissension after the meeting is over. This dissension can be considered disruptive behavior. Any team member who witnesses or hears of another member with an after-meeting agenda is responsible for directing the member to vocalize the issue during the meeting or bringing the issue up on the member's behalf at the next session. The previous guideline specifies what could happen to a member who continues to persist with after-meeting agendas

- Feedback will be communicated within the mutually agreed-upon guidelines. The team members' objective in giving constructive feedback should be to provide guidance by supplying information in a useful manner, either to support effective behavior (and thus take away common performance anxiety) or to guide a team member back on the track toward successful performance or team standards of conduct.[5] The team may develop a format to assist with communication of the guidelines. Exhibit 2 shows a sample feedback format with an example

Exhibit 3 shows a sample of a basic covenant.

The organization's interpersonal relations will undergo many changes during the transition period. Team members may resist changing to the team concept (i.e., not trusting or relying upon other members, learning new skills, or assuming additional responsibilities). These issues can be resolved through consistent and frequent meetings, adhesion to the covenant guidelines, improving communication, and attending training meetings.

Training

Training is an essential component to implement the teamwork program. It is an investment in the teamwork program, as well as a basic investment in human resources. Training can be a response to counter the reasons people leave organizations—boredom with the job and limited opportunities for advancement. As an employee's knowledge and skills increase, so will the possibilities for internal advancement and career opportunities.

Training and development skills can be divided into three types: social interaction, quality action, and technical job skills. Social interactions skills could also be referred to as human relations skills. The interaction skills encompass training topics, such as listening and feedback, gender sensitivity, handling conflict, and participating in meetings. These skills provide a mutual base from which individuals can compare and contrast different communication styles and progress forward as a united team. Gender differences seem subtle yet represent vast dissimilarities in the way that men and women communicate. "Men usually interrupt more, talk for longer periods of time, and focus more on outcome than on process. Women tend to speak more politely, talk about a wider range of topics and make better eye contact while speaking. The training reduces the tendency for people to work within preferred comfort zones—men working only with men and women working only with women."[6] Experiences in childhood and adolescence can affect social skills as adults. For example, if a person grew up with parents who were constantly arguing, as an adult the individual may yield in discussions to avoid dissension or a unnecessary, unpleasant argument. Conflict training helps the individuals vocalize questions and statements in a nonthreatening, constructive manner.

Individuals can learn to listen to someone's point of view without interrupting, acknowledge the similarities between viewpoints, and objectively discuss the differences. Working in groups will require that individuals learn to prepare an agenda, lead a meeting, focus the participants on agenda issues, and manage conflict and dissension. The training teaches how to praise individuals for positive contributions, such as a low telephone call abandonment rate, or provide constructive feedback, such as language terms to summarize a conversation that a service representative could use to lower the abandonment rate in the future.

Quality action skills include many of the analysis techniques used for total quality management and quality improvement. Quality skills encompass training topics, such as clarifying customer (internal and external) requirements, identifying improvement opportunities, developing and selecting solutions, planning the improvement, and measuring ongoing quality. For example, review of the weekly telephone call records showed that newly enrolled customers called to request identification cards. In reviewing the situation, the team discovered that the customers were receiving the welcoming kits but had difficulty locating the identification card because it was a small card placed in the back of the packet. The team suggested a new envelope with slits in the front pocket, to prominently display the card for easy location. The new envelopes were obtained at the same price as the previous type and the change reduced the incoming telephone calls to the customer service department and eliminated potential customer hassle with a time-consuming telephone call.

Technical job skills include daily techniques necessary to perform the responsibilities of a customer service representative. The job skills encompass training topics, such as telephone etiquette for customer service, equipment operations, reporting functions, and work processes. Telephone etiquette for communicating with customers could vary among geographic areas. For example, customers in low-social-economic areas may not be well educated on healthcare benefits and may be confused on how to access medical care. The customer service representative may have to speak at a slower rate, repeat the message more than once, or use simplified language. Speaking at a slower rate allows the customer time to absorb the message. Repeating the message more than one time can be used to assure the customer's understanding of the information. Simplified language, such as "personal doctor" instead of "primary care physician" or "gatekeeper, " translates insurance terminology into an expression more familiar to the customer.

Telephone equipment training can be important considering the complexity of the new systems. Customer service representatives should learn the technical features thoroughly to avoid negative experiences for the customer, such as losing a call during a transfer or having difficulty arranging a multiparty conference call.

Work processes such as interviewing potential team members and team member evaluations will require training. The team members should eventually have the responsibility of selecting new or replacement members for the team. These individuals will require training on questions to ask during an interview that would comply with Equal Employment Opportunity Commission and the Americans with Disabilities Act guidelines. Eventually, team members should assume the responsibilities for conducting performance reviews. Team reviews could include such criteria as the individual's contribution to team performance goals, innovative problem solving, recognition of outstanding contributions, and the identification of new directions for the team to pursue. The criteria also may be included as part of the team's covenant. The team members' assessments of other members' daily performance may better reflect the actual performance than the infrequent or irregular observations by management. Team evaluations can require extensive time to implement; this is because a solid foundation of trust, commitment, and communication is necessary for the evaluation to be conducted in an appropriate manner.

Each of the three training areas is important during the transition to effective teams. Management, in conjunction with the team members, will need to assess the status of social, quality, and technical skills, and prioritize the training. Surveys to inventory the skills of current personnel should be conducted. Based on the survey results, training sessions would be scheduled in the areas that are most critically needed. An overall training schedule should be developed outlining the topics and the availability of the sessions, so the teams may arrange for members to receive training.

Summary

The transition process from a traditional management structure to team programs takes into consideration organization philosophy and managerial commitment, group composition, meeting schedule, group dynamics, and training. Managers will need to demonstrate support throughout the transition process to build and maintain trust and commitment among team members. The transition from the traditional management hierarchy to the team structure can be summarized in an analogy of a parent teaching a child to ride a bicycle.

The child can grasp the concept of what learning to ride a bicycle is about: the excitement in learning something new, the independence, the ability to go to previously traveled places more quickly and efficiently than before, new opportunities because of increased abilities, and being with people who have learned the skill and who offer camaraderie. Training expertise and guidance are important, as are instructional aids such as training wheels. The student who masters the experience will become the teacher to assist others with learning these new skills.

As the parent prepares for the experience, it is known that patience and commitment are essential for both parties and that learning the skills will take time and practice. Providing this opportunity has risks; the parent will have to trust the child to make decisions and exercise independence wisely. Along the way the child will experience accidents and pitfalls, which will require the parent's wisdom to help overcome the incident and encouragement to continue the process. The parent can offer helpful hints to aid in the experience, but in the end the child must do the learning.

All participants in the program can benefit, as individuals and as a collective group, from the transition to teamwork. Healthcare organizations must be responsive to the changing environment and be innovative with their employees and operations. Teamwork can empower customer service representatives to deliver exceptional service that delights customers and creates a work culture that retains service-oriented representatives. Innovation through a teamwork program provides the organization with a means to differentiate itself from the competitors for the organization's long-term success.

NOTES

1. Robert Half International, Inc., *Survey of 150 Executives from the Nation's 1,000 Largest Companies* (Robert Half International Inc., October, 1994).

2. D. Keith Denton, PhD, "The Service Imperative," *Personnel Journal* (March, 1990).

3. R. S. Wellins, W. C. Byham, and J. M. Wilson, *Empowered Teams* (San Francisco: Jossey-Bass Publishers, 1991).

4. Career Track, *Implementing Self-Directed Work Teams* (Boulder: Career Track, Inc., 1994).

5. Zenger Miller, Inc., "Giving Constructive Feedback," *Frontline Leadership,* 1990.

6. J. J. Laabs, "Kinney Narrows the Gender Gap," *Personnel Journal* (August, 1994).

EXHIBIT 1
Teamwork program feasibility survey

The purpose of this survey is to determine if the work environment is ready for the implementation of a teamwork program. Using the scale below, indicate a response number for each statement. Indicate a "5" if you strongly agree with the statement or a "1" if you strongly disagree with the statement. Indicate a "4" if you agree more than you disagree with the statement or a "2" if you disagree more than you agree with the statement.

1. Management has an established, positive track record for meeting commitments and keeping promises. _____

2. Management believes that frontline employees should make the majority of decisions that affect how they conduct their work. _____

3. Management understands that developing the team is a lengthy, time-consuming, and labor- and financially intensive process. _____

4. Management and the organization are willing and able to make the necessary investments. _____

5. Management is willing to shift responsibility downward and significantly change traditional roles. _____

6. Management listens to what frontline employees have to say about the work conditions, product or service delivery, and customer feedback. _____

7. Management appreciates and understands individual viewpoints and demonstrates respect for the person and ideas. _____

8. Management will view this as a cultural shift rather than just a new program. _____

9. Management will commit the organization to provide a stable time period for the team to develop. _____

10. Frontline employees would be interested or willing to organize into a team. _____

EXHIBIT 2
Feedback format

Concept

Indicate the purpose by stating what you would like to cover, why it's important, what you've observed, and describe your reaction.

Discussion

Sandy: "Jon, I'd like to discuss an issue that affects the service to our customers. I noticed that you have been arriving in the office 10 to 15 minutes late each day. This means that you are not available to answer telephone calls at the start of the business day. With one less representative to answer calls the customer has to wait on hold longer, and the rest of us have to handle more telephone calls and deal with the customer's issue more quickly. I feel this places an unfair stress on me and the other team members and is not the best service to our customers."

Consider yourself in the individual's situation. Consider possible reasons for the situation. (Is this situation controllable or uncontrollable by individual member or by team?)

1. Have personal problems at home, car trouble, or children's day care, that makes it difficult to get to work
2. Burned out from job; not motivated to get to work on time
3. Other issues?

Give the team member an opportunity to respond.

Sandy: "Jon, what is your view of the situation? What do you think should be done to address the situation?"

Be prepared to offer specific suggestions or desired outcomes.

1. Carpool with other coworkers
2. Rotate job responsibilities; create new on-the-job challenges; pursue career development/advancement
3. Set alarm earlier in morning

Summarize feedback and express your support to achieve desired outcomes.

If the lateness situation were due to burnout, the summary and support of desired outcome could be as follows:

Sandy: "Jon, I'm glad we had an opportunity to discuss the lateness situation. I appreciate you sharing your feelings of burnout about customer service. A new challenge and responsibility could be assumed by you if you took a class in spreadsheet functions. This skill would provide for some variation in the day-to-day responsibilities and something new to tackle. The team understands and wants to assist you, yet meet our obligation to deliver the best customer service. We are pleased that you have agreed to arrive on time to answer the customer calls in a supportive team effort."

EXHIBIT 3
Sample covenant

We the team members of this group, a.k.a. the Smarter Bears, will operate on a mutually agreeable foundation and abide by the following terms:

- Each individual will be supportive and respectful of the other team members' personalities, beliefs, and ideas. There will be no bias based on ethnicity, gender, or other differences.

- The team presently consists of five members. The agreement level for group decision making will be at 80 percent (i.e., decisions will be approved when three of our five-person group reach consensus).

- Each individual is expected to participate consistently. Individuals are expected to be prepared for discussion of scheduled and unscheduled issues. Positive and constructive input is required from each individual.

- Individuals who are unable to contribute in a constructive manner or who demonstrate demoralizing behavior can be voted out of the team by the other members. The decision to remove an individual from the team may be made with or without management intervention.

- There will be no "after-meeting" agendas by team members. Any pursuit of a topic in a negative manner outside the group forum will be redirected to the next meeting either by the dissenting participant with the issue or by another team member on the other participant's behalf.

- Feedback will be communicated through the "Feedback Format" guidelines.

- As changes occur, the guidelines will be reviewed and revised accordingly.

Our signatures on this covenant symbolize our commitment to these team guidelines. We also understand these team guidelines may be used as a performance measure on our yearly performance reviews.

_____   _____
Sandy Smith   Ned Turner

_____   _____
Jon Sequers   Dan Mason

_____
Monique Myers

_____
Date

37

Training a multiskilled workforce

Donald Eggleston
Director of Staff Development

Susan Peters
Nursing Education Coordinator
St. Mary's Health Center
St. Louis, Missouri

T HE STAFF DEVELOPMENT DEPARTMENT at St. Mary's Health Center was responsible for cross-training staff for the implementation of patient-focused care (PFC). The enormity of the commitment, effort, and resources necessary for success was realized as the training and implementation progressed. The initial training of the multiskilled worker proved to be a challenge, as well as a learning experience, for the educators and the management staff.

Background

St. Mary's Health Center (SMHC) is a 70-year-old, 411-bed health center located in St. Louis, Missouri. While the health center campus is undergoing a significant redesign to enable St. Mary's to better serve patients, physicians, and other customers, a major renovation is occurring in how St. Mary's employees care for patients on a daily basis.

With the pressure for better access, improved quality, and lower healthcare costs in an extremely competitive healthcare market, St. Mary's has turned to PFC. The traditional delivery of healthcare at the hospital had been wasteful:

- 52 percent of expenditures went to payroll, yet only 25 percent of the employees' time was spent with patients

- 75 percent of hospital employees' time was spent on forms, scheduling, documenting, and waiting for others

- On average, 58 different employees saw one patient during a three-day stay

- Staff was fragmented—350 different job classes exist in a typical hospital with an average of six people in each class

- Same-day surgery patients admitted to St. Mary's were required to be seen in five different departments before undergoing surgery

- Routine procedures in diagnostic areas could require 30 or more steps

With the implementation of PFC, the hope was to overcome the compartmentalization of people and equipment and instead have most of the staff spend the majority of its time working with patients. The executive vice president of the hospital wanted to save money, but at the same time tried to improve the quality of services by eliminating unnecessary work. The current organization added costs and wasted resources.

Work redesign for a seamless workforce

PFC is designed to organize resources and personnel around patients, and not around central departments. The patient is number one. This is not to indicate that healthcare delivery has not always been focused on the patient—hospitals have historically attempted to improve efficiency by redesigning processes or procedures. However, seldom has the entire system been evaluated and restructured. A PFC hospital restructures the entire delivery system to offer seamless care to its patients. Restructuring for PFC includes deployment of services, work redesign, and physical or geographical reorganization and cross-training workers. With the implementation of PFC, all staff jobs are different: no employee is exempt.

At SMHC, a steering team was appointed to coordinate all PFC activities. The executive vice president chaired the team using advice and recommendations from a consulting group. Members included representatives from administration, human services, staff development, planning and marketing, and information systems. The team met weekly for a minimum of four hours to discuss and suggest designs and implementation methods. Concurrently, functional design teams developed the three new roles: clinical, administrative, and service associates. The steering team discussed and approved recommendations from the functional design teams. Any decision requiring approval from senior management was presented to the administrative council by the appropriate member of the steering team.

It quickly became apparent that this would be a slow and tedious undertaking. Making decisions often required considering a multitude of issues: equipment, system, and facility recommendations were evaluated. Center-based activities were assessed for potential shareability among the associates. Activities from central departments were considered for redesign. Preliminary job descriptions were developed with information developed by focus groups. The functional design teams documented their initial thoughts about central department redesign. Decisions from the functional design teams were evaluated and approved by the steering team or administrative council.

Patient care center design teams

Once recommendations from the functional design teams had been approved, the information was funneled to the center design teams, which were composed of the patient care center administrator, managers, staff members, and physicians. The functional design teams and the center design teams can be compared to a person building a home. The carpenters build the home (functional design team) but the home owner (center design team) designs the interior of each individual room. The six center design teams took the recommendations for deployment, job descriptions, and shareability of tasks and finalized the decisions for their specific center design and activities. Staffing requirements for the patient care center were also determined. Each design team developed a business and implementation plan for their center.

CARE OF PEOPLE AND COMMUNICATIONS SUBTEAMS

Several subteams worked with all of the teams during the time of design and implementation. The care of people (COPS) and communications subteams worked with the steering team to communicate information about the design process to the staff in a timely manner. An important aspect of the steering team is to deal with employee concerns. Change was disconcerting to the staff, and resulting fear and uncertainty needed to be addressed in a timely and honest manner. The steering team began each weekly session by addressing organizational concerns—the rumor of the week and people's questions and concerns. COPS was developed to keep employees informed, articles were included in the hospital newspaper, and a PFC hot line was established. COPS also held workshops on interviewing techniques for new job positions. The communications subteam disseminated information to employees as well as to physicians, universities, and managed care affiliations.

HUMAN RESOURCE SUBTEAM

Another team, the human resource subteam, assisted the functional design teams in standardizing job descriptions that reflected the service and administrative associate positions. Personnel policies on applications, transferring to new positions, and performance plans were revised to integrate PFC. A wage-and-salary survey was completed to determine a fair wage-and salary-structure for the new positions. Communication was of prime importance when new positions became available. The application and interviewing time frame was indicated clearly to all possible applicants.

CENTRALIZED VERSUS DEPLOYED SERVICES

PFC required moving services and personnel closer to the point of their use, thus minimizing the time spent transporting the patient around the hospital. Decisions were based on the individual center's needs, volume, and technical support required, and costs involved. The majority of deployed activities were high-volume, low-tech services. Complex activities such as computerized axial tomography (CAT scan) and blood banking procedures that required high-tech equipment, environment, and personnel remained centralized. Activities that were moved to a patient care center were performed by either a professional assigned to the center or a cross-trained associate, depending on the licensure requirements for performing the activity.

During the design phase, all centralized activities were considered for possible deployment. Activities remaining centralized were examined for possible streamlining and turnaround time improvement. Transferral of activities to care centers created many questions that needed to be addressed: What were the staffing needs of the central department? Could individuals be cross-trained on the remaining functions? Was it feasible that two similar departments consolidate?

As activities and personnel were moved to patient care centers, several departments had large numbers of staff going to training sessions and transferring to a patient care center. As the new associates learned their jobs, the central departments were expected to continue to function as usual during this transition period. During this phase, central departments needed to develop a plan to ensure an effective transition. This plan included using temporary personnel or employees in training to work on the evening shifts. Once the new associates completed their training and had accepted responsibilities for new activities on the patient care centers, the central department workload decreased. When the new workload for the central departments was determined, staffing requirements for the remaining activities were projected. Everyone's job status was affected.

PATIENT CARE CENTERS

To ensure that deployment decisions are economically feasible, there must be enough patients in a center who require the services. Patients with similar needs must be grouped together. Patient groupings can be based on diagnosis, physician services, or general services required. At SMHC, PFC centers were established by diagnosis, which also identified the general services. There are six patient care centers (PCC). The women's and infant's center provides obstetrical and gynecological services including normal and high-risk newborn care. Other inpatient services include the cardiovascular/medicine, surgery/oncology, orthopedic/neurology/rehabilitation, and behavioral medicine PCCs. The ambulatory care PCC provides outpatient services.

Patient groupings increase efficiency by eliminating unnecessary equipment and personnel support. Grouping patients also provides a basis for staffing and establishing care teams. For example, care centers with patients requiring varied respiratory treatments and ventilator use would want a sufficient number of respiratory care practitioners (RCP) in their center. The RCP could be included as part of the care team. In contrast, a center with a minimal need for respiratory care could deploy a cross-trained RCP for all the center's responsibilities.

Staffing roles

Three distinct roles evolved at SMHC during the PFC design process. Clinical associates include professionals involved in patient care as well as technical support services such as EKG technicians, certified nursing assistants, and phlebotomists. Administrative associates are responsible for admissions, medical record deficiency analysis, unit clerk functions, supply maintenance, and receptionist duties. Service associates are responsible for cleaning, transporting patients and specimens, delivering trays, ordering supplies, and basic maintenance. Certain tasks are shared functions and include basic patient care, assisting visitors, answering the phone and call lights, safety, and CPR (see Figure 1). As deployment

FIGURE 1
Sharing responsibility

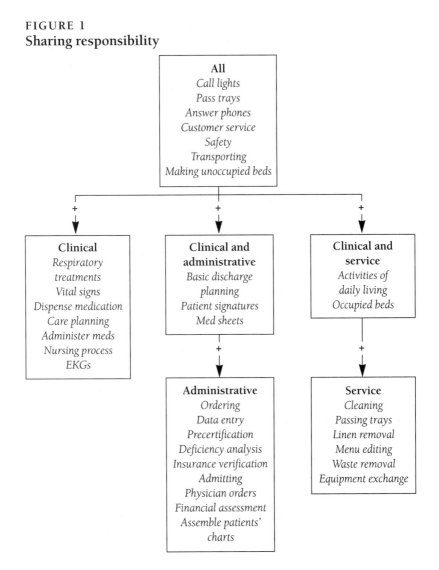

decisions and staffing requirements were decided, so too were shareability issues. These decisions bring in to reality a basic premise of PFC,
never hand off any task you can complete yourself. Never again in a PFC
environment should an employee hear, "that's not my job" in regard to a
shareable task. Not only did associates share tasks but they were cross-
trained within their roles. For example, an RN (a clinical associate) may
be cross-trained to perform EKGs and respiratory treatments, depending
on the deployment decisions and activities in an individual care center.

Some clinical responsibilities require professional licensure and are
strictly regulated by outside agencies such as the Joint Commission on
Accreditation of Health Care Organizations (JCAHO). Therefore, the
clinical associate job description delineated who may perform activities
regulated and limited by licensure. Some of these regulations impacted
the feasibility of some initial deployment decisions. The success of the
cross-training and the shareability aspect of PFC was crucial in achieving the goal of seamless care.

TRAINING RESPONSE

The biggest challenge of PFC was cross-training new associates. The transition to PFC required tremendous change and upheaval for employees.
Removing workers from jobs they have performed competently for years
and putting them into other positions that require them to learn and perform multiple new tasks can seem like an overwhelming expectation.

In a traditional healthcare setting, the training department is typically
the minimal staff needed to accomplish orientations and other employee
programs. Most ongoing education opportunities are available primarily to the professional staff. Restructuring and training multiskilled
workers at SMHC required a shift in focus to include all employees. This
audience presented new challenges to instructors. Many individuals
from ancillary departments had not experienced success in previous academic settings and had low expectations of future success. Staff able to
function in roles with repetitive tasks were required to learn and function at a new skill level. Current employees selected for cross-training
were frequently not as motivated as new employees seeking the same
positions, perhaps because they viewed their new positions as forced
transfers in which they had to give up their existing peer groups.
Employees who had peripheral responsibilities in patient care areas
would work directly with patients, which can be frightening for the

untrained person. All of these challenges could have become obstacles if they were not acknowledged and addressed.

COACH-EDUCATORS AS TRAINERS

It was determined early in the planning process that the existing training department staff was not adequate. A decision was subsequently made to select eight individuals to serve as "coach-educators" to provide the training and to support employees who were selected for the new centers. The coach-educators were selected according to the following requirements:

- Understanding of patient-focused care concept

- Leadership experience

- Functional expertise in several operational areas

- Customer orientation

- Instructional and coaching skills

The group of coach-educators (proclaimed the "energizers") had previously been directors or members of several hospital departments (i.e., respiratory therapy, IV therapy, occupational medicine, central supply, patient transport, social service, admitting, and same-day surgery). The coach-educators were temporary employees of the staff development department.

The first step was to bring the coach-educators through an "empowerment" program to develop tools for effective communication, conflict resolution, coaching, team building, creative problem solving, presentation skills, instructional design, and other skills.

Working with the patient center managers, the coach-educators identified the curriculum for the new associates (see Table 1). Training modules included a core curriculum as well as the primary job duties. Prior to the onset of each training session, it was necessary to customize for each specific center because some of the basic duties are performed differently depending on the clientele (e.g., transferring and transporting an orthopedic patient with a hip or knee replacement is very different when compared to the transferring techniques used in the women's and infant's centers).

The shared element of basic patient care was also designed specifically

TABLE 1
Training modules

Core curriculum for administrative and service associates
Mission, values, and partnership
Patient-focused care overview
Service and administrative role
Dealing with loss and change
Medical terminology/abbreviations
Interpersonal communication skills
Teamwork
Problem solving
Premier customer service
Basic patient care
Safety
Infection control
Transporting patients, equipment, and specimens
Call lights
Military time conversion
Introduction to computers

Administrative associates
Managing the patient's record
Deficiency analysis
Reservations
Precertification
Insurance verification
Registration
Financial assessment
Processing and entering physician's orders
Reception
Office supplies

Service associates
Patient-area cleaning
Patient-center cleaning
Menu editing
Linen management
Materials management
Central services management

for each center. The intent was not to have the new associates assume the role traditionally held by the nursing assistant but to train additional personnel to provide the very basic care that some patients require (e.g., answering call lights, passing out water, and giving a bedpan). In the past, an individual cleaning a patient room was not allowed to provide any type of hands-on care. Yet, this group of individuals, whose jobs require that they spend blocks of time in patient rooms, could provide some basic care. Training was designed to transition new associates to work directly with the patients by teaching them basic care activities. As associates become more comfortable and skilled in their new roles, additional patient care functions may be added to their job duties.

When training associates for basic patient care, there are many additional skills and principles to include. For example, if associates are expected to pass out water and trays and transport patients, they must be able to interpret medical terminology and military time (the 24-hour clock); proper body mechanics is imperative for protection of the patient and the employee involved in transporting; infection control principles and safety are paramount for individuals required to handle blood and body fluids; and confidentiality must be stressed for associates with access to information in medical records. Modules covering these topics were included in the core curriculum.

Concern arose among patients and their families that the person cleaning the room and assisting the patient to the bathroom was now also responsible for serving the patient's meals. These were also examples of activities of daily living that would be required in the home and more than likely would be accomplished by one caretaker. In view of this, it is important to stress infection control principles in the patient's room before and after each care activity.

Service associates, previously assigned from a centralized department, were now expected to contribute and communicate as team members. In response to this need, team building, problem solving, and communication skills were included in the curriculum to prepare the associate for their team involvement.

Considering the instructors' past experience and area of expertise, coach-educators were assigned specific materials to develop. While most of the instructors were able to work within their area of expertise, several had to learn new information. For example, a trainer with extensive experience in social work designed the module on medical record deficiency analysis. However, coach-educators who were assigned modules where they had no past experience actually were able to address the work in new ways. Since old ideas were not entrenched, they explored new ideas and techniques.

The training modules were developed over a two-month period. Coach-educators spent time observing the work process in a number of central departments such as medical records, admitting, and dietary to develop their skills and knowledge. They were assisted in designing materials by the staff in these departments. Periodic meetings were held with center administrators and managers to keep them abreast of training issues.

Materials were evaluated for literacy requirements. Fortunately, SMHC had a workplace skills program in place to assist in the evaluation. Step-by-step instructions were developed for each task. A proficiency checklist (see Figure 2) was developed for each skill, allowing for evaluation of the associate during on-the-job training and providing the manager with tools for future evaluation. Coach-educators were mentored and coached throughout the design process by members of the staff development department.

Staff development and functional experts evaluated the presentation skills of the coach-educators during several practice sessions. These sessions provided opportunity for the energizers to cross-train. It was expected that the coach-educators would develop several areas of expertise to facilitate supervision of the new associates during on-the-job training. Decisions were made regarding resources (e.g., audio-visual equipment, computers, and classrooms) and support (functional experts) required for training. The length of the classes and the degree of overlap between sessions was finalized.

Supplemental teaching tools and audiovisuals were designed—flash cards for medical terminology and military time were provided for self-study with peers. A video was filmed for use in the medical emergency class. Sample charts and physician order sheets were compiled for the administrative associates. Numerous slides and overheads were produced. Several practice labs were set up for inventories and dietary activities. Mock patient rooms were available for practice cleaning, patient transfers, and patient positioning. A computer lab was set up with the actual program utilized for admissions, billings, and physician orders. In teaching new skills, it is important to allow practice with the actual materials and equipment. This valuable practice time allows for a smooth transfer of learning from classroom to actual clinical activities.

In addition to the tools, a self-assessment of the employees' current skills, strengths, and weaknesses was compiled. The assessment, which would be completed the first day of training, emphasized the students' competencies and allowed for customization of training for each group (see Figure 3). An evaluation tool was developed. Daily evaluations of

FIGURE 2

Administrative competency inventory reservations

Associate name _____

At the completion of training and orientation, the associate will perform the following:

	Meets standard	Does not meet	Comments
1. Obtain necessary patient demographics, diagnosis, and other physician requests to initiate the reservations process			
2. Access master patient index (MPI) to obtain correct patient and medical record number for patients having prior admits			
3. Assess special patient needs such as hearing impaired with need for special hearing device for patient telephone			
4. Assess with admitting internist, the need or desire for placement in a teaching or nonteaching bed			
5. Discern need to refer to case management for appropriateness of admission type (inpatient or outpatient observation system)			
6. Obtain admission orders from physician's office and enter into the computer			
7. Initiate precertification with physician's office and follow up to ensure patient's admission has been approved by the insurance company			
8. Select and enter appropriate admitting, referring, and primary care MD			
9. Enter appropriate outpatient observation system identifiers			
10. Enter data correctly into computer to facilitate preadmission or admission process when patient arrives at the health center			
11. Assign bed and room in accordance with patient and physician needs and request			

Comments:

Signature _____ Date: _____
                    Manager

Signature _____ Date: _____
                    Associate

presentations provided valuable feedback for updating and modifying training materials.

The training for all associates was scheduled for eight weeks: a four-week classroom session and four weeks of on-the-job training. Two coach-educators were designated to coordinate each eight-week session. All associates from a center were assigned to the same training session. Having associates from one center together facilitated the presentation of the customized materials and provided opportunities for associates to become acquainted with their new coworkers. When one group completed the four-week didactic portion and moved on to on-the-job training, a second group began classroom sessions. Coach-educators were responsible for inviting the new associates to training and informing them of the time and place.

FIGURE 3
Service associate skills check

Name: _____   Date: _____

This form is to be completed on the first day of your training classes. This information will allow the instructors to see and record the areas that you already have been trained in and can perform. Please check in the appropriate column below:

	Past work experience		
	Have never done	*Have basic experience*	*Have average experience*
Minor maintenance			
Giving/taking bedpans and/or urinals			
Operating a bed			
Changing light bulbs (fluorescent)			
Transporting patients			
Transporting specimens			
Housekeeping			
Ordering supplies from central service			
Menu editing			
Passing and collecting trays			
Call lights			
CPR			

Please list any additional personal skills: _____

_____

Your greatest strength: _____
Your greatest weakness: _____

During the time the training was being developed, a team from the staff development department began a program to prepare the clinical associates on the patient care centers to receive the new employees. Even though numerous information sessions had been conducted and written information had been disseminated, many individuals still were unprepared for the transition. A four-hour "receivership" program was mandatory for all clinical associates. Employees were scheduled to attend prior to the deployment of their patient care center. The program was presented several times each week over a five-month period. Content consisted of an overview of PFC (including the design and implementation), a review of job descriptions for the new associates, and the shareability aspect. Patient center administrators and the PFC coordinator participated in these sessions and addressed questions and concerns. The curriculum and time

	Training		Comments
Have a lot of experience	*No training*	*Past training*	

frame for the training sessions were outlined. The medical emergency curriculum and video were shared with the participants so they would be aware of what the new associates were being taught. For many, the receivership program served as a confirmation that PFC redesign was really going to happen.

ISSUES

As the training process unfolded, it became evident that like all valuable training initiatives, the PFC effort at SMHC would have to address a number of issues to sustain momentum and strongly support a successful change effort. Some of these issues were anticipated, some were not. The issues that surfaced include

- *The lack of a reference point for the new roles of service and administrative associate.* These were new positions with new work teams that had manager-leaders who were themselves unfamiliar with the PFC design. These jobs simply did not exist previously and it took time for all affected parties to understand their new roles and how all of these jobs complement each other. The manager-leaders were themselves on a learning curve that restricted their abilities to provide direction for their new associates. A positive outcome of this uncertainty, however, was the willingness to improve and fine-tune in terms of staffing and training. There was also a begrudging acceptance that there would be no quick fix for some daily operational issues (e.g., problems in transporting patients in a more timely manner and failure to share certain tasks) and that many issues would have to be resolved and integrated over time. It was difficult to maintain vision and focus at these times because problems kept appearing. When problems arose, the training response was deliberate and focused on correcting problems in performing the tasks

- *A tendency to blame any and all problems, incidents, and concerns on the new way of delivering patient care.* It became common to associate any lapses in delivery of services (e.g., the development of a hematoma from a phlebotomy or the failure to promptly answer a call light) on PFC, when a review of quality assurance reports would verify that such problems had already existed

- *An attitude among the staff that redesign was simply a phase that would eventually pass.* Numerous employees were quick to assure their peers that SMHC had undergone major changes in the past and that the best response was to simply wait it out. This was evident in the refusal of some employees to apply for positions in the new patient care centers; it was necessary to convince some of the employees that their current jobs were being eliminated and they definitely needed to apply for new positions. However, behind this resistance were legitimate concerns. Job security was the biggest concern. While guarantees were not made, SMHC was able to reduce the number of jobs through attrition, early retirements, and internal hiring. Another concern involved the level of training that would be available to learn the new skills required. Training has been one of the largest expenses in the PFC process. SMHC has allowed some employees two opportunities to complete the classroom and on-the-job training, and additional coaching-tutoring has been offered when appropriate. Ten employees were unsuccessful in the training process and were offered centralized positions or opted to leave the organization

- *The complexity of the new tasks for new associates.* In addition to being expected to perform a wide range of duties, some employees found it difficult to prioritize tasks, work without direction, and perform problem-solving steps. To address these issues, SMHC participated in a grant from the U.S. Department of Education to deliver workplace skills assessment and training for employees who were struggling to learn. Also, the coach-educators were directed to assist the employees as concretely as possible with their problems in learning the new tasks. Finally, the steering team agreed to provide temporary support staff (e.g., housekeeping, patient transport, and admitting) to help lessen the inefficiencies experienced as people learned new skills. Their commitment to temporary staff has been more extensive and costly than anticipated; it has simply been necessary to buy time to allow the training demands to be met

- *Connecting the training effort to the observations of the leadership teams of each center.* It was critical for the training staff to be promptly notified of performance shortfalls. Requests for training from the staff development department increased by 10 percent in each of the first three quarters of the implementation time frame. These requests ranged from medical terminology and telephone courtesy to stress management and managing change, with the training response usually following within two days of the initial request. Finally, it was important that leader-managers and the training staff work closely to distinguish training issues from employee accountability issues

Lessons learned

As patient-focused care progressed, many lessons were learned. The restructuring challenged SMHC to become a learning organization. Some of these lessons were anticipated, while others arose unexpectedly.

Lesson 1: In undertaking a project of this magnitude, do not underestimate the training function. The administration must recognize the substantial amount of time and money that must be committed for a successful training program. The training staff must consist of educators with various areas of expertise (e.g., patient care, admitting, and medical records). Those charged with leading the training function must be flexible, receptive to feedback, and committed to success.

Lesson 2: Training is never complete. Strive to develop a workforce that is more versatile. It will be even more important to provide ongoing education (i.e., new skills and technology and annual validation of skills) for all the staff. In the near future, healthcare facilities such as SMHC will be asked by accrediting bodies, such as JCAHO, to standardize both continuous quality control and PFC training. Employee recruitment, orientation, and continuing education will need to respond to these trends.

Lesson 3 : Do not attempt to teach everything at once. SMHC delayed the training of a new information system to allow breathing room for the administrative associates who were already learning a multitude of new tasks. It is not advisable to force too much on a group faced with such intense learning.

Lesson 4: Customize as much of the training as is possible. The self-assessment of skills, experiences, limitations, and strengths were conducted and utilized in customizing training. Frequent juggling of classroom and on-the-job training was required.

Lesson 5: Despite all the best efforts, restructuring will not happen overnight. Employees often assume that redesign means that previous work has been inadequate. Also, the changes in the work processes seem overwhelming. There is a tremendous difference between discussing concepts in a classroom and putting the concepts to work on a PCC.

Thus, the training function must be in concert with strong leadership from upper management and an organizational willingness to take risks in the cause of delivering exemplary patient care.

As the PCCs evolve into autonomous teams providing seamless care, so too will multiskilled workers. Assessing educational needs and developing appropriate training will be an ongoing process. Maintaining skills, remaining current with technology, and competency assessment are areas that must be continually addressed. Organizational restructuring and training of the multiskilled worker will continue to provide numerous opportunities and challenges for the training department.

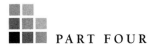

PART FOUR

Information systems and
information technology

38

Restructuring organizations through IS/IT innovation

O. John Kralovec
Vice President
First Consulting Group
Mt. Laurel, New Jersey

T HE FUNDAMENTAL PREMISE of reengineering is that significant advances in information systems and information technology (IS/IT) enable radically new organizational structures. New approaches to organization redesign and restructuring are now possible because IS/IT innovations allow new and different ways to communicate, coordinate, and conduct business. Traditional managerial hierarchies can be dismantled by new technologies. The result is that activities are centralized and decentralized to support innovative use of multiskilled, multitasking employees and work teams. The relationship between IS/IT and reengineering is the driving factor in the j"new industrial revolution." This chapter explores the IS/IT/reengineering relationship and provides a representative case study.

Reengineering is a widely discussed and frequently deployed management concept, both in organizations competing for industry dominance and in those struggling for survival. Many healthcare executives believe that reengineering enables almost every aspect of the organization to be restructured, resulting in better service and reduced costs. Increasingly, organizations committed to long-term success have initiated or considered some type of reengineering effort. These organizations recognize that it is no longer business as usual.

Despite the rapidly growing interest in reengineering concepts and intensified reengineering implementation activities, fundamental misconceptions still persist. Consequently, many organizations will be surprised to learn that significant reengineering investments may result in unmet expectations, limited success, or disappointing outcomes.

To avoid any disappointment, it is important to address the most common misperceptions about reengineering. For many organizations, the essential role of IS/IT often goes unrecognized in reengineering. But once decision makers fully understand key issues, progress toward reengineering success can be made.

Reengineering is unequivocally IS/IT-based. An organization cannot reengineer without understanding that a successful effort is focused from the start on IS/IT's role. Reengineering the delivery of healthcare to move from independent provider-based, fee-for-service medicine to integrated delivery networks (IDNs) under capitation is possible only through advanced technologies. Community health information networks (CHINs) work because they leverage the capabilities of network technology to support IDNs. New database and client-server architectures provide the tools for clinical analysis, utilization review, and outcomes tracking—all essential to successful capitation. IS/IT support is integral to new delivery models.

The power of technology and leverage gained through the deployment of IS/IT during a reengineering initiative is even more obvious when reviewing operational improvements that do not take advantage of IS/IT. Traditional operations improvement efforts using management engineering tools and techniques, as well as TQM/CQI, show that some improvement in operation methods, work flows, task distribution, and organization structure is possible without a significant IS/IT component. But many organizations are disappointed with the incremental improvements achieved by these approaches.

Real change in healthcare delivery systems requires more than incremental improvements. Organization approaches that worked from 1970 to 1980 do not work today. Old models built around control mechanisms need to be restructured to provide flexibility, and those built around a predictable business climate must be adapted to respond effectively to the unprecedented pace of change. Traditional healthcare organization models must be redesigned to respond to ongoing pressures to reduce costs, improve cycle time, and sustain and enhance quality. Rethinking this process requires examining how IS/IT is used and realizing that IS/IT is a key strategic enabler.

The new business environment is driving new forms of work organization, often enabled by technology-supported reengineering. Such future organization structures include

- *Networked organizations.* Independent operating clusters coordinated through IS/IT links

- *Widespread participation.* Greater employee involvement at all levels through open access to information

- *Self-management.* Less supervisory and management intervention as a result of IS/IT-supported feedback on-line, real time

- *Cross-functional teams.* Using IS/IT to link work activities that cross traditional departmental boundaries

Each of these forms structural components of evolving organizations. These evolving organizations require a number of new elements, including information handling, communication flows, organizational interdependencies, reporting relationships (both formal and informal), and IS/IT structures to support them.

New organization structures will push managers to deploy technology in innovative ways. As technology progresses, continued advances in evolving organization structures will be possible, which, in turn, will expand the limits of existing technology. Organization structure and information systems are then inextricably linked.

Strategic perspective

From a reengineering perspective, customer requirements and expectations drive business strategy. This strategy frames issues to be addressed by organization structure and design. IS/IT then provides the infrastructure to support the model required to achieve primary strategic initiatives. Properly developing and defining strategic issues before creating new organization models and determining IS/IT needs is essential.

A number of management tools have improved understanding of key relationships and critical links in the reengineering process. These tools include the external business model, strategic process model, case for action, and IS/IT profile. The following description provides an overview of these key elements.

EXTERNAL BUSINESS MODEL

The external business model presents the business's key customers, partners, and stakeholders in graphs (see Figure 1). Drawing on information from executive interviews, customer requirement documentation, and the strategic plan, the model highlights essential issues, concerns, expectations, and requirements. This picture sets the stage to confirm strategic priorities, assess the degree of alignment within the executive team, and provide the proper context for the reengineering effort. While the model does not typically reveal any surprising or unexpected information, it has proven valuable to assist organizations to maintain focus and direction.

STRATEGIC PROCESS MODEL

The strategic process model partitions the organization into core business processes, usually seven to nine. This model shifts organizational focus away from departments and functions onto broad, integrated operational activities. These functions are then mapped back to the external business model to determine if and how well they support the strategic objectives. The reengineering team evaluates current strengths, weaknesses, and significant operational characteristics to determine high-priority areas, specific reengineering opportunities, and potential benefits. As a result, the business makes all reengineering decisions in the context of its strategic imperatives aligning the needs of its primary customers.

FIGURE 1
External business model

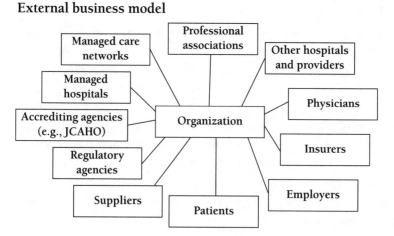

CASE FOR ACTION

The case for action is a concise, unambiguous statement of the compelling reasons for undertaking a reengineering effort. The cases present strategic factors driving the need for reengineering, such as shifting competitive pressures, eroding market share, changing customer expectations or demands, and increasing costs for providing services. Impacts of these factors are presented in ways all employees can understand. Resistance to change is frequently the greatest obstacle organizations must overcome, so the case must identify the issues and their impact in a way that will provide motivation for change.

IS/IT BASELINE

As the key strategic issues are confirmed, core processes evaluated, and the case for action developed, current IS/IT capabilities must be addressed, including these key questions:

- What IS/IT support is needed to achieve the strategic objectives?

- What IS/IT support is needed to enable new organization structures and operating models?

- Will current systems allow the organization to do what is needed to effect change?

- What financial resources are needed to develop the IS/IT infrastructure?

- Will the organization be able to move quickly enough?

Redesigned plans developed in isolation from technological realities will create tremendous frustration and duplication of effort.

Technology and new organization models

Once the strategic impact issues and focus have been addressed, attention can then be directed to redesign and restructuring activities. The term "organizational architecture" describes the structure within which an organization operates and the context in which reengineering and organization change occur. Continuing with this architectural analogy, just as steel girders and reinforced concrete enabled new building techniques, evolving information infrastructure capabilities allow very different organization models. IS/IT becomes the new structural material supporting the organization's architecture. The future organization's foundation is information, and information is the defining element in new organization models.

With IS/IT as a fundamental building block, new business models require new process configurations that depend on the availability and flow of information. Reengineering not only provides the tools and techniques to think "out-of-the-box," it also positions the organization to exploit new and existing information and communication technologies.

IS/IT is supporting organization structures that were impossible just a few years ago. IS/IT-enabled networks, joint ventures, and other alliances are being managed using advanced communications and network technologies. For example, providers are now electronically linked with vendors to improve purchasing processes, control inventory costs, and ensure supply or equipment availability. Multiple organizations functioning within emerging IDNs are able to access critical financial and clinical information on-line, real time. This IS/IT-enabled information sharing on-line, real time among providers, managed care organizations, employers, and payers is breaking down traditional geographic and organizational barriers at an unprecedented rate and degree. The blurring of organizational barriers now allows executive teams from multiple organizations to work together remotely as a "virtual corporation."

In operations, IS/IT advances enable very different models as well. Advances in database design, client/server architecture, graphical user interfaces, and data storage devices allow organizations to realize new structures with flat hierarchies, self-directed and self-managed work teams, and networked organization units. Technology-supported collaboration (i.e., using IS/IT to coordinate and support the work of multiple individuals and groups) and hybrid process design (i.e., new organization structures replacing old departmental models) increasingly characterize the new organization.

Through IS/IT it is now possible to integrate tasks in very different ways. For example

- Many organizations are now using IS/IT to restructure and combine scheduling, admitting registration, financial counseling, and clinical screening into a new function—arrange care. Arrange care integrates multiple activities previously performed independently by several different and uncoordinated departments

FIGURE 2
Process-focused organization

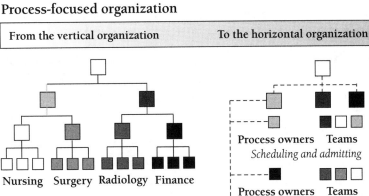

New models for patient care delivery decentralize "hotel service" activities to nursing units or care centers using distributed IS/IT capabilities. These activities include purchasing, receiving, inventory control, material supply logistics, preventive maintenance, and routine engineering activities

- Sophisticated clinical databases (i.e., data repositories) and widespread access to clinical data through IS/IT networks allow measurement tasks associated with managed care. This includes on-line, real-time case management and concurrent review, which helps providers avoid delays that may increase length of stay. Case management and concurrent review can reduce overutilization and improve medical practice

ENABLING NEW ORGANIZATION MODELS

To successfully implement a reengineering process, there are five primary project phases. These include

1. Evaluate current processes and determine current performance capabilities and future performance requirements—starting with a documentation of current performance metrics (e.g., process flows, response time, quality attributes, service levels, costs, and functional

interdependencies) and preliminary targets for performance enhancements (e.g., response time reduced by 50 percent, quality indices improved by 30 percent, costs reduced by 20 percent)

2. Develop a new vision of the ideal process starting with a clean sheet of paper. If we were going to start over today and design the perfect process, without past constraints or limitations, what would it look like?

3. Challenge the rules and assumptions to determine how things are done and determine new rules to support the new vision. Does it add value, do we need to do in the same way, how would we do it differently in the ideal process?

4. Apply reengineering principles to test and ensure the new design incorporates the most effective trends in work restructuring such as parallel processing of activities, new approaches to centralizing or decentralizing tasks, cross-trained, multiskilled individuals, and technology-enhanced work activities. These principles all represent trends that should be closely evaluated to finalize new process designs

5. Identify the primary technology enablers required to support the new process design, such as current information-based and technology-dependent process activities, innovative and creative technology uses, and technology-related process scenarios and implications

Because the IS/IT component is critical to successful reengineering efforts, the tasks in phase five create the need for additional activities for information systems managers.

- Evaluate information-based process activities to determine the IS/IT implications of

  1. *Data capturing.* Where are data captured and who inputs data into the system?

  2. *Data processing.* What are the key decision-making activities and who makes the decisions?

  3. *Data storage.* Where are data stored and what information is key?

  4. *Data movement.* How are data transmitted?

5. *Data presentation.* What is the ultimate purpose of the information? What is the value-added component?

- Examine each new organization model and process thoroughly to determine if the current IS/IT capabilities can effectively support the new process design or if additional IS/IT capabilities are required

- Determine positive and negative implications of new process and component scenarios

- Identify new technology benefits and uses

- Determine IS/IT requirements and document preliminary technological recommendations

- Prepare IS/IT cost/benefit analysis and assess the overall impact of technology acquisition against the IS/IT strategic plan

- Determine any potential drawbacks to implement new IS/IT enablers to support redesigned processes and address any unanswered issues, such as the value of potential change

The role of IS/IT in reengineering is not limited to current or prospective needs. IS/IT are fundamental components of a reengineering effort, and act as primary enablers of process redesign. Information systems managers support the redesign process by helping to evaluate the potential impact of new technology, to assess the impact of current technology, and to illuminate future technology requirements for supporting the redesigned activities. If information systems managers successfully assess the technology component of the reengineering effort, numerous business processes may be redefined.

ROLE OF IS/IT PROFESSIONALS

Because of the diverse functions of IS/IT, the information systems departments can play two distinct roles within the reengineering process: directing and supporting.

IT directing reengineering

In some organizations, IT executives and managers are called to direct organizationwide reengineering efforts, assuming the responsibilities of a reengineering czar. However, the organization's chief executive needs to be viewed as the primary sponsor of the reengineering effort, sending a strong message of the importance of the initiative and commitment at the top. The senior executive becomes responsible for overall planning, coordinating, managing, and evaluating the initiative. In this role, the IT executive chairs a reengineering steering committee and ensures the appropriate topics and issues are addressed in a timely and thorough manner.

IT supporting reengineering

Even if not involved in direct responsibility for overseeing an enterprise-wide effort, IT executives and managers will support a reengineering effort as facilitator, team leader, or member. The following highlights the responsibilities in each of the three roles.

Team facilitator. The team facilitator is responsible for coaching and teaching the team reengineering techniques. The facilitator ensures that all team members have an opportunity to contribute, the team charter and ground rules are followed, and the interpersonal dynamics of the team are positive and productive. The facilitator works with the team leader to evaluate the effectiveness of each team session, identify areas where meetings can be more productive, ensure the team is progressing adequately, and assist in preparation for the next meeting. The facilitator also shares responsibility for helping the team leader develop group process facilitation, conflict resolution, and consensus-building skills and to increase the leader's ability to work effectively with the team. The facilitator often plays a staff role (not part of the organization unit being redesigned) and generally will facilitate multiple teams over time.

Team leader. The team leader is accountable for enabling the team to complete its project. The team leader, typically part of the organization being redesigned, chairs team meetings, serves as the primary liaison with the reengineering steering committee, guides the team through the reengineering activities, and ensures that team activities are coordinated with organization priorities. A successful team leader has strong inter-personal skills, can work effectively with a team, demonstrates good analytical ability, has sound judgment, and can think out of the box. The team leader must have no conflict that would disrupt the team and must work in an open, participative, and congenial manner. The team leaders and facilitator must be able to work closely together throughout the reengineering effort.

Team member. Members participate in the reengineering process by assessing current operations, determining areas for improvement, and developing a new vision of what the process should look like. They challenge existing rules and assumptions about how the process works, apply redesign principles in developing new models, and determine the IS/IT enablers to support the new process design. Team members must be able to think out of the box, be comfortable with making change, and willing to make recommendations that may upset the status quo. Team members must be comfortable working in a group setting to reach consensus on new operational models, and they must be willing to express their ideas and opinions openly. They typically represent different disciplines, departments, sections, or stages of the process that is being reengineered.

IT executives and managers are the single most important technical resource to ensure all technology-related issues are adequately and thoroughly addressed. Moreover, they help identify appropriate technology requirements and integrate current and future IS/IT plans. The IT manager's role is to identify practical and realistic solutions for achieving new business concepts and work processes, potential constraints of existing technology, and budget and capital expenditure issues. The latter includes costs to enhance or upgrade current systems, acquire new systems, or build new IS/IT capabilities.

One of the major challenges for IT professionals engaged in reengineering is to find creative ways to leverage existing technology to support the restructured process. Existing IT platforms and architecture generally will not be adequate and budget constraints will be encountered. Innovative ways to use existing technology, protect previous technology investments to the extent possible, and propose cost-effective solutions are essential.

IT AND IMPLEMENTATION

Once IS/IT issues are identified and discussed, an implementation plan must be drafted to refine the reengineering transition. The implementation plan should address all aspects of the transition to ensure that all organizational initiatives are carefully integrated into the reengineering effort and that potential roadblocks can be addressed. Specific steps to do this are as follows:

Step one: Formulating a transition strategy

A transition strategy should be formulated in several steps to identify who will be affected and how (e.g., which jobs will change, how staffing patterns will be altered, differences in information flow, and new technology enablers). A pilot implementation project should also be designed to respond to any unforeseen variables and obstacles including modified operational activities that need further improvement, unanticipated areas of resistance, and limitations of existing infrastructure to support changes (e.g., testing recommended staffing models, testing entry and retrieval of data on new information systems, and evaluating support for new reporting relationships). Education and training programs should be developed to augment the strategy and to orient those involved about the direction and focus of the redesign process (e.g., clearly specifying new tasks, summarizing changes in the scope and sequence of activities, communicating new reporting relationships, and providing orientation to new technologies). A detailed tactical implementation plan can then be laid out and applied.

Step two: Implementing the new process

The implementation plan should be phased in, starting with high-benefit areas—areas demonstrating potential for service improvement, cost reduction, or quality enhancement. Successful pilots should be used as models for future implementation activities. In some cases, implementation will focus initially on benefits that are quickly and easily achieved (e.g., consolidating similar activities or eliminating unnecessary tasks that will improve service levels or reduce costs quickly through improved staff utilization) in order to demonstrate success, build commitment, and provide a mechanism for early payback. In other cases, focus may be placed on areas with high benefit potential that may not produce immediate payback but may position the organization to realize major long-term gains in reducing costs, improving cycle time, and enhancing service levels (e.g., redesigning a service delivery process that does not result in reduced staff or lower operating costs but that does improve customer satisfaction in ways that will eventually improve market share and enhance competitive positioning).

Step three: Implementing supporting infrastructure

Supporting activities and management structures are key components to a successful implementation project. When organization structures are changed and jobs redesigned, the supporting infrastructure must also be addressed. Physical space and layout may be affected as employees are moved or clustered into new areas. Computers, work stations, telephone systems, and facsimile machines may need to be reconfigured. Reengineered processes must be fully supported with appropriate infrastructure.

Step four: Continually evaluating the effectiveness of the redesigned process

Regardless of the reengineering team's performance, improvements to new operational models will be necessary. Day-to-day work activities must be fine-tuned and the basic premises of continuous improvement applies at this stage. As organizational and operational changes are made, progress needs to be monitored carefully and action taken to enhance or refine methods and procedures taken promptly.

Step five: Realizing the initial benefits

The benefits achieved by the new design should be monitored and measured against preliminary benefit estimates. The achievement of benefits must be carefully managed or the desired result will not be achieved. The organization will need to clearly specify the methods to monitor and analyze the impact of the new process and the resulting decreases in costs, improvements in cycle time, or enhancements in service levels (e.g., automated tracking of improvement in wait times, measuring customer satisfaction levels through questionnaires or focus groups, documenting payroll reductions, and calculation of operating expense reductions). An established plan should be developed to address, manage, and evaluate the realization of tangible, quantifiable benefits.

Conclusion

The reengineering process forces all employees to examine the work process as a whole, rather than from individual departmental perspectives. The main goals and functions of the institution become the focus instead of specific areas or divisions. Thus, work activities are streamlined, conflicts more easily resolved, and the outcome or result takes priority over the activities currently being performed.

Therefore, the IS/IT department's role is critical. Because profit margins are shrinking, IS/IT must demonstrate its tangible value. Increasing pressure will be placed on IS/IT professionals to link and align technology with business strategies and objectives. Technology will be challenged to solve and satisfy business problems and requirements rather than technological problems and requirements.

Information technology and systems provide guidance, direction, and support for reengineering at all stages from analysis through implementation. The role of information technology in reengineering is vital and multifaceted. Since information systems enable specific reengineered processes, the IS/IT function itself can realize a new and more important role as information technology capabilities increase, new technologies emerge, and enhanced IS/IT resources are better able to support new process designs.

Businesses undergoing a reengineering effort must be aware of the diverse avenues available through employing technology. Network technology, client-server capabilities, database architectures, and applications software are becoming essential components of successful process reengineering. By fully using appropriate resources an enterprise can reorganize for long-term competitiveness.

Case study

The following highlights the high-level IS/IT recommendations from a team chartered to reengineer clinical and diagnostic services for a 450-bed medical center that had previously redesigned patient care delivery processes. The clinical and diagnostic service team, with representatives from laboratory, radiology, pharmacy, and other clinical and diagnostic areas, focused on two objectives: improving clinical and diagnostic support for the newly redesigned patient care areas and developing a new approach to addressing increasing ambulatory and outpatient activities.

Using the approach presented in this chapter, the team developed a vision of the new clinical and diagnostic processes, documented the rules and assumptions guiding the new processes, and tested the emerging process modes against proven work restructuring principles. The new process models developed by the team replaced the old department structures with clinical and diagnostic clusters to address specific patient needs (e.g., a cluster for women's services, a "fast track" lab/EKG cluster for high-volume outpatient procedures, as well as core lab-radiology-EKG cluster to support inpatient patient centers and more complex outpatient procedures). At this stage, the team identified the key technology enablers required to support the new process design. Several technology enablers for the new organization and operational models emerged as key elements of the redesigned processes:

- Clinical/diagnostic areas are to be linked to all medical center area terminals and printers through the medical center's wide area network (WAN), providing access to all pertinent clinical, operational, and financial data enterprisewide. Automated scanners are used to facilitate patient processing. Voice data collection devices and media digitizers will be used to support key clinical activities. These areas have on-line, real-time access to scheduling, medical records, billing, and patient-tracking information as well as report generator capabilities

- In addition to the requirements for physician offices, clinical diagnostic areas, and inpatient centers/satellites, the following IS/IT capabilities were identified by the team:

  Report generator: The report generator receives downloaded information from the clinical/diagnostic systems (including lab, radiology, and pharmacy systems). The system has capability for digitized media, digitized voice, and electronic signatures and compiles information into a uniform report structure and includes performance tracking and work-in-progress tracking

  Performance tracking: This system receives and tracks all performance statistics and quality indicators for use in assessing production parameters and system compliance. The system will automatically flag any activity or indicator where statistical abnormalities are occurring

Computerized patient record: This system will eventually contain all patient medical data in a uniform, retrievable, intelligent format. Outpatient records will be stored on a short-term bulletin board (for report access), then transferred to long-term storage

"ICE" scheduling system: Information captured through the centralized information capture and encounter (ICE) expert scheduling system will be used for scheduling, registration, billing, and patient record purposes

Billing/financial: The system generates professional and technical charges with electronic transfer to third parties. Additionally, payments will be electronically transferred from the medical center to the institution's bank

"Greeter" self-registration: Terminals at patient entrances will be used to confirm patient arrivals and to register patients that have not been "ICEed" at the physician's office

Resource inventory: This system calculates and tracks the resource consumption (e.g., supplies, personnel, equipment utilization) for the entire medical center and projects future demand based on the scheduled activities

Critical pathways database: This system maintains current and historic definitions of the critical paths and allows charting by exception. The system automatically flags any critical path where exception reporting frequency exceeds an acceptable threshold

Inventory and purchasing: This system maintains the inventory levels of all supplies within the medical center and automatically reorders, through electronic data interchange, when inventory restocking points are reached, or when levels are projected to reach that level through the resource inventory system

Preventive maintenance/scheduling: The preventive maintenance (PM) system tracks all maintainable equipment and other service technician performed work (e.g., housekeeping) and generates weekly work lists. The system also tracks any repairs to determine if PM activity should be included on the PM schedule due to the frequency of the repairs

- All inpatient centers, clinical and diagnostic clusters, and satellite provider sites will have PCs and printers connected to the WAN, ensuring enterprisewide access to all pertinent clinical, operational, and financial data. Users will have access to scheduling, medical records, billing, patient tracking, and other bulletin board functions

- Physician offices are connected to the medical center's WAN with access to all internal systems controlled by office passwords. With this accessibility, the physician's office becomes an extension of the medical center with information collected and transmitted in both directions. The system provides flexibility to add or delete components for each office through password controls. Each office has a terminal and printer connected to the WAN (solid connection or modem) that provides access to scheduling, medical records, billing, and other bulletin board functions

39

Conducting an IT reengineering project

Joseph M. DeLuca, FACHE
Founder and President

Rebecca Enmark Cagan, MLIS
Research Associate

Gemma Mata Tayao
Manager Associate
JDA
San Francisco, California

OVER THE PAST DECADE, advances in information technology (IT) have given healthcare providers tools to adapt to the changing medical, business, and regulatory environments. Through developing a rapid and flexible IT capability, provider organizations are able to support operational activity as well as long-term access to data and information. IT can be used operationally and strategically as a

- Cost-reducing measure

- Productivity enhancer

- Data collection and analysis tool, enabling cost/quality comparisons

- Vehicle to support fundamental and extreme organizational change activities (reengineering)

As a vehicle for reengineering, IT raises complex business and technological implications. Almost universally accepted as an enabling tool in reengineering projects, IT is often viewed as the driving force allowing fundamental change. At a minimum, reengineered processes must be supported by IT. Support may come from different technologies such as information and data systems (i.e., "traditional" systems such as patient administration or financial); voice and PBX systems (e.g., automated call processing, local or intercampus access); or local, wide, or metropolitan area networks, allowing the distribution and access of data directly at the point of need.

In spite of the strong involvement of technology in reengineering efforts, information systems (IS) departments at many healthcare organizations are not well structured to handle the additional complexities created by reengineering. The implications of reengineering projects on the department are often not systematically reviewed and can result in departmental chaos. Prior to any organization or enterprisewide reengineering effort, reengineering, redesign, and implementation of total quality management or continuous quality improvement initiatives in the IS department should be conducted.

Done effectively, IT reengineering can support the success of other improvement efforts as well as work to reduce costs, increase the effectiveness of all information systems, and improve satisfaction levels of both caregivers and patient populations.

This chapter is designed to educate readers on the forces and principles driving IT reengineering in healthcare and to provide a methodology for conducting an IT reengineering project. Three critical questions will be addressed.

1. How can IT professionals recognize the signs that reengineering is needed, rather than incremental work flow analysis and modification?

2. What are the critical process steps in IT reengineering projects? What questions must be clearly answered in the reengineering process?

3. What are the common failures in reengineering projects, and how can an organization take steps to avoid them?

Driving forces

The forces behind reengineering are numerous and disparate in nature. Changes in the practice and focus of healthcare—patient-focused care, managed care, the shift to ambulatory, rather than inpatient, encounters—have transformed the information needs of practitioners and management. Technology continues to evolve rapidly and fundamental changes in the business world of IT vendors—business failures, acquisitions, mergers, and partnerships—have created a favorable atmosphere for providers looking to maximize their technology return on investment.

Historically, the role of the IS/IT department has been analogous to that of a wheel—important to keeping the car running smoothly, but ultimately replaceable with a little effort. Today, IT goals and corporate objectives are symbiotically intertwined with clinical users and executive strategists. IT and the IS department must incorporate this way of thinking. Rather than a wheel, IT is now the engine that provides power to drive the car where it needs to go.

CHANGING PRACTICE AND FOCUS

The demand for and performance pressure on IT have increased significantly as a result of many factors. They include

- Increasing movement to integrated delivery systems (IDSs)

- Rapidly expanding community health information networks (CHINs)

- Continued market growth of managed care and capitation

- Continued shift to ambulatory services, rather than inpatient care

Provider organizations across the continuum of care are consolidating, regionalizing, and focusing on the management of patient or enrollee populations. As a result of these changes, provider data requirements have shifted from being focused primarily on inpatient care to a more comprehensive set of service offerings.

IDS executives must have information from clinic, home care, skilled nursing, and multiple inpatient settings to evaluate accurately the cost of care in the delivery system. To measure and maintain the quality of care, providers must have access to patient records from throughout the treatment continuum. Patients and enrollees must experience uniform and consistent scheduling, registration, and business office functions.

As with an IDS, a CHIN creates increased demand for information and IT. Unlike an IDS, a CHIN faces the added complexity of linking

TABLE 1
Demand for IT

	Traditional use of IT by single facility or provider group	New use of IT to support multiple groups and facilities (e.g., IDSs, CHINs)
Orientation:	*Departmental*	*Patient centered*
Access requirement:	Extensive for separate and/ or financial application; shallow need for others	Immediate access for knowledge processing
Integration architecture:	Point-to-point interfaces	Interface engines and relational databases
Communications network:	Local, point-to-point	Distributed, intelligent
Implementation:	Departmental	Distributed
User interface:	Menu	Graphical
Processing:	Data	Data, voice, image, text
Benefits:	Productivity improvement	Quality improvement
Perception of IT use:	A necessity	A competitive asset

nonaffiliated providers as well as nontraditional healthcare groups. CHINs are extending the need for central data repositories, accessible by various providers, payers, employers, and researchers.

Table 1 illustrates how the focus of IT for IDs systems and CHINs differs from more traditional models of care delivery.

As managed care and capitation become more prominent, the use of IT to meet information collection and analysis needs will expand as well. The increasingly common use of capitation and risk-sharing arrangements in reimbursement demands greater sophistication in financial analysis tools. The rapid rise in the development and adoption of clinical outcome measures has resulted in many IT vendors incorporating some level of tracking or analysis capability into their systems.

The volume of healthcare services provided in the inpatient hospital setting is shrinking as more and more care delivery assumes an ambulatory focus. What does this shift mean for IT? As ambulatory volumes increase, IT must focus on the capture and dissemination of information to more points of service. Communications and networking technologies thus become critical links in the provision and outcome of care.

Recognizing the signs

Reengineering is not a small undertaking, and not every IT department or facility needs such a fundamental overhaul. There are a number of key indicators that may signal the need for a complete rethinking of IT functions:

- A recent or upcoming major change in business structure (e.g., merger, affiliation, or physician-hospital organization or management service organization formation)

- Recent, ongoing, or upcoming rapid shifts in the local healthcare market (e.g., entrance or exit of a large competing organization, passage of state or local healthcare reform)

- Significant dissatisfaction with IT support

- Proliferation of new IT-driven reengineering projects

Whenever multiple organizations combine—whether through affiliation, merger, or outright acquisition—the timing is right for examining and restructuring more efficient ways of doing business. Key considerations include

1. Types of organizations involved

   - Two similar organizations may combine and find that IT departments now play redundant roles and must be combined as well

   - A hospital acquired by a large chain may need to incorporate its IT function into the corporate culture and administrative practices of the acquirer

   - A health system acquiring a physician practice must incorporate the needs of that practice, particularly if they are not addressed in the current IT structure

2. Similarity of current IT functions

   - If the current IT functions and technology are similar or complementary, only minimal restructuring may be necessary. If, however, the fundamental architecture or approach is different, it may be more effective to reengineer IT development strategy and infrastructure suited to the needs of all organizations involved

Many of the changes occurring in healthcare today require basic shifts in the collection and application of data. Managed care, particularly with its emphasis on at-risk contracting and capitation, requires advanced data analysis capabilities.

Another change in the local market may include the entrance or emergence of a large, well-structured IDS. This competition can drive other healthcare organizations to evaluate their internal structures and processes, as well as their ability to provide quality, low-cost care.

Success in capitation, and effective contract negotiation, requires that clear and accurate pricing, outcome data, and utilization statistics be available to decision makers.

Satisfaction levels with IT support are often difficult to measure quantitatively. Table 2 lists conditions that may support the need for an IT reengineering project.

A large number of reengineering projects occurring throughout the organization may indicate the current IT structures and services are not effectively supporting the needs of the organization. Reengineering IT across the organization may help alleviate or even solve problems identified in other areas.

In either case, any reengineering project must be supported effectively, both during the process and upon completion, by the organization's IT.

Return on investment is a primary management concern when reviewing any proposed plan of action. In proposing an IT reengineering project, the following information will help support the overall worth of the idea, as well as present a solid focus and vision for the overall project.

- Vision of the organization

- Projected time line to achieve this vision

TABLE 2
Indications of organizational or executive dissatisfaction with IT

1. IT is not perceived as a strategic weapon
2. IT is not represented on other reengineering projects
3. The long-range IT plan is not directly tied to the organizational long-range plan, or there may be no long-range IT plan
4. IT staffing and budget levels are not commensurate with other organizations of comparable size, volumes, and service lines
5. There is a large backlog of IT projects
6. There is a proliferation of PCs functioning as stand-alone systems, or departments are maintaining redundant databases or functionality (e.g., multiple patient accounting, patient registration systems)
7. The organization is in financial or regulatory trouble
8. Executives perceive low return on IT investments

- Tangible objectives to measure attainment of this vision

- Assessed needs of the organization

- Effectiveness of current IT to address these needs

- Resource requirements (i.e., time, money) for achieving IT objectives

- Benefits derived from this IT investment, quantified in terms of extended life cycles, better customer service, and better outcomes measurement

Reengineering design

Once the decision has been made to begin a reengineering effort, the steps flow in the sequence depicted in Figure 1. By conducting a series of activities, grouped by these steps, any organization can make a radical change in the way its IT is structured, perceived, or managed.

The following section offers a step-by-step review of this methodology, together with a discussion of important issues to address and resolve. The first three steps to reengineering involve the collection and organization of data about existing and projected capabilities, activities, and services at the provider organization.

FIGURE 1
Process of reengineering IT

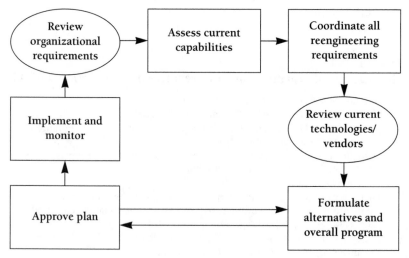

STEP ONE: REVIEW GLOBAL REQUIREMENTS

Once an organization makes a commitment to reengineering, the first step is to examine the organization as a whole. IT can only offer effective support for an organization's needs if those needs have been clearly identified.

Commonly, input and approval are generated from critical user groups and decision makers through a steering committee. Representation on the committee should, at a minimum, include

- Executive management such as the CEO, CFO or other person(s) with final power to approve the project scope, size, and budget

- The chief IT executive at the organization

- Representatives from each major type of IS (i.e., patient accounting, business office, and clinical staff, including laboratory, pharmacy, radiology, medical records). This group should include system users as well as administrators. Depending on the size of the organization and the scope of existing ISs, this group may be large or small

- User and technical liaisons. These members, typically not at the executive level, are often able to inject reality to the process, as well as offer valuable perspective about the situation under discussion

- Representatives from other reengineering projects

This committee may already exist if there are reengineering projects currently under way at the organization.

At this early stage, reviewing the medical service requirements and organizational structure of the healthcare provider, the reengineering project team should particularly examine

- The stated mission of the organization

- The existing business lines, as well as those projected in the organizational long-range plan

- The current service requirements of the organization

- The current "depth" of IS/IT

Table 3 depicts a relatively common business objective, together with some strategies for its achievement.

TABLE 3
Organizational business objective

Business objective	Strategy to achieve objective
Manage the growth of managed care and capitation	Identify and eliminate duplicative, overlapping services
	Migrate toward prevention and wellness of covered population; manage toward a "cost of covered lives" structure
	Analyze population to identify "at-risk" characteristics and strategize to reduce "covered lives" risk
	Measure and evaluate quality and outcomes

STEP TWO: ASSESS CURRENT CAPABILITIES

Once the objectives of the organization are clear (i.e., business and medical service needs), the next step is to conduct a baseline assessment of how the IT structure and services support those objectives.

Key characteristics to examine include

1. *Basic structure of the IT department.* What are the staffing levels and scope of services offered by the department (i.e., is the department confined to IS, or does it hold responsibility for IT-related functions such as telecommunications)? With what budget is the department expected to carry out its responsibilities? Are there multiple IT departments across facilities? What are the opportunities to consolidate and reduce redundant overhead?

2. *Current services offered.* Is the department confined primarily to computer and network support, or are staff involved in other IT-related functions such as telecommunications? Is IT represented on other hospital committees? At what executive level is the top IT staff member—middle or senior management?

3. *Current output and productivity levels*

4. *Customer satisfaction indicators.* How well does IT support organizational staff? Does IT generally improve or decrease patient satisfaction with the healthcare experience?

5. *Current ISs.* How old are the systems? What financial investment is needed to keep them up and running?

TABLE 4
IT support of organizational long-range goals

Business objective	Strategy to achieve objective	Systems implications	Current IT support	IT as critical success factor
Manage the growth of managed care and capitation	Migrate toward prevention and wellness of covered population; manage toward a "cost of covered lives" structure	Flexible reporting databases allow customized clinical program and management analyses	?	Medium
		Independent cost determination and management systems to provide accurate unit cost information and determine contract profitability	?	High
		Systems must be able to provide capability to measure PMPM performance by service and provider	?	High

6. *Current IT environment.* What is the current systems architecture? What is the primary vendor environment—a single vendor supporting organizational needs or many fragmented vendors offering partial solutions?

7. *Current data exchange capabilities*

8. *Benefits the current IT structure provides to the organization*

A key indicator of the value IT provides is how well IT services support organizational long-range goals. Table 4 illustrates the process by which business objectives and strategies translate into IT evaluation and planning.

STEP THREE: COORDINATE ALL REENGINEERING REQUIREMENTS

In reviewing ongoing reengineering efforts, there are numerous questions to consider, including

1. Is each effort striving to support the overall goals and objectives of the organization?

2. Are project initiatives redundant? If several projects are striving to meet common or similar goals, how can they be consolidated to reduce cost or achieve objectives?

3. How might any parallel or ongoing efforts support each other?

4. How might the efforts affect each other? If projects rely on inputs or outputs from areas or people not directly involved in the initiative, will those inputs or outputs remain static?

5. What are the potential economic benefits from each individual effort?

STEP FOUR: REVIEW CURRENT TECHNOLOGIES AND VENDORS

In planning IT reengineering, organizations must evaluate the state of their current technology to determine if the systems and structure in place are truly inadequate or simply utilized incorrectly or inefficiently.

When reviewing the current structure and IS, a number of issues should be considered:

1. Is this organization using one of the most current releases of the software from each vendor? Is the software in use more than two to three years old? Many vendors are issuing new and updated versions several times per year to keep up with the rapidly changing needs of the market

2. How old is the technology (i.e., how many years of use are still available)? How current are the data access and storage mechanisms embedded in the technology?

3. Have staff received adequate training on current systems? Consider the orientation that new hires receive on the system, as well as refresher training provided to current employees. If training is inadequate, the capabilities of application software may be underutilized

4. How much coordination occurs between systems? Commonly used data, particularly administrative patient information, is often collected at multiple points of care. Using interfaces, or feeder mechanisms, to pass such data between and across systems impacts convenience for staff and patients, as well as the accuracy of the information

5. What types of development projects are vendors involved in, outside of the organization? How might that work be leveraged to assist ongoing reengineering efforts?

STEP FIVE: FORMULATE ALTERNATIVES
AND OVERALL PROGRAM

After completing steps one through three, the focus of reengineering turns to formulating a plan—specific to the organization—with input from all participants important to the success of the effort. At a minimum, the plan should contain the project's mission, scope and objectives, resources required for implementation, projected budgets, projected time lines, and evaluation mechanisms (i.e., specifics as to how the project will be judged a success or failure).

Steps five and six (detailed below) form an iterative loop. Upon completion of step six, a viable plan with buy-in from all important participants should be ready for implementation.

STEP SIX: APPROVE PLAN

Approval of the final reengineering plan draws participation and review from a wide variety of organization members and leaders. End-users as well as departmental and organizational leadership should ultimately affirm overall goals and objectives as well as operational requirements.

Rapid advances in technology and ongoing price fluctuations in the market make long-term budget projections uncertain. Throughout planning review and approval cycles, this uncertainty should be taken into consideration. A typical reengineering plan may contain approved versions of its five-year concept and vision, three-year operational objectives, and two-year budgetary guidelines.

STEP SEVEN: IMPLEMENT AND MONITOR

Even a well-planned project can fail if the realities of implementation are not considered. Organizations should form quality action teams, groups of individuals given the task of making a specific part of the reengineering effort become a reality.

Each team should mandate and identify its roles and responsibilities; it should also lay out meeting obligations, reports or investigations to be completed, and the estimated duration of service. It is important to remember that such teams are not designed to continue forever. Assigned a very specific part of the implementation plan, the team should last only as long as it takes to complete that part of the plan. To extend participation indefinitely risks reducing members' effective span of participation, as well as adding a layer of unnecessary bureaucracy to their work lives.

STEP EIGHT: REVIEW ORGANIZATIONAL REQUIREMENTS

Once the project is complete, it is important to perform at least a basic evaluation of the project and its success or failure. Were the objectives attained? What kind of return on the reengineering investment has been realized? Were customer service goals met? This type of evaluative process might entail

1. Revisiting the original goals and objectives of the project. Were objectives met? Did those objectives lead to their corresponding goals?

2. Evaluating the benefits of the new systems or structures against those that were projected

3. Assessing individuals' involvement in the project. How critical was each person's contribution to the success of the project? How critical was each person's role in the project's failure?

4. Assessing if quality action teams were a useful mechanism for implementation

5. Reevaluating the organization (step one). Does the current IT structure now fit business objectives?

Key boosts and barriers

Many positive and negative factors commonly influence the outcome of reengineering projects. These relate primarily to cultural, planning, and leadership issues. Any of these issues can have a lasting and powerful impact on the success or failure of IT reengineering. Most issues revolve around the following key determinants:

- Corporate culture

- Project leadership

- IT and corporate harmony

- Reaction to change; change management ability

- Organizational knowledge, preparation, and core skills

- Multilayer management commitment

IT and corporate harmony, organizational knowledge, preparation, and core skills, and multilayer management commitment become particularly important issues to examine because of the complex technical and data questions facing IT reengineering. Failure to actively address each of them will almost certainly ensure project failure.

IT AND CORPORATE HARMONY

Successful implementation of any reengineering effort requires a careful marriage of IT and corporate planning. Even after reaching consensus on a strategic IT plan, organizations find it challenging to implement a reengineering plan.

Staff-level employees and managers may intellectually understand the organization's need to address new business requirements yet may be insecure and apprehensive when faced with change. Common reactions may be: "let somebody else take the lead" or "the risks are too great in being a pioneer" or "we cannot afford to be the beta site." These reactions, left unchecked, can escalate into outright resistance to planned changes, jeopardizing the entire reengineering project.

As the reengineering effort unfolds, progress on meeting corporate objectives must be continually evaluated.

ORGANIZATIONAL KNOWLEDGE, PREPARATION, AND CORE SKILLS

Successful IT strategies require technical expertise to implement and integrate disparate software applications and systems to work together smoothly. Organizations must determine if they have the right IT team to take on these tasks or consider hiring outside expertise for lacking technical or management skills. An objective assessment should be made of the available resources within the corporation and a balance of various skill mixes must be considered.

MULTILAYER MANAGEMENT COMMITMENT

Management commitment to IT reengineering is often tested when funding sources change or diminish. As staff cuts are being made, organizations must be sensitive to the staff whose focus for cost-cutting may be targeted to the new system or technology. It is easy to blame any hurdles or initial setbacks on IT rather than identifying the originating point of project difficulties. If finger pointing or constant turnover at the project management level occurs, employees will inevitably lose faith in the project itself. Furthermore, the strategic plan will be impacted and organizations may not be able to recapture the lost time and opportunity.

Conclusion

Reengineering is not an end goal in itself. Focusing on the reengineering process, with its associated constant upheaval and change, inevitably causes frustration and disillusionment for those involved. The key to succeeding is to understand the importance and difficulties involved in reengineering but not to lose sight of the main goal: system and process improvement with demonstrable goals and measurable results.

▚ 40

Using computer modeling and simulation approaches

Charles E. Saunders, MD
Manager
A. T. Kearney, Inc.
San Francisco, California

Busi ness process reengineering (BPR) involves the fundamental restructuring of business processes across an organization's functional boundaries. If accomplished successfully, dramatic performance gains are achievable. However, barriers to success often challenge even the most technically effective redesign effort. Among these challenges is the enormous cultural change that may be required within an organization, plus the potential for layoffs, job retraining, and acclimation to new tools, work sites, and practices. Because of this, BPR can often be a high-stakes gamble where mistakes can be both costly and painful. Therefore, before implementation it is important to understand and anticipate the behavior, resource requirements, and performance of a process redesign of an organization. Understanding and predicting how a process will behave is technically challenging but can be simplified through the use of specialized approaches called modeling and simulation. The widespread availability of powerful microcomputers along with advances in computer software has made computer modeling and simulation highly accessible.

This chapter highlights the use of modeling and computer simulation in BPR and illustrates the roles these techniques can play in gaining a better understanding of processes and forecasting the impact of proposed process changes.

Systems thinking

Predicting a new process behavior or performance may be easier said than done. Many business processes are part of a system, or larger set of interrelated processes. A change in one process can influence another in unexpected ways, like the proverbial pebble that when dropped in the ocean causes a ripple that leads to a tidal wave on a faraway shore. For this reason, it is often useful to view the reengineering process from a systems perspective. The behavior of complex processes and systems is dependent on many interrelated variables; it is also dynamic—changing moment to moment as a result of the changing state of these variables and the influence of these forces. "Systems thinking" is simply an approach to BPR where processes are considered dynamically in terms of interrelationships between events.[1]

Modeling

Systems thinking is aided by reducing the complexities of real processes into simplified conceptual models. There are several types: descriptive models are those in which components of a system are represented in iconic form, such as a flight simulator, architectural model, pictorial flow diagram, or animation. An understanding of the model's behavior is gained through visual and tactile interaction and the real-life system reference is intuitive. Symbolic models are those in which components in the system are represented by mathematical or statistical expressions of relationships between variables. It is symbolic modeling that allows quantitative prediction of the model's behavior and lends itself to computer simulation.[2]

Symbolic models can be further characterized by their time relationship either as static, where time is not a factor, or dynamic, where system variables are expressed as a function of time. Examples of static models used in BPR are spreadsheets and queuing models. Familiarity with spreadsheet modeling is now widespread and commonly used to represent financial variables. In healthcare, a queuing model can be used effectively to predict waiting times, patient throughput times (cycle time from patient entry to exit), and resource utilization for a given number of resources, patient rates arrivals, and resource service rates.[3]

Queuing models are appealing in BPR for several reasons. Business processes usually involve sequential tasks performed on entities flowing through the system (e.g., patients, records, specimens). It takes time to perform each task. If the time between arriving entities is shorter than the time to provide service to each entity, then queuing (waiting) occurs. Queuing models have advantages: they are fast and inexpensive to create and provide a good first approximation of the behavior of each stage of a process. They also have disadvantages; they are simple, idealized models and not well suited for modeling complex systems with interrelated tasks or random events with complex distributions.

A queuing approach to BPR is shown in Figure 1. The flow diagram represents a typical emergency room triage/registration station with long waiting lines.

A hypothetical redesigned process with expanded hours for primary care and an urgent care clinic is created as shown in Figure 2, which redirects some nonemergency patients away from the emergency room (ER), reducing total ER patient visits. A queuing model is then used to represent the new process and predict waiting times and triage nurse utilization.

Under the new model, fewer triage nurses are needed and former ER patients are now treated in a lower-cost setting, resulting in cost savings. The queuing approach quickly and easily provides a first-approximation view of the behavior of a simplified system of flows and services processes. The mathematics involved in queuing models can be cumbersome, however. Fortunately, inexpensive computer programs exist that are easy to use.[4] Input variables typically include the arrival rate of entities, the service rate (the inverse of service time), and the number of servers. The outputs include average waiting time, average number waiting, and server utilization fraction.

Simulation

Static models, such as spreadsheeting and queuing, that are based on abstract formulas, provide little insight into relationships between events and cannot model the detail and complexity of many real-life systems. A dynamic model that is able to represent a complex system in detail is a simulation model. The two main types of simulation are continuous and discrete-event simulation. Continuous simulations are based on mathematical equations that yield continuously changing results over time. These are often used in modeling chemical processes.

FIGURE 1
Typical ER triage/registration station with long waiting lines

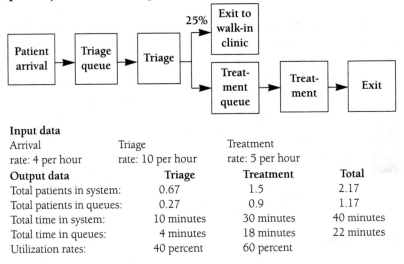

Input data

Arrival	Triage	Treatment
rate: 4 per hour	rate: 10 per hour	rate: 5 per hour

Output data	Triage	Treatment	Total
Total patients in system:	0.67	4.0	4.67
Total patients in queues:	0.27	3.2	3.47
Total time in system:	10 minutes	60 minutes	70 minutes
Total time in queues:	4 minutes	48 minutes	52 minutes
Utilization rates:	40 percent	80 percent	

FIGURE 2
Hypothetical redesigned process with expanded hours for primary care and an urgent care clinic

Input data

Arrival	Triage	Treatment
rate: 4 per hour	rate: 10 per hour	rate: 5 per hour

Output data	Triage	Treatment	Total
Total patients in system:	0.67	1.5	2.17
Total patients in queues:	0.27	0.9	1.17
Total time in system:	10 minutes	30 minutes	40 minutes
Total time in queues:	4 minutes	18 minutes	22 minutes
Utilization rates:	40 percent	60 percent	

Discrete event simulation creates discrete entities that "flow" through a sequence of events in time. These are more commonly used for materials handling, manufacturing, and other types of job processing (including the flow of patients, specimens, and information). In discrete-event simulation, the arrival of entities and their interaction with events can be either stochastic (i.e., random) or deterministic (i.e., preestablished according to some rule or historical data).

CONTINUOUS SIMULATION

An elegant and fairly simple continuous simulation system that is finding application in healthcare BPR is available in a software application called *ithink* on both Apple Macintosh and PC platforms.[5] *ithink* uses symbol elements to represent relationships between events through a metaphor of stocks, to represent accumulations of entities, and flows, to represent operations. Linkages can be drawn between elements to represent influences of a modifying entity or of feedback loops.

Using this approach, a computer model of a hypothetical ER can easily be constructed with multiple queues and service stages, such as triage and treatment. Patients flow along the model's symbolic "pipes" and accumulate in queues while they wait for service. The mathematical expressions of operations or linkages are accessible by clicking a mouse button on a given element that can be modified at will. When the model is run for a period of time, system variables change dynamically and are represented both visually on the model diagram and in various graphs.

A BPR effort may involve the redesign of the ER process (e.g., the introduction of the requirement that the patient first must contact a high-level telephone advice service that involves a primary care physician who can redirect nonemergency patients to a scheduled office visit the next day or solve the problem by telephone without an ER visit). The new process can easily be redesigned by making modifications to the base model. Using the same input data as the base model, but assuming that 25 percent of patients will be redirected, the waiting times, queue sizes, and average number of patients in the ER drop to almost zero. Both the queuing model and the computer model using *ithink* accomplish the same objective, but the *ithink* model provides greater insight and more detailed and complex models, shows interrelationships between events, and is dynamic. It is also fairly intuitive and easy to use; complete models can be developed rapidly (within hours), rudimentary animation is possible, and state variables can be changed in real time by the user, allowing immediate and dynamic visualization of results.

DISCRETE-EVENT SIMULATION

Although the *ithink* software can, with some modifications, approximate a discrete-event simulation, it has limitations and is best suited for high-level modeling. If greater detail is required, the process to be modeled is complex, or more sophisticated animation is desired, then discrete-event simulation will be required. The traditional approach to this type of simulation has been through programming, by building a model with computer codes using one of several computer simulation languages.[6] For example, a typical code sequence for a patient entering an ER might be simplified as

Create patient	(Poisson distribution, five-minute interval)
Queue for triage nurse	(first in, first out)
Sieze triage nurse	(nurse = one)
Delay to do triage	(exponential distribution, two minutes)
Release triage nurse	(nurse = one)
Queue for ER room	(first in, first out)

Real code is actually more arcane, with numerous arguments and parameters, and can be tedious to write and debug, especially if the simulation is complex. Development time for a complex model can be lengthy (several days or weeks or more). A more recent innovation can be found with any of several simulators that are essentially shell applications that serve as interfaces between the user and the code through icons, buttons, and menus.[7] Simulators simplify the task of model building, reduce the model development time, and are visually oriented, intuitive, and many contain integrated animation. On the down side, some flexibility is given up. For example, nonstandard queuing behaviors, resource scheduling, use of system variables and statistics, and methods of organizing output data may follow preprogrammed defaults or conventions and be less amenable to customization without resorting to programming.

Although simulation systems can be expensive (e.g., from $10,000 to $20,000), new innovative and inexpensive alternatives are beginning to appear. One such recent application is Process Charter, by Scitor Corporation.[8] Process Charter is a flowcharting drawing program that is also a discrete-event simulator. It uses drag-and-drop functionality to create realistic process-flow diagrams that can then be parameterized through pop-up dialog boxes. A typical simulation model, which can be built in a matter of a few minutes to a few hours, includes rudimentary animation as well as built-in activity-based cost analysis, all for a few hundred dollars. As one might expect with a highly simplified system, some tradeoffs in flexibility and the ability to model complexity must be accepted.

There are many cases in which discrete-event simulation has been used to analyze and design a healthcare process.[9] Using the ER again as an example, discrete-event simulation allows more of the true complexity of the patient-flow process to be accurately modeled, allows realistic resource scheduling, and can better replicate the intricate decision-tree logic inherent in patient-flow scenarios. For example, using actual data from the ER for patient arrivals, service cycle times, and resource levels, a base simulation can be constructed and validated based on its ability to represent the actual process (comparison of model output to actual observations). Then design options can be introduced by making changes in the model and repeating the simulation. With this information, a reconfiguration of the ER can be more accurately rendered, complete with staffing and space requirements, that optimizes both resource utilization and patient flow. (See endnote number nine's first listing for a discrete-event simulation model of an ER written in SIMAN IV, a robust, high-level discrete-event computer simulation language that can be used to create realistic models of complex processes. Models in SIMAN IV are constructed through lines of programming code, and may be animated through special animation tools.)

With many simulation systems, animation is available either as an integrated feature of the software or with a compatible add-on application. While not essential to the simulation, animation is a powerful avenue through which insights can be gained into the dynamics of the process being modeled; it also helps laypersons understand and accept the model and aids in the debugging process.

Use of simulation in BPR

The most appropriate place to involve simulation is in the innovation or redesign phase of the reengineering effort. Depending on the simulation approach used, the development time and expense involved to create a simulation model can be significant. For example, a simulation model using an analytical tool such as *ithink,* or a model-builder such as Pro-Model can be developed in a matter of hours if the process is simple and most data are either available or can be accurately estimated. However, it may take days or even weeks if the process is more complex, especially if data must be collected. (Regardless of whether simulation is employed, data collection is normally required in a BPR effort to quantify performance and activity-based costs; however, the use of simulation often requires more detailed and accurate data.) The model must then be validated by client operations staff, tested for accuracy, and debugged if necessary. Validation and debugging can usually be accomplished in a few days but can take longer for a complex model. If a more robust modeling approach is taken using discrete-event simulation requiring programming, the modeling effort can take weeks. Writing code is time-consuming and tedious to debug. Because the use of simulation languages is generally reserved for more complex models, there is usually more data required, hence the added time for data collection. As a general rule, one should expect to spend a minimum of one week creating and validating a low- to moderate-complexity simulation model using a model-builder and two to three weeks using a programming approach. Add one to two more weeks if any significant manual data collection is required (i.e., by direct time and motion study). If the model is large or complex, requiring a detailed simulation or using a simulation language, it can take four to eight weeks to create and validate the model.

The effort required for detailed simulation of the current process may not be well spent if the current process is likely to be abolished or substantially altered. To fully anticipate its behavior and optimize resources, the investment is best reserved for the proposed redesigned process. The best approach is one in which the level of detail is sufficient, but not greater than that needed to explore critical elements of the process at a minimum investment in development time. Once the reengineering work team has designed a new process, then staff with appropriate technical skills must create a working simulation model of the new process and present it to the work group for validation and experimentation. This sequence of events can take from days to weeks as described above.

A simulation is best viewed as an experiment that tests a proposed business process' hypothesis. As such, a sound experimental method should be used—the design must be sufficient to prove or disprove the hypothesis, and the results should be statistically valid with sufficient replications to achieve statistical validity. In general, simulation involves several steps, as shown in Table 1. If necessary, animation can be created

TABLE 1
Steps involved in conducting a simulation

Step	Description
Define the problem	Define the question to be answered by simulation (e.g., what is the patient throughput time of the proposed process?)
Develop a conceptual model	Use flow diagrams to map the new process and identify key performance variables
Design the simulation experiment	Design the simulation approach, methodology, and experiment (i.e., what is simulated, by what approach, using what data)
Collect input data	Collect or estimate input data for service and arrival rates and frequency distributions
Create the computer model	Develop the computer model and write computer code
Verify and validate the model	Confirm the model does what it is supposed to do (verify) and that the results are believable in reference to the real world (validate)
Conduct the experiment	Conduct the simulation experiment with a base case, sufficient replications, sensitivity, and perturbation analysis (i.e., systematically vary input parameters to determine their effect on output variables)
Analyze the results	Include statistical analysis, graphing, and transient phase corrections

to help debug and validate the simulation and to demonstrate the proposed process to the work group or oversight body.

Advantages and disadvantages of computer simulation

The types of reengineering processes that are amenable to simulation are wide and varied. Computer simulation's main advantage is that it allows experimentation with systems without the cost, time, and disruption inherent in trial and error or pilot studies (see Table 2).

Computer simulation does have disadvantages, mostly related to greater effort and technical requirements in conducting it compared with simpler modeling techniques and to the "black box" nature of the simulation approach. In many cases, it is sufficient to take a high-level view with a tool such as *ithink,* or to simplify the system around its critical components and use a spreadsheet, queuing, or statistical (e.g., benchmarking) model first. However, for modeling complex systems,

TABLE 2
Advantages and disadvantages to computer simulation in BPR

Advantages	Disadvantages
Performance of a newly designed business process, operating characteristics, flow times, and bottlenecks can be predicted	Computer simulation requires sophisticated technical expertise
Resource needs of newly designed business processes can be determined and optimized	Computer simulation approaches are sometimes seen as a "black box" and approached with skepticism
Existing and proposed processes can be compared side by side	Detailed or complex simulations can be time-consuming to create and debug
Relationships between components and variables can be explored and demonstrated	With most processes, there is usually one critical step that can easily be modeled with simple approaches, such as queuing, which may be sufficient
The newly designed process can be fine-tuned before implementation, thus reducing the chance for error and costly mistakes	In many cases, a "walk-through" or "lab" is less costly, quicker, and provides more realistic insights
Computer simulation is less costly and time-consuming than a pilot implementation	Simulation software can be expensive
Staff can gain comfort with new process by observing its simulated system behavior	
Compared with other modeling techniques, discrete-event simulation can model the greatest level of complexity and detail	

where stakes are high and errors can be costly and painful, discrete-event computer simulation provides unique value. With the use of the new simulators, the simulation development time can be dramatically reduced, in some cases, to a matter of hours. Through animation key insights and understanding often can be gained.

NOTES

1. P. Senge, A. Kleiner, and C. Roberts, *The Fifth Discipline Fieldbook* (New York: Currency Doubleday, 1994).

2. C. D. Pegden, R. E. Shannon, and R. P. Sadowski, *Introduction to Simulation Using SIMAN* (New York: McGraw-Hill, 1990).

3. J. A. Payne, *Introduction to Computer Simulation: Programming Techniques and Methods of Analysis* (New York: McGraw-Hill, 1982); and J. K. Cooper, "Estimating Bed Needs by Means of Queuing Theory," *NEJM* 291(1974): 404–5.

4. T. L. Dennis and L. B. Dennis, *Microcomputer Models for Management Decision-Making* (St. Paul: West Publishing Company, 1988).

5. High Performance Systems, Inc., Hanover, N.H.

6. SIMAN IV, Systems Modeling Corporation, Sewickley, Pa.; GPSS/H, Wolverine Software Corporation, Annandale, Va.; GPSS World, Minuteman Software, Stow, Mass.; SLAM II, Pritsker Corporation, Indianapolis, Ind.; SIMSCRIPT II.5, CACI Products Company, La Jolla, Calif.

7. ProModel/MedModel, PROMODEL Corporation, Orem, Utah; AUTOMOD, AutoSimulations, Bountiful, Utah; SIMFACTORY, CACI Products Company, La Jolla, Calif.; ARENA, Systems Modeling Corporation, Sewickley, Pa.

8. Process Charter, Scitor Corp., Menlo Park, Calif.

9. C. E. Saunders, P. K. Makens and L. J. LeBlanc, "Modeling Emergency Department Operations Using Advanced Computer Simulation Systems," *Ann Emerg Med* 18 (1989): 134–38; and C. G. Dankbar, "The use of simulation to evaluate automated equipment for a clinical processing laboratory"; J. C. Lowery, "Simulation of a hospital's surgical suite and critical care area"; and M. A. Draeger, "An emergency department simulation model used to evaluate alternative nurse staffing and patient population scenarios," from *Proceedings of the 1992 Winter-Simulation Conference,* ed. J. J. Swain et al. (Washington, DC: WSC, 1992); M. A. Coffin et al., "A simulation model of an x-ray facility"; M. Ritondo and R. W. Freedman, "The effect of procedure scheduling on emergency room throughput: A simulation study," *Simulation in Health Sciences and Services,* ed. J. G. Anderson and M. Katzper (San Diego: Simulation Councils, 1993); R. W. Freedman, "Reduction of average length of stay in the emergency room using discrete simulation," *Simulation in the Health Sciences,* ed. J. G. Anderson and M. Katzper (San Diego: Simulation Councils, 1994).

Contributors

Editor

Peter Boland, PhD
President and Publisher
Boland Healthcare, Inc.
Berkeley, California

A consistently thought-provoking commentator and nationally recognized authority on managed care, Peter Boland forecasts industry trends and develops publications to improve healthcare management. He is the editor and publisher of The Capitation Sourcebook and *Redesigning Healthcare Delivery*, coeditor of *Physician Profiling and Risk Adjustment,* and was the principal author and editor of *Making Managed Healthcare Work* and *The New Healthcare Market.* He was also the founding editor of *Managed Care Quarterly.*

He received a PhD from the University of California, Los Angeles, a master's degree from the University of Michigan, and a postgraduate certificate from Harvard University's executive program in health policy and management. Often quoted in trade and news media, he frequently challenges the conventional wisdom and speaks regularly at industry conferences.

Authors

Saad Allawi
Senior Principal
William M. Mercer Provider Consulting Practice
New York, New York

Saad Allawi leads the firm's efforts in applying reengineering practices in healthcare organizations. He was director of operations focusing on cost reduction and organizational redesign at APM and a consultant for McKinsey and Company.

He has an MBA with an emphasis in operations research and international business from Columbia Business School and frequently speaks on process redesign, business reinvention, and organization transformation.

John L. Aitken, PhD
Principal
Ernst & Young, LLP
Kansas City, Missouri

John Aitken concentrates on reengineering, business process improvement, strategic planning, and knowledge management. He held a number of senior executive positions at Marion Merrell Dow including vice president of performance improvement and vice president of human resources.

He has a degree in industrial engineering from GMI Institute of Engineering and Management and a PhD in organizational behavior from Case Western Reserve University.

Linda Andrews
Assistant for CEO Communications
Group Health Cooperative of Puget Sound
Seattle, Washington

Linda Andrews is a communications specialist.

She has a master of fine arts degree from the University of Washington and has published extensively in healthcare trade magazines such as the *Journal of Healthcare Resource Management* and the *Journal of Health Care Benefits*.

Wendy L. Baker
Business Manager, Primary Care Network
University of Michigan Health System
Ann Arbor, Michigan

Wendy Baker facilitates the purchase and management of primary care practices for network development. She was the director of patient care innovation at Vanderbilt University Hospital and Clinic and project manager for the Robert Wood Johnson/Pew Charitable Trust program to improve patient care by strengthening hospital nursing. She was a clinical nurse specialist in critical care and trauma care. She was also a Kellogg National Fellow and worked on organizational leadership and transformation.

She has a master's degree in nursing from the University of Michigan.

Donna L. Bertram
Senior Vice President and Chief Operating Officer
Penrose–St. Francis Health System
Colorado Springs, Colorado

Donna Bertram oversees operations for two acute care hospitals, an Alzheimer's center, an urgent care facility, and a health center. She teaches healthcare administration at Regis University in Denver.

She received an MBA from the University of Dallas Graduate School of Management and a nursing degree from the University of Texas at Arlington. She is a fellow in the American Academy of Nursing; has published on financial management, nursing delivery systems, and personnel issues; and served on the editorial board of *Heart and Lung, the Journal of Critical Care*.

Walter J. Besecker
Director, Medical Care Cost Recovery
Department of Veterans Affairs
Washington, DC

Walter Besecker leads a national program to recover the cost of healthcare provided to Veterans Administration patients from insurers. He was director of strategic management and led automation efforts in patient registration, clinical data capture, billing, collection, and utilization review.

He has a master's degree from Kent State University.

John J. Byrnes, MD
Vice President of Quality Improvement
Lovelace Health Systems
Albuquerque, New Mexico

John Byrnes directs clinical practice improvement, disease management, and organizational reengineering for the health system. He has published and presented extensively on these topics.

He received a medical degree from the University of Missouri in Kansas City, completed his residency training through the University of Texas in Houston, and is board certified in anesthesiology with special emphasis in critical care medicine and quality improvement.

Rebecca Enmark Cagan
Research Associate
JDA
San Francisco, California

Rebecca Enmark Cagan specializes in healthcare information technology research, particularly product functionality and vendor support.

She has a master's degree in information management from the University of California, Berkeley. She is coauthor of the forthcoming *Getting the Most From Your Healthcare Information System: Management Strategies* and acted as research manager for *Quality Measurement Systems: Strategies, Product Profiles and Healthcare Information Systems Capabilities.* She previously coordinated research and library development for a state-based computerized career information system.

Tim Coan
President
Aslex, Inc.
Denver, Colorado

Tim Coan specializes in strategic transformation and works with companies to redefine how value will be added to customers through redesigning the total organization. He previously was a leader in the change management practice of an international consulting firm and worked in human resource management for a large tertiary hospital.

He has a master's degree in industrial/organizational psychology from the University of Tulsa, has authored articles in *Healthcare Forum Journal* and *Quality Management in Healthcare,* and is on the faculty of the University of Denver's graduate healthcare program.

Carol A. Craft, DNS
Program Director, St. Louis Continuing Education Center
Department of Veterans Affairs
St. Louis, Missouri

Carol Craft manages professional continuing education activities and coordinates the reengineering pilot project on medical care cost recovery for the Veterans Administration.

She has a nursing doctorate from St. Louis University and is associate clinical professor of nursing at St. Louis University.

Connie R. Curran, EdD
President
CurranCare
North Riverside, Illinois

Connie Curran directs consulting projects on patient care services and focuses on operations improvement and work restructuring programs. She directed a comprehensive reform initiative for the Province of Manitoba, Canada, and served as dean at the Medical College of Wisconsin and as director of the City University of New York's Health Profession's Institute. She was vice president of the American Hospital Association and the senior scholar in residence at the Institute of Medicine.

She has a doctorate in education from Northern Illinois University and a master's degree in nursing from De Paul University. She is a fellow of the American Academy of Nursing and the editor of *Nursing Economics*.

James Cyr
Director of Cardiovascular Medical Services
University of Massachusetts Medical Center
Worcester, Massachusetts

James Cyr oversees operations in the coronary care unit, cardiac short stay unit, cardiac telemetry unit, the electrophysiology laboratories and the heart station.

He has an MBA from Nichols College School of Business and a master's degree in nursing management and administration from the University of Massachusetts. He has published in various journals and presents widely on many clinical topics.

Joseph M. DeLuca
Founder and President
JDA
San Francisco, California

Joseph DeLuca specializes in information systems planning, particularly for integrated delivery systems. He has managed healthcare facilities, as well as planned and managed information systems product development.

He has an MBA in health services administration from the University of Wisconson, Madison, and is a fellow in the American College of Healthcare Executives. He coauthored *Health Care Information Systems: An Executive's Guide for Successful Management* and the forthcoming *Getting the Most From Your Healthcare Information Systems: Management Strategies*.

Marilyn Dubree
Director, Patient Care Services
Vanderbilt University Hospital
Nashville, Tennessee

Marilyn Dubree most recently served as the director of operational improvement at Vanderbilt University Hospital. In this role, she provided leadership and support of the task forces and design teams involved in work redesign and implementation of the housewide integrated patient care delivery model. She has held positions in clinical nursing, nursing education, and nursing administration. She was the project director for the Orthopedic Work Redesign Project at Vanderbilt University Hospital and directed the planning and implementation of this program. Prior to this appointment, she was the associate director of surgical nursing at Vanderbilt University Hospital.

She has a master's degree in nursing from Vanderbilt University School of Nursing.

Donald Eggleston
Director of Staff Development
St. Mary's Health Center
St. Louis, Missouri

Donald Eggleston directs the training and development function with particular emphasis on nursing and clinical training, continuous quality improvement, leadership development, and workplace basic skills enhancement. He is also responsible for facilitating educational support for several rural hospitals within the network. He was previously coordinator of community education for a metropolitan hospital with a focus on developing prevention wellness models.

He received a master's degree in education from the University of Missouri, St. Louis, and a master of divinity degree from Kenrick Seminary.

Moira G. Feingold
Vice President
Oncology Resource Consultants, Inc.
Santa Monica, California

Moira Feingold develops and administers hospital and community oncology programs, cancer data collection and analysis, and hospital medical staff and quality management issues. She was formerly vice president of medical affairs at a large urban hospital and served as administrative director of a community hospital oncology program funded by the National Cancer Institute.

She has a master's degree in public administration from the University of Southern California.

Victoria P. Gaw
Quality Management Coordinator
University of Massachusetts Medical Center
Worcester, Massachusetts

Victoria Gaw serves as a facilitator for clinical process redesign teams at the medical center, in the areas of ventilator weaning, community-acquired pneumonia, craniotomy, and stroke. She was formerly a nursing and staff educator and project coordinator for the medical center's Breast Cancer Screening Project, a community intervention study to increase mammography utilization and quality.

She is a registered nurse and has a master's degree from Anna Maria College. She has coauthored publications in *QRB* and *Journal of Cancer Education*.

> Mary Gelinas, EdD
> *Managing Director*
> *Gelinas James Akiyoshi*
> *Oakland, California*

Mary Gelinas specializes in collaborative approaches to complex change. She was a principal of an international consulting firm, served as director of operations for a research and development company, and managed a team of consultants for a national training and consulting center.

She has a doctorate of education in organization development from the University of Massachusetts and is the coauthor of *Collaborative Organization Design—Consultant Guide* and *Workbook and Consulting Skills—Bringing Your Authentic Self Forward.*

> William A. Golomski
> *President*
> *W. A. Golomski & Associates*
> *Chicago, Illinois*

William Golomski consults on total quality management, corporate growth strategies, and research and development management for corporations as well as local and national governments. He is a senior lecturer in business policy and quality management at the University of Chicago's Graduate School of Business.

He is the past president of the American Society of Quality Control as well as recipient of the American Deming Medal. He is a fellow of the American Association for the Advancement of Science, the founding editor of the *Quality Management Journal,* and author of numerous books, including *A Quality Revolution in Manufacturing.*

> Margaret Gunter, PhD
> *Vice President and Executive Director*
> *Lovelace Clinic Foundation*
> *Albuquerque, New Mexico*

Margaret Gunter administers the Lovelace Clinical Foundation, a nonprofit healthcare delivery research institute affiliated with Lovelace Health Systems. She has been an active participant in the development of the Episode of Care Disease Management Program at Lovelace and presents widely at national conferences on outcomes research and disease management. Dr. Gunter is currently chair of the National Steering Committee of the American Group Practice Association's 60-clinic Outcomes Measurement Consortia.

She has a PhD in medical sociology from the University of Pittsburgh.

Tami Hechtel
Director, Organizational Development
The Bradford Group
Niles, Illinois

Tami Hechtel is an organizational development specialist with an emphasis in implementing large system changes.

She has a master's degree in health education from Illinois State University and is a certified health education specialist. She has published in professional journals representing human resources as well as training and development. She also presents reengineering topics to healthcare industry conferences.

Michael E. Henry
President and Chief Executive Officer
CAPP CARE
Newport Beach, California

Michael Henry heads a national managed care organization with 4,000,000 members in 40 states. He was president and chief executive officer of General Med HMO, senior vice president of HealthCare USA, and assistant commissioner of the California Department of Corporations responsible for the licensing and regulation of health plans. He was also president of the National Association of HMO Regulators for two terms and held positions within the Blue Cross Association in Chicago where he ran its National Alternative Delivery Systems.

He has an MBA in health administration from the University of North Carolina.

Roger Hite, PhD
Executive Vice President and Chief Operating Officer
Dominican Santa Cruz Hospital
Santa Cruz, California

Roger Hite heads the daily operations of a 300-bed, two-campus, general acute care hospital and rehabilitation center and is responsible for leading the transformation of traditional management operations into a new customer-driven management system involving 22 interdisciplinary teams. He was the vice president for business development and strategic planning at Mercy Health Care, as well as staff development director, director of planning, and assistant administrator at Mercy General Hospital in Sacramento.

He has a PhD in speech and communications from the University of Oregon.

Roger G. James, EdD
Managing Director
Gelinas James Akiyoshi
Oakland, California

Roger James focuses on developing high-performance, high-commitment organizations through large-scale redesign activities. He was the director of organization development at Pacific Gas and Electric Company.

He has a doctorate in education from the University of Massachusetts and is a graduate of Columbia University's advanced program in organizational development. He is a coauthor of *Collaborative Organization Design—Consultant Guide* and *Workbook and Consulting Skills—Bringing Your Authentic Self Forward.*

> Margaret Jordan
> *President and Chief Executive Officer*
> *Dallas Medical Resources*
> *Dallas, Texas*

Margaret Jordan, prior to joining Dallas Medical Resources, was responsible for redesigning Southern California Edison's healthcare system and driving necessary changes through the transition. She has served with the U.S. Public Health Service, was a senior regional manager with Kaiser Foundation Health Plans in Dallas and Atlanta, and served on the executive board of the American Public Health Association and the Council on Health Promotion and Disease Prevention of the U.S. Department of Health and Human Services.

She is a registered nurse with a master's degree in public health from the University of California, Berkeley, and frequently testifies before Congress.

> Matt Kelliher
> *Executive Director, Health Care Division*
> *Blue Cross and Blue Shield of Massachusetts*
> *Farmington, Massachusetts*

Matt Kelliher directs the operations of an integrated delivery system with nine health centers. He was formerly vice president of quality management at Harvard Community Health Plan and director of management systems engineering at the University of California, San Diego.

He has an MBA from Roosevelt University and has published widely in the healthcare field.

> Mark Kimmel, PhD
> *President*
> *Kimmel and Associates*
> *Berkeley, California*

Mark Kimmel consults on organizational development and specializes in strategic planning, redesign, and team development.

He has an PhD from the California School of Professional Psychology and coauthored The American Society for Training and Development's *Quality* monograph.

> Brian Klapper
> *Principal*
> *Mercer Management Consulting*
> *New York, New York*

Brian Klapper specializes in developing and implementing business strategies for companies in healthcare, consumer products, and financial services. He also consults on process development, redesign, and implementation.

He has an MBA from the Wharton Graduate School of Business at the University of Pennsylvania.

O. John Kralovec
Vice President
First Consulting Group
Mt. Laurel, New Jersey

John Kralovec heads the reengineering practice with responsibility for design and development of methodologies. He focuses on operations enhancement, performance improvement, and IS/IT benefits realization. He was formerly an executive with Ernst & Young.

He has published in *Journal of Healthcare Information Management, Nursing Administration Quarterly,* and *Healthcare Forum Journal.* He is a frequent lecturer for professional trade associations.

Anthony J. Kubica
Executive Manager, Integrated Delivery Networks Practice
Superior Consultant Company
Farmington Hills, Michigan

Anthony Kubica specializes in reengineering, change management, as well as strategic/tactical planning for healthcare oraganizations and physician groups. He was vice president of hospital services for a large teaching hospital.

He has a master's degree in pharmacy and an MBA in healthcare administration from the University of Connecticut and is a diplomate of the American College of Healthcare Executives. He has served as an issues editor of *Topics in Hospital Pharmacy Management* and has published widely in professional journals.

Nancy Lakier
Operations Strategist
Scripps Memorial Hospital
La Jolla, California

Nancy Lakier leads the clinical redesign process for five hospital facilities. She also directs a consulting company specializing in clinical process redesign, Care Tracs and clinical pathways, case management, and standardization of operating systems.

She has an MBA from the University of Nebraska and a nursing degree from Creighton University. She has published in *Healthcare Forum and Surgical Services Management* and presents widely to healthcare systems, hospitals, and clinical professional groups.

J. Philip Lathrop
Vice President
Booz-Allen & Hamilton, Inc.
Chicago, Illinois

Philip Lathrop specializes in market strategy, finance, and operations restructuring for large hospitals, healthcare systems, and managed care organizations.

He has an MBA in hospital administration from the University of Chicago, is the author of *Restructuring Health Care—The Patient-Focused Paradigm,* and is a frequent writer and speaker on hospital restructuring.

William J. Leander
Cofounder and Director
PFCA
Atlanta, Georgia

William Leander specializes in structural work and process redesign across clinical and nonclinical services for inpatient, outpatient, and emergency settings. Client work focuses on performance management programs and automated redesign tools.

He has an MBA from Carnegie-Mellon University, is coauthor of *Patients First: Experiences of a Patient-Focused Pioneer,* and speaks frequently on redesign issues and results.

Stephen E. Leichtman
Assistant Vice President, Organization Effectiveness
Tufts Health Plan
Waltham, Massachusetts

Steven Leichtman leads efforts to strengthen the alignment between the health plan's strategy, processes, administrative structure, and culture. He was previously with Mercer Management Consulting and specialized in process and organization design and strategic management of human resources. He also was a consultant at Bain and Company, where he focused on strategic planning and implementation issues.

He has an MBA with a specialization in marketing and international management from the Sloan School of Management at the Massachusetts Institute of Technology and has published in *Human Resource Professional.*

Steven J. Lewis
Senior Associate
Ronning Management Group
Mammoth Lakes, California

Steven Lewis focuses on planning, strategy development, technology, and program management, with an emphasis on cardiovascular and neuroscience services. He served on the coordinating committee for the National Heart, Lung, and Blood Institute's Heart Attack Alert Program.

He has a master's degree in health administration from Duke University, has published on service line management and the impact of technology on healthcare services, and was on the editorial board of the *Journal of Cardiovascular Management.*

John Lucas, MD
President and Chief Executive Officer
Lovelace Health Systems
Albuquerque, New Mexico

John Lucas leads a fully integrated, managed healthcare organization and champions the development of clinical practice improvement programs nationally.

He has a medical degree from the University of Alberta and a master's in public health from Harvard University.

Rick Martin
Senior Vice President, Operations
St. Charles Medical Center
Bend, Oregon

Rick Martin directs overall internal operations at a 181-bed, acute care, rural referral center and leads reengineering efforts. He was previously director of human resources and director of medical services at the hospital. He is active in community boards and spearheaded the recent restructuring at St. Charles.

He speaks at conferences and assemblies and has contributed to COR Healthcare Resources publications.

Melissa McCanna
Assistant Director, National Media Development Center
Department of Veterans Affairs
St. Louis, Missouri

Melissa McCanna coordinates educational media and produces videotapes and training programs on medical and administrative topics for Veterans Administration facilities across the country.

She has a master of fine arts degree from Southern Illinois University.

Roselyn J. Meier
Senior Program Manager, Patient Flow Management
Legacy Health System
Portland, Oregon

Roselyn Meier manages reengineering activities for an integrated healthcare system with two tertiary care hospitals, two suburban hospitals, and one home health and ambulatory care agency.

She has a master's degree in education from Springfield College and speaks on reengineering methodologies to industry trade groups.

John W. Meyer
Principal
Ronning Management Group
Mammoth Lakes, California

John Meyer specializes in strategic planning, marketing strategy development, and program service development with a focus on cardiovascular, oncology, neuroscience, and orthopedic services. He was director of planning and director of marketing for community, tertiary, nonprofit, and proprietary hospitals.

He has a master's degree in hospital administration from the University of California, Berkeley, and is a fellow of the American College of Healthcare Executives. He has published and lectured extensively.

Kurt Miller
Partner, Director of Care Delivery Solution Team
Andersen Consulting
Pittsburgh, Pennsylvania

Kurt Miller directs the company's medical management and care delivery reengineering engagements. He assists large managed care organizations and integrated delivery systems by creating and implementing business strategies to reduce medical costs, improve health outcomes, and enhance customer service.

He recently chaired the implementation subcommittee of the HL-7 standards organization and is a frequent guest speaker at healthcare conferences. He is coauthor of *Changing Health Care* and a contributor to industy publications such as *Modern Health Care, Health Systems Review,* and *Report on Quality Management.*

Milan Moravec
President
Moravec and Associates
Walnut Creek, California

Milan Moravec specializes in diagnosing, transforming, and revitalizing organizations. He consults with organizations and conducts workshops on managing change.

He has an MBA from the University of Western Ontario. He coauthored *From Downsizing to Recovery: Strategic Transition Options for Organizations and Individuals* and contributes to numerous management journals.

Judy Morton, PhD
Vice President, Quality Resources
Premera
Seattle, Washington

Judy Morton develops and implements strategies to improve health and satisfaction outcomes. Her responsibilities include policy analysis and development, quality measurement and reporting, and education and human resources. She was formerly quality-of-service director at Group Health Cooperative of Puget Sound and director of organizational development for the group practice at Pacific Medical Center.

She has a PhD in education and business from the University of Washington, has published in *Managed Care Quarterly,* and coauthored two books for healthcare professionals: *Dental Teamwork Strategies* and *Building Assertive Skills.*

Richard J. Nierenberg, MD
Associate Director, Emergency Services
Yale–New Haven Hospital
New Haven, Connecticut

Richard Nierenberg specializes in emergency medicine and has participated extensively in hospital redesign efforts.

He has a medical degree from the University of Southern California School of Medicine and is certified in critical care, internal medicine, and emergency medicine. He has published in social science and clinical medicine journals.

Phil Nudelman, PhD
President and Chief Executive Officer
Group Health Cooperative of Puget Sound
Seattle, Washington

Phil Nudelman manages the nation's sixth largest nonprofit HMO, with 2 hospitals, 6 specialty centers, and 30 primary care medical centers. He was previously a hospital administrator and registered pharmacist.

He has an MBA and PhD from Pacific Western University.

Kathryn Payne
Independent Consultant
Associated with Gemini Consulting
Houston, Texas

Kathryn Payne directs change programs for healthcare organizations using strategic planning, business process reengineering, information technology, and organization and people development. Her particular emphasis is translating market trends into organizational action and leadership roles.

She has an MBA from the University of Houston, has published in *Management Review*, and presents widely to healthcare organizations on the creation of market-focused organizations and managing alliances.

Vincent Pelote
Senior Quality Advisor, Quality Management Services
University of Massachusetts Medical Center
Worcester, Massachusetts

Vince Pelote is responsible for providing organizational support for the redesign of clinical and operational practices at the medical center. He founded Value Added Performance in 1990 as a consulting collaborative to support the organizational and performance needs of organizations.

He has an MBA, is a senior examiner for the Massachusetts Quality Award, and is on the National Board of Directors for the TQM Network. He has published in various journals and presents at national conferences.

Susan Peters
Nursing Education Coordinator
St. Mary's Health Center
St. Louis, Missouri

Susan Peters is responsible for coordinating nursing education for an acute care facility, served on the steering team for the design of patient-focused care, and mentored and coached the educators responsible for conducting the training. She was formerly a nursing instructor responsible for designing and implementing educational materials for nursing fundamentals, medical-surgical nursing, pediatrics, and pharmacology.

She received a master's degree in education from Washington University and is a registered nurse.

Ann Gillespie Pietrick, JD
Vice President and General Counsel
The Scheur Management Group, Inc.
Newton, Massachusetts

Ann Gillespie Pietrick provides legal counsel and guidance on organizational structure and operations to integrated delivery systems and was executive director of the Illinois Association Health Maintenance Organizations. She was a senior associate at Gardner, Carton & Douglas and legal counsel to ANCHOR HMO and Access Health (now Rush–Prudential Health Plans). She has served as chair of the Illinois HMO Guaranty Association.

She received a law degree from DePaul University and presents at industry conferences.

William Reeves
Partner, Managed Healthcare Consulting Practice
Price Waterhouse
St. Louis, Missouri

William Reeves leads client projects in strategic, organizational, and technological change and is a member of the firm's worldwide change integration leadership group.

He has an MBA from the University of Chicago and is coauthor of *Better Change, Best Practices for Transforming Your Organization* and *The Paradox Principles, How High Performance Companies Manage Chaos, Complexity and Contradiction to Achieve Superior Results.*

Cheryl Robbins
Partner
Deloitte & Touche Consulting Group
Los Angeles, California

Cheryl Robbins consults in the areas of managed care, hospital restructuring, and reengineering patient care delivery for inpatient and outpatient services. She has been a hospital administrator and a respiratory therapist.

She has an MBA from the Anderson School at the University of California, Los Angeles.

Sharon Roggy
Vice President, Strategic Planning and Business Development
Penrose–St. Francis Health System
Colorado Springs, Colorado

Sharon Roggy leads planning and marketing efforts for two hospital systems and was the director of strategic planning for the Penrose Health System.

She has a master's degree in educational research from the University of Massachusetts and has published on mergers and organizational change in *Health Care Strategic Management* and *Physician Executive.*

Charles E. Saunders, MD
Manager
A.T. Kearney, Inc.
San Francisco, California

Charles Saunders heads the integrated delivery segment of the healthcare consulting practice and focuses on business, operations, and systems planning, as well as process reengineering. He was previously an associate professor of medicine at the University of California, San Francisco, and executive director of the PHO at San Francisco General Hospital.

He received a medical degree from Johns Hopkins University and is board certified in internal medicine and emergency medicine. He has conducted academic studies involving process analysis and modeling healthcare operations and has numerous publications.

Paulette Seymour
Director of Cardiovascular Surgical Services
University of Massachusetts Medical Center
Worcester, Massachusetts

Paulette Seymour is the coleader for the CARB redesign team at the medical center. She serves as a member of the University Hospital Consortium National CABG Benchmarking Committee. She is an associate faculty member of the Graduate School of Nursing at the University of Massachusetts, Worcester.

She has a master's degree from Boston College and is currently a PhD candidate concentrating on quality management, in the nursing program at the University of Massachusetts, Amherst.

Michael Shainline
Director, Quality Control
Lovelace Health Systems
Albuqueque, New Mexico

Michael Shainline focuses on patient satisfaction surveys, outcomes management, physician profiling, and the application of total quality management within the healthcare industry. He was the director of outcomes management, and director of marketing research at the health plan. He has also been a planner, program evaluator, and researcher for public education.

He has an MBA from the University of Phoenix and received a master's degree in vocational rehabilitation from the University of Arizona with an emphasis on measurement and statistics.

Mark K. Shishida
Vice President
Fox Systems, Inc.
Scottsdale, Arizona

Mark Shishida concentrates on developing system requirements and designing systems to accommodate new business needs and assessing the impact on the organization's operational procedures. Information engineering concepts, joint application design techniques, and computer-assisted software engineering tools are used to develop model system requirements.

John J. Skalko
Assistant Vice President, Operations Improvement
Lee Memorial Health System
Fort Myers, Florida

John Skalko directs reengineering and performance improvement initiatives and was instrumental in developing a horizontal strategy for broad-based reengineering. He is also an advisor to Health Care Resource Group, specializing in health system reengineering and operations improvement.

He has a master's degree in industrial management from Georgia Institute of Technology and is a diplomate in the American College of Healthcare Executives. He coauthored *Reengineering Health Care, A Vision for the Future* and has published widely in healthcare journals.

Glenn H. Snyder
Manager
Deloitte & Touche Consulting Group
San Francisco, California

Glenn Snyder specializes in developing healthcare operating strategies, with a focus on reengineering services across integrated delivery networks, implementing patient-focused concepts, and improving physician network capability.

He has an MBA from the Wharton School of Business at the University of Pennsylvania and a master's degree from the University of Southern California.

Steven L. Strongwater, MD
Associate Chief Medical Officer, Clinical System
University of Massachusetts Medical Center
Worcester, Massachusetts

Steven Strongwater directs quality management, clinical resource management, and utilization management activities. He is the physician leader in developing and implementing the institution's clinical process redesign methodology. He also serves on the Council on Evaluative Science and Clinical Information Management Steering Committees of the University Hospitals Consortium and the Hospital/Health Plan Information Partnership Executive Committee of the Massachusetts Rate Setting Commission.

He has a medical degree from the State University of New York Upstate Medical Center. He completed a fellowship in rheumatology at the University of Michigan Medical Center. He is editor of the *Healthcare Quality Alliance Newsletter.*

Mark A. Swift
President
M. A. Swift and Associates
Chicago, Illinois

Mark Swift focuses on new business start-ups and reengineering healthcare manufacturers, payers, and providers. He also works with buyers and sellers to find, evaluate, and structure mergers and acquisitions.

He has an MBA from the University of Chicago, where he is a guest lecturer, and speaks to industry groups on reengineering, quality management, and organizational efficiency.

Gemma Mata Tayao
Manager Associate
JDA
San Francisco, California

Gemma Mata Tayao works with physicians and medical groups on maintaining and redesigning their business office practices. She was director of patient accounting for Loma Linda University's Faculty Medical Group, assistant director for medical group business services at the University of California, San Francisco, and a practice management consultant focusing on expense reduction through process analysis and redesign.

Adrian Tibbetts, PhD
Director of Service Innovation
AvMed-Santa Fe HealthCare
Gainesville, Florida

Adrian Tibbets directs the development and implementation of new concepts for "best-in-class" customer service and directed an AvMed regional member service department. She was formerly a managed care coordinator with Anthem Insurance Companies specializing in provider recruitment, reimbursement and contract negotiations, and network maintenance.

She has a PhD in Management from California Coast University and an MBA from the University of South Florida and is a faculty instructor at Webster College.

Gennaro J. Vasile, PhD
Vice President
Gemini Consulting
Morristown, New Jersey

Gennaro Vasile is the North American leader of the company's global healthcare practice. His expertise is in planning and implementation of strategic management and operations improvements for hospitals and health services. He was executive vice president at the Johns Hopkins Hospital, chief executive officer of United Health Services, and chief executive officer of Strong Memorial Hospital.

He has a PhD in health services management from the University of Iowa and an MBA in hospital administration from Xavier University. He is an associate professor at Johns Hopkins University where he teaches strategic management.

Diana Weaver, DNS
Senior Vice President for Patient Services
Yale–New Haven Hospital
New Haven, Connecticut

Diana Weaver directs nursing, ambulatory care, emergency services, pharmacy, and social services. She was instrumental in the organization's redesign efforts and cochaired the team that developed the overall care philosophy. She is the past president of the American Organization of Nurse Executives and speaks frequently on leadership and change.

She has a nursing doctorate from Indiana University, and is a fellow of American Academy of Nursing.

Timothy E. Weddle
Independent Consultant
Chicago, Illinois

Timothy Weddle focuses on information system strategic planning, decision support, and clinical documentation systems for teaching hospitals. He was the director for decision support services at Loyola University Medical Center and implemented organizationwide total quality management activities.

He received an MBA from the University of Michigan and lectures on organizational performance, physician hospital collaboration, and customer-driven improvement plans.

Index